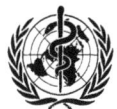

WORLD HEALTH ORGANIZATION

INTERNATIONAL AGENCY FOR RESEARCH ON CANCER

IARC MONOGRAPHS

ON THE

EVALUATION OF CARCINOGENIC

RISKS TO HUMANS

Some Antiviral and Antineoplastic Drugs, and Other Pharmaceutical Agents

VOLUME 76

This publication represents the views and expert opinions
of an IARC Working Group on the
Evaluation of Carcinogenic Risks to Humans,
which met in Lyon,

12–19 October 1999

2000

IARC MONOGRAPHS

In 1969, the International Agency for Research on Cancer (IARC) initiated a programme on the evaluation of the carcinogenic risk of chemicals to humans involving the production of critically evaluated monographs on individual chemicals. The programme was subsequently expanded to include evaluations of carcinogenic risks associated with exposures to complex mixtures, life-style factors and biological and physical agents, as well as those in specific occupations.

The objective of the programme is to elaborate and publish in the form of monographs critical reviews of data on carcinogenicity for agents to which humans are known to be exposed and on specific exposure situations; to evaluate these data in terms of human risk with the help of international working groups of experts in carcinogenesis and related fields; and to indicate where additional research efforts are needed.

The lists of IARC evaluations are regularly updated and are available on Internet: http://www.iarc.fr/, under Publications.

This project was supported by Cooperative Agreement 5 UO1 CA33193 awarded by the United States National Cancer Institute, Department of Health and Human Services. Additional support has been provided since 1986 by the European Commission, since 1993 by the United States National Institute of Environmental Health Sciences and since 1995 by the United States Environmental Protection Agency through Cooperative Agreement Assistance CR 824264.

©International Agency for Research on Cancer, 2000

Distributed by IARC*Press* (Fax: +33 4 72 73 83 02; E-mail: press@iarc.fr)
and by the World Health Organization Distribution and Sales, CH-1211 Geneva 27
(Fax: +41 22 791 4857; E-mail: publications@who.int)

Publications of the World Health Organization enjoy copyright protection in accordance with the provisions of Protocol 2 of the Universal Copyright Convention.

All rights reserved. Application for rights of reproduction or translation, in part or *in toto*, should be made to the International Agency for Research on Cancer.

IARC Library Cataloguing in Publication Data

Some antiviral and antineoplastic drugs, and other pharmaceutical agents /
    IARC Working Group on the Evaluation of Carcinogenic Risks to Humans
    (2000 : Lyon, France).

(IARC monographs on the evaluation of carcinogenic risks to humans ; 76)

1. Carcinogens – congresses 2. Drugs – congresses
I. IARC Working Group on the Evaluation of Carcinogenic Risks to Humans
II. Series

ISBN 92 832 1276 2   (NLM Classification: W1)
ISSN 1017-1606

PRINTED IN FRANCE

CONTENTS

NOTE TO THE READER 1

LIST OF PARTICIPANTS 3

PREAMBLE 9
   Background 9
   Objective and Scope 9
   Selection of Topics for Monographs 10
   Data for Monographs 11
   The Working Group 11
   Working Procedures 11
   Exposure Data 12
   Studies of Cancer in Humans 14
   Studies of Cancer in Experimental Animals 17
   Other Data Relevant to an Evaluation of Carcinogenicity
      and its Mechanisms 20
   Summary of Data Reported 22
   Evaluation 23
   References 27

GENERAL REMARKS 33

THE MONOGRAPHS 43

   Antiretroviral agents 45
      Aciclovir 47
      Zidovudine (AZT) 73
      Zalcitabine 129
      Didanosine 153

   DNA topoisomerase II inhibitors 175
      Etoposide 177
      Teniposide 259
      Mitoxantrone 289
      Amsacrine 317

Other pharmaceutical agents 345
    Hydroxyurea 347
    Phenolphthalein 387
    Vitamin K substances 417

SUMMARY OF FINAL EVALUATIONS 487

CUMULATIVE INDEX TO THE MONOGRAPHS SERIES 489

NOTE TO THE READER

The term 'carcinogenic risk' in the *IARC Monographs* series is taken to mean the probability that exposure to an agent will lead to cancer in humans.

Inclusion of an agent in the *Monographs* does not imply that it is a carcinogen, only that the published data have been examined. Equally, the fact that an agent has not yet been evaluated in a monograph does not mean that it is not carcinogenic.

The evaluations of carcinogenic risk are made by international working groups of independent scientists and are qualitative in nature. No recommendation is given for regulation or legislation.

Anyone who is aware of published data that may alter the evaluation of the carcinogenic risk of an agent to humans is encouraged to make this information available to the Unit of Carcinogen Identification and Evaluation, International Agency for Research on Cancer, 150 cours Albert Thomas, 69372 Lyon Cedex 08, France, in order that the agent may be considered for re-evaluation by a future Working Group.

Although every effort is made to prepare the monographs as accurately as possible, mistakes may occur. Readers are requested to communicate any errors to the Unit of Carcinogen Identification and Evaluation, so that corrections can be reported in future volumes.

IARC WORKING GROUP ON THE EVALUATION OF CARCINOGENIC RISKS TO HUMANS: SOME ANTIVIRAL AND ANTINEOPLASTIC DRUGS, AND OTHER PHARMACEUTICAL AGENTS

Lyon, 12–19 October 1999

LIST OF PARTICIPANTS

Members

D.E. Barker, The CORE Center for Infectious Diseases, Cook County Hospital, Division of Infectious Diseases, 2020 W. Harrison Street, Chicago, IL 60612, United States

T.A. Dragani, Istituto Nazionale dei Tumori, via G. Venezian 1, 20133 Milan, Italy

J.K. Dunnick, National Institute of Environmental Health Sciences, PO Box 12233, Research Triangle Park, NC 27709, United States

C.A. Felix, Division of Oncology, The Children's Hospital of Philadelphia, Abramson Pediatric Research Center, Room 902B, 3516 Civic Center Boulevard, Philadelphia, PA 19104-4318, United States

L.R. Ferguson, Auckland Cancer Society Research Centre, Faculty of Medical and Health Science, The University of Auckland, Private Bag 92019, Auckland 1000, New Zealand

S.P. Joel, Medical Oncology, St Bartholomew's Hospital, West Smithfield, London EC1A 7BE, United Kingdom

R. von Kries, Institute for Social Pediatrics and Adolescent Medicine, Ludwig-Maximilians University, Heiglhofstrasse 63, 81377 Munich, Germany

F.E. van Leeuwen, Department of Epidemiology, The Netherlands Cancer Institute, Plesmanlaan 121, 1066 CX Amsterdam, The Netherlands

J. Little, Institute of Medical Sciences, Department of Medicine & Therapeutics, University of Aberdeen Medical School, Polwarth Building, Foresterhill, Aberdeen AB9 2ZD, United Kingdom

S. Olin, International Life Sciences Institute, Risk Science Institute, 1126 Sixteenth Street NW, Washington, DC 20036, United States

J.H. Olsen, Danish Cancer Society, Institute of Cancer Epidemiology, Box 839, 2100 Copenhagen Ø, Denmark

M.C. Poirier, Carcinogen–DNA Interactions Section, National Cancer Institute, Building 37, Room 2A05, 37 Convent Drive, Bethesda, MD 20892-4255, United States (*Chairperson*)

M.J. Shearer, The Vitamin K Research Unit of the Haemophilia Centre, The Rayne Institute, 4th Floor Lambeth Wing, St Thomas's Hospital, London SE1 7EH, United Kingdom

W. Slikker, Jr, Division of Neurotoxicology, National Center for Toxicological Research, Food and Drug Administration, Jefferson, AR 72079-9502, United States

F.M. Sullivan, Harrington House, 8 Harrington Road, Brighton, East Sussex BN1 6RE, United Kingdom

V. Turusov, Blokhin Cancer Research Centre, Russian Academy of Medical Sciences, Kashirskoye Shosse 24, 115478 Moscow, Russian Federation

V.E. Walker, Wadsworth Center for Laboratories and Research, New York State Department of Health, Empire State Plaza, PO Box 509, Albany, NY 12201-0509, United States

Representative/Observer
Representative of the National Cancer Institute
S.M. Sieber, Division of Cancer Epidemiology and Genetics, National Cancer Institute, Executive Plaza North, 6100 Executive Boulevard, Rockville, MD 20852, United States

Secretariat
E. Heseltine (*Editor*), Lajarthe, 24290 St Léon-sur-Vézère, France

IARC
R. Baan, Unit of Carcinogen Identification and Evaluation
P. Brennan, Unit of Environmental Cancer Epidemiology
M. Friesen, Unit of Gene–Environment Interactions
Y. Grosse, Unit of Carcinogen Identification and Evaluation
V. Krutovskikh, Unit of Multistage Carcinogenesis
C. Malaveille, Unit of Endogenous Cancer Risk Factors
D. McGregor, Unit of Carcinogen Identification and Evaluation
C. Partensky, Unit of Carcinogen Identification and Evaluation
J. Rice, Unit of Carcinogen Identification and Evaluation (*Head of Programme*)
J. Wilbourn, Unit of Carcinogen Identification and Evaluation (*Responsible Officer*)

Technical assistance
M. Lézère
A. Meneghel
D. Mietton
J. Mitchell

PARTICIPANTS

E. Perez
S. Reynaud
J. Thévenoux

PREAMBLE

IARC MONOGRAPHS PROGRAMME ON THE EVALUATION OF CARCINOGENIC RISKS TO HUMANS

PREAMBLE

1. BACKGROUND

In 1969, the International Agency for Research on Cancer (IARC) initiated a programme to evaluate the carcinogenic risk of chemicals to humans and to produce monographs on individual chemicals. The Monographs programme has since been expanded to include consideration of exposures to complex mixtures of chemicals (which occur, for example, in some occupations and as a result of human habits) and of exposures to other agents, such as radiation and viruses. With Supplement 6 (IARC, 1987a), the title of the series was modified from *IARC Monographs on the Evaluation of the Carcinogenic Risk of Chemicals to Humans* to *IARC Monographs on the Evaluation of Carcinogenic Risks to Humans*, in order to reflect the widened scope of the programme.

The criteria established in 1971 to evaluate carcinogenic risk to humans were adopted by the working groups whose deliberations resulted in the first 16 volumes of the *IARC Monographs series*. Those criteria were subsequently updated by further ad-hoc working groups (IARC, 1977, 1978, 1979, 1982, 1983, 1987b, 1988, 1991a; Vainio *et al.*, 1992).

2. OBJECTIVE AND SCOPE

The objective of the programme is to prepare, with the help of international working groups of experts, and to publish in the form of monographs, critical reviews and evaluations of evidence on the carcinogenicity of a wide range of human exposures. The *Monographs* may also indicate where additional research efforts are needed.

The *Monographs* represent the first step in carcinogenic risk assessment, which involves examination of all relevant information in order to assess the strength of the available evidence that certain exposures could alter the incidence of cancer in humans. The second step is quantitative risk estimation. Detailed, quantitative evaluations of epidemiological data may be made in the *Monographs*, but without extrapolation beyond the range of the data available. Quantitative extrapolation from experimental data to the human situation is not undertaken.

The term 'carcinogen' is used in these monographs to denote an exposure that is capable of increasing the incidence of malignant neoplasms; the induction of benign neoplasms may in some circumstances (see p. 19) contribute to the judgement that the exposure is carcinogenic. The terms 'neoplasm' and 'tumour' are used interchangeably.

Some epidemiological and experimental studies indicate that different agents may act at different stages in the carcinogenic process, and several mechanisms may be involved. The aim of the *Monographs* has been, from their inception, to evaluate evidence of carcinogenicity at any stage in the carcinogenesis process, independently of the underlying mechanisms. Information on mechanisms may, however, be used in making the overall evaluation (IARC, 1991a; Vainio *et al.*, 1992; IARC, 1995; Kane *et al.*, 1996; Capen *et al.*, 1999; see also pp. 25–27).

The *Monographs* may assist national and international authorities in making risk assessments and in formulating decisions concerning any necessary preventive measures. The evaluations of IARC working groups are scientific, qualitative judgements about the evidence for or against carcinogenicity provided by the available data. These evaluations represent only one part of the body of information on which regulatory measures may be based. Other components of regulatory decisions vary from one situation to another and from country to country, responding to different socioeconomic and national priorities. **Therefore, no recommendation is given with regard to regulation or legislation, which are the responsibility of individual governments and/or other international organizations.**

The *IARC Monographs* are recognized as an authoritative source of information on the carcinogenicity of a wide range of human exposures. A survey of users in 1988 indicated that the *Monographs* are consulted by various agencies in 57 countries. About 3000 copies of each volume are printed, for distribution to governments, regulatory bodies and interested scientists. The Monographs are also available from IARC*Press* in Lyon and via the Distribution and Sales Service of the World Health Organization in Geneva.

3. SELECTION OF TOPICS FOR MONOGRAPHS

Topics are selected on the basis of two main criteria: (a) there is evidence of human exposure, and (b) there is some evidence or suspicion of carcinogenicity. The term 'agent' is used to include individual chemical compounds, groups of related chemical compounds, physical agents (such as radiation) and biological factors (such as viruses). Exposures to mixtures of agents may occur in occupational exposures and as a result of personal and cultural habits (like smoking and dietary practices). Chemical analogues and compounds with biological or physical characteristics similar to those of suspected carcinogens may also be considered, even in the absence of data on a possible carcinogenic effect in humans or experimental animals.

The scientific literature is surveyed for published data relevant to an assessment of carcinogenicity. The IARC information bulletins on agents being tested for carcinogenicity (IARC, 1973–1996) and directories of on-going research in cancer epidemiology (IARC, 1976–1996) often indicate exposures that may be scheduled for future meetings. Ad-hoc working groups convened by IARC in 1984, 1989, 1991, 1993 and 1998 gave recommendations as to which agents should be evaluated in the IARC Monographs series (IARC, 1984, 1989, 1991b, 1993, 1998a,b).

As significant new data on subjects on which monographs have already been prepared become available, re-evaluations are made at subsequent meetings, and revised monographs are published.

4. DATA FOR MONOGRAPHS

The *Monographs* do not necessarily cite all the literature concerning the subject of an evaluation. Only those data considered by the Working Group to be relevant to making the evaluation are included.

With regard to biological and epidemiological data, only reports that have been published or accepted for publication in the openly available scientific literature are reviewed by the working groups. In certain instances, government agency reports that have undergone peer review and are widely available are considered. Exceptions may be made on an ad-hoc basis to include unpublished reports that are in their final form and publicly available, if their inclusion is considered pertinent to making a final evaluation (see pp. 25–27). In the sections on chemical and physical properties, on analysis, on production and use and on occurrence, unpublished sources of information may be used.

5. THE WORKING GROUP

Reviews and evaluations are formulated by a working group of experts. The tasks of the group are: (i) to ascertain that all appropriate data have been collected; (ii) to select the data relevant for the evaluation on the basis of scientific merit; (iii) to prepare accurate summaries of the data to enable the reader to follow the reasoning of the Working Group; (iv) to evaluate the results of epidemiological and experimental studies on cancer; (v) to evaluate data relevant to the understanding of mechanism of action; and (vi) to make an overall evaluation of the carcinogenicity of the exposure to humans.

Working Group participants who contributed to the considerations and evaluations within a particular volume are listed, with their addresses, at the beginning of each publication. Each participant who is a member of a working group serves as an individual scientist and not as a representative of any organization, government or industry. In addition, nominees of national and international agencies and industrial associations may be invited as observers.

6. WORKING PROCEDURES

Approximately one year in advance of a meeting of a working group, the topics of the monographs are announced and participants are selected by IARC staff in consultation with other experts. Subsequently, relevant biological and epidemiological data are collected by the Carcinogen Identification and Evaluation Unit of IARC from recognized sources of information on carcinogenesis, including data storage and retrieval systems such as MEDLINE and TOXLINE.

For chemicals and some complex mixtures, the major collection of data and the preparation of first drafts of the sections on chemical and physical properties, on analysis, on production and use and on occurrence are carried out under a separate contract funded by the United States National Cancer Institute. Representatives from industrial associations may assist in the preparation of sections on production and use. Information on production and trade is obtained from governmental and trade publications and, in some cases, by direct contact with industries. Separate production data on some agents may not be available because their publication could disclose confidential information. Information on uses may be obtained from published sources but is often complemented by direct contact with manufacturers. Efforts are made to supplement this information with data from other national and international sources.

Six months before the meeting, the material obtained is sent to meeting participants, or is used by IARC staff, to prepare sections for the first drafts of monographs. The first drafts are compiled by IARC staff and sent before the meeting to all participants of the Working Group for review.

The Working Group meets in Lyon for seven to eight days to discuss and finalize the texts of the monographs and to formulate the evaluations. After the meeting, the master copy of each monograph is verified by consulting the original literature, edited and prepared for publication. The aim is to publish monographs within six months of the Working Group meeting.

The available studies are summarized by the Working Group, with particular regard to the qualitative aspects discussed below. In general, numerical findings are indicated as they appear in the original report; units are converted when necessary for easier comparison. The Working Group may conduct additional analyses of the published data and use them in their assessment of the evidence; the results of such supplementary analyses are given in square brackets. When an important aspect of a study, directly impinging on its interpretation, should be brought to the attention of the reader, a comment is given in square brackets.

7. EXPOSURE DATA

Sections that indicate the extent of past and present human exposure, the sources of exposure, the people most likely to be exposed and the factors that contribute to the exposure are included at the beginning of each monograph.

Most monographs on individual chemicals, groups of chemicals or complex mixtures include sections on chemical and physical data, on analysis, on production and use and on occurrence. In monographs on, for example, physical agents, occupational exposures and cultural habits, other sections may be included, such as: historical perspectives, description of an industry or habit, chemistry of the complex mixture or taxonomy. Monographs on biological agents have sections on structure and biology, methods of detection, epidemiology of infection and clinical disease other than cancer.

For chemical exposures, the Chemical Abstracts Services Registry Number, the latest Chemical Abstracts Primary Name and the IUPAC Systematic Name are recorded; other synonyms are given, but the list is not necessarily comprehensive. For biological agents, taxonomy and structure are described, and the degree of variability is given, when applicable.

Information on chemical and physical properties and, in particular, data relevant to identification, occurrence and biological activity are included. For biological agents, mode of replication, life cycle, target cells, persistence and latency and host response are given. A description of technical products of chemicals includes trade names, relevant specifications and available information on composition and impurities. Some of the trade names given may be those of mixtures in which the agent being evaluated is only one of the ingredients.

The purpose of the section on analysis or detection is to give the reader an overview of current methods, with emphasis on those widely used for regulatory purposes. Methods for monitoring human exposure are also given, when available. No critical evaluation or recommendation of any of the methods is meant or implied. The IARC published a series of volumes, *Environmental Carcinogens: Methods of Analysis and Exposure Measurement* (IARC, 1978–93), that describe validated methods for analysing a wide variety of chemicals and mixtures. For biological agents, methods of detection and exposure assessment are described, including their sensitivity, specificity and reproducibility.

The dates of first synthesis and of first commercial production of a chemical or mixture are provided; for agents which do not occur naturally, this information may allow a reasonable estimate to be made of the date before which no human exposure to the agent could have occurred. The dates of first reported occurrence of an exposure are also provided. In addition, methods of synthesis used in past and present commercial production and different methods of production which may give rise to different impurities are described.

Data on production, international trade and uses are obtained for representative regions, which usually include Europe, Japan and the United States of America. It should not, however, be inferred that those areas or nations are necessarily the sole or major sources or users of the agent. Some identified uses may not be current or major applications, and the coverage is not necessarily comprehensive. In the case of drugs, mention of their therapeutic uses does not necessarily represent current practice, nor does it imply judgement as to their therapeutic efficacy.

Information on the occurrence of an agent or mixture in the environment is obtained from data derived from the monitoring and surveillance of levels in occupational environments, air, water, soil, foods and animal and human tissues. When available, data on the generation, persistence and bioaccumulation of the agent are also included. In the case of mixtures, industries, occupations or processes, information is given about all agents present. For processes, industries and occupations, a historical description is also given, noting variations in chemical composition, physical properties and levels of occupational exposure with time and place. For biological agents, the epidemiology of infection is described.

Statements concerning regulations and guidelines (e.g., pesticide registrations, maximal levels permitted in foods, occupational exposure limits) are included for some countries as indications of potential exposures, but they may not reflect the most recent situation, since such limits are continuously reviewed and modified. The absence of information on regulatory status for a country should not be taken to imply that that country does not have regulations with regard to the exposure. For biological agents, legislation and control, including vaccines and therapy, are described.

8. STUDIES OF CANCER IN HUMANS

(a) Types of studies considered

Three types of epidemiological studies of cancer contribute to the assessment of carcinogenicity in humans—cohort studies, case–control studies and correlation (or ecological) studies. Rarely, results from randomized trials may be available. Case series and case reports of cancer in humans may also be reviewed.

Cohort and case–control studies relate the exposures under study to the occurrence of cancer in individuals and provide an estimate of relative risk (ratio of incidence or mortality in those exposed to incidence or mortality in those not exposed) as the main measure of association.

In correlation studies, the units of investigation are usually whole populations (e.g. in particular geographical areas or at particular times), and cancer frequency is related to a summary measure of the exposure of the population to the agent, mixture or exposure circumstance under study. Because individual exposure is not documented, however, a causal relationship is less easy to infer from correlation studies than from cohort and case–control studies. Case reports generally arise from a suspicion, based on clinical experience, that the concurrence of two events—that is, a particular exposure and occurrence of a cancer—has happened rather more frequently than would be expected by chance. Case reports usually lack complete ascertainment of cases in any population, definition or enumeration of the population at risk and estimation of the expected number of cases in the absence of exposure. The uncertainties surrounding interpretation of case reports and correlation studies make them inadequate, except in rare instances, to form the sole basis for inferring a causal relationship. When taken together with case–control and cohort studies, however, relevant case reports or correlation studies may add materially to the judgement that a causal relationship is present.

Epidemiological studies of benign neoplasms, presumed preneoplastic lesions and other end-points thought to be relevant to cancer are also reviewed by working groups. They may, in some instances, strengthen inferences drawn from studies of cancer itself.

(b) Quality of studies considered

The Monographs are not intended to summarize all published studies. Those that are judged to be inadequate or irrelevant to the evaluation are generally omitted. They may be mentioned briefly, particularly when the information is considered to be a useful supplement to that in other reports or when they provide the only data available. Their inclusion does not imply acceptance of the adequacy of the study design or of the analysis and interpretation of the results, and limitations are clearly outlined in square brackets at the end of the study description.

It is necessary to take into account the possible roles of bias, confounding and chance in the interpretation of epidemiological studies. By 'bias' is meant the operation of factors in study design or execution that lead erroneously to a stronger or weaker association than in fact exists between disease and an agent, mixture or exposure circumstance. By 'confounding' is meant a situation in which the relationship with disease is made to appear stronger or weaker than it truly is as a result of an association between the apparent causal factor and another factor that is associated with either an increase or decrease in the incidence of the disease. In evaluating the extent to which these factors have been minimized in an individual study, working groups consider a number of aspects of design and analysis as described in the report of the study. Most of these considerations apply equally to case–control, cohort and correlation studies. Lack of clarity of any of these aspects in the reporting of a study can decrease its credibility and the weight given to it in the final evaluation of the exposure.

Firstly, the study population, disease (or diseases) and exposure should have been well defined by the authors. Cases of disease in the study population should have been identified in a way that was independent of the exposure of interest, and exposure should have been assessed in a way that was not related to disease status.

Secondly, the authors should have taken account in the study design and analysis of other variables that can influence the risk of disease and may have been related to the exposure of interest. Potential confounding by such variables should have been dealt with either in the design of the study, such as by matching, or in the analysis, by statistical adjustment. In cohort studies, comparisons with local rates of disease may be more appropriate than those with national rates. Internal comparisons of disease frequency among individuals at different levels of exposure should also have been made in the study.

Thirdly, the authors should have reported the basic data on which the conclusions are founded, even if sophisticated statistical analyses were employed. At the very least, they should have given the numbers of exposed and unexposed cases and controls in a case–control study and the numbers of cases observed and expected in a cohort study. Further tabulations by time since exposure began and other temporal factors are also important. In a cohort study, data on all cancer sites and all causes of death should have been given, to reveal the possibility of reporting bias. In a case–control study, the effects of investigated factors other than the exposure of interest should have been reported.

Finally, the statistical methods used to obtain estimates of relative risk, absolute rates of cancer, confidence intervals and significance tests, and to adjust for confounding should have been clearly stated by the authors. The methods used should preferably have been the generally accepted techniques that have been refined since the mid-1970s. These methods have been reviewed for case–control studies (Breslow & Day, 1980) and for cohort studies (Breslow & Day, 1987).

(c) *Inferences about mechanism of action*

Detailed analyses of both relative and absolute risks in relation to temporal variables, such as age at first exposure, time since first exposure, duration of exposure, cumulative exposure and time since exposure ceased, are reviewed and summarized when available. The analysis of temporal relationships can be useful in formulating models of carcinogenesis. In particular, such analyses may suggest whether a carcinogen acts early or late in the process of carcinogenesis, although at best they allow only indirect inferences about the mechanism of action. Special attention is given to measurements of biological markers of carcinogen exposure or action, such as DNA or protein adducts, as well as markers of early steps in the carcinogenic process, such as proto-oncogene mutation, when these are incorporated into epidemiological studies focused on cancer incidence or mortality. Such measurements may allow inferences to be made about putative mechanisms of action (IARC, 1991a; Vainio *et al.*, 1992).

(d) *Criteria for causality*

After the individual epidemiological studies of cancer have been summarized and the quality assessed, a judgement is made concerning the strength of evidence that the agent, mixture or exposure circumstance in question is carcinogenic for humans. In making its judgement, the Working Group considers several criteria for causality. A strong association (a large relative risk) is more likely to indicate causality than a weak association, although it is recognized that relative risks of small magnitude do not imply lack of causality and may be important if the disease is common. Associations that are replicated in several studies of the same design or using different epidemiological approaches or under different circumstances of exposure are more likely to represent a causal relationship than isolated observations from single studies. If there are inconsistent results among investigations, possible reasons are sought (such as differences in amount of exposure), and results of studies judged to be of high quality are given more weight than those of studies judged to be methodologically less sound. When suspicion of carcinogenicity arises largely from a single study, these data are not combined with those from later studies in any subsequent reassessment of the strength of the evidence.

If the risk of the disease in question increases with the amount of exposure, this is considered to be a strong indication of causality, although absence of a graded response is not necessarily evidence against a causal relationship. Demonstration of a decline in risk after cessation of or reduction in exposure in individuals or in whole populations also supports a causal interpretation of the findings.

Although a carcinogen may act upon more than one target, the specificity of an association (an increased occurrence of cancer at one anatomical site or of one morphological type) adds plausibility to a causal relationship, particularly when excess cancer occurrence is limited to one morphological type within the same organ.

Although rarely available, results from randomized trials showing different rates among exposed and unexposed individuals provide particularly strong evidence for causality.

When several epidemiological studies show little or no indication of an association between an exposure and cancer, the judgement may be made that, in the aggregate, they show evidence of lack of carcinogenicity. Such a judgement requires first of all that the studies giving rise to it meet, to a sufficient degree, the standards of design and analysis described above. Specifically, the possibility that bias, confounding or misclassification of exposure or outcome could explain the observed results should be considered and excluded with reasonable certainty. In addition, all studies that are judged to be methodologically sound should be consistent with a relative risk of unity for any observed level of exposure and, when considered together, should provide a pooled estimate of relative risk which is at or near unity and has a narrow confidence interval, due to sufficient population size. Moreover, no individual study nor the pooled results of all the studies should show any consistent tendency for the relative risk of cancer to increase with increasing level of exposure. It is important to note that evidence of lack of carcinogenicity obtained in this way from several epidemiological studies can apply only to the type(s) of cancer studied and to dose levels and intervals between first exposure and observation of disease that are the same as or less than those observed in all the studies. Experience with human cancer indicates that, in some cases, the period from first exposure to the development of clinical cancer is seldom less than 20 years; latent periods substantially shorter than 30 years cannot provide evidence for lack of carcinogenicity.

9. STUDIES OF CANCER IN EXPERIMENTAL ANIMALS

All known human carcinogens that have been studied adequately in experimental animals have produced positive results in one or more animal species (Wilbourn *et al.*, 1986; Tomatis *et al.*, 1989). For several agents (aflatoxins, 4-aminobiphenyl, azathioprine, betel quid with tobacco, bischloromethyl ether and chloromethyl methyl ether (technical grade), chlorambucil, chlornaphazine, ciclosporin, coal-tar pitches, coal-tars, combined oral contraceptives, cyclophosphamide, diethylstilboestrol, melphalan, 8-methoxypsoralen plus ultraviolet A radiation, mustard gas, myleran, 2-naphthylamine, nonsteroidal oestrogens, oestrogen replacement therapy/steroidal oestrogens, solar radiation, thiotepa and vinyl chloride), carcinogenicity in experimental animals was established or highly suspected before epidemiological studies confirmed their carcinogenicity in humans (Vainio *et al.*, 1995). Although this association cannot establish that all agents and mixtures that cause cancer in experimental animals also cause cancer in humans, nevertheless, **in the absence of adequate data on humans, it is biologically plausible and prudent to regard agents and mixtures for which there is *sufficient evidence* (see p. 24) of carcinogenicity in experimental animals as if they presented a carcinogenic risk to humans**. The possibility that a given agent may cause cancer through a species-specific mechanism which does not operate in humans (see p. 27) should also be taken into consideration.

The nature and extent of impurities or contaminants present in the chemical or mixture being evaluated are given when available. Animal strain, sex, numbers per group, age at start of treatment and survival are reported.

Other types of studies summarized include: experiments in which the agent or mixture was administered in conjunction with known carcinogens or factors that modify carcinogenic effects; studies in which the end-point was not cancer but a defined precancerous lesion; and experiments on the carcinogenicity of known metabolites and derivatives.

For experimental studies of mixtures, consideration is given to the possibility of changes in the physicochemical properties of the test substance during collection, storage, extraction, concentration and delivery. Chemical and toxicological interactions of the components of mixtures may result in nonlinear dose–response relationships.

An assessment is made as to the relevance to human exposure of samples tested in experimental animals, which may involve consideration of: (i) physical and chemical characteristics, (ii) constituent substances that indicate the presence of a class of substances, (iii) the results of tests for genetic and related effects, including studies on DNA adduct formation, proto-oncogene mutation and expression and suppressor gene inactivation. The relevance of results obtained, for example, with animal viruses analogous to the virus being evaluated in the monograph must also be considered. They may provide biological and mechanistic information relevant to the understanding of the process of carcinogenesis in humans and may strengthen the plausibility of a conclusion that the biological agent under evaluation is carcinogenic in humans.

(a) *Qualitative aspects*

An assessment of carcinogenicity involves several considerations of qualitative importance, including (i) the experimental conditions under which the test was performed, including route and schedule of exposure, species, strain, sex, age, duration of follow-up; (ii) the consistency of the results, for example, across species and target organ(s); (iii) the spectrum of neoplastic response, from preneoplastic lesions and benign tumours to malignant neoplasms; and (iv) the possible role of modifying factors.

As mentioned earlier (p. 11), the *Monographs* are not intended to summarize all published studies. Those studies in experimental animals that are inadequate (e.g., too short a duration, too few animals, poor survival; see below) or are judged irrelevant to the evaluation are generally omitted. Guidelines for conducting adequate long-term carcinogenicity experiments have been outlined (e.g. Montesano *et al.*, 1986).

Considerations of importance to the Working Group in the interpretation and evaluation of a particular study include: (i) how clearly the agent was defined and, in the case of mixtures, how adequately the sample characterization was reported; (ii) whether the dose was adequately monitored, particularly in inhalation experiments; (iii) whether the doses and duration of treatment were appropriate and whether the survival of treated animals was similar to that of controls; (iv) whether there were adequate numbers of animals per group; (v) whether animals of each sex were used; (vi) whether animals were allocated randomly to groups; (vii) whether the duration of observation was adequate; and (viii) whether the data were adequately reported. If available, recent data on the incidence of specific tumours in historical controls, as well as in concurrent controls, should be taken into account in the evaluation of tumour response.

When benign tumours occur together with and originate from the same cell type in an organ or tissue as malignant tumours in a particular study and appear to represent a stage in the progression to malignancy, it may be valid to combine them in assessing tumour incidence (Huff *et al.*, 1989). The occurrence of lesions presumed to be preneoplastic may in certain instances aid in assessing the biological plausibility of any neoplastic response observed. If an agent or mixture induces only benign neoplasms that appear to be end-points that do not readily progress to malignancy, it should nevertheless be suspected of being a carcinogen and requires further investigation.

(b) *Quantitative aspects*

The probability that tumours will occur may depend on the species, sex, strain and age of the animal, the dose of the carcinogen and the route and length of exposure. Evidence of an increased incidence of neoplasms with increased level of exposure strengthens the inference of a causal association between the exposure and the development of neoplasms.

The form of the dose–response relationship can vary widely, depending on the particular agent under study and the target organ. Both DNA damage and increased cell division are important aspects of carcinogenesis, and cell proliferation is a strong determinant of dose–response relationships for some carcinogens (Cohen & Ellwein, 1990). Since many chemicals require metabolic activation before being converted into their reactive intermediates, both metabolic and pharmacokinetic aspects are important in determining the dose–response pattern. Saturation of steps such as absorption, activation, inactivation and elimination may produce nonlinearity in the dose–response relationship, as could saturation of processes such as DNA repair (Hoel *et al.*, 1983; Gart *et al.*, 1986).

(c) *Statistical analysis of long-term experiments in animals*

Factors considered by the Working Group include the adequacy of the information given for each treatment group: (i) the number of animals studied and the number examined histologically, (ii) the number of animals with a given tumour type and (iii) length of survival. The statistical methods used should be clearly stated and should be the generally accepted techniques refined for this purpose (Peto *et al.*, 1980; Gart *et al.*, 1986). When there is no difference in survival between control and treatment groups, the Working Group usually compares the proportions of animals developing each tumour type in each of the groups. Otherwise, consideration is given as to whether or not appropriate adjustments have been made for differences in survival. These adjustments can include: comparisons of the proportions of tumour-bearing animals among the effective number of animals (alive at the time the first tumour is discovered), in the case where most differences in survival occur before tumours appear; life-table methods, when tumours are visible or when they may be considered 'fatal' because mortality rapidly follows tumour development; and the Mantel-Haenszel test or logistic regression, when occult tumours do not affect the animals' risk of dying but are 'incidental' findings at autopsy.

In practice, classifying tumours as fatal or incidental may be difficult. Several survival-adjusted methods have been developed that do not require this distinction (Gart *et al.*, 1986), although they have not been fully evaluated.

10. OTHER DATA RELEVANT TO AN EVALUATION OF CARCINOGENICITY AND ITS MECHANISMS

In coming to an overall evaluation of carcinogenicity in humans (see pp. 25–27), the Working Group also considers related data. The nature of the information selected for the summary depends on the agent being considered.

For chemicals and complex mixtures of chemicals such as those in some occupational situations or involving cultural habits (e.g. tobacco smoking), the other data considered to be relevant are divided into those on absorption, distribution, metabolism and excretion; toxic effects; reproductive and developmental effects; and genetic and related effects.

Concise information is given on absorption, distribution (including placental transfer) and excretion in both humans and experimental animals. Kinetic factors that may affect the dose–response relationship, such as saturation of uptake, protein binding, metabolic activation, detoxification and DNA repair processes, are mentioned. Studies that indicate the metabolic fate of the agent in humans and in experimental animals are summarized briefly, and comparisons of data on humans and on animals are made when possible. Comparative information on the relationship between exposure and the dose that reaches the target site may be of particular importance for extrapolation between species. Data are given on acute and chronic toxic effects (other than cancer), such as organ toxicity, increased cell proliferation, immunotoxicity and endocrine effects. The presence and toxicological significance of cellular receptors is described. Effects on reproduction, teratogenicity, fetotoxicity and embryotoxicity are also summarized briefly.

Tests of genetic and related effects are described in view of the relevance of gene mutation and chromosomal damage to carcinogenesis (Vainio *et al.*, 1992; McGregor *et al.*, 1999). The adequacy of the reporting of sample characterization is considered and, where necessary, commented upon; with regard to complex mixtures, such comments are similar to those described for animal carcinogenicity tests on p. 18. The available data are interpreted critically by phylogenetic group according to the end-points detected, which may include DNA damage, gene mutation, sister chromatid exchange, micronucleus formation, chromosomal aberrations, aneuploidy and cell transformation. The concentrations employed are given, and mention is made of whether use of an exogenous metabolic system *in vitro* affected the test result. These data are given as listings of test systems, data and references. The Genetic and Related Effects data presented in the *Monographs* are also available in the form of Graphic Activity Profiles (GAP) prepared in collaboration with the United States Environmental Protection Agency (EPA) (see also

Waters *et al.*, 1987) using software for personal computers that are Microsoft Windows® compatible. The EPA/IARC GAP software and database may be downloaded free of charge from *www.epa.gov/gapdb*.

Positive results in tests using prokaryotes, lower eukaryotes, plants, insects and cultured mammalian cells suggest that genetic and related effects could occur in mammals. Results from such tests may also give information about the types of genetic effect produced and about the involvement of metabolic activation. Some end-points described are clearly genetic in nature (e.g., gene mutations and chromosomal aberrations), while others are to a greater or lesser degree associated with genetic effects (e.g. unscheduled DNA synthesis). In-vitro tests for tumour-promoting activity and for cell transformation may be sensitive to changes that are not necessarily the result of genetic alterations but that may have specific relevance to the process of carcinogenesis. A critical appraisal of these tests has been published (Montesano *et al.*, 1986).

Genetic or other activity manifest in experimental mammals and humans is regarded as being of greater relevance than that in other organisms. The demonstration that an agent or mixture can induce gene and chromosomal mutations in whole mammals indicates that it may have carcinogenic activity, although this activity may not be detectably expressed in any or all species. Relative potency in tests for mutagenicity and related effects is not a reliable indicator of carcinogenic potency. Negative results in tests for mutagenicity in selected tissues from animals treated *in vivo* provide less weight, partly because they do not exclude the possibility of an effect in tissues other than those examined. Moreover, negative results in short-term tests with genetic end-points cannot be considered to provide evidence to rule out carcinogenicity of agents or mixtures that act through other mechanisms (e.g. receptor-mediated effects, cellular toxicity with regenerative proliferation, peroxisome proliferation) (Vainio *et al.*, 1992). Factors that may lead to misleading results in short-term tests have been discussed in detail elsewhere (Montesano *et al.*, 1986).

When available, data relevant to mechanisms of carcinogenesis that do not involve structural changes at the level of the gene are also described.

The adequacy of epidemiological studies of reproductive outcome and genetic and related effects in humans is evaluated by the same criteria as are applied to epidemiological studies of cancer.

Structure–activity relationships that may be relevant to an evaluation of the carcinogenicity of an agent are also described.

For biological agents—viruses, bacteria and parasites—other data relevant to carcinogenicity include descriptions of the pathology of infection, molecular biology (integration and expression of viruses, and any genetic alterations seen in human tumours) and other observations, which might include cellular and tissue responses to infection, immune response and the presence of tumour markers.

11. SUMMARY OF DATA REPORTED

In this section, the relevant epidemiological and experimental data are summarized. Only reports, other than in abstract form, that meet the criteria outlined on p. 11 are considered for evaluating carcinogenicity. Inadequate studies are generally not summarized: such studies are usually identified by a square-bracketed comment in the preceding text.

(a) Exposure

Human exposure to chemicals and complex mixtures is summarized on the basis of elements such as production, use, occurrence in the environment and determinations in human tissues and body fluids. Quantitative data are given when available. Exposure to biological agents is described in terms of transmission and prevalence of infection.

(b) Carcinogenicity in humans

Results of epidemiological studies that are considered to be pertinent to an assessment of human carcinogenicity are summarized. When relevant, case reports and correlation studies are also summarized.

(c) Carcinogenicity in experimental animals

Data relevant to an evaluation of carcinogenicity in animals are summarized. For each animal species and route of administration, it is stated whether an increased incidence of neoplasms or preneoplastic lesions was observed, and the tumour sites are indicated. If the agent or mixture produced tumours after prenatal exposure or in single-dose experiments, this is also indicated. Negative findings are also summarized. Dose–response and other quantitative data may be given when available.

(d) Other data relevant to an evaluation of carcinogenicity and its mechanisms

Data on biological effects in humans that are of particular relevance are summarized. These may include toxicological, kinetic and metabolic considerations and evidence of DNA binding, persistence of DNA lesions or genetic damage in exposed humans. Toxicological information, such as that on cytotoxicity and regeneration, receptor binding and hormonal and immunological effects, and data on kinetics and metabolism in experimental animals are given when considered relevant to the possible mechanism of the carcinogenic action of the agent. The results of tests for genetic and related effects are summarized for whole mammals, cultured mammalian cells and nonmammalian systems.

When available, comparisons of such data for humans and for animals, and particularly animals that have developed cancer, are described.

Structure–activity relationships are mentioned when relevant.

For the agent, mixture or exposure circumstance being evaluated, the available data on end-points or other phenomena relevant to mechanisms of carcinogenesis from studies in humans, experimental animals and tissue and cell test systems are summarized within one or more of the following descriptive dimensions:

(i) Evidence of genotoxicity (structural changes at the level of the gene): for example, structure–activity considerations, adduct formation, mutagenicity (effect on specific genes), chromosomal mutation/aneuploidy

(ii) Evidence of effects on the expression of relevant genes (functional changes at the intracellular level): for example, alterations to the structure or quantity of the product of a proto-oncogene or tumour-suppressor gene, alterations to metabolic activation/inactivation/DNA repair

(iii) Evidence of relevant effects on cell behaviour (morphological or behavioural changes at the cellular or tissue level): for example, induction of mitogenesis, compensatory cell proliferation, preneoplasia and hyperplasia, survival of premalignant or malignant cells (immortalization, immunosuppression), effects on metastatic potential

(iv) Evidence from dose and time relationships of carcinogenic effects and interactions between agents: for example, early/late stage, as inferred from epidemiological studies; initiation/promotion/progression/malignant conversion, as defined in animal carcinogenicity experiments; toxicokinetics

These dimensions are not mutually exclusive, and an agent may fall within more than one of them. Thus, for example, the action of an agent on the expression of relevant genes could be summarized under both the first and second dimensions, even if it were known with reasonable certainty that those effects resulted from genotoxicity.

12. EVALUATION

Evaluations of the strength of the evidence for carcinogenicity arising from human and experimental animal data are made, using standard terms.

It is recognized that the criteria for these evaluations, described below, cannot encompass all of the factors that may be relevant to an evaluation of carcinogenicity. In considering all of the relevant scientific data, the Working Group may assign the agent, mixture or exposure circumstance to a higher or lower category than a strict interpretation of these criteria would indicate.

(a) Degrees of evidence for carcinogenicity in humans and in experimental animals and supporting evidence

These categories refer only to the strength of the evidence that an exposure is carcinogenic and not to the extent of its carcinogenic activity (potency) nor to the mechanisms involved. A classification may change as new information becomes available.

An evaluation of degree of evidence, whether for a single agent or a mixture, is limited to the materials tested, as defined physically, chemically or biologically. When the agents evaluated are considered by the Working Group to be sufficiently closely related, they may be grouped together for the purpose of a single evaluation of degree of evidence.

(i) Carcinogenicity in humans

The applicability of an evaluation of the carcinogenicity of a mixture, process, occupation or industry on the basis of evidence from epidemiological studies depends on the variability over time and place of the mixtures, processes, occupations and industries. The Working Group seeks to identify the specific exposure, process or activity which is considered most likely to be responsible for any excess risk. The evaluation is focused as narrowly as the available data on exposure and other aspects permit.

The evidence relevant to carcinogenicity from studies in humans is classified into one of the following categories:

Sufficient evidence of carcinogenicity: The Working Group considers that a causal relationship has been established between exposure to the agent, mixture or exposure circumstance and human cancer. That is, a positive relationship has been observed between the exposure and cancer in studies in which chance, bias and confounding could be ruled out with reasonable confidence.

Limited evidence of carcinogenicity: A positive association has been observed between exposure to the agent, mixture or exposure circumstance and cancer for which a causal interpretation is considered by the Working Group to be credible, but chance, bias or confounding could not be ruled out with reasonable confidence.

Inadequate evidence of carcinogenicity: The available studies are of insufficient quality, consistency or statistical power to permit a conclusion regarding the presence or absence of a causal association between exposure and cancer, or no data on cancer in humans are available.

Evidence suggesting lack of carcinogenicity: There are several adequate studies covering the full range of levels of exposure that human beings are known to encounter, which are mutually consistent in not showing a positive association between exposure to the agent, mixture or exposure circumstance and any studied cancer at any observed level of exposure. A conclusion of 'evidence suggesting lack of carcinogenicity' is inevitably limited to the cancer sites, conditions and levels of exposure and length of observation covered by the available studies. In addition, the possibility of a very small risk at the levels of exposure studied can never be excluded.

In some instances, the above categories may be used to classify the degree of evidence related to carcinogenicity in specific organs or tissues.

(ii) *Carcinogenicity in experimental animals*

The evidence relevant to carcinogenicity in experimental animals is classified into one of the following categories:

Sufficient evidence of carcinogenicity: The Working Group considers that a causal relationship has been established between the agent or mixture and an increased incidence of malignant neoplasms or of an appropriate combination of benign and malignant neoplasms in (a) two or more species of animals or (b) in two or more independent studies in one species carried out at different times or in different laboratories or under different protocols.

Exceptionally, a single study in one species might be considered to provide sufficient evidence of carcinogenicity when malignant neoplasms occur to an unusual degree with regard to incidence, site, type of tumour or age at onset.

Limited evidence of carcinogenicity: The data suggest a carcinogenic effect but are limited for making a definitive evaluation because, e.g. (a) the evidence of carcinogenicity is restricted to a single experiment; or (b) there are unresolved questions regarding the adequacy of the design, conduct or interpretation of the study; or (c) the agent or mixture increases the incidence only of benign neoplasms or lesions of uncertain neoplastic potential, or of certain neoplasms which may occur spontaneously in high incidences in certain strains.

Inadequate evidence of carcinogenicity: The studies cannot be interpreted as showing either the presence or absence of a carcinogenic effect because of major qualitative or quantitative limitations, or no data on cancer in experimental animals are available.

Evidence suggesting lack of carcinogenicity: Adequate studies involving at least two species are available which show that, within the limits of the tests used, the agent or mixture is not carcinogenic. A conclusion of evidence suggesting lack of carcinogenicity is inevitably limited to the species, tumour sites and levels of exposure studied.

(b) *Other data relevant to the evaluation of carcinogenicity and its mechanisms*

Other evidence judged to be relevant to an evaluation of carcinogenicity and of sufficient importance to affect the overall evaluation is then described. This may include data on preneoplastic lesions, tumour pathology, genetic and related effects, structure–activity relationships, metabolism and pharmacokinetics, physicochemical parameters and analogous biological agents.

Data relevant to mechanisms of the carcinogenic action are also evaluated. The strength of the evidence that any carcinogenic effect observed is due to a particular mechanism is assessed, using terms such as weak, moderate or strong. Then, the Working Group assesses if that particular mechanism is likely to be operative in humans. The strongest indications that a particular mechanism operates in humans come from data on humans or biological specimens obtained from exposed humans. The data may be considered to be especially relevant if they show that the agent in question has caused changes in exposed humans that are on the causal pathway to carcinogenesis. Such data may, however, never become available, because it is at least conceivable that certain compounds may be kept from human use solely on the basis of evidence of their toxicity and/or carcinogenicity in experimental systems.

For complex exposures, including occupational and industrial exposures, the chemical composition and the potential contribution of carcinogens known to be present are considered by the Working Group in its overall evaluation of human carcinogenicity. The Working Group also determines the extent to which the materials tested in experimental systems are related to those to which humans are exposed.

(c) *Overall evaluation*

Finally, the body of evidence is considered as a whole, in order to reach an overall evaluation of the carcinogenicity to humans of an agent, mixture or circumstance of exposure.

An evaluation may be made for a group of chemical compounds that have been evaluated by the Working Group. In addition, when supporting data indicate that other, related compounds for which there is no direct evidence of capacity to induce cancer in humans or in animals may also be carcinogenic, a statement describing the rationale for this conclusion is added to the evaluation narrative; an additional evaluation may be made for this broader group of compounds if the strength of the evidence warrants it.

The agent, mixture or exposure circumstance is described according to the wording of one of the following categories, and the designated group is given. The categorization of an agent, mixture or exposure circumstance is a matter of scientific judgement, reflecting the strength of the evidence derived from studies in humans and in experimental animals and from other relevant data.

Group 1 —The agent (mixture) is carcinogenic to humans.
The exposure circumstance entails exposures that are carcinogenic to humans.

This category is used when there is *sufficient evidence* of carcinogenicity in humans. Exceptionally, an agent (mixture) may be placed in this category when evidence of carcinogenicity in humans is less than sufficient but there is *sufficient evidence* of carcinogenicity in experimental animals and strong evidence in exposed humans that the agent (mixture) acts through a relevant mechanism of carcinogenicity.

Group 2

This category includes agents, mixtures and exposure circumstances for which, at one extreme, the degree of evidence of carcinogenicity in humans is almost sufficient, as well as those for which, at the other extreme, there are no human data but for which there is evidence of carcinogenicity in experimental animals. Agents, mixtures and exposure circumstances are assigned to either group 2A (probably carcinogenic to humans) or group 2B (possibly carcinogenic to humans) on the basis of epidemiological and experimental evidence of carcinogenicity and other relevant data.

Group 2A—The agent (mixture) is probably carcinogenic to humans.
The exposure circumstance entails exposures that are probably carcinogenic to humans.

This category is used when there is *limited evidence* of carcinogenicity in humans and *sufficient evidence* of carcinogenicity in experimental animals. In some cases, an agent (mixture) may be classified in this category when there is *inadequate evidence* of carcinogenicity in humans, *sufficient evidence* of carcinogenicity in experimental animals and strong evidence that the carcinogenesis is mediated by a mechanism that also operates in humans. Exceptionally, an agent, mixture or exposure circumstance may be classified in this category solely on the basis of *limited evidence* of carcinogenicity in humans.

Group 2B—The agent (mixture) is possibly carcinogenic to humans The exposure circumstance entails exposures that are possibly carcinogenic to humans.

This category is used for agents, mixtures and exposure circumstances for which there is *limited evidence* of carcinogenicity in humans and less than *sufficient evidence* of carcinogenicity in experimental animals. It may also be used when there is *inadequate evidence* of carcinogenicity in humans but there is *sufficient evidence* of carcinogenicity in experimental animals. In some instances, an agent, mixture or exposure circumstance for which there is *inadequate evidence* of carcinogenicity in humans but *limited evidence* of carcinogenicity in experimental animals together with supporting evidence from other relevant data may be placed in this group.

Group 3—The agent (mixture or exposure circumstance) is not classifiable as to its carcinogenicity to humans.

This category is used most commonly for agents, mixtures and exposure circumstances for which the *evidence of carcinogenicity* is *inadequate* in humans and *inadequate* or *limited* in experimental animals.

Exceptionally, agents (mixtures) for which the *evidence of carcinogenicity is inadequate* in humans but *sufficient* in experimental animals may be placed in this category when there is strong evidence that the mechanism of carcinogenicity in experimental animals does not operate in humans.

Agents, mixtures and exposure circumstances that do not fall into any other group are also placed in this category.

Group 4—The agent (mixture) is probably not carcinogenic to humans.

This category is used for agents or mixtures for which there is *evidence suggesting lack of carcinogenicity* in humans and in experimental animals. In some instances, agents or mixtures for which there is *inadequate evidence* of carcinogenicity in humans but *evidence suggesting lack of carcinogenicity* in experimental animals, consistently and strongly supported by a broad range of other relevant data, may be classified in this group.

References

Breslow, N.E. & Day, N.E. (1980) *Statistical Methods in Cancer Research*, Vol. 1, *The Analysis of Case–Control Studies* (IARC Scientific Publications No. 32), Lyon, IARC*Press*

Breslow, N.E. & Day, N.E. (1987) *Statistical Methods in Cancer Research*, Vol. 2, *The Design and Analysis of Cohort Studies* (IARC Scientific Publications No. 82), Lyon, IARC*Press*

Capen, C.C., Dybing, E., Rice, J.M. & Wilbourn, J.D., eds (1999) Species Differences in Thyroid, Kidney and Urinary Bladder Carcinogenesis (IARC Scientific Publications No. 147), Lyon, IARC*Press*

Cohen, S.M. & Ellwein, L.B. (1990) Cell proliferation in carcinogenesis. *Science*, **249**, 1007–1011

Gart, J.J., Krewski, D., Lee, P.N., Tarone, R.E. & Wahrendorf, J. (1986) *Statistical Methods in Cancer Research*, Vol. 3, *The Design and Analysis of Long-term Animal Experiments* (IARC Scientific Publications No. 79), Lyon, IARC*Press*

Hoel, D.G., Kaplan, N.L. & Anderson, M.W. (1983) Implication of nonlinear kinetics on risk estimation in carcinogenesis. *Science*, **219**, 1032–1037

Huff, J.E., Eustis, S.L. & Haseman, J.K. (1989) Occurrence and relevance of chemically induced benign neoplasms in long-term carcinogenicity studies. *Cancer Metastasis Rev.*, **8**, 1–21

IARC (1973–1996) *Information Bulletin on the Survey of Chemicals Being Tested for Carcinogenicity/Directory of Agents Being Tested for Carcinogenicity*, Numbers 1–17, Lyon, IARC*Press*

IARC (1976–1996), Lyon, IARC*Press*

Directory of On-going Research in Cancer Epidemiology 1976. Edited by C.S. Muir & G. Wagner

Directory of On-going Research in Cancer Epidemiology 1977 (IARC Scientific Publications No. 17). Edited by C.S. Muir & G. Wagner

Directory of On-going Research in Cancer Epidemiology 1978 (IARC Scientific Publications No. 26). Edited by C.S. Muir & G. Wagner

Directory of On-going Research in Cancer Epidemiology 1979 (IARC Scientific Publications No. 28). Edited by C.S. Muir & G. Wagner

Directory of On-going Research in Cancer Epidemiology 1980 (IARC Scientific Publications No. 35). Edited by C.S. Muir & G. Wagner

Directory of On-going Research in Cancer Epidemiology 1981 (IARC Scientific Publications No. 38). Edited by C.S. Muir & G. Wagner

Directory of On-going Research in Cancer Epidemiology 1982 (IARC Scientific Publications No. 46). Edited by C.S. Muir & G. Wagner

Directory of On-going Research in Cancer Epidemiology 1983 (IARC Scientific Publications No. 50). Edited by C.S. Muir & G. Wagner

Directory of On-going Research in Cancer Epidemiology 1984 (IARC Scientific Publications No. 62). Edited by C.S. Muir & G. Wagner

Directory of On-going Research in Cancer Epidemiology 1985 (IARC Scientific Publications No. 69). Edited by C.S. Muir & G. Wagner

Directory of On-going Research in Cancer Epidemiology 1986 (IARC Scientific Publications No. 80). Edited by C.S. Muir & G. Wagner

Directory of On-going Research in Cancer Epidemiology 1987 (IARC Scientific Publications No. 86). Edited by D.M. Parkin & J. Wahrendorf

Directory of On-going Research in Cancer Epidemiology 1988 (IARC Scientific Publications No. 93). Edited by M. Coleman & J. Wahrendorf

Directory of On-going Research in Cancer Epidemiology 1989/90 (IARC Scientific Publications No. 101). Edited by M. Coleman & J. Wahrendorf

Directory of On-going Research in Cancer Epidemiology 1991 (IARC Scientific Publications No.110). Edited by M. Coleman & J. Wahrendorf

Directory of On-going Research in Cancer Epidemiology 1992 (IARC Scientific Publications No. 117). Edited by M. Coleman, J. Wahrendorf & E. Démaret

Directory of On-going Research in Cancer Epidemiology 1994 (IARC Scientific Publications No. 130). Edited by R. Sankaranarayanan, J. Wahrendorf & E. Démaret

Directory of On-going Research in Cancer Epidemiology 1996 (IARC Scientific Publications No. 137). Edited by R. Sankaranarayanan, J. Wahrendorf & E. Démaret

IARC (1977) *IARC Monographs Programme on the Evaluation of the Carcinogenic Risk of Chemicals to Humans*. Preamble (IARC intern. tech. Rep. No. 77/002), Lyon, IARC*Press*

IARC (1978) *Chemicals with Sufficient Evidence of Carcinogenicity in Experimental Animals—IARC Monographs Volumes 1–17* (IARC intern. tech. Rep. No. 78/003), Lyon, IARC*Press*

IARC (1978–1993) *Environmental Carcinogens. Methods of Analysis and Exposure Measurement*, Lyon, IARC*Press*

    Vol. 1. Analysis of Volatile Nitrosamines in Food (IARC Scientific Publications No. 18). Edited by R. Preussmann, M. Castegnaro, E.A. Walker & A.E. Wasserman (1978)

    Vol. 2. Methods for the Measurement of Vinyl Chloride in Poly(vinyl chloride), Air, Water and Foodstuffs (IARC Scientific Publications No. 22). Edited by D.C.M. Squirrell & W. Thain (1978)

    Vol. 3. Analysis of Polycyclic Aromatic Hydrocarbons in Environmental Samples (IARC Scientific Publications No. 29). Edited by M. Castegnaro, P. Bogovski, H. Kunte & E.A. Walker (1979)

    Vol. 4. Some Aromatic Amines and Azo Dyes in the General and Industrial Environment (IARC Scientific Publications No. 40). Edited by L. Fishbein, M. Castegnaro, I.K. O'Neill & H. Bartsch (1981)

    Vol. 5. Some Mycotoxins (IARC Scientific Publications No. 44). Edited by L. Stoloff, M. Castegnaro, P. Scott, I.K. O'Neill & H. Bartsch (1983)

    Vol. 6. N-Nitroso Compounds (IARC Scientific Publications No. 45). Edited by R. Preussmann, I.K. O'Neill, G. Eisenbrand, B. Spiegelhalder & H. Bartsch (1983)

    Vol. 7. Some Volatile Halogenated Hydrocarbons (IARC Scientific Publications No. 68). Edited by L. Fishbein & I.K. O'Neill (1985)

    Vol. 8. Some Metals: As, Be, Cd, Cr, Ni, Pb, Se, Zn (IARC Scientific Publications No. 71). Edited by I.K. O'Neill, P. Schuller & L. Fishbein (1986)

    Vol. 9. Passive Smoking (IARC Scientific Publications No. 81). Edited by I.K. O'Neill, K.D. Brunnemann, B. Dodet & D. Hoffmann (1987)

    Vol. 10. Benzene and Alkylated Benzenes (IARC Scientific Publications No. 85). Edited by L. Fishbein & I.K. O'Neill (1988)

    Vol. 11. Polychlorinated Dioxins and Dibenzofurans (IARC Scientific Publications No. 108). Edited by C. Rappe, H.R. Buser, B. Dodet & I.K. O'Neill (1991)

    Vol. 12. Indoor Air (IARC Scientific Publications No. 109). Edited by B. Seifert, H. van de Wiel, B. Dodet & I.K. O'Neill (1993)

IARC (1979) *Criteria to Select Chemicals for IARC Monographs* (IARC intern. tech. Rep. No. 79/003), Lyon, IARC*Press*

IARC (1982) *IARC Monographs on the Evaluation of the Carcinogenic Risk of Chemicals to Humans, Supplement 4, Chemicals, Industrial Processes and Industries Associated with Cancer in Humans* (IARC Monographs, Volumes 1 to 29), Lyon, IARC*Press*

IARC (1983) *Approaches to Classifying Chemical Carcinogens According to Mechanism of Action* (IARC intern. tech. Rep. No. 83/001), Lyon, IARC*Press*

IARC (1984) *Chemicals and Exposures to Complex Mixtures Recommended for Evaluation in IARC Monographs and Chemicals and Complex Mixtures Recommended for Long-term Carcinogenicity Testing* (IARC intern. tech. Rep. No. 84/002), Lyon, IARC*Press*

IARC (1987a) *IARC Monographs on the Evaluation of Carcinogenic Risks to Humans*, Supplement 6, *Genetic and Related Effects: An Updating of Selected* IARC Monographs *from Volumes 1 to 42*, Lyon, IARC*Press*

IARC (1987b) *IARC Monographs on the Evaluation of Carcinogenic Risks to Humans*, Supplement 7, *Overall Evaluations of Carcinogenicity: An Updating of* IARC Monographs *Volumes 1 to 42*, Lyon, IARC*Press*

IARC (1988) *Report of an IARC Working Group to Review the Approaches and Processes Used to Evaluate the Carcinogenicity of Mixtures and Groups of Chemicals* (IARC intern. tech. Rep. No. 88/002), Lyon, IARC*Press*

IARC (1989) *Chemicals, Groups of Chemicals, Mixtures and Exposure Circumstances to be Evaluated in Future IARC Monographs, Report of an ad hoc Working Group* (IARC intern. tech. Rep. No. 89/004), Lyon, IARC*Press*

IARC (1991a) *A Consensus Report of an IARC Monographs Working Group on the Use of Mechanisms of Carcinogenesis in Risk Identification* (IARC intern. tech. Rep. No. 91/002), Lyon, IARC*Press*

IARC (1991b) *Report of an ad-hoc* IARC Monographs *Advisory Group on Viruses and Other Biological Agents Such as Parasites* (IARC intern. tech. Rep. No. 91/001), Lyon, IARC*Press*

IARC (1993) *Chemicals, Groups of Chemicals, Complex Mixtures, Physical and Biological Agents and Exposure Circumstances to be Evaluated in Future* IARC Monographs, *Report of an ad-hoc Working Group* (IARC intern. Rep. No. 93/005), Lyon, IARC*Press*

IARC (1995) *Peroxisome Proliferation and its Role in Carcinogenesis, Views and Expert Opinions of an IARC Working Group, Lyon 7–9 December 1994* (IARC Tech. Rep. No. 24), Lyon, IARC*Press*

IARC (1998a) *Report of an ad-hoc* IARC Monographs *Advisory Group on Physical Agents* (IARC Internal Report No. 98/002), Lyon, IARC*Press*

IARC (1998b) *Report of an ad-hoc* IARC Monographs *Advisory Group on Priorities for Future Evaluations* (IARC Internal Report No. 98/004), Lyon, IARC*Press*

Kane, A.B., Boffetta, P., Saracci, R. & Wilbourn, J.D., eds (1996) *Mechanisms of Fibre Carcinogenesis* (IARC Scientific Publications No. 140), Lyon, IARC*Press*

McGregor, D.B., Rice, J.M. & Venitt, S., eds (1999) *The Use of Short and Medium-term Tests for Carcinogens and Data on Genetic Effects in Carcinogenic Hazard Evaluation* (IARC Scientific Publications No. 146), Lyon, IARC*Press*

Montesano, R., Bartsch, H., Vainio, H., Wilbourn, J. & Yamasaki, H., eds (1986) *Long-term and Short-term Assays for Carcinogenesis—A Critical Appraisal* (IARC Scientific Publications No. 83), Lyon, IARC*Press*

Peto, R., Pike, M.C., Day, N.E., Gray, R.G., Lee, P.N., Parish, S., Peto, J., Richards, S. & Wahrendorf, J. (1980) Guidelines for simple, sensitive significance tests for carcinogenic effects in long-term animal experiments. In: *IARC Monographs on the Evaluation of the Carcinogenic Risk of Chemicals to Humans*, Supplement 2, *Long-term and Short-term Screening Assays for Carcinogens: A Critical Appraisal*, Lyon, IARC*Press*, pp. 311–426

Tomatis, L., Aitio, A., Wilbourn, J. & Shuker, L. (1989) Human carcinogens so far identified. *Jpn. J. Cancer Res.*, **80**, 795–807

Vainio, H., Magee, P.N., McGregor, D.B. & McMichael, A.J., eds (1992) *Mechanisms of Carcinogenesis in Risk Identification* (IARC Scientific Publications No. 116), Lyon, IARC*Press*

Vainio, H., Wilbourn, J.D., Sasco, A.J., Partensky, C., Gaudin, N., Heseltine, E. & Eragne, I. (1995) *Identification of human carcinogenic risk in IARC Monographs. Bull. Cancer,* **82**, 339–348 (in French)

Waters, M.D., Stack, H.F., Brady, A.L., Lohman, P.H.M., Haroun, L. & Vainio, H. (1987) Appendix 1. Activity profiles for genetic and related tests. In: *IARC Monographs on the Evaluation of Carcinogenic Risks to Humans*, Suppl. 6, *Genetic and Related Effects: An Updating of Selected IARC Monographs from Volumes 1 to 42*, Lyon, IARC*Press*, pp. 687–696

Wilbourn, J., Haroun, L., Heseltine, E., Kaldor, J., Partensky, C. & Vainio, H. (1986) Response of experimental animals to human carcinogens: an analysis based upon the IARC Monographs Programme. *Carcinogenesis*, **7**, 1853–1863

GENERAL REMARKS

GENERAL REMARKS ON THE SUBSTANCES CONSIDERED

This seventy-sixth volume of *IARC Monographs* comprises evaluations of some pharmaceutical agents, including some antiviral agents (aciclovir, zidovudine, zalcitabine and didanosine), some DNA topoisomerase II inhibitors (teniposide, etoposide, mitoxantrone and amsacrine), and others (hydroxyurea, phenolphthalein and vitamin K substances). These agents have not been evaluated by previous IARC working groups.

For several compounds evaluated in this volume, no data were available on carcinogenicity in experimental animals, and this limited the possibility of a comprehensive evaluation of their carcinogenic risks to humans. Although they may not have been tested for carcinogenicity, the Working Group suspected that studies might have been conducted by pharmaceutical companies but never published. The Working Group encourages pharmaceutical companies and cognizant governmental agencies to make available all studies of carcinogenesis that have been, or will be, carried out on pharmaceutical agents in the form of publications or technical reports.

Two chemicals were tested for carcinogenicity in genetically engineered mice which are particularly susceptible to induction of tumours at certain sites through specific mechanisms. The use of such animals for evaluation of the carcinogenicity of chemicals has been reviewed (McGregor *et al.*, 1999). Some, but not all, of these transgenic ('knockout') models can be considered the laboratory counterparts of certain rare human genetic syndromes, and the models may be particularly useful for testing drugs to be administered to individuals with such syndromes. Also, genetically engineered mice that lack one copy of an essential tumour suppressor gene, such as *p53*, model the situation in which a functioning copy of the suppressor gene has been lost in the somatic cells of a normal individual through a stochastic process. The transgenic models may therefore also be useful for studying the mechanism or mode of action of chemicals and, in particular, to test genetic targets of carcinogenicity. Because of the limited database on the responses of particular genetically engineered mice to chemical carcinogens, however, the results of bioassays with these animals must be interpreted with caution.

1. Antiretroviral agents

Although studies on three antiretroviral agents (zidovudine, zalcitabine and didanosine) and on one agent used in adjunctive therapy (hydroxyurea) are reviewed in this volume, numerous drugs are approved for the treatment of human immunodeficiency virus (HIV) infections. Furthermore, the anti-herpesvirus drug, aciclovir, is often given to patients with HIV infections. The drugs evaluated in this volume are usually combined with other nucleoside reverse transcriptase inhibitors, protease inhibitors and/or non-nucleoside reverse transcriptase inhibitors in order to constitute a regimen likely to suppress HIV replication fully. Combination regimens have been proven repeatedly to be superior to therapy with single drugs for effective and durable treatment of HIV infection (Graham *et al.*, 1996; Hammer, 1996; Englund *et al.*, 1997; Hammer *et al.*, 1997; Phillips *et al.*, 1998). In two large, well-conducted trials, initial therapy with multiple drugs followed by simplification of the regimen in a maintenance phase has been shown to be less effective than continued multi-agent therapy (Havlir *et al.*, 1998; Pialoux *et al.*, 1998).

The field of HIV therapy continues to evolve rapidly, and guidelines are available (e.g. Centers for Disease Control and Prevention, 1998; Gazzard & Moyle, 1998) on the goals of combination therapy, monitoring and recommended combinations. Recent revisions of treatment and prevention guidelines are available on-line from the HIV AIDS treatment information service (http://www.hivatis.org/atisinfo.html).

Data on the possible carcinogenic effects of antiretroviral agents in humans have been obtained predominantly in studies in developed countries, where HIV-1 is the main agent in HIV infection. In this volume, therefore, the term HIV should be assumed to refer to HIV-1.

The incidence of non-Hodgkin lymphoma is greatly increased in persons with HIV infection (IARC, 1996), and in AIDS patients the rate may be increased at least 100-fold. The vast majority of AIDS-related non-Hodgkin lymphomas are B-cell neoplasms. No substantial variation in risk by mode of transmission has been observed. The association appears to be mediated by HIV-related immune dysregulation and to involve Epstein-Barr virus (human herpesvirus 4) infection, which is widely prevalent (IARC, 1997). The risk for Kaposi sarcoma of persons infected with HIV is much higher than that of uninfected persons (IARC, 1996), and, in developed countries, homosexual and bisexual men have a 5-10-fold greater risk for Kaposi sarcoma than other groups infected with HIV. There is now evidence that this neoplasm results from co-infection with another herpesvirus, human herpesvirus 8 (IARC, 1997). Effective combination therapy in HIV-infected patients can result in improved immuno-competence, which has led to reduced viraemia and decreased incidences of opportunistic malignancies, especially Kaposi sarcoma and to a lesser extent B-cell lymphomas (Rabkin *et al.*, 1999). These beneficial results may, however, mask potential carcinogenic effects of the antiviral agents.

Much of the evidence on the possible carcinogenic effects of antiretroviral agents in humans is derived from trials designed to evaluate the efficacy of these agents in the treatment of patients with immunosuppression of varying severity. Many of the studies are based on data from a time when these drugs were used singly for treatment of HIV infection. In consequence, the survival of infected patients was relatively poor and the opportunity for long-term follow-up to assess cancer risk was limited.

Difficulties were encountered in seeking to evaluate cancer risk from most of these studies, which was not their primary objective, because the length of follow-up was too short, the numbers of participants were too small, and there was insufficient information about the severity of immunodeficiency. In addition, the occurrence of cancer may have been underascertained, and in many of the studies, no formal, appropriate analyses of cancer rates were presented.

Transplacental exposure to single or combinations of antiretroviral drugs, given during pregnancy to prevent maternal transmission of HIV, may constitute a carcinogenic risk for the children. This inference is based on the transplacental carcinogenicity of zidovudine (AZT), the most widely used such agent, in mice. Approximately 7000 HIV-positive women in the USA become pregnant yearly (Mofenson, 1998), and most receive antiretroviral therapy during pregnancy. While the situation is similar in other developed countries, most developing countries are currently unable to offer these therapies because of their cost.

The number and complexity of antiretroviral drug regimens given to HIV-positive pregnant women is increasing, and the potential carcinogenic risk to children exposed *in utero* may become apparent only many years after birth. The remarkable success of the antiretroviral treatments in saving the lives of thousands of children born annually to HIV-infected women supports continuing use of these drugs during pregnancy, but data from experimental studies suggest that long-term surveillance of these children for cancer risk would be appropriate.

2. DNA topoisomerase II inhibitors

DNA topoisomerase II is a nuclear enzyme that transiently cleaves and re-ligates double-stranded DNA, thereby changing its topology. The structure and biological functions of DNA topoisomerase II have been reviewed (Baguley & Ferguson, 1998; Berger, 1998; Burden & Osheroff, 1998; Isaacs *et al.*, 1998; Nitiss, 1998). Type II DNA topoisomerases are located at the base of chromosomal scaffolds during mitosis, but can also be detected free in the cell throughout the cell cycle. The topological changes mediated by these enzymes are important for chromosomal replication and condensation, and disruption of their function may prevent accurate chromosomal segregation and increase recombination. DNA topoisomerase II-catalysed cleavage is necessary to separate the multiply intertwined daughter DNA strands after DNA replication and before or during the progressive chromatin condensation that precedes mitosis.

The DNA topoisomerase II inhibitors that are evaluated in this volume of the *Monographs* trap the DNA topoisomerase II reaction intermediate at the point where the enzyme has formed a double-strand break in DNA and is covalently bound to the 5' ends of the broken strands (Woynarowski *et al.*, 1994). This decreases the rate of re-ligation catalysed by the enzyme and has the overall effect of enhancing DNA strand cleavage. Especially during replication, enhanced DNA strand cleavage leads to accumulation of DNA–protein cross-links and double-stranded DNA breaks

(Pommier et al., 1985), which may be relevant to translocations. It is important to note that the drugs that target DNA topoisomerase II which are evaluated in this volume are not classical inhibitors in the enzymological sense, inasmuch as they do not inhibit the activity of the free enzyme but rather decrease the rate of re-ligation. Although widely referred to as DNA topoisomerase II inhibitors they are more strictly DNA topoisomerase II poisons (Corbett & Osheroff, 1993).

Antineoplastic treatment of patients with regimens that include DNA topoisomerase II inhibitors has been associated with the occurrence of acute myeloid leukaemia (AML) and other forms of leukaemia. The subtypes of AML are classified according to the French–American–British (FAB) system (Bennett et al., 1985; Cheson et al., 1990), which is summarized in Table 1. The types associated with exposure to DNA topoisomerase II inhibitors are typically acute myelomonocytic (FAB subtype M4) and monoblastic (FAB subtype M5a) leukaemias, but other AML subtypes, myelodysplastic syndrome, acute lymphoblastic leukaemia and chronic myeloid leukaemia have also been described.

Table 1. French–American–British (FAB) classification of acute myeloid leukaemia subtypes

Subtype	Morphology
M0	Acute undifferentiated leukaemia
M1	Acute undifferentiated myeloid leukaemia
M2	Acute differentiated myeloid leukaemia
M3	Acute promyelocytic leukaemia
M4	Acute myelomonocytic leukaemia
M5a	Acute monoblastic leukaemia
M5b	Acute differentiated monocytic leukaemia
M6	Acute erythroleukaemia
M7	Acute megakaryoblastic leukaemia

The term 'secondary leukaemia' indicates that the disease did not develop spontaneously or de novo (Larson et al., 1996). Leukaemia preceded by myelodysplastic syndrome was recognized as a risk associated with anti-cancer chemotherapy with alkylating agents long before the association of DNA topoisomerase II inhibitors with leukaemias was described. The leukaemias seen after alkylating agent therapy are characterized by antecedent myelodysplastic syndrome, a mean latency of 5–7 years and deletion of chromosomes 5 or 7, while those associated with administration of DNA topoisomerase II inhibitors have a mean latency of 2 years and certain balanced chromosomal translocations, usually but not always involving the MLL gene at chromosome 11q23 (Felix et al., 1998). The particular mechanisms of DNA damage by these different agents may underlie differences in the chromosomal aberrations with which they are associated. Leukaemias associated with translocations involving *MLL* have a propensity to express both myeloid- and lymphoid-associated phenotypic cell-surface markers. The translocation process seems central to leukaemogenesis, and translocations involving *MLL* are associated with progression to leukaemia over a short interval.

The *MLL* gene undergoes rearrangement by fusion with various partner genes in the course of specific chromosomal rearrangements which, with few exceptions, are involved in both therapy-related and *de novo* cases. Although hyperleukocytosis and extramedullary disease occur less often in treatment-related cases, the clinical features, FAB types and immunophenotypes are otherwise similar to those of *de novo* cases. These similarities between *de novo* and treatment-related leukaemias may sometimes make it difficult to ascribe the leukaemia to the treatment; however, most *de novo* leukaemias associated with *MLL* gene translocations occur in infants and young children (reviewed by Felix & Lange, 1999), in whom the translocations have been shown to occur *in utero* (Ford *et al.*, 1993; Gill-Super *et al.*, 1994; Gale *et al.*, 1997; Megonigal *et al.*, 1998).

DNA topoisomerase II inhibitors are usually used in combination chemotherapy regimens that may include alkylating agents or other DNA topoisomerase II inhibitors, which themselves may be leukaemogenic. Such combinations may confound analysis of the association of specific agents with leukaemia. Furthermore, in some studies in which patients were treated with etoposide and/or teniposide, the authors used various empirical conversion factors to derive an 'equivalent dose' of etoposide from that of teniposide. The conversions were based, however, on the therapeutic effects rather than on metabolic considerations or on possible leukaemogenic potency at a given dose. Such studies do not allow evaluation of the carcinogenicity of either compound as a single agent.

Additional chromosomal and genetic changes may occur in secondary leukaemias (Corral *et al.*, 1996). Certain individuals may be at higher risk for secondary leukaemia because they have a DNA repair deficiency or another heritable predisposition such as polymorphisms in the gene encoding cytochrome P450 3A4, an important drug-metabolizing enzyme (Felix *et al.*, 1998). Some individuals with the form of leukaemia associated with anti-tumour treatment with alkylating agents have germ-line mutations in the *TP53* cell cycle checkpoint gene as a predisposing factor (Felix *et al.*, 1996).

There are close structural homologies between the DNA topoisomerase II enzymes in higher eukaryotes, but bacterial gyrase and topoisomerase IV play the relevant role in bacteria (Levine *et al.*, 1998). Inhibitors of mammalian DNA topoisomerase II are not necessarily effective inhibitors of these bacterial enzymes and, as a result, may not be detected in microbial assays for mutagenic and clastogenic effects.

A number of drugs target DNA topoisomerase I, a different enzyme, which introduces transient single-stranded nicks into DNA. These drugs are not considered in this volume.

References

Baguley, B.C. & Ferguson, L.R. (1998) Mutagenic properties of topoisomerase-targeted drugs. *Biochim. biophys. Acta*, **1400**, 213–222

Bennett, J.M., Catovsky, D., Daniel, M.T., Flandrin, G., Galton, D.A., Gralnick, H.R. & Sultan, C. (1985) Proposed revised criteria for the classification of acute myeloid leukemia, a report of the French–American–British cooperative group. *Ann. intern. Med.*, **103**, 620–629

Berger, J.M. (1998) Structure of DNA topoisomerases. *Biochim. biophys. Acta*, **1400**, 3–18

Burden, D.A. & Osheroff, N. (1998) Mechanism of action of eukaryotic topoisomerase II and drugs targeted to the enzyme. *Biochim. biophys. Acta*, **1400**, 139–154

Centers for Disease Control and Prevention (1998) Guidelines for the use of antiretroviral agents in HIV-infected adults and adolescents. *Morb. Mortal. wkly Rep.*, **47** (RR-5), 42–82

Cheson, B.D., Cassileth, P.A., Head, D.R., Schiffer, C.A., Bennett, J.M., Bloomfield, C.D., Brunning, R., Gale, R.P., Grever, M.R., Keating, M. J., Sawitzky, A., Stass, S., Weinstein, H. & Woods, W.G. (1990) Report of the National Cancer Institute-sponsored workshop on definitions of diagnosis and response in acute myeloid leukemia. *J. clin. Oncol.*, **8**, 813–819

Corbett, A.H. & Osheroff, N. (1993) When good enzymes go bad: Conversion of topoisomerase II to a cellular toxin by antineoplastic drugs. *Chem. Res. Toxicol.*, **6**, 585–597

Corral, J., Lavenir, I., Impey, H., Warren, A.J., Forster, A., Larson, T.A., Bell, S., McKenzie, A.N., King, G. & Rabbitts, T.H. (1996) An *Mll-AF9* fusion gene made by homologous recombination causes acute leukemia in chimeric mice: A method to create fusion oncogenes. *Cell*, **85**, 853–861

Englund, J.A., Baker, C.J., Raskino, C., McKinney, R.E., Petrie, B., Fowler, M.G., Pearson, D., Gershon, A., McSherry, G.D., Abrams, E.J., Schliozberg, J. & Sullivan, J.L. (1997) Zidovudine, didanosine, or both as the initial treatment for symptomatic HIV-infected children. AIDS Clinical Trials Group (ACTG) Study 152 Team. *New Engl. J. Med.*, **24**, 1704–1712

Felix, C. & Lange, B. (1999) Leukemia in infants. *Oncologist*, **4**, 225–240

Felix, C.A., Hosler, M.R., Provisor, D., Salhany, K., Sexsmith, E.A., Slater, D.J., Cheung, N.K., Winick, N.J., Strauss, E.A., Heyn, R., Lange, B.J. & Malkin, D. (1996) The *p53* gene in pediatric therapy-related leukemia and myelodysplasia. *Blood*, **87**, 4376–4381

Felix, C.A., Walker, A.H., Lange, B.J., Williams, T.M., Winick, N.J., Cheung, N.K., Lovett, B.D., Nowell, P.C., Blair, I.A. & Rebbeck, T.R. (1998) Association of CYP3A4 genotype with treatment-related leukemia. *Proc. natl Acad. Sci. USA*, **95**, 13176–13181

Ford, A.M., Ridge, S.A., Cabrera, M.E., Mahmoud, H., Steel, C.M., Chan, L.C. & Greaves, M. (1993) In utero rearrangements in the trithorax-related oncogene in infant leukaemias. *Nature*, **363**, 358–360

Gale, K., Ford, A., Repp, R., Borkhardt, A., Keller, C., Eden, O.B. & Greaves, M.F. (1997) Backtracking leukemia to birth: Identification of clonotypic gene fusion sequences in neonatal bloodspots. *Proc. natl Acad. Sci. USA*, **94**, 13950–13954

Gazzard, B. & Moyle, G. (1998) 1998 Revision to the British HIV Association guidelines for antiretroviral treatment of HIV seropositive individuals. BHIVA Guidelines Writing Committee. *Lancet*, **352**, 314–316

Gill-Super, H.J., Rothberg, P.G., Kobayashi, H., Freeman, A.I., Diaz, M.O. & Rowley, J.D. (1994) Clonal, nonconstitutional rearrangements of the *MLL* gene in infant twins with acute lymphoblastic leukemia: *in utero* chromosome rearrangement of 11q23. *Blood*, **83**, 641–644

Graham, N.M., Hoover, D.R., Park, L.P., Stein, D.S., Phair, J.P., Mellors, J.W., Detels, R. & Saah, A.J. (1996) Survival in HIV-infected patients who have received zidovudine: Comparison of combination therapy with sequential monotherapy and continued zidovudine monotherapy. Multicenter AIDS Cohort Study Group. *Ann. intern. Med.*, **124**, 1031–1038

Hammer, S.M. (1996) Advances in antiretroviral therapy and viral load monitoring. *AIDS*, **Suppl. 3**, S1–S11

Hammer, S.M., Squires, K.E., Hughes, M.D., Grimes, J.M., Demeter, L.M., Currier, J.S., Eron, J.J., Jr, Feinberg, J.E., Balfour, H.H., Jr, Deyton, L.R., Chodakewitz, J.A. & Fischl, M.A. (1997) A controlled trial of two nucleoside analogues plus indinavir in persons with human immunodeficiency virus infection and CD4 cell counts of 200 per cubic millimeter or less. AIDS Clinical Trials Group 320 Study Team. *New Engl. J. Med.*, **337**, 725–733

Havlir, D.V., Marschner, I.C., Hirsch, M.S., Collier, A.C., Tebas, P., Bassett, R.L., Ioannidis, J.P., Holohan, M.K., Leavitt, R., Boone, G. & Richman, D.D. (1998) Maintenance antiretroviral therapies in HIV infected patients with undetectable plasma HIV RNA after triple-drug therapy. AIDS Clinical Trials Group Study 343 Team. *New Engl. J. Med.*, **339**, 1261–1268

IARC (1996) *IARC Monographs on the Evaluation of Carcinogenic Risks to Humans*, Vol. 67, *Human Immunodeficiency Viruses and Human T-cell Lymphotropic Viruses*, Lyon, IARC*Press*

IARC (1997) *IARC Monographs on the Evaluation of Carcinogenic Risks to Humans*, Vol. 70, *Epstein-Barr Virus and Kaposi's Sarcoma Herpesvirus/Human Herpesvirus 8*, Lyon, IARC*Press*

Isaacs, R.J., Davies, S.L., Sandri, M.I., Redwood, C., Wells, N.J. & Hickson, I.D. (1998) Physiological regulation of eukaryotic topoisomerase II. *Biochim. biophys. Acta*, **1400**, 121–138

Larson, R.A., LeBeau, M.M., Vardiman, J.W. & Rowley, J.D. (1996) Myeloid leukemia after hematotoxins. *Environ. Health Perspectives*, **104**, 1303–1307

Levine, C., Hiasa, H. & Marians, K.J. (1998) DNA gyrase and topoisomerase IV: Biochemical activities, physiological roles during chromosome replication, and drug sensitivities. *Biochim. biophys. Acta*, **1400**, 29–43

McGregor, D.B., Rice, J.M. & Venitt, S., eds (1999) *The Use of Short- and Medium-term Tests for Carcinogens and Data on Genetic Effects in Carcinogenic Hazard Evaluation* (IARC Scientific Publications No. 146), Lyon, IARC*Press*

Megonigal, M.D., Rappaport, E.F., Jones, D.H., Williams, T.M., Lovett, B.D., Kelly, K.M., Lerou, P.H., Moulton, T., Budarf, M.L. & Felix, C.A. (1998) t(11;22)(q23;q11.2) in acute myeloid leukemia of infant twins fuses *MLL* with hCDC*rel*, a cell division cycle gene in the genomic region of deletion in DiGeorge and velocardiofacial syndromes. *Proc. natl Acad. Sci. USA*, **95**, 6413–6418

Mofenson, L.M. (1998) Antiretroviral therapy and interruption of HIV perinatal transmission. *Immunol. Allergy Clin. N. Am.*, **18**, 441–463

Nitiss, J.L. (1998) Investigating the biological functions of DNA topoisomerases in eukaryote cells. *Biochim. biophys. Acta*, **1400**, 63–82

Phillips, A.N., Katlama, C., Barton, S., Vella, S., Blaxhult, A., Clotet, B., Goebel, F.D., Hirschel, B., Pedersen, C. & Lundgren, J.D. (1998) Survival in 2367 zidovudine-treated patients according to use of other nucleoside analogue drugs. The EuroSIDA Study Group. *J. acquir. Immune Defic. Syndrome hum. Retrovirol.*, **17**, 239–244

Pialoux, G., Raffi, F., Brun-Vezinet, F., Meiffredy, V., Flandre, P., Gastaut, J.A., Dellamonica, P., Yeni, P., Delfraissy, J.F. & Aboulker, J.P. (1998) A randomized trial of three maintenance regimens given after three months of induction therapy with zidovudine, lamivudine, and indinavir in previously untreated HIV-1-infected patients. Trilege (Agence Nationale de Recherches sur le SIDA 072) Study Team. *New Engl. J. Med.*, **339**, 1269–1276

Pommier, Y., Minford, J.K., Schwartz, R.E., Zwelling, L.A. & Kohn, K.W. (1985) Effects of the DNA intercalators 4'-(9-acridinylamino)methanesulfon-m-anisidide and 2-methyl-9-hydroxyellipticinium on topoisomerase II mediated DNA strand cleavage and strand passage. *Biochemistry*, **24**, 6410–6416

Rabkin, C.S., Testa, M.A., Huang, J. & Von Roenn, J.H. (1999) Kaposi's sarcoma and non-Hodgkin's lymphoma incidence in AIDS clinical trial group study participants. *J. acquir. Immune Defic. Syndrome*, **21** (Suppl. 1), S31–S33

Woynarowski, J.M., McCarthy, K., Reynolds, B., Beerman, T.A. & Denny, W.A. (1994) Topoisomerase II mediated DNA lesions induced by acridine-4-carboxamide and 2-(4-pyridyl)quinoline-8-carboxamide. *Anticancer Drug Des.*, **9**, 9–24

THE MONOGRAPHS

ANTIRETROVIRAL AGENTS

ACICLOVIR

1. Exposure Data

1.1 Chemical and physical data

1.1.1 *Nomenclature*

Aciclovir

Chem. Abstr. Serv. Reg. No.: 59277-89-3
Chem. Abstr. Name: 2-Amino-1,9-dihydro-9-[(2-hydroxyethoxy)methyl]-6*H*-purin-6-one
IUPAC Systematic Name: 9-[(2-Hydroxyethoxy)methyl]guanine
Synonyms: ACV; acycloguanosine; acyclovir; BW-248U; 9-(2-hydroxyethoxymethyl)guanine

Aciclovir sodium

Chem. Abstr. Serv. Reg. No.: 69657-51-8
Chem. Abstr. Name: 2-Amino-1,9-dihydro-9-[(2-hydroxyethoxy)methyl]-6*H*-purin-6-one, sodium salt
IUPAC Systematic Name: 9-[(2-Hydroxyethoxy)methyl]guanine, monosodium salt
Synonyms: Acycloguanosine sodium; acyclovir sodium; acyclovir sodium salt; sodium acyclovir

1.1.2 *Structural and molecular formulae and relative molecular mass*

Aciclovir

$C_8H_{11}N_5O_3$ Relative molecular mass: 225.21

Aciclovir sodium

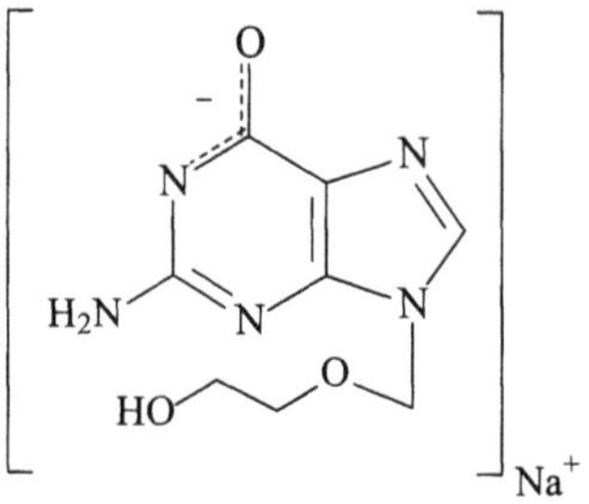

$C_8H_{10}N_5NaO_3$ Relative molecular mass: 247.19

1.1.3   *Chemical and physical properties of the pure substances*

Aciclovir

  (*a*) *Description*: White, crystalline powder (American Hospital Formulary Service, 1999)
  (*b*) *Melting-point*: 256.5–257 °C (Budavari, 1996)
  (*c*) *Spectroscopy data*: Infrared spectral data have been reported (British Pharmacopoeial Commission, 1993).
  (*d*) *Solubility*: Slightly soluble in water (1.3 mg/mL at 25 °C); very slightly soluble in ethanol (0.2 mg/mL); soluble in dilute aqueous solutions of alkali hydroxides and mineral acids; freely soluble in dimethyl sulfoxide (American Hospital Formulary Service, 1999; Royal Pharmaceutical Society of Great Britain, 1999)
  (*e*) *Dissociation constants*: pK_a, 2.27 and 9.25 (American Hospital Formulary Service, 1999)

Aciclovir sodium

  (*a*) *Description*: White, crystalline, lyophilized powder (American Hospital Formulary Service, 1999)
  (*b*) *Solubility*: Soluble in water (> 100 mg/mL at 25 °C); but at pH 7.4 and 37 °C, the drug is almost completely un-ionized and has a maximum solubility of 2.5 mg/mL (American Hospital Formulary Service, 1999)

1.1.4   *Technical products and impurities*

Aciclovir is available as 200, 400- and 800-mg tablets, a 200-mg capsule, a 200-mg/5 mL suspension, a 500- or 1000-mg lyophilized powder for intravenous injection, a 50-mg/g (5% w/w) cream in a water-miscible base, a 3% (30 mg/g) ophthalmic ointment in petrolatum and a 5% (50 mg/g) ointment in a polyethylene glycol or soft paraffin base. The tablets may also contain aluminium–magnesium trisilicate, cellulose, copolyvidon, corn starch, FD&C Blue No. 2, hypromellose, indigocarmine, indigotine, lactose, macrogol, magnesium stearate, methylhydroxypropylcellulose, microcrystalline cellulose, poly(*O*-carboxymethyl)–starch sodium salt, povidone, red iron oxide, silicon dioxide, sodium starch glycolate and titanium dioxide. The capsules may also contain corn starch, lactose, magnesium stearate and sodium lauryl sulfate; the capsule shell may also contain gelatin, FD&C Blue No. 2, one or more parabens and titanium dioxide. The suspension may also contain carboxymethylcellulose sodium, flavours (banana, orange), glycerol, methyl 4-hydroxybenzoate, microcrystalline cellulose, propyl 4-hydroxybenzoate, sorbitol and vanillin. The powder may also contain sodium hydroxide. The cream may also contain cetostearyl alcohol, glycerol monostearate, liquid paraffin, macrogol stearate, petroleum jelly, poloxamer 407, polyoxyethylene fatty acid, propylene glycol, sodium lauryl sulfate and soft white paraffin. Dimeticon was added in the past.

Aciclovir sodium is available as a powder for injection or intravenous infusion in dosages of 25 and 50 mg/mL. After reconstitution with sterile water for injection, aciclovir sodium solutions containing 50 mg/mL aciclovir, have a pH of approximately 11 (10.5–11.7) and are clear and colourless (Gennaro, 1995; American Hospital Formulary Service, 1997; Canadian Pharmaceutical Association, 1997; British Medical Association/Royal Pharmaceutical Society of Great Britain, 1998; Editions du Vidal, 1998; LINFO Läkemedelsinformation AB, 1998; Rote Liste Sekretariat, 1998; Thomas, 1998; Medical Economics Data Production, 1999).

The following impurities are limited by the requirements of the British and European pharmacopoeias: 2-amino-9-{[2-(acetyloxy)ethoxy]methyl]}-1,9-dihydro-6*H*-purin-6-one; 2-amino-1,7-dihydro-6*H*-purin-6-one; 2-amino-7-{[2-hydroxyethoxy]methyl}-1,7-dihydro-6*H*-purin-6-one; 2-amino-9-{[2-(benzoyloxy)ethoxy]methyl}-1,9-dihydro-6*H*-purin-6-one; 6-amino-9-{[2-hydroxyethoxy]methyl}-1,3-dihydro-2*H*-purin-2-one; 2-acetamido-9-{[2-hydroxyethoxy]methyl}-1,9-dihydro-6*H*-purin-6-one; 2-acetamido-9-{[2-(acetyloxy)ethoxy]methyl}-1,9-dihydro-6*H*-purin-6-one; and 2-acetamido-9-{[2-(benzoyloxy)ethoxy]methyl}-1,9-dihydro-6*H*-purin-6-one (British Pharmacopoeial Commission, 1996; Council of Europe, 1998).

Trade names for aciclovir include Acerpes, Acic, Aciclin, Aciclobene, Aciclobeta, Aciclosina, Aciclostad, Aciclovir, Aciclovir 1A Pharma, Aciclovir AL, Aciclovir Allen, Aciclovir Alonga, Aciclovir-Austropharm, Aciclovir Brahms, Aciclovir Cream BP 1998, Aciclovir Dorom, Aciclovir Ebewe, Aciclovir Eye Ointment BP 1998, Aciclovir Filaxis, Aciclovir Heumann, Aciclovir Oral Suspension BP 1998, Aciclovir NM Pharm, Aciclovir-ratiopharm, Aciclovir-Sanorania, Aciclovir Tablets BP 1998, aciclovir von ct, Acic-Ophtal, Aciklovir, Aciklovir Norcox, Acipen Solutab, Aci-Sanorania, Aciviran Pomata, Aclovir, Activar, Activir, Acyclo-V, Acyclovir, Acyclovir Alpharma, Acyclovir Capsules USP 23, Acyclovir-Cophar, Acyclovir for Injection USP 23, Acyclovir-Mepha, Acyclovir Ointment USP 23, Acyclovir Oral Suspension USP 23, Acyclovir Tablets USP 23, Acyl, Acyrax, Acyvir, Aklovir, Alovir, Antiherpes Creme, Antivir, Apo-Acyclovir, Asiviral, Aviclor, Aviral, Avirase, Avirax, Avix, Avyclor, Avyplus, Awirol, Cevirin, Cicloferon, Cicloviral, Citivir, Clonorax, Cusiviral,

Cyclivex, Cyclovir, Cycloviran, Dravyr, Efriviral, Esavir, Exviral, Geavir, Hermixsofex, Hermocil, Hernovir, Herpesin, Herpetad, Herpex, Herpofug, Herpotern, Herpoviric, Klovireks-L, Lisovyr, Mapox, Maynar, Milavir, Neviran, Nycovir, Orivir, Poviral, Rexan, Sifiviral, Simplex, Soothelip, Supravilab, Supraviran, Virasorb, Virax, Virax-Puren, Virherpes, Virmen, Virocul, Virolex, Virosil, Virovir, Virupos, Viruseen, Xiclovir, Zoliparin, Zoviplus, Zovirax and Zyclir (Royal Pharmaceutical Society of Great Britain, 1999; Swiss Pharmaceutical Society, 1999). Those that have been discontinued include Acicloftal, Aciviran, Clovix, Viclocir, Vipral and Zovir.

Trade names for aciclovir sodium include Acic, Aciclovir Alonga, Aciclovir-Austropharm, Aciclovir Biochemie, Aciclovir Brahms i.v., Aciclovir Ebewe, Aciclovir Filaxis, Aciclovir Genthon, Aciclovir Intravenous Infusion BP 1998, Aciclovir-ratiopharm p.i., Aciclovir-Sanorania, Aciclovir Tyrol Pharma, Acivir, Acyclovir Alpharma, Cicloviral i.v., Cusiviral, Geavir, Herpesin, Herpotern, Heviran, Mapox, Maynar, Nycovir, Supraviran, Supraviran i.v., Virherpes, Virmen, Virolex, Zovir, Zovirax, Zovirax for Injection and Zyclir (Royal Pharmaceutical Society of Great Britain, 1999; Swiss Pharmaceutical Society, 1999). The name Viclovir has been discontinued.

1.1.5 *Analysis*

Several international pharmacopoeias specify infrared absorption spectrophotometry with comparison to standards, thin-layer chromatography and liquid chromatography as the methods for identifying aciclovir; potentiometric titration with perchloric acid and liquid chromatography are used to assay its purity. In pharmaceutical preparations (capsule, cream, eye ointment, intravenous infusion, oral suspension, tablet), aciclovir is identified by ultraviolet absorption spectrophotometry and liquid chromatography; ultraviolet absorption spectrophotometry, ultraviolet fluorescence and liquid chromatography are used to assay for aciclovir content (British Pharmacopoeial Commission, 1993, 1994; US Pharmacopeial Convention, 1994; British Pharmacopoeial Commission, 1996; Council of Europe, 1998; US Pharmacopeial Convention, 1998).

1.2 Production

Aciclovir can be prepared by alkylating guanine with 2-(chloromethoxy)ethyl benzoate and hydrolysing the resulting ester to aciclovir (Gennaro, 1995). Approximately 7.5 tonnes of aciclovir were produced worldwide in 1984 and production has increased significantly since then (Glaxo Wellcome, Inc., 1999).

Information available in 1999 indicated that aciclovir and aciclovir sodium were manufactured and/or formulated in 46 and 22 countries, respectively (CIS Information Services, 1998; Royal Pharmaceutical Society of Great Britain, 1999; Swiss Pharmaceutical Society, 1999).

1.3 Use

Aciclovir and its sodium salt are active against herpes simplex viruses (HSV-1 and HSV-2), varicella-zoster infections, and Epstein-Barr virus. Aciclovir is an acyclic nucleoside analogue, and it is incorporated into viral DNA inside an infected cell where it interferes with viral replication (King, 1988; Gennaro, 1995; see section 4.1 for a more complete description of the mechanism of action of aciclovir).

The first new drug application for aciclovir was filed in 1981, and it was first approved for general systemic clinical use in the United Kingdom and the USA in 1982 (King, 1988). By 1988, aciclovir had been licensed in more than 40 countries, and it was estimated that intravenous and oral preparations had already been used in over 10 million courses of treatment (Tilson, 1988).

Aciclovir is used intravenously in the treatment of severe initial and recurrent mucocutaneous infections caused by HSV-1, HSV-2 and varicella-zoster virus (chickenpox virus) in adults and children. It is also the drug of choice for treatment of herpes simplex encephalitis (American Hospital Formulary Service, 1997; Medical Economics Data Production, 1999).

Aciclovir is frequently given orally in the management of first and recurrent episodes of mucocutaneous herpes in selected patients, for the acute treatment of herpes zoster (shingles) and for the treatment of chickenpox in adults and children. Aciclovir is also used topically in the treatment of mucocutaneous HSV infections, although it is substantially less effective than systemic therapy (American Hospital Formulary Service, 1999).

The oral doses of aciclovir for adults range from 200 mg every 4 h (while awake) to 800 mg three times a day for 5–10 days. For chronic suppression of recurrent infections, the dose is 400 mg twice a day. The oral dose for treatment of chickenpox and herpes zoster is 800 mg aciclovir every 4 h for 5–10 days. Topical treatment of the affected skin or mucous membrane (not conjunctival) with 5% ointment or cream is given up to every 3 h. For ocular herpes simplex keratitis, a 3% ointment may be applied five times daily up to every 4 h until 3 days after healing (Gennaro, 1995; American Hospital Formulary Service, 1999; Royal Pharmaceutical Society of Great Britain, 1999).

In young children, aciclovir is given intravenously at 250–500 mg/m^2 of body-surface area every 8 h. In older children and adults, intravenous injections are given at 5–10 mg/kg bw every 8 h (Thomas, 1998; Royal Pharmaceutical Society of Great Britain, 1999).

Doses of aciclovir should be reduced in patients with renal impairment (American Hospital Formulary Service, 1999; Royal Pharmaceutical Society of Great Britain, 1999).

1.4 Occurrence

Aciclovir is not known to occur as a natural product. No data on occupational exposures were available to the Working Group.

1.5 Regulations and guidelines

Aciclovir is listed in the British, European, French, German, Swiss and US pharmacopoeias (Royal Pharmaceutical Society of Great Britain, 1999; Swiss Pharmaceutical Society, 1999).

2. Studies of Cancer in Humans

Kaplowitz *et al.* (1991) conducted a prospective study of 1146 patients (mean age, 34 years) in 24 treatment centres in the USA who had a history of recurrent genital herpes simplex infection confirmed by culture. The patients were treated with aciclovir at various doses, continously and/or for five-day periods for treatment of episodes of infection. No cancers were reported after a follow-up of three years. In 389 patients who were still under treatment and active surveillance five years after the beginning of the first study, one cancer each of the thyroid, pancreas (resulting in death) and ovary and one malignant melanoma were observed (Goldberg *et al.*, 1993). [The Working Group noted that neither the initial study nor the subsequent follow-up was designed to investigate cancer incidence. Thus, the numbers of cancers that were expected were not given, and the relative risk could not be calculated. Furthermore, the low age of the patients, indicating a small expected number of cancers, resulted in poor statistical power to identify an effect. The Working Group also noted the high rate of loss to follow-up.]

In the study of Pluda *et al.* (1990, 1993), described in the monograph on zidovudine, three of eight patients receiving aciclovir plus zidovudine for treatment of symptomatic HIV infection (see IARC, 1996) developed a high-grade, B-cell non-Hodgkin lymphoma. [The Working Group noted that the risk is difficult to interpret in the absence of a suitable reference group consisting of AIDS patients with a similar degree of immunosuppression.]

3. Studies of Cancer in Experimental Animals

3.1 Oral administration

3.1.1 Mouse

Groups of 100 male and 100 female CD-1 Swiss mice [age not specified] were treated with aciclovir [purity not specified] suspended in 0.25% sterile agar at doses of 0, 50, 150 or 450 mg/kg bw by gavage, once daily for 126 (males) and 111 (females) weeks, when the group size was about 20% of that at the beginning of the study. Tissues from control animals and those at the high dose were evaluated histologically. The mean body weights of females at the intermediate and high doses were 2 g higher than those of the control group ($p < 0.01$). Treatment did not affect survival in males, and females at the two higher doses had significantly ($p < 0.05$, log-rank test) longer survival rates than controls. The incidences of benign and malignant tumours were not increased (Tucker et al., 1983a). [The Working Group noted that data on specific tumour incidences were not reported].

3.1.2 Rat

Groups of 85 male and 85 female Sprague-Dawley rats [age not specified] were treated with aciclovir [purity not specified] suspended in 0.25% sterile agar at doses of 0 (control), 50, 150 or 450 mg/kg bw by gavage once daily for 110 (males) and 122 (females) weeks, when the group size was about 20% of that at the beginning of the study. Tissues from control animals and those at the high dose were evaluated by microscopy. Ten male and 10 female rats from each group were killed at 30 and 52 weeks. Treatment did not affect survival rates, except that of females at the intermediate dose, which was significantly shorter than that of control females ($p < 0.05$, log-rank test). No increase in the incidence of benign or malignant tumours was observed (Tucker et al., 1983a). [The Working Group noted that data on specific tumour incidences were not reported.]

4. Other Data Relevant to an Evaluation of Carcinogenicity and its Mechanisms

Aciclovir is active against viruses by virtue of its phosphorylation, incorporation into DNA and the consequent chain termination (Brigden & Whiteman, 1983; Elion, 1983; Laskin, 1984). This series of events occurs readily in herpesvirus-infected tissues but poorly in normal tissues, since the initial phosphorylation is accomplished mainly by a herpesvirus-specific deoxynucleoside (thymidine) kinase (Elion, 1983; Laskin, 1984; King, 1988). Subsequent phosphorylations, to form the aciclovir di- and triphosphates, occur through the action of host cellular enzymes (King, 1988). The aciclovir triphosphate is formed readily and is more persistent than the parent compound, remaining for several hours in cultured cells. The viral polymerase is capable of incorporating aciclovir triphosphate into the growing DNA chain but becomes trapped when attempting to extend the chain with an additional nucleotide, because it is unable to separate from the replication complex (Elion, 1993). Therefore, aciclovir is effective not only because it becomes incorporated into DNA but also because it traps the viral DNA polymerase. The drug is primarily effective for the treatment of HSV-1 and -2 and is less effective against varicella-zoster and Epstein-Barr viruses (Gnann et al., 1983; King, 1988).

4.1 Absorption, distribution, metabolism and excretion

4.1.1 Humans

The absorption, distribution, metabolism and excretion of aciclovir in adults have been reviewed extensively (Laskin, 1983; de Miranda & Blum, 1983; Rogers & Fowle, 1983; Brigden & Whiteman, 1985; O'Brien & Campoli-Richards, 1989; Vergin et al., 1995). When taken orally, the drug is poorly absorbed from the gastrointestinal tract, with a reported bioavailability of 15–30%, owing to its limited solubility in an aqueous environment; therefore, intravenous dosing is considered more effective (O'Brien & Campoli-Richards, 1989). The drug is widely distributed throughout the body and has been found in plasma, kidney, lung, liver, heart, vagina, brain, cerebrospinal fluid, aqueous humor, saliva and skin (Laskin, 1983; de Miranda & Blum, 1983; Rogers & Fowle, 1983; Brigden & Whiteman, 1985; O'Brien & Campoli-Richards, 1989; Vergin et al., 1995). After oral doses of 200 mg taken four to five times daily or 400 mg taken two to three times daily, the peak plasma concentration is about 2 μmol/L (0.49 μg/mL) (Brigden & Whiteman, 1983). After oral administration, the amount of aciclovir in the kidney and lung was actually higher than that in plasma, while the concentration in cerebrospinal fluid was half of that in plasma (Blum et al., 1982; O'Brien & Campoli-Richards, 1989) and the concentration in tear fluid reached 18% of that in plasma (O'Brien & Campoli-Richards, 1989). After topical administration, the epidermal concentration of aciclovir was enhanced 48-fold over that observed after oral dosing, but the delivery of the drug to viruses replicating in the basal epidermis was considerably less efficient (Parry et al., 1992).

The pharmacokinetics of intravenously administered aciclovir has been described best by a two-compartment open model (Laskin, 1983; Rogers & Fowle, 1983; O'Brien & Campoli-Richards, 1989). The binding of aciclovir to plasma protein has been reported to be 9–33%; the peak concentrations in plasma are typically achieved within 1.5–3.2 h, and the half-time for drug removal from plasma is about 3 h (Laskin, 1983; de Miranda & Blum, 1983; Rogers & Fowle, 1983; O'Brien & Campoli-

Richards, 1989; Vergin et al., 1995). The pharmacokinetics is stable over a wide dose range (Rogers & Fowle, 1983).

After intravenous dosing with aciclovir, 45–75% of the drug is excreted in the urine as unchanged compound, but after oral dosing this percentage is reduced to 14–22%, with a large fraction appearing in the faeces (Laskin, 1983; de Miranda & Blum, 1983; Vergin et al., 1995). Two minor urinary metabolites, 9-carboxymethoxy-methylguanine and 8-hydroxy-9-(2-hydroxyethyl)guanine, have been reported to constitute 8–14% and about 0.2% of the total dose, respectively (de Miranda & Blum, 1983; Rogers & Fowle, 1983; Brigden & Whiteman, 1985; O'Brien & Campoli-Richards, 1989; Vergin et al., 1995). Active renal clearance occurs by glomerular filtration and renal tubular secretion, with a half-time of 2–3 h (Laskin, 1983; O'Brien & Campoli-Richards, 1989) and a clearance rate of 3.8–4.9 mL/min per kg of body weight (Rosenberry et al., 1982). In patients with renal impairment, the mean elimination half-time can be extended to 20 h, and the total body clearance rate can be decreased 10-fold; it is therefore necessary to reduce the dose accordingly (de Miranda & Blum, 1983; Rogers & Fowle, 1983; Brigden & Whiteman, 1985; O'Brien & Campoli-Richards, 1989).

Transplacental pharmacokinetics

A 39-year-old pregnant woman, presumed to be at 30 weeks of gestation, was treated with aciclovir (350 mg, or 15 mg/kg bw) intravenously every 8 h throughout the remainder of gestation. At 38–53 h after the last dose, aciclovir was found at a concentration of 0.2–2.8 μg/mL in the urine of the infant, delivered by caesarean section (Greffe et al., 1986).

Beginning at week 38 of gestation and continuing until delivery, seven women were treated orally with 200 mg aciclovir every 8 h and eight with 400 mg aciclovir every 8 h. With 200 mg aciclovir, the maternal plasma concentrations at delivery were 0.65–3.5 μmol/L, and the cord plasma concentrations were 0.59–2.2 μmol/L. The maternal:cord plasma ratio ranged from 1.1 to 1.9. With 400 mg aciclovir, the maternal plasma concentrations at delivery were 0–4.1 μmol/L, the cord plasma concentrations were 0–3.4 μmol/L, and the maternal:cord plasma ratio ranged from 0.83 to 1.4. No adverse effects were reported in the newborn infants (Frenkel et al., 1991).

4.1.2 *Experimental systems*

The absorption, distribution, metabolism and excretion of aciclovir have been determined in several species. The drug appears to be taken up efficiently by many tissues, including the brain and skin (de Miranda et al., 1982; Good et al., 1983; Rogers & Fowle, 1983; Fujioka et al., 1991; Bando et al., 1997). The proportion of drug excreted unchanged in the urine is 3.7% for monkeys, 19% for rats, 43% for mice and 75% for dogs (de Miranda et al., 1982). The major urinary metabolite,

9-carboxymethoxymethylguanine, comprised about 5% of the excreted dose in rats, mice and dogs and about 40% in rabbits, guinea-pigs and rhesus monkeys. Like humans, dogs, rats and rhesus monkeys show a biphasic decline in the plasma concentration of aciclovir, indicating a two-compartment open model, with a half-time of 1–3 h (de Miranda *et al.*, 1982; Gnann *et al.*, 1983).

Rats aged 1–8 weeks received aciclovir by gavage at a dose of 20 mg/kg bw. Gastrointestinal absorption was poor in the 8-week-old rats, with a bioavailability of 7.3%, while rats aged 1–3 weeks had greater intestinal membrane permeability and higher drug bioavailability. Absorption of aciclovir in the gastrointestinal tracts of the young rats was shown to occur by an efficient passive diffusion process, which apparently becomes inefficient at the time of weaning (Fujioka *et al.*, 1991).

Beagle dogs given 20 mg/kg bw aciclovir had a mean peak plasma concentration of 42 μmol/L (10 mg/L) by 1.3–2.2 h, and 30% of the dose was bound to plasma. The mean plasma clearance time was 2.4 h, and 75% of the dose was recovered in urine. The body clearance was similar to the glomerular filtration rate, indicating the absence of active tubular secretion (de Miranda *et al.*, 1982).

As HSV lesions are primarily external (mouth, genitals), transdermal administration of aciclovir was studied *in vivo* and *in vitro* in Wistar rats. Skin absorption occurred by a first-order process which resulted in excretion of about 0.24% of the administered drug in the urine as parent drug; no metabolites were found (Bando *et al.*, 1997).

4.2   Toxic effects

4.2.1   Humans

A summary of the safety of aciclovir, compiled from case reports (about 20 million individuals) and epidemiological studies (about 50 000 patients) during the first 10 years of its use demonstrated that it rarely has adverse effects in healthy individuals. In the USA, 923 adverse events were reported among > 10 million persons, and 129 of these were classified as serious (Tilson *et al.*, 1993). When aciclovir is given orally, the doses are typically low and serious adverse events are extremely rare (Goldberg *et al.*, 1986; Mertz *et al.*, 1988); however, it is given at higher doses intravenously to individuals with serious illnesses, and is associated with more frequent toxic effects (Tilson *et al.*, 1993). The commonest adverse effects include nausea (2.7–8%), vomiting (2.5%), diarrhoea (1.5–2.4%), inflammation at the injection site (9%) and headache (0.6–5.9%) (Ernst & Franey, 1998). The commonest serious effects are neurotoxicity (Adair *et al.*, 1994) and nephrotoxicity (Whitley *et al.*, 1990).

(*a*)   *Neurotoxicity*

Intravenous dosing with aciclovir is commonly associated with neurotoxicity in renally compromised patients, since the drug clearance rates are considerably reduced under such conditions (Rashiq et al., 1993; Tilson et al., 1993; Adair et al., 1994; Kitching et al., 1997). Oral dosing is less frequently neurotoxic but was reported to induce acute disorientation in four patients, three of whom had renal insufficiency (MacDiarmaid-Gordon et al., 1992). Renal dysfunction is not an absolute requirement for aciclovir-induced neurotoxicity; but, apart from age and neurotoxic medications (Rashiq et al., 1993), other definite predisposing factors have not been defined (Ernst & Franey, 1998). The neurotoxicity induced by aciclovir manifests primarily as tremor (28–30%), myclonus (30%), confusion (30–43%), lethargy (17–30%), agitation (27–33%) and hallucination (20–26%) (Rashiq et al., 1993; Ernst & Franey, 1998). Less frequent manifestations (3–17%) include dysarthia, asterixis, ataxia, hemiparesthaesia and seizures (Ernst & Franey, 1998). Neurotoxicity typically occurs during the first 24–72 h of drug administration, and discontinuation of the drug results in a complete return to normal by about 15 days (Rashiq et al., 1993; Ernst & Franey, 1998). Haemodialysis has been shown to attenuate aciclovir-induced neurotoxicity effectively in symptomatic patients (Krieble et al., 1993; Adair et al., 1994).

(b) *Nephrotoxicity*

Intravenous infusion of large doses of aciclovir can occasionally cause crystallization of the drug in the renal tubules (Peterslund et al., 1988) and, rarely, tubular necrosis (Whitley et al., 1990). In patients receiving high doses of aciclovir, reversible increases in serum creatinine concentrations can occur (Kumor et al., 1988; Whitley et al., 1990; Becker & Schulman, 1996). The existence of compromised renal function, use of other nephrotoxic drugs, rapid infusion of large doses, advanced age and dehydration can all contribute to aciclovir-induced nephrotoxicity (Rosenberry et al., 1982; Becker & Schulman, 1996). Like aciclovir-induced neurotoxicity, the nephrotoxic effects are typically transient and rapidly ameliorated by haemodialysis (Whitley et al., 1990; Krieble et al., 1993; Adair et al., 1994; Johnson et al., 1994; Vachvanichsanong et al., 1995).

(c) *Other toxic effects*

Rare effects of intravenous and oral treatment with aciclovir include colitis (Wardle et al., 1997) and reversible, mild abnormalities of haematological and clinical chemical parameters (Mindel et al., 1988; Goldberg et al., 1993). Topical administration may be associated with pain, burning or rash (Rosenberry et al., 1982; Gnann et al., 1983).

Aciclovir, like other anti-HIV nucleoside analogues, has been associated with a rare (1 in 10^5 to 1 in 10^6 patients) idiosyncratic syndrome of a progressive increase in the activity of liver enzymes in serum, fulminating hepatic steatosis and lactic acidosis. Failure to discontinue the drug can lead to death (US Food and Drug Administration Antiviral Advisory Committee, 1993).

4.2.2 *Experimental systems*

(a) Rodents

Aciclovir is relatively non-toxic in rodents. The main effect observed is related to kidney function but is dependent on dose, animal strain and route of administration. Wistar rats given three subcutaneous injections of 15 mg/kg bw aciclovir per day for five days (a total of 45 mg/kg bw per day) showed no significant changes (Hannemann *et al.*, 1997), but intraperitoneal injection of 100 mg/kg bw aciclovir daily for seven days caused polyuria, increased blood urea nitrogen concentration and fractional excretion of sodium and potassium, suggesting damage to the renal proximal tubules (Campos *et al.*, 1992). Obstructive nephropathy, caused by crystalline precipitation of the drug in the renal tubules and collecting ducts, was observed in Long-Evans rats given intravenous injections of 20, 40 or 80 mg/kg bw aciclovir daily for three weeks. These changes were accompanied by increased water consumption, urine output, blood urea nitrogen concentration and kidney weight (Tucker *et al.*, 1983b). All of the nephrotoxic effects of aciclovir resolved within two weeks after drug discontinuation. In Sprague-Dawley rats given 50, 150 or 450 mg/kg bw aciclovir per day by gavage for 25 months, no treatment-related toxic effects were observed (Tucker *et al.*, 1983a). Taken together, these studies suggest that nephrotoxicity is much more likely to result from intravenous than from oral dosing with aciclovir. Parallel clinical observations support the notion that oral dosing is less toxic than intravenous infusion in humans.

No signs of toxicity were observed in CD-1 mice given aciclovir by gavage at a dose of 50, 150 or 450 mg/kg bw per day for one month (Tucker *et al.*, 1983b) or in Swiss mice treated identically for 15 months (Tucker *et al.*, 1983a).

(b) Dogs

As in rodents, high doses of aciclovir given to dogs by infusion over a short time were more nephrotoxic than lower doses given over a longer time. Beagle dogs given rapid intravenous injections of 10, 20, 25, 50 or 100 mg/kg bw aciclovir twice a day for one month showed marked dose-related toxic effects, including death, at the two higher doses. At doses of 20–50 mg/kg bw, decreased ability to concentrate urine, increased blood urea nitrogen concentration and renal tubular damage were observed (Tucker *et al.*, 1983b).

Labrador retrievers infused with 210 mg/kg bw/day aciclovir via constant infusion for 43 h and with 15 mg/kg bw aciclovir three times daily for 28 days had significantly decreased glomerular filtration rates and urine concentrating capacity at the higher dose. The authors concluded that continuous infusion of the high dose of aciclovir was more detrimental than intermittent administration of the lower dose (Kimes *et al.*, 1989).

In a one-year study of toxicity, aciclovir was given orally to beagle dogs at a dose of 15, 45 or 150 mg/kg bw per day. Because of vomiting, diarrhoea and weight loss, the two higher doses were reduced to 60 and 30 mg/kg bw early in the study. The only other reported toxic effects were sore paws due to erosion of the footpads and splitting of the nails at the two higher doses (Tucker et al., 1983a).

(c) *Other species*

Ophthalmic and cutaneous testing of aciclovir in guinea-pigs and rabbits preceded topical application and ophthalmic use in patients. Ointments containing 5 and 10% aciclovir were tested on shaved, abraded or intact skin of guinea-pigs for 24 days with no sign of dermal toxicity. In New Zealand white rabbits, corneal applications of 1 and 3% aciclovir in petrolatum ointment for 21 days had no effect, whereas ointments containing 5 and 6% aciclovir produced mild conjunctival irritation when applied to the eyes (Tucker et al., 1983c).

4.3 Reproductive and prenatal effects

4.3.1 *Humans*

The Acyclovir in Pregnancy Registry was established to gather data on prenatal exposure to aciclovir between 1 June 1984 and 30 June 1990 and comprised information on 312 women exposed to aciclovir and on their children. Most of the women (> 81%) had taken aciclovir orally at doses of 200–1000 mg per day (3.3–17 mg/kg bw assuming a body weight of 60 kg) for 1 to 39 days during pregnancy. No increase in the number of birth defects was found when compared with that expected in the general population (Andrews et al., 1992). [The Working Group noted that the cases accumulated to 30 June 1990 represent a sample of insufficient size for a reliable conclusion about the safety of aciclovir for pregnant women and their developing fetuses.]

4.3.2 *Experimental systems*

In a two-generation study of reproduction and fertility, groups of 15 mature male and 15 female CD-1 mice were treated once each day by gavage with a 0.25% agar vehicle containing 0, 50, 150 or 450 mg/kg bw aciclovir, beginning 64 days before mating for males and 15 days before mating for females and continuing until day 13 of gestation or through day 21 of lactation. No treatment-related alterations in fertility indices, weight gain, pup survival or body weight were reported for the F_0, F_1 or F_2 generation [no data shown] (Moore et al., 1983).

Groups of 21–27 pregnant Sprague-Dawley rats were treated subcutaneously with a 0.9% saline vehicle containing 0, 12, 25 or 50 mg/kg bw per day aciclovir on days 6–15 of gestation. No signs of maternal or fetal toxicity were reported. The mean concentration of aciclovir in fetal homogenate was dose-related: 0, 0.70, 0.96 and 1.95 µg/g wet weight at the four doses, respectively (Moore et al., 1983).

Nineteen pregnant Wistar rats were treated subcutaneously with three doses of 100 mg/kg bw aciclovir on day 10 of gestation, given at 7:00, 12:00 and 17:00 h. Nine control pregnant rats were treated with the vehicle (0.1 mol/L NaCl) only. Maternal weight gain was reduced by aciclovir during pregnancy, but this was attributed to reduced gravid uterine weight and not to maternal toxicity. Various reproductive and developmental effects were reported in the aciclovir-treated group, including an increased rate of resorptions to implantations, skull anomalies and gross structural anomalies of the vertebral column and tail (Chahoud *et al.*, 1988). [The Working Group noted that limited statistical analysis was reported and only one dose was tested.]

Pregnant Wistar rats were treated subcutaneously at 7:00, 12:00 and/or 17:00 h on day 10 or on days 9, 10 and 11 of gestation with either 50, 100 or 200 mg/kg bw aciclovir. On day 11.5 of gestation, the dams were killed and the embryos were evaluated. Dose-related reductions in embryonic growth and increased incidences of abnormalities were observed at the higher doses and with the larger number of doses. Maternal plasma concentrations of aciclovir > 19 mg/mL were associated with embryonic effects (Stahlmann *et al.*, 1988). [The Working Group noted that the number of pregnant dams was not defined but probably ranged from 3 to 10 litters.]

Pregnant Wistar rats were treated subcutaneously with a single dose of 100 mg/kg bw aciclovir or three doses of 100 mg/kg bw at 7:00, 12:00 and 17:00 h on day 10 of gestation and were allowed to deliver their pups. At 12 weeks, both groups of male offspring exposed *in utero* had reduced body weight, liver weight (high dose only) and reduced thymus weight and increased spleen weight. The only significant change in organ weights in female offspring was reduced relative (to body weight) weight of the liver. Aciclovir-exposed offspring showed an impaired immune response, as judged from host resistance to *Trichinella spiratis* and immunoglobulin titres (Stahlmann *et al.*, 1992). [The Working Group noted that the number of dams exposed per group in the test for immune response was not clear.]

Twelve pregnant EPM-I Wistar rats were treated subcutaneously with saline or 60 mg/kg bw aciclovir on days 1–20 of gestation and were killed on day 20. Treatment severely reduced the weight gain of the dams throughout gestation, increased the ratio of resorptions to implantations and decreased the number of viable fetuses (Mamede *et al.*, 1995).

Pregnant New Zealand white rabbits were treated subcutaneously with a 0.9% saline vehicle containing 0, 12, 25 or 50 mg/kg bw aciclovir on days 6–18 of gestation. Five to seven samples of fetal homogenate collected on day 18 of gestation showed mean concentrations of aciclovir of 0, 0.16, 0.21 and 0.32 µg/g at the four doses, respectively. No signs of maternal or fetal toxicity were reported in the fetuses on day 18 or in samples collected on day 29 of gestation from 15–18 additional dams (Moore *et al.*, 1983).

Fertilized eggs ($n = 37$–47) from white Leghorn chickens were incubated at 37.5 ± 0.5 °C and the yolk sac was dosed with 30–1000 µg aciclovir or the 0.01 N sodium hydroxide vehicle as a single dose before and after 24 h of incubation. In another experiment, the embryos in 37–39 fertilized eggs were dosed directly with 3–100 µg aciclovir or 0.01 N sodium hydroxide after two, three or four days of incubation. At evaluation on day 8 of incubation, a dose-related increase in the rate of abnormal development was reported in both series (Heinrich-Hirsch & Neubert, 1991).

Male and female rat embryos collected from pregnant Wistar rats on day 9.5 of gestation were cultured for 48 h in 10–200 µmol/L (2.2–45 µg/mL) aciclovir. Retarded development of the ear anlagen was observed at 25 µmol/L aciclovir, and gross structural abnormalities, especially in the brain, were found at concentrations ≥ 50 µmol/L. Aciclovir at 100 µmol/L resulted in major deformities of the telencephalon and ventricles. No alterations were observed in mouse limb bud explants taken from 11-day-old mouse embryos and exposed to aciclovir at concentrations ≤ 500 µmol/L (Klug et al., 1985).

4.4 Genetic and related effects

4.4.1 *Humans*

No data were available to the Working Group.

4.4.2 *Experimental systems*

Studies of the genotoxicity of aciclovir have yielded largely negative results, and high concentrations of the compound were generally required to produce a positive result or to induce sufficient cytotoxicity to make a negative result valid (Table 1). The genotoxic effects of aciclovir are related primarily to its clastogenicity. Clive *et al.* (1983) provided a review of the genetic activity profile of this drug.

Aciclovir was not genotoxic in various prokaryotic and lower eukaryotic systems. It did not induce reverse mutation in *Salmonella typhimurium* at concentrations of 0.1 µg to 300 mg/plate, with or without exogenous metabolic activation, in a modified plate assay and in the preincubation assay, with five standard strains of *S. typhimurium*. There was no evidence of differential or absolute killing in the *Escherichia coli polA$^+$/polA$^-$* repair assay by aciclovir at concentrations up to 10 mg per well, with or without exogenous metabolic activation. Clive *et al.* (1983) noted that strict proof that aciclovir does not induce *polA*-repairable DNA damage is lacking, but no evidence of lethal damage was found. Aciclovir did not induce gene conversion in *Saccharomyces cerevisiae* strain D5 over the standard dose range in the presence or absence of exogenous activation.

In cultured mammalian cells, aciclovir was not mutagenic at the *Oua* or *Hprt* locus of mouse lymphoma L5178Y cells or at the *Oua*, *Hprt* or *Aprt* locus of Chinese hamster ovary cells, but it was mutagenic in the *Tk* gene of lymphoma cells and this effect was unambiguous, reproducible and dose-related at concentrations ≥ 400 µg/mL. The occurrence of primarily small-type *Tk* mutant colonies in aciclovir-

Table 1. Genetic and related effects of aciclovir

Test system	Result[a]		Dose[b] (LED/HID)	Reference
	Without exogenous metabolic system	With exogenous metabolic system		
Escherichia coli pol A/W3110-P3478, differential toxicity (spot test)	–	–	10 000 µg/plate	Clive *et al.* (1983)
Salmonella typhimurium TA100, TA1535, TA1537, TA1538, TA98, reverse mutation	–	–	300 mg/plate	Clive *et al.* (1983)
Saccharomyces cerevisiae, gene conversion	–	–	500 µg/plate	Clive *et al.* (1983)
Gene mutation, Chinese hamster ovary cells *in vitro*, *Hprt* locus	–	–	3000	Clive *et al.* (1983)
Gene mutation, Chinese hamster ovary cells *in vitro*, *Aprt* locus	–	–	3000	Clive *et al.* (1983)
Gene mutation, Chinese hamster ovary cells *in vitro*, *Oua* locus	–	–	3000	Clive *et al.* (1983)
Gene mutation, Chinese hamster ovary cells *in vitro*, *Hprt* locus	–	NT	22.5	Pizer *et al.* (1987)
Gene mutation, mouse lymphoma L5178Y cells, *Tk* locus *in vitro*	+	+	400	Clive *et al.* (1983)
Gene mutation, mouse lymphoma L5178Y cells, *Hprt* locus *in vitro*	–	–	2400	Clive *et al.* (1983)
Gene mutation, mouse lymphoma L5178Y cells, *Oua* locus *in vitro*	–	–	2400	Clive *et al.* (1983)
Sister chromatid exchange, Chinese hamster cells *in vitro*	(+)	NT	90	Thust *et al.* (1996)
Chromosomal aberrations, Chinese hamster cells *in vitro*	(+)	NT	135	Thust *et al.* (1996)
Cell transformation, BALB/c 3T3 mouse cells	+	NT	50	Clive *et al.* (1983)
Cell transformation, C3H 10T1/2 mouse cells	–	NT	64	Clive *et al.* (1983)
Sister chromatid exchange, human lymphocytes *in vitro*	–	NT	200	De Clercq & Cassiman (1986)
Chromosomal aberrations, human lymphocytes *in vitro*	+	NT	250	Clive *et al.* (1983)
Micronucleus formation, mouse cells *in vivo*	+		122 iv × 2	Haynes *et al.* (1996)
Chromosomal aberrations, rat bone-marrow cells *in vivo*	–		100 iv × 1	Clive *et al.* (1983)

Table 1 (contd)

Test system	Result[a]		Dose[b] (LED/HID)	Reference
	Without exogenous metabolic system	With exogenous metabolic system		
Chromosomal aberrations, Chinese hamster bone-marrow cells in vivo	+		500 ip × 1	Clive et al. (1983)
Dominant lethal mutation, mice	−		50 ip × 5	Clive et al. (1983)

[a] +, positive; (+), weak positive; −, negative; NT, not tested
[b] LED, lowest effective dose; HID, highest ineffective dose; in-vitro tests, µg/mL; in-vivo tests, mg/kg bw per day; d, day; iv, intravenous; ip, intraperitoneal

treated lymphoma cells is consistent with a clastogenic response associated with DNA chain termination.

Aciclovir was found to transform BALB/c-3T3 cells at the highest dose tested (50 μg/mL) applied for 72 h, but did not transform similarly exposed C3H/10T1/2 cells. The apparent discrepancy between the two systems may be ascribed in part to the fact that the C3H cells were exposed for shorter times and few cells were used. An effort to normalize these factors between the two assays suggests that the results with the BALB/c cells would have paralleled those of the C3H cells had the exposures been identical [no reason was given for the use of different conditions] (Clive et al., 1983).

Aciclovir is clastogenic in mammalian cells both in vitro and in vivo. Chinese hamster strain V79-E cells were evaluated for the frequencies of sister chromatid exchange and chromosomal aberrations after exposure to 0.0073–2.0 mmol/L of aciclovir and judged to show borderline increases in the frequency of chromosomal aberrations. The authors (Thust et al., 1996) did not perform a statistical analysis of these results but used a doubling of the background frequency to assign significance to changes in the frequency of chromosomal aberrations. This fact is important because the increase in chromosomal aberration frequency was due to chromatid gaps and chromatid breaks [although the authors did not discuss these findings]. Exposure of cultured human lymphocytes to 250 and 500 μg/mL aciclovir in the absence of exogenous metabolic activation caused a linear increase in the frequency of chromosomal aberrations, due mainly to chromatid breaks. [The Working Group considered the borderline increase in frequency and the nature of the chromosomal aberrations observed to indicate the clastogenicity of aciclovir at high doses.]

Male CD-1 mice were given two intravenous doses of aciclovir at 0 and 24 h and the frequencies of micronucleated polychromatic erythrocytes were evaluated 48 h after exposure. The frequency of micronucleated cells increased in a dose-related fashion.

When groups of four female and four male CD rats were given intravenous doses of aciclovir up to and including the maximum tolerated dose of 100 mg/kg bw, no increase in the frequency of chromosomal aberrations in bone marrow was found in either sex at any of three sacrifice times. A single intravenous dose of 80 mg/kg bw resulted in a peak plasma concentration of 87 ± 16 μg/mL, however, which is lower than the concentration that caused clastogenic effects in assays for chromosomal aberrations in vitro.

In groups of three female Chinese hamsters, intraperitoneal injections of ≤ 100 mg/kg bw aciclovir had no effect, while 500 mg/kg bw caused a very high frequency of chromosomal aberrations 24 h after exposure. For example, one treated hamster had chromosome breaks in 99 of 108 cells scored, and 97 of these 99 breaks occurred at the centromere of a single one of the six intermediate size metacentric chromosomes. The mean concentration of aciclovir in human plasma is 0.2 μg/mL after topical administration, 1.0 μg/mL after intravenous administration and 0.6 μg/mL after oral administration, while the peak plasma concentration found after intraperitoneal administration of 500 mg/kg bw to Chinese hamsters was 611 ± 91 μg/mL, which is well above the minimum required to cause a clastogenic effect *in vitro*. The authors (Clive *et al.*, 1983) noted that the natural bases and their nucleosides are clastogenic at a concentration of about 1 mmol/L and that the clastogenicity of aciclovir in hamsters occurred at roughly comparable concentrations of the natural bases and their nucleosides.

4.5 Mechanistic considerations

Aciclovir has little toxicity in either humans or experimental animals, but there is convincing evidence that it can induce genetic changes in a number of mammalian cellular systems, both *in vitro* and *in vivo*. Structural chromosomal aberrations were observed in cultured Chinese hamster fibroblasts and human lymphocytes and in the bone-marrow cells of Chinese hamsters dosed *in vivo*. In addition, an increased frequency of micronucleated cells was observed in mice dosed *in vivo*. These effects are probably consequential to the DNA chain termination activity of aciclovir. It should be noted that the doses required to produce a clastogenic response were much higher than those to which people and experimental animals are exposed. Furthermore, the doses of up to 450 mg/kg bw per day that were given to mice and rats by gavage during the two-year tests for carcinogenicity, in which treatment-related tumours did not develop, are unlikely to have produced peak plasma concentrations sufficient to precipitate a clastogenic response. The lowest clastogenic doses were 250 µg/mL in cultured human lymphocytes and 540 µmol/kg bw in mouse bone marrow after intravenous administration. The latter dose would have resulted in an extremely high plasma concentration. The peak plasma concentration in humans receiving a typical dosing regime is about 2 µmol/L, or 0.5 µg/mL.

5. Summary of Data Reported and Evaluation

5.1 Exposure data

Aciclovir is an acyclic nucleoside analogue which was first approved for use as an antiviral agent in 1982. It is used in the treatment of herpes simplex, varicella and herpes zoster viral infections. Oral and topical forms of aciclovir are very widely used for mucocutaneous infections. Intravenous preparations are widely used for some infections including encephalitis associated with herpes simplex viral infection and neonatal herpesvirus infection.

5.2 Human carcinogenicity data

The results of one prospective study and an extended observational follow-up indicated no increased risk for cancer among patients with recurrent herpes simplex infection given aciclovir orally, but, as the studies were not designed to investigate cancer, no conclusion can be drawn.

5.3 Animal carcinogenicity data

Aciclovir was tested for carcinogenicity in one experiment in mice and one experiment in rats by oral administration. The tumour incidence was not increased in either species.

5.4 Other relevant data

The pharmacokinetics of intravenously administered aciclovir in humans is stable over a wide dose range. The bioavailability of orally administered aciclovir is 15–30%. It is widely distributed, can cross the placenta and is, relative to many other antiviral drugs, slowly removed from plasma. More than half the administered drug is excreted unchanged, while the metabolite 9-carboxymethoxymethylguanine constitutes 8–14% of the dose. Urinary excretion can be markedly reduced in patients with impaired renal function. The pharmacokinetics of aciclovir in dogs is similar to that in humans, but the drug is removed more rapidly from the plasma of rats. Virtually all of the drug is recovered unchanged from dosed rats.

Adverse effects of aciclovir have been reported extremely rarely in people who have received oral or topical formulations. Higher doses are given intravenously in cases of serious illness, and most of the side-effects have been reported after such usage. The most common serious adverse effects are neurotoxicity and nephrotoxicity. Dogs and rats also show nephrotoxicity when treated at high doses.

Insufficient human data were available on the reproductive and prenatal effects of aciclovir. No developmental toxicity was reported in mice, rats or rabbits given doses over several days during gestation.

The available mutagenicity data indicate that aciclovir is primarily clastogenic at high concentrations, consistent with its action as a DNA chain terminator.

5.5 Evaluation

There is *inadequate evidence* in humans for the carcinogenicity of aciclovir.

There is *inadequate evidence* in experimental animals for the carcinogenicity of aciclovir.

Overall evaluation

Aciclovir is *not classifiable as to its carcinogenicity to humans (Group 3)*.

6. References

Adair, J.C., Gold, M. & Bond, R.E. (1994) Acyclovir neurotoxicity: Clinical experience and review of the literature. *South. med. J.*, **87**, 1227–1231

American Hospital Formulary Service (1997) *AHFS Drug Information® 97*, Bethesda, MD, American Society of Health-System Pharmacists, pp. 440–449, 2678–2680

American Hospital Formulary Service (1999) *AHFS Drug Information® 99*, Bethesda, MD, American Society of Health-System Pharmacists [AHFSfirst MedAxon CD-ROM]

Andrews, E.B., Yankaskas, B.C., Cordero, J.F., Schoeffler, K., Hampp, S. & the Acyclovir in Pregnancy Registry Advisory Committee (1992) Acyclovir in pregnancy registry: Six years' experience. *Obstet. Gynecol.*, **79**, 7–13

Bando, H., Sahashi, M., Yamashita, F., Takakura, Y. & Hashida, M. (1997) *In vivo* evaluation of acyclovir prodrug penetration and metabolism through rat skin using a diffusion/bio-conversion model. *Pharm. Res.*, **14**, 56–62

Becker, B.N. & Schulman, G. (1996) Nephrotoxicity of antiviral therapies. *Curr. Opin. Nephrol. Hyperten.*, **5**, 375–379

Blum, M.R., Liao, S.H.T. & de Miranda, P. (1982) Overview of acyclovir pharmacokinetics disposition in adults and children. *Am. J. Med.*, **73** (Suppl. 1A), 186–192

Brigden, D. & Whiteman, P. (1983) The mechanism of action, pharmacokinetics and toxicity of acyclovir—A review. *J. Infect.*, **6** (Suppl. 1), 3–9

Brigden, D. & Whiteman, P. (1985) The clinical pharmacology of acyclovir and its prodrugs. *Scand. J. infect. Dis.*, **47**, 33–39

British Medical Association/Royal Pharmaceutical Society of Great Britain (1998) *British National Formulary*, No. 36, London, pp. 275–276, 452, 509

British Pharmacopoeial Commission (1993) *British Pharmacopoeia 1993*, London, Her Majesty's Stationery Office, Vol. I, p. 24, S5

British Pharmacopoeial Commission (1994) *British Pharmacopoeia 1993, Addendum 1994*, London, Her Majesty's Stationery Office, pp. 1402–1404

British Pharmacopoeial Commission (1996) *British Pharmacopoeia 1993, Addendum 1996*, London, Her Majesty's Stationery Office, pp. 1712–1713

Budavari, S., ed. (1996) *The Merck Index*, 12th Ed., Whitehouse Station, NJ, Merck & Co., p. 27

Campos, S.B., Seguro, A.C., Cesar, K.R. & Rocha, A.S. (1992) Effects of acyclovir on renal function. *Nephron*, **62**, 74–79

Canadian Pharmaceutical Association (1997) *CPS Compendium of Pharmaceuticals and Specialties*, 32nd Ed., Ottawa, pp. 147–148, 1811–1815

Chahoud, I., Stahlmann, R., Bochert, G., Dillmann, I. & Neubert, D. (1988) Gross-structural defects in rats after acyclovir application on day 10 of gestation. *Arch. Toxicol.*, **62**, 8–14

CIS Information Services (1998) *Worldwide Bulk Drug Users Directory 1997/98 Edition*, Dallas, TX [CD-ROM]

Clive, D., Turner, N.T., Hozier, J., Batson, A.G. & Tucker, W.E., Jr (1983) Preclinical toxicology studies with acyclovir: Genetic toxicity tests. *Fundam. appl. Toxicol.*, **3**, 587–602

Council of Europe (1998) *European Pharmacopoeia*, 3rd Ed., *Supplement 1998*, Strasbourg, pp. 164–165

De Clercq, E. & Cassiman, J.-J. (1986) Mutagenic potential of anti-herpes agents. *Life Sci.*, **38**, 281–289

Editions du Vidal (1998) *Dictionnaire Vidal 1998*, 74th Ed., Paris, OVP, pp. 2048–2051

Elion, G.B. (1983) The biochemistry and mechanism of action of acyclovir. *J. antimicrob. Chemother.*, **12** (Suppl. B), 9–17

Elion, G.B. (1993) Acyclovir: Discovery, mechanism of action, and selectivity. *J. med. Virol.*, **1**, 2–6

Ernst, M.E. & Franey, R.J. (1998) Acyclovir- and ganciclovir-induced neurotoxicity. *Ann. Pharmacother.*, **32**, 111–113

Frenkel, L.M., Brown, Z.A., Bryson, Y.J., Corey, L., Unadkat, J.D., Hensleigh, P.A., Arvin, A.M., Prober, C.G. & Connor, J.D. (1991) Pharmacokinetics of acyclovir in the term human pregnancy and neonate. *Am. J. Obstet. Gynecol.*, **164**, 569–576

Fujioka, Y., Mizuno, N., Morita, E., Motozono, H., Takahashi, K., Yamanaka, Y. & Shinkuma, D. (1991) Effect of age on the gastrointestinal absorption of acyclovir in rats. *J. pharm. Pharmacol.*, **43**, 465–469

Gennaro, A.R. (1995) *Remington: The Science and Practice of Pharmacy*, 19th Ed., Easton, PA, Mack Publishing, Vol. II, pp. 1332–1333

Glaxo Wellcome, Inc. (1999) Department of Infectious Diseases and Hepatitis, Research Triangle Park, NC, USA

Gnann, J.W., Barton, N.H. & Whitley, R.J. (1983) Acyclovir: Mechanism of action, pharmacokinetics, safety and clinical applications. *Pharmacotherapy*, **3**, 275–283

Goldberg, L.H., Kaufman, R.H., Conant, M.A., Sperber, J., Allen, M.L., Illeman, M. & Chapman, S. (1986) Oral acyclovir for episodic treatment of recurrent genital herpes. *J. Am. Acad. Dermatol.*, **15**, 256–264

Goldberg, L.H., Kaufman, R.H., Kurtz, T.O., Conant, M.A., Eron, L.J., Batenhorst, R.L., Boone, G.S. & the Acyclovir Study Group (1993) Continuous five-year treatment of patients with frequently recurring genital herpes simplex virus infection with acyclovir. *J. med. Virol.*, **Suppl. 1**, 45–50

Good, S.S., Krasny, H.C., Elion, G.B. & de Miranda, P. (1983) Disposition in the dog and the rat of 2,6-diamino-9-(2-hydroxyethoxymethyl)purine (A134U), a potential prodrug of acyclovir. *J. Pharmacol. exp. Ther.*, **227**, 644–651

Greffe, B.S., Dooley, S.L., Deddish, R.B. & Krasny, H.C. (1986) Transplacental passage of acyclovir. *J. Pediatr.*, **108**, 1020–1021

Hannemann, J., Wunderle, W., Yousif, T., Krüger, S. & Baumann, K. (1997) Toxic effect of concomitant administration of cylcosporin A and acyclovir on renal function and morphology in rats. *Arch. Toxicol.*, **71**, 556–562

Haynes, P., Lambert, T.R. & Mitchell, I. de G. (1996) Comparative in-vivo genotoxicity of antiviral nucleoside analogues; penciclovir, acyclovir, ganciclovir and the xanthine analogue, caffeine, in the mouse bone marrow micronucleus assay. *Mutat. Res.*, **369**, 65–74

Heinrich-Hirsch, B. & Neubert, D. (1991) Effects of aciclovir on the development of the chick embryo in ovo. *Arch. Toxicol.*, **65**, 402–408

IARC (1996) *IARC Monographs on the Evaluation of Carcinogenic Risks to Humans*, Vol. 67, *Human Immunodeficiency Viruses and Human T-cell Lymphotropic Viruses*, Lyon, IARC*Press*, pp. 31–259

Johnson, G.L., Limon, L., Trikha, G. & Wall, H. (1994) Acute renal failure and neurotoxicity following oral acyclovir. *Ann. Pharmacother.*, **28**, 460–463

Kaplowitz, L.G., Baker, D., Gelb, L., Blythe, J., Hale, R., Frost, P., Crumpacker, C., Rabinovich, S., Peacock, J.E., Jr, Herndon, J., Davis, L.G. & the Acyclovir Study Group (1991) Prolonged continuous acyclovir treatment of normal adults with frequently recurring genital herpes simplex virus infection. *J. Am. med. Assoc.*, **265**, 747–751

Kimes, A.S., Kumor, K., McCullough, K., Holtzclaw, D., Teller, D., Dobyan, D. & Spector, D. (1989) Effects of acute and chronic acyclovir on canine renal function. *J. Pharmacol. exp. Ther.*, **249**, 483–491

King, D.H. (1988) History, pharmacokinetics, and pharmacology of acyclovir. *J. Am. Acad. Dermatol.*, **18**, 176–179

Kitching, A.R., Fagg, D., Hay, N.M., Hatfield, P.J. & Macdonald, A. (1997) Neurotoxicity associated with acyclovir in end stage renal failure. *N.Z. med. J.*, **110**, 167–169

Klug, S., Lewandowski, C., Blankenburg, G., Merker, H.-J. & Neubert, D. (1985) Effect of acyclovir on mammalian embryonic development in culture. *Arch. Toxicol.*, **58**, 89–96

Krieble, B.F., Rudy, D.W., Glick, M.R. & Clayman, M.D. (1993) Case report: Acyclovir neurotoxicity and nephrotoxicity—The role for hemodialysis. *Am. J. med. Sci.*, **305**, 36–39

Kumor, K., Conklin, R., Woo, J., Katz, L. & Strocchia, C. (1988) Renal function studies during intravenous acyclovir treatment of immune suppressed patients including renal transplantation. *Am. J. Nephrol.*, **8**, 35–39

Laskin, O.L. (1983) Clinical pharmacokinetics of acyclovir. *Clin. Pharmacokinet.*, **8**, 187–201

Laskin, O.L. (1984) Acyclovir. Pharmacology and clinical experience. *Arch. intern. Med.*, **144**, 1241–1246

LINFO Läkemedelsinformation AB (1998) *FASS 1998 Läkemedel i Sverige*, Stockholm, pp. 97–100, 1289–1292

MacDiarmaid-Gordon, A.R., O'Connor, M., Beaman, M. & Ackrill, P. (1992) Neurotoxicity associated with oral acyclovir in patients undergoing dialysis. *Nephron*, **62**, 280–283

Mamede, J.A.V., Simões, J.d.J., Novo, N.F., Juliano, Y., Oliveira-Filho, R.M. & Kulay, L., Jr (1995) Chronic effects of azidothymidine and acyclovir on pregnant rats. *Gen. Pharmacol.*, **26**, 523–526

Medical Economics Data Production (1999) *PDR®: Physicians' Desk Reference*, 53rd Ed., Montvale, NJ, pp. 1272–1277

Mertz, G.J., Jones, C.C., Mills, J., Fife, K.H., Lemon, S.M., Stapleton, J.T., Hill, E.L., Davis, L.G. & the Acyclovir Study Group (1988) Long-term acyclovir suppression of frequently recurring genital herpes simplex virus infection. *J. Am. med. Assoc.*, **260**, 201–206

Mindel, A., Carney, O., Ferris, M., Faherty, A., Patou, G. & Williams, P. (1988) Dosage and safety of long-term suppressive acyclovir therapy for recurrent genital herpes. *Lancet*, **i**, 926–928

de Miranda, P. & Blum, M.R. (1983) Pharmacokinetics of acyclovir after intravenous and oral administration. *J. antimicrob. Chemother.*, **12** (Suppl. B), 29–37

de Miranda, P., Krasny, H.C., Page, D.A. & Elion, G.B. (1982) Species differences in the disposition of acyclovir. *Am. J. Med.*, **73**, 31–35

Moore, H.L., Jr, Szczech, G.M., Rodwell, D.E., Kapp, R.W., Jr, de Miranda, P. & Tucker, W.E., Jr (1983) Preclinical toxicology studies with acyclovir: Teratologic, reproductive and neonatal tests. *Fundam. appl. Toxicol.*, **3**, 560–568

O'Brien, J.J. & Campoli-Richards, D.M. (1989) Acyclovir. An updated review of its antiviral activity, pharmacokinetic properties and therapeutic efficacy. *Drugs*, **37**, 233–309

Parry, G.E., Dunn, P., Shah, V.P. & Pershing, L.K. (1992) Acyclovir bioavailability in human skin. *J. invest. Dermatol.*, **98**, 856–863

Peterslund, N.A., Larsen, M.L. & Mygind, H. (1988) Acyclovir crystalluria. *Scand. J. infect. Dis.*, **20**, 225–228

Pizer, L.I., Mitchell, D.H., Bentele, B., & Betz, J.L. (1987) A mammalian cell line designed to test the mutagenic activity of anti-herpes nucleosides. *Int. J. Cancer*, **40**, 114–121

Pluda, J.M., Yarchoan, R., Jaffe, E.S., Feuerstein, I.M., Solomon, D., Steinberg, S.M., Wyvill, K.M., Raubitschek, A., Katz, D. & Broder, S. (1990) Development of non-Hodgkin lymphoma in a cohort of patients with severe human immunodeficinecy virus (HIV) infection on long-term antiretroviral therapy. *Ann. intern. Med.*, **113**, 276–282

Pluda, J.M., Venzon, D.J., Tosato, G., Lietzau, J., Wyvill, K., Nelson, D.L., Jaffe, E.S., Karp, J.E., Broder, S. & Yarchoan, R. (1993) Parameters affecting the development of non-Hodgkin's lymphoma in patients with severe human immunodeficiency virus infection receiving antiretroviral therapy. *J. clin. Oncol.*, **11**, 1099–1107

Rashiq, S., Briewa, L., Mooney, M., Giancarlo, T., Khatib, R. & Wilson, F.M. (1993) Distinguishing acyclovir neurotoxicity from encephalomyelitis. *J. intern. Med.*, **234**, 507–511

Rogers, H.J. & Fowle, A.S.E. (1983) The clinical pharmacology of acyclovir. *J. clin. Hosp. Pharm.*, **8**, 89–102

Rosenberry, K.R., Bryan, C.K. & Sohn, C.A. (1982) Acyclovir: Evaluation of a new antiviral agent. *Clin. Pharm.*, **1**, 399–406

Rote Liste Sekretariat (1998) *Rote Liste 1998*, Frankfurt, Rote Liste Service GmbH, pp. 10-398–10-439, 32-060–32-074, 32-078–32-079, 32-083–32-084, 32-091–32-092, 68-218, 68-222–68-224

Royal Pharmaceutical Society of Great Britain (1999) *Martindale, The Extra Pharmacopoeia*, 13th Ed., London, The Pharmaceutical Press [MicroMedex CD-ROM]

Stahlmann, R., Klug, S., Lewandowski, C., Bochert, G., Chahoud, I., Rahm, U., Merker, H.-J. & Neubert, D. (1988) Prenatal toxicity of acyclovir in rats. *Arch. Toxicol.*, **61**, 468–479

Stahlmann, R., Korte, M., Van Loveren, H., Vos, J.G., Thiel, R. & Neubert, D. (1992) Abnormal thymus development and impaired function of the immune system in rats after prenatal exposure to aciclovir. *Arch. Toxicol.*, **66**, 551–559

Swiss Pharmaceutical Society, ed. (1999) *Index Nominum, International Drug Directory*, 16th Ed., Stuttgart, Medpharm Scientific Publishers [MicroMedex CD-ROM]

Thomas, J., ed. (1998) *Australian Prescription Products Guide*, 27th Ed., Victoria, Australian Pharmaceutical Publishing, Vol. 1, pp. 239–241, 261–263, 3035–3044

Thust, R., Schacke, M. & Wutzler, P. (1996) Cytogenetic genotoxicity of antiherpes virostatics in Chinese hamster V79-E cells. I. Purine nucleoside analogues. *Antiviral Res.*, **31**, 105–113

Tilson, H.H. (1988) Monitoring the safety of antivirals. *Am. J. Med.*, **85** (Suppl. 2A), 116–122

Tilson, H.H., Engle, C.R. & Andrews, E.B. (1993) Safety of acyclovir: A summary of the first 10 years experience. *J. med. Virol.*, **Suppl. 1**, 67–73

Tucker, W.E., Jr, Krasny, H.C., de Miranda, P., Goldenthal, E.I., Elion, G.B., Hajian, G. & Szczech, G.M. (1983a) Preclinical toxicology studies with acyclovir: Carcinogenicity bioassays and chronic toxicity tests. *Fundam. appl. Toxicol.*, **3**, 579–586

Tucker, W.E., Jr, Macklin, A.W., Szot, R.J., Johnston, R.E., Elion, G.B., de Miranda, P. & Szczech, G.M. (1983b) Preclinical toxicology studies with acyclovir: Acute and subchronic tests. *Fundam. appl Toxicol.*, **3**, 573–578

Tucker, W.E., Jr, Johnston, R.E., Macklin, A.W., Szot, R.J., Elion, G.B., de Miranda, P. & Szczech, G.M. (1983c) Preclinical toxicology studies with acyclovir: Ophthalmic and cutaneous tests. *Fundam. appl. Toxicol.*, **3**, 569–572

US Food and Drug Administration Antiviral Drugs Advisory Committee (1993) *Mitochondrial Damage Associated with Nucleoside Analogues*, Rockville, MD

US Pharmacopeial Convention (1994) *The 1995 US Pharmacopeia*, 23rd Rev./*The National Formulary*, 18th Rev., Rockville, MD, pp. 35–36

US Pharmacopeial Convention. (1998) *The 1995 US Pharmacopeia*, 23rd Rev./*The National Formulary*, 18th Rev., Supplement 9, Rockville, MD, pp. 4514–4516

Vachvanichsanong, P., Patamasucon, P., Malagon, M. & Moore, E.S. (1995) Brief report. Acute renal failure in a child associated with acyclovir. *Pediatr. Nephrol.*, **9**, 346–347

Vergin, H., Kikuta, C., Mascher, H. & Metz, R. (1995) Pharmacokinetics and bioavailability of different formulations of aciclovir. *Arzneim.-Forsch./Drug Res.*, **45**, 508–515

Wardle, T.D., Finnerty, J.P., Swale, V. & Beer, T. (1997) Acyclovir-induced colitis. *Alim. Pharmacol. Ther.*, **11**, 415–417

Whitley, R.J., Middlebrooks, M. & Gnann, J.W., Jr (1990) Acyclovir: The past ten years. *Adv. exp. Med. Biol.*, **278**, 243–253

ZIDOVUDINE (AZT)

1. Exposure Data

1.1 Chemical and physical data

Zidovudine is an analogue of thymidine in which the 3-hydroxyl group is replaced by an azido group.

1.1.1 Nomenclature

Chem. Abstr. Serv. Reg. No.: 30516-87-1
Chem. Abstr. Name: 3′-Azido-3′-deoxythymidine
IUPAC Systematic Name: 3′-Azido-3′-deoxythymidine
Synonyms: 1-(3-Azido-2,3-dideoxy-β-D-ribofuranosyl)-5-methylpyrimidine-2,4-(1*H*,3*H*)-dione; azidothymidine; 3′-azidothymidine; AZT; 3′-deoxy-3′-azidothymidine; ZDV
[Note: The abbreviation AZT is also used for another drug, azathioprine (Royal Pharmaceutical Society of Great Britain, 1999).]

1.1.2 Structural and molecular formulae and relative molecular mass

$C_{10}H_{13}N_5O_4$ Relative molecular mass: 267.25

1.1.3 Chemical and physical properties of the pure substance

(*a*) *Description*: White to off-white crystals or needles (Gennaro, 1995; American Hospital Formulary Service, 1997)

(b) *Melting-point*: 106–112 °C (from petroleum ether); 120–122 °C (from water) (Budavari, 1996)
(c) *Spectroscopy data*: Infrared, ultraviolet, nuclear magnetic resonance (proton) and mass spectral data have been reported (National Cancer Institute, 1989).
(d) *Solubility*: Soluble in water (25 mg/mL at 25 °C) and ethanol (67 mg/mL) (Gennaro, 1995; Budavari, 1996)
(e) *Optical rotation*: $[\alpha]_D^{25}$, +99° (c = 0.5 in water) (Budavari, 1996)
(f) *Dissociation constant*: pK_a, 9.68 (Gennaro, 1995)

1.1.4 Technical products and impurities

Zidovudine is available as a 300-mg tablet, a 100- or 250-mg capsule, a 50-mg/5 mL syrup and a 200-mg/20 mL injection solution; it is also available as a tablet in combination with lamivudine. The tablets may also contain macrogol, magnesium stearate, microcrystalline cellulose, povidone, sodium carboxymethyl starch and titanium dioxide. The capsules may also contain corn starch, gelatin, indigo carmine (CI 73015), indigotine, magnesium stearate, microcrystalline cellulose, polysorbate 80, sodium starch glycollate, starch–maize, sulfites, iron oxides and titanium dioxide. The syrup may also contain anhydrous citric acid, flavourings, glycerol, maltitol solution, saccharin sodium, sodium benzoate, sodium hydroxide and sucrose. The injection solution may also contain hydrochloric acid or sodium hydroxide (Gennaro, 1995; Canadian Pharmaceutical Association, 1997; British Medical Association/Royal Pharmaceutical Society of Great Britain, 1998; Editions du Vidal, 1998; LINFO Läkemedelsinformation AB, 1998; Rote Liste Sekretariat, 1998; Thomas, 1998; US Pharmacopeial Convention, 1998a). The oral solution containing 50 mg/5 mL zidovudine is colourless to pale yellow and has a pH of 3–4; the oral solution contains sodium benzoate as a preservative and may contain sodium hydroxide to adjust the pH. The injection for intravenous infusion has a pH of approximately 5.5 and contains no preservatives, but hydrochloric acid and/or sodium hydroxide may be added during manufacture to adjust the pH (American Hospital Formulary Service, 1997).

The following impurities are limited by the requirements of the British and European pharmacopoeias: 1-[(2R,5S)-5-hydroxymethyl-2,5-dihydro-2-furyl]-5-methylpyrimidine-2,4(1H,3H)-dione; 1-(3-chloro-2,3-dideoxy-β-D-ribofuranosyl)-5-methylpyrimidine-2,4(1H,3H)-dione; thymine; and triphenylmethanol (British Pharmacopoeia Commission, 1996; Council of Europe, 1997).

Trade names for zidovudine include Apo-Zidovudine, Azitidin, Azoazol, Azotine, Azovir, AZT Filaxis, Crisazet, Enper, Exovir, Novo-AZT, Retrovir, Virustat, Zidosan, Zidovir, Zidovudina Combino Pharm, Zidovudina Lazar and Zidovudine Asofarma (Swiss Pharmaceutical Society, 1999).

1.1.5 *Analysis*

Several international pharmacopoeias specify infrared absorption spectrophotometry with comparison to standards and liquid chromatography as the methods for identifying zidovudine; liquid chromatography is used to assay its purity. In pharmaceutical preparations, zidovudine is identified by ultraviolet absorption spectrophotometry, thin-layer chromatography and liquid chromatography; liquid chromatography is used to assay for zidovudine content (British Pharmacopoeia Commission, 1996; Council of Europe, 1997; US Pharmacopeial Convention, 1998b).

A simple, rapid method by high-performance liquid chromatography (HPLC) for zidovudine in plasma with a reversed-phase column and detection at 265 nm has been reported. The detection limits in plasma and urine were 20 and 200 ng/mL, respectively. Quantification of zidovudine in serum, milk and tissues by isocratic HPLC has been reported. A colorimetric method of assay has been developed for anti-human immunodeficiency virus (HIV) agents, including zidovudine. Simultaneous quantification of zidovudine and its metabolites in serum and urine by HPLC with a column-switching technique has been reported. The concentration of zidovudine in serum has been measured by the enzyme-linked immunosorbent assay and by the time-resolved fluoroimmunoassay. Paper and thin-layer chromatography of nucleoside derivatives including zidovudine have also been used (Sethi, 1991).

1.2 Production

Zidovudine was first synthesized in 1964. It was prepared by mesylation of 1'-(2'-deoxy-5'-O-trityl-β-D-lyxosyl)thymine to the sulfonate, which was treated with lithium azide in *N,N*-dimethylformamide to form 3'-azido-3'-deoxythymidine (Sethi, 1991). Other synthesis methods have been reported (Glinski *et al.*, 1973; Chu *et al.*, 1988).

Information available in 1999 indicated that zidovudine was manufactured and/or formulated in 35 countries (CIS Information Services, 1998; Royal Pharmaceutical Society of Great Britain; 1999; Swiss Pharmaceutical Society, 1999).

1.3 Use

Zidovudine was originally synthesized in the 1960s as a possible anti-cancer agent, but was found to be ineffective. In 1985, it was found to be active against HIV-1 *in vitro* (Hoetelmans *et al.*, 1996). It was approved as the first anti-HIV agent in 1987 and remains a widely prescribed mainstay of HIV therapy. Zidovudine has additive or synergistic activity with almost all other antiretroviral agents except the chemically related stavudine (3',5'-didehydrodideoxythymidine) with which it is antagonistic. Zidovudine alone provides only transient benefit (Graham *et al.*, 1992; Concorde Coordinating Committee, 1994; Vella *et al.*, 1994) owing to the development of genotypic changes within the virus that result in relative resistance to zidovudine (Larder &

Kemp, 1989; Larder *et al.*, 1989). Prolonged administration of zidovudine as part of a regimen which does not suppress HIV replication can lead to selection of strains of HIV that contain mutations which confer broad cross-resistance to all nucleoside reverse transcriptase inhibitors (Shafer *et al.*, 1995; Venturi *et al.*, 1999).

Zidovudine is frequently included in a variety of highly active antiretroviral regimens such as with lamivudine and indinavir (a protease inhibitor), with lamivudine and nevirapine or efavirenz, and with lamivudine and abacavir (Hammer *et al.*, 1997; Staszewski *et al.*, 1998; Barry *et al.*, 1999). Zidovudine plus didanosine is one of the most potent, extensively studied nucleoside regimens (Husson *et al.*, 1994; Henry *et al.*, 1998; Montaner *et al.*, 1998), although it is not superior to didanosine plus 3′,5′-didehydroxydideoxythimidine (Raffi *et al.*, 1998).

Perhaps the most dramatic use of zidovudine was that of the Pediatric AIDS Clinical Trials Group in its protocol 076, which showed that giving zidovudine alone during the last two trimesters of pregnancy, intravenously intrapartum and to the newborn orally could decrease the incidence of vertical transmission of HIV by two-thirds (Connor *et al.*, 1994; Simonds *et al.*, 1998). Subsequent studies have demonstrated that shorter durations and simpler all-oral regimens still provide substantial benefits (Wade *et al.*, 1998; Dabis *et al.*, 1999; Shaffer *et al.*, 1999; Wiktor *et al.*, 1999). Several studies have demonstrated that administration to pregnant women of zidovudine-containing combinations that reduce maternal HIV viral loads to near zero is highly likely to prevent vertical transmission (Garcia *et al.*, 1999; Mofenson *et al.*, 1999). The US Public Health Service has published guidelines for the treatment of HIV in pregnancy (Centers for Disease Control and Prevention, 1998a).

Zidovudine is also used in combination with other agents for the prevention of HIV after exposure to the virus (Tokars *et al.*, 1993; Katz & Gerberding, 1997; Centers for Disease Control and Prevention, 1998b).

It appears to be effective in the prevention and possibly the treatment of AIDS dementia complex and paediatric HIV developmental disability (Pizzo *et al.*, 1988; Portegies *et al.*, 1989; Bacellar *et al.*, 1994; Baldeweg *et al.*, 1995). It is also effective in HIV-related thrombocytopenia (Hirschel *et al.*, 1988).

1.4 Occurrence

Zidovudine is not known to occur as a natural product. No data on occupational exposure were available to the Working Group.

1.5 Regulations and guidelines

Zidovudine is listed in the British, European, French, German, Swiss and US pharmacopoeias (Swiss Pharmaceutical Society, 1999).

2. Studies of Cancer in Humans

2.1 Ecological studies

Coté and Biggar (1995) linked data from AIDS and cancer registries in several parts of the USA to compare the risk for non-Hodgkin lymphoma among people with AIDS before and after introduction of zidovudine. Each patient was followed-up for a maximum of 3.5 years. The standardized incidence ratios for non-Hodgkin lymphoma among patients with AIDS relative to that of the background population without AIDS were 222 (95% confidence interval [CI], 190–260) in 1981–86 and slightly lower (193; 95% CI, 176–212) in 1988–90 when zidovudine and other antiretroviral agents were on the market. [The Working Group noted that information on the treatment received by the patients was not available, but it has been estimated that 30–50% of those treated in the latter era would have received zidovudine (Gail *et al.*, 1990).]

2.2 Cohort studies

Pluda *et al.* (1990) examined the records of 55 patients with AIDS or severe AIDS-related complex (defined as having either oral candidiasis, oral hairy leukoplasia (Pluda *et al.*, 1993) or weight loss of > 10% of total body weight) who during 1985–87 were entered into phase I studies, in the Clinical Oncology Program of the National Cancer Institute, USA, of zidovudine alone ($n = 29$), zidovudine with simultaneously administered aciclovir ($n = 8$) or zidovudine alternated with zalcitabine ($n = 18$). All patients had fewer than 350 CD4 cells/µL plasma at the time of entry. Patients were followed for a minimum of 0.5 years and a maximum of 3.1 years, during which time eight patients developed a high-grade non-Hodgkin lymphoma of the B-cell type (three out of 29 in the group receiving zidovudine alone, three out of eight receiving zidovudine plus aciclovir and two out of 18 receiving zidovudine alternated with zalcitabine). When the follow-up was extended by another 1.7 years to a maximum of 4.8 years (Pluda *et al.*, 1993), no additional cases of lymphoma were seen. The estimated cumulative risk of developing non-Hodgkin lymphoma by 24 months of therapy was 12% (95% CI, 4.7–27%; Kaplan-Meier method), increasing to 29% (95% CI, 15–49%) by 36 months. The median CD4 cell count at initiation of antiretroviral therapy in the lymphoma patients was 26 cells/µL (range, 8–135) (Pluda *et al.*, 1990).

In a randomized, placebo-controlled trial, Fischl *et al.* (1990) included 711 subjects with mildly symptomatic HIV infection diagnosed at one of 29 treatment centres in the USA during the period 1987–89. Of these, 351 subjects were assigned to receive placebo and 360 were assigned to receive 200 mg zidovudine orally every 4 h (six did not receive zidovudine). All subjects had to have a mean pretreatment CD4 count of > 200 but < 800 cells/µL plasma. The median duration of follow-up was 11 months (range, 0.3–23 months), during which time one case of non-Hodgkin lymphoma of the B-cell type was seen in each group, and three cases of Kaposi sarcoma were seen in the group given placebo and two in the group given zidovudine.

Moore et al. (1991a) analysed data from a prospective, observational multicentre study at 12 clinical sites in the USA of 1030 patients with AIDS or advanced AIDS-related complex (at least one of five symptoms of HIV infection: oral thrush, weight loss of ≥ 10%, unexplained fever, diarrhoea or herpes zoster). All the patients had a CD4 cell count of no more than 250 cells/μL plasma at the time of entry. All patients were treated with zidovudine only at a daily dose of 1200 mg (85% of patients) or 600 mg (15%). Data collection was completed at baseline, i.e. during the period 1987–88, and every two months for two years or until death (median time, 1.5 years). Twelve patients had non-Hodgkin lymphoma, and two additional patients were suspected of having developed the disease before the date of start of zidovudine treatment and were excluded from the analysis. Twenty-four patients developed non-Hodgkin lymphoma after the start of treatment; the latter observation was equivalent to a rate of 1.6 cases of non-Hodgkin lymphoma per 100 person–years of therapy. The cumulative risk for non-Hodgkin lymphoma over the two years of zidovudine therapy showed a linear increase of 0.8% for each additional six months of therapy. Neither the proportion of time during the study that zidovudine was received by the patients nor the average daily dose was associated with non-Hodgkin lymphoma. [The Working Group noted that the power of the study to detect differences between the two dose groups was very low.]

In an international, randomized trial in 175 centres in several countries between 1992 and 1994, the Delta Coordinating Committee (1996) allocated 3207 individuals with antibodies to HIV who had symptoms of infection or a CD4 count of < 350 cells/μL plasma to treatment with either zidovudine at 600 mg per day ($n = 1055$), zidovudine (same dose) plus didanosine at 400 mg per day ($n = 1080$) or zidovudine (same dose) plus zalcitabine at 2.25 mg per day ($n = 1072$). The patients were followed up to September 1995 for a median of 2.5 years (range, 1.8–2.9), during which time 14 deaths due to cancer [not further specified] occurred; five of the deaths occurred in the group treated with zidovudine alone, five in the group treated with zidovudine plus didanosine and four in the group treated with zidovudine plus zalcitabine. [The Working Group noted that these trials were designed to evaluate the efficacy of zidovudine in the treatment of patients with various degrees of severity of immunosuppression. For the purposes of evaluating cancer risk, therefore, the numbers of participants were too small and the length of follow-up too short, cancer incidence may have been under-ascertained, and cancer rates could not be analysed adequately.]

In a study of 2627 HIV-infected homosexual men who were followed prospectively in four sites in the USA during 1985–91, Muñoz et al. (1993) examined the effects of severity of immunosuppression, assessed by CD4 cell counts, and anti-retroviral therapy, mainly zidovudine, on the incidence of Kaposi sarcoma and non-Hodgkin lymphoma, whenever these malignancies constituted the AIDS-defining disease. On the basis of a total of 194 cases of Kaposi sarcoma and 34 non-Hodgkin lymphomas observed among the AIDS-free seropositive individuals, the authors found a strong inverse relationship between the CD4 cell count and the risk for Kaposi sarcoma and a moderate inverse relationship between this cell count and the risk for non-Hodgkin lymphoma. In a further multivariate analysis with adjustment for severity of immunosuppression and other factors, the authors observed non-significantly decreased relative risks for Kaposi sarcoma (relative risk, 0.83) and non-Hodgkin lymphoma (relative risk, 0.47) associated with prophylactic use of antiretroviral agents. [The Working Group noted that the type of antiretroviral therapy used is not specified, although it would have been predominantly zidovudine.]

Forseter *et al.* (1994) conducted a prospective, observational study of 60 health-care workers treated at one institution in New York City, USA, between 1989 and 1992, who had percutaneous or permucosal exposures to blood or body fluids of HIV-infected patients. Although study subjects were recommended a 42-day course of therapy with 200 mg zidovudine every 4 h, starting from 30 min to three days after exposure, only 21 completed the course. Among the 42 subjects followed for three months or longer (mean, 7.8 months; range, three months to 2.7 years), none had undergone HIV antibody seroconversion. One 23-year-old health-care worker reported the development of Hodgkin disease (nodular sclerosing variety, stage 3A) 1.5 years after completion of the 42-day course of zidovudine therapy. [The Working Group noted the anecdotal nature of the report.]

2.3 Case–control studies

Levine *et al.* (1995) reported the results of a population-based case–control study of 112 cases of intermediate or high-grade non-Hodgkin lymphoma diagnosed in 1989–92 among HIV-infected homosexual or bisexual men living in Los Angeles County, USA. The cases were identified in 1431 patients notified with an intermediate- or high-grade lymphoma during the period to the population-based cancer registry of Los Angeles. Of these, 658 died before an interview could be conducted. Of the remaining cases, 527 participated in the study of non-Hodgkin lymphoma, and each gave a blood sample for determination of HIV status. Personal interviews were conducted with a structured questionnaire to obtain information on the subjects' lifetime history of use of medications ever taken for at least a month, including zidovudine and other antiretroviral agents, medical history and selected personal habits and lifestyle factors. For each of the 112 HIV-positive homosexual or bisexual men who provided information about zidovudine, one matched HIV-positive asymptomatic control subject was selected from a County- or University-affiliated clinic in the community. The matching criteria were year of birth (within three years), race and ethnic group, sex, language of interview and mode of transmission of initial HIV infection. Data on zidovudine use and the other factors investigated were obtained from controls in a similar way to cases. The reference period for cases was up to 12 months before the time of diagnosis, and for controls up to 12 months before the time of diagnosis of the matched case. Forty-four men with lymphoma reported a history of zidovudine use for at least a month (mean duration, 19 months; SD, 13 months) compared with 24 controls (21%: mean duration, 12.6 months; SD, 10.5 months). The matched odds ratio for lymphoma associated with use of zidovudine was 1.6 (95% CI, 0.94–2.9). The authors noted that until around 1990 zidovudine use was primarily restricted to patients with AIDS or symptomatic HIV disease, whereas after that time it became accepted practice to use this drug in asymptomatic HIV-positive subjects with fewer than 500 CD4 cells/μL. Therefore, it is possible that the comparison of cases with asymptomatic controls may have provided a misleading estimate of association. For this reason, zidovudine use by 49 men with AIDS-associated lymphoma was compared with use of the drug by individually matched controls in whom AIDS was diagnosed in the same period but who did not have a lymphoma. These controls were identified from the records of one treatment centre; the same matching criteria were used as described for the comparison with asymptomatic controls. Twelve (about 25%) of these men had used zidovudine (mean duration, 13 months; SD, 10.5 months) compared with 20 controls (41%; mean duration, 11 months; SD, 7.1 months). The matched odds ratio was 0.43 (95% CI, 0.17–1.1). [The Working Group noted that the proportion of patients with lymphoma who were HIV-positive and died before interview was unknown, and this may have have biased the association with reported zidovudine use. The participation rate among control subjects was not specified. Although CD4 counts were not available, restriction of the analysis to AIDS cases was an attempt to address this limitation.]

2.4   Childhood cancer

The medical records of prospectively followed HIV-exposed infants with known exposure to zidovudine *in utero* and/or neonatallly were reviewed by Hanson *et al.* (1999) for the development of tumours. The HIV-infected pregnant mothers were enrolled from various treatment centres across the USA during 1989–96, and 727 live-born children, of whom 115 were also included in the study of Sperling *et al.* (1998), described in section 4.3, were followed from date of birth onwards, for a mean of 1.2 or 3.2 years (range, one month to six years). No tumours of any type were reported in the 727 zidovudine-exposed infants; however, on the basis of the incidence rates for cancer in the general childhood population in the USA the authors calculated an upper 95% CI of 18. [The Working Group noted that a substantially increased risk could not be excluded.]

In two studies described in detail in section 4.3, no tumours were observed in the children of mothers given zidovudine during pregnancy. The length of follow-up was 1.5 years in one study (Sperling *et al.*, 1998) and 4.2 years in the other (Culnane *et al.*, 1999).

3. Studies of Cancer in Experimental Animals

3.1 Oral administration

3.1.1 Mouse

Groups of 100 male and 100 female CD-1 mice, seven weeks of age, were given zidovudine free base [purity not specified] in 0.5% methylcellulose once daily by gavage at a dose of 30, 60 or 120 mg/kg bw per day. Twenty-five to 40 mice from each group were used only for haematological examinations and for determinations of the plasma concentration of the drug. At day 91, anaemia was seen in animals at the intermediate and high doses, and the doses were lowered to 20, 30 and 40 mg/kg bw per day. Two separate groups of 85 male and 85 female mice were left untreated or were given the vehicle alone. The study was terminated at 19 and 22 months for male and female mice, respectively. Tissues from all mice in the untreated, vehicle control and high-dose groups were examined microscopically. In addition, the vaginas from all mice at the low and intermediate doses were examined. Treatment with zidovudine did not affect the survival rate in either sex, and the rate at 18 months was 50%. Body weight was unaffected by treatment in either sex. The incidences of vaginal squamous-cell carcinomas were 0/60, 0/60, 0/60, 0/60 and 5/60 [$p = 0.06$, Fisher's exact test] in untreated controls, vehicle controls and at the three doses, respectively. One squamous-cell papilloma of the vagina was seen at the intermediate dose and one at the high dose. Squamous-cell hyperplasia of the vaginal epithelium was seen in all groups of mice, including the controls, and the incidence of moderate to severe hyperplasia was dose-relatedly increased in mice given the intermediate or high dose of zidovudine. Treatment did not affect the incidence of any other benign or malignant tumour in any tissue or organ examined [specific tumour incidences not reported] (Ayers et al., 1996a).

Groups of 95 male and 95 female B6C3F$_1$ mice, seven to eight weeks of age, were treated with zidovudine (~98% pure) in 0.5% methylcellulose by gavage at a daily dose of 0, 30, 60 or 120 mg/kg bw, administered as two equal doses at least 6 h apart, on five days per week for 105 weeks. Each group of 95 animals of each sex comprised 50 animals of each sex for evaluation of carcinogenic response, 30 animals of each sex for evaluation of haematological end-points and bone-marrow cellularity, and 15 animals of each sex from which blood was drawn for determination of the plasma concentrations of zidovudine at week 54. The survival and mean body weights of mice exposed to zidovudine were similar to those of the vehicle control groups. Squamous-cell carcinomas or papillomas (combined) of the vagina occurred in 0/50, 0/49, 5/45 ($p = 0.028$) and 11/49 ($p < 0.001$) animals in the control group and at the three doses, respectively ($p < 0.001$, trend test), and epithelial hyperplasia of the vagina was observed in 0/50, 3/49, 4/45 and 11/49 ($p < 0.01$) mice in those groups, respectively. Three renal tubular adenomas and one renal tubular carcinoma were observed in male mice receiving the high dose, and the combined incidence in this group exceeded the range in historical controls: 2/365 (range, 0–4%). The incidences of Harderian gland tumours in male mice were 3/50, 5/50, 2/50 and 10/50 ($p = 0.059$) in the four groups, respectively ($p = 0.027$, trend test) (National Toxicology Program, 1999). [The Working Group noted that the incidence of squamous-cell vaginal tumours in unexposed mice is very rare.]

3.1.2 Rat

Groups of 60 male and 60 female CD rats, six weeks of age, were given zidovudine [purity not specified] in 0.5% methylcellulose once daily by gavage at a dose of 80, 220 or 600 mg/kg bw. At day 91, the high dose was lowered to 450 mg/kg bw per day because of the occurrence of anaemia. Progression of anaemia led to a further reduction of the high dose to 300 mg/kg bw per day on day 278. Two separate groups of 60 male and 60 female rats were left untreated or were given the vehicle alone. The study was terminated at 24 and 22 months for male and female rats, respectively. Tissues from all rats in the untreated, vehicle control and high-dose groups were examined microscopically. In addition, the vaginas from all female rats at the low and intermediate doses were examined. Treatment with zidovudine did not affect the survival rate in either of the sexes, and the rate at 18 months was 50% or greater. Body weight was unaffected by treatment in either sex. Two squamous-cell carcinomas of the distal vagina were observed in females at the high dose, but no vaginal tumours occurred in the other groups, or in the untreated or vehicle control groups. Treatment with zidovudine did not affect the incidence of any other benign or malignant tumour in any tissue or organ examined [specific tumour incidences not reported] (Ayers *et al.*, 1996a). [The Working Group noted that the occurrence of squamous-cell vaginal tumours in unexposed rats is exceedingly rare.]

3.2 Transplacental exposure

Mouse: Groups of 60 female CD-1 mice, 79 days of age, were mated with male CD-1 mice and given zidovudine [purity not specified] in 0.5% methylcellulose once daily by gavage at 20 or 40 mg/kg bw per day, beginning on day 10 of gestation and throughout gestation, parturition and lactation. At weaning, zidovudine was administered to the offspring at the same doses in the drinking-water for 17–35 days and then by gavage for 24 months. Two additional groups were treated similarly with 40 mg/kg bw per day, but one group was treated only until day 21 of lactation and the second by gavage for 90 days after birth. Two groups each of 60 female mice were either untreated or were given the vehicle, beginning on day 10 of gestation and throughout gestation, parturition and lactation, and then in the drinking-water for 17–35 days, followed by daily gavage for 24 months. The study was designed to give a total of 70 male and 70 female progeny in each dose group. All animals were killed at 24 months. Fifty separate tissues and organs [not specified] were taken for microscopic examination, and the vaginas from all females were examined microscopically. There was no treatment-related effect on survival rates or body weight. No treatment-related increase in the incidence of neoplastic or non-neoplastic lesions was observed in males [specific tumour incidences not reported]. In females, vaginal squamous-cell carcinomas were found in 11 ($p = 0.0002$) mice at the high dose, in two mice at the low dose and in one mouse given the high dose by gavage for 90 days after birth. No vaginal tumours were seen in the other groups (Ayers et al., 1997).

Groups of female CD-1 Swiss mice [age unspecified] were mated with male CD-1 mice, and 45 pregnant mice were given zidovudine (purity, > 99.8%) by gavage at doses of 0 (17 litters), 12.5 (13 litters) or 25 (15 litters) mg/mouse (approximately 210 and 420 mg/kg bw for the low and high dose, respectively) on days 12–18 of gestation. The pups were delivered normally and were kept without further treatment. Ten pups of each sex from each group were killed 13, 26 and 52 weeks after delivery. At week 52, the observation of lung and liver tumours prompted the authors to kill additional mice and to report the results. The numbers of mice in each group were 31 male controls and 23 and 26 at the low and high doses and 30 female controls and 22 and 24 at the low and high doses. In the two sexes combined, the incidence of lung carcinomas was 3% in controls, 7% at the low dose and 14% at the high dose ($p = 0.037$, Cochran-Armitage trend test). The multiplicity of lung tumours was 0.10 in male controls and 0.13 and 0.50 at the low and high doses ($p = 0.014$, trend test) and 0.13 in female controls and 0.14 and 0.38 at the low and high doses ($p = 0.15$, trend test). Neoplasms of the ovary, uterus and vagina were seen in 0% of controls, 14% at the low dose and 17% at the high dose ($p = 0.033$, trend test). The incidence of hepatocellular tumours (mainly adenomas) was increased in males, being about 13% in controls, 30% at the low dose and 52% at the high dose; the multiplicity of hepatocellular tumours was 0.23 in controls, 0.48 at the low dose and 0.79 at the high dose ($p = 0.013$, trend test) (Olivero et al., 1997).

In a study involving prenatal initiation and postnatal promotion, groups of pregnant CD-1 Swiss mice were given 0 or 25 mg/mouse (approximately 420 mg/kg bw) zidovudine (purity, > 99.8%) by gavage once daily on days 12–18 of gestation. Groups of 16 male and 14 female control pups and 13 male and 17 female pups of zidovudine-treated dams were selected randomly at five weeks of age for topical treatment with 12-O-tetradecanoylphorbol 13-acetate (TPA) on the dorsal skin at a dose of 2 μg twice a week for 17 weeks and then 5 μg twice a week in weeks 18–35. The experiment was terminated 41 weeks after the start of TPA promotion, at which time the offspring were 46 weeks of age. At the end of the experiment, about 96% of the mice given zidovudine plus TPA had developed skin tumours. The effect was more pronounced in females: 5/14 (35%) female mice given TPA and 15/17 (88%) given zidovudine plus TPA had skin tumours ($p < 0.05$). The average numbers of tumours per mouse was 0.57 ± 0.13 (mean ± SE) in the group given TPA alone and 1.44 ± 0.36 in that given zidovudine plus TPA ($p = 0.006$). Most (82%) of the skin tumours were papillomas; the rest (18%) were keratoacanthomas (Zhang et al., 1998).

3.3 Intravaginal administration

Mouse: Groups of 50 female CD-1 mice, seven weeks of age, were given zidovudine [purity not specified] in 0.9% saline intravaginally twice daily approximately 6 h apart at a dose of 2 or 8 mg/day. Two additional groups of 50 female mice were either left untreated or were given the vehicle intravaginally. The study was terminated at 24 months. The vagina and cervix from animals in all groups were examined microscopically. Vaginal squamous-cell carcinomas were observed in 2/50 mice at the low dose and 13/50 at the high dose [$p < 0.001$]. Vaginal epithelial-cell tumours were not seen in either control group (Ayers *et al.*, 1996a).

3.4 Administration with other agents

Mouse: Groups of 50 male and 50 female B6C3F$_1$ mice, seven to eight weeks of age, were treated with zidovudine (~98% pure) in 0.5% aqueous methyl cellulose by gavage at a daily dose of 0 (control), 30, 60 or 120 mg/kg bw in two equal doses on five days per week for 105 weeks. All groups also received subcutaneous injections of 500 or 5000 U α-interferon three times per week for 105 weeks. Survival rates and body weights were similar in treated and vehicle control groups. The incidences of squamous-cell carcinoma of the vagina in the groups receiving 500 U α-interferon were 0/49, 0/44, 5/48 ($p = 0.030$) and 6/48 ($p = 0.011$, logistic regression test), in the control group and at the three doses, respectively ($p < 0.001$, trend test). Epithelial hyperplasia of the vagina was seen in 0/49 controls and 4/44, 8/48 and 12/48 at the three doses, respectively ($p = 0.047$, trend test). In the groups receiving 5000 U α-interferon, the incidences of squamous-cell carcinoma or papilloma (combined) of the vagina were 1/50, 1/48, 5/48 and 4/50 ($p = 0.047$, trend test), and those of epithelial hyperplasia of the vagina were 1/50, 4/48, 8/48 and 15/50 ($p < 0.01$, trend test) in controls and at the three doses, respectively. There was no significant increase in the incidence of tumours at other sites (National Toxicology Program, 1999).

4. Other Data Relevant to an Evaluation of Carcinogenicity and its Mechanisms

4.1 Absorption, distribution, metabolism and excretion

4.1.1 *Humans*

The pharmacokinetics of zidovudine has been reviewed and summarized extensively (Morse *et al.*, 1993; Dudley, 1995; Acosta *et al.*, 1996; Hoetelmans *et al.*, 1996), and large inter- and intra-individual variations have been observed (Mentré *et al*, 1993; Dudley, 1995; Acosta *et al.*, 1996; Hoetelmans *et al.*, 1996). The peak plasma concentrations of zidovudine after a dose of 200 mg have been reported to be 3.2–10.8 µmol/L [0.86–2.9 mg/L], and are reached after 30–60 min (Dudley, 1995; Hoetelmans *et al.*, 1996). The half-time for removal of the drug from plasma is about 1 h, and the clearance rate is 5–12.5 L/h (Morse *et al.*, 1993; Dudley, 1995). In one study of HIV-negative individuals given an intravenous dose of 2.5 mg/kg bw zidovudine, the integrated area under the curve of plasma concentration–time was 22% of the total for zidovudine, 72% for 3'-azido-3'-deoxy-5'-*O*-α-D-glucopyranosyl-thymidine and 5% for 3'-amino-3'-deoxythymidine, and the half-time for removal was 1.2 h for zidovudine, 1.7 h for 3'-azido-3'-deoxy-5'-*O*-α-D-glucopyranosyl-thymidine and 2.7 h for 3'-amino-3'-deoxythymidine (Stagg *et al.*, 1992). The renal clearance rate has been reported to be about 12 L/h for zidovudine and 18 L/h for 3'-azido-3'-deoxy-5'-*O*-α-D-glucopyranosyl-thymidine (Morse *et al.*, 1993). These values are reduced in patients with compromised renal function (Dudley, 1995; Acosta *et al.*, 1996). In patients with normal kidney and liver function, the pharmacokinetics of zidovudine is similar after the first dose and during long-term dosing (Gallicano *et al.*, 1993), but significant changes may occur in the presence of hepatic or renal compromise (Dudley, 1995; Acosta *et al.*, 1996; Hoetelmans *et al.*, 1996). The pharmacokinetics of zidovudine in cerebrospinal fluid has been reported (Rolinski *et al.*, 1997); the drug penetrated the cerebrospinal fluid slowly, the peak concentration being achieved at 2 h, an area under the curve that was about 75% of that in plasma and a half-time of about 3 h.

The absorption, distribution, metabolism and excretion of zidovudine in adults with and without HIV infection have been reviewed extensively (Kamali, 1993; Morse *et al.*, 1993; Dudley, 1995; Stretcher, 1995; Acosta *et al.*, 1996; Hoetelmans *et al.*, 1996). Oral dosing was used in the majority of these studies, and absorption was significantly altered by the presence of food in the stomach (Acosta *et al.*, 1996). About 64% of an oral dose is bioavailable, although zidovudine binds poorly to plasma proteins (~25%) and is distributed to cells by passive diffusion (Kamali, 1993; Dudley, 1995; Acosta *et al.*, 1996). The drug is distributed throughout the body and has been found in plasma, saliva, semen, breast milk and cerebrospinal fluid, although the concentration in the last may be only 15% of that in plasma (Morse *et al.*, 1993; Dudley, 1995; Acosta *et al.*, 1996).

Zidovudine is metabolized primarily along three separate pathways (Figure 1), and about 95% of a total dose is recovered in the urine, with 15–20% as unchanged drug (Stagg *et al.*, 1992; Morse *et al.*, 1993; Dudley, 1995). The major pathway is first-pass glucuronidation with renal excretion and results in the elimination of about 65–75% of the total dose. The urinary glucuronide metabolite, 3'-azido-3'-deoxy-5'-*O*-α-D-glucopyranosyl-thymidine, is formed by the action of uridine 5'-diphosphoglucuronyl transferase and was first characterized chemically by Good *et al.* (1990). In plasma and urine, the 3'-azido-3'-deoxy-5'-*O*-α-D-glucopyranosyl-thymidine:zidovudine ratio is typically 3 or 4, although large interindividual variation has been reported (Acosta *et al.*, 1996).

Figure 1. Metabolic pathways of zidovudine

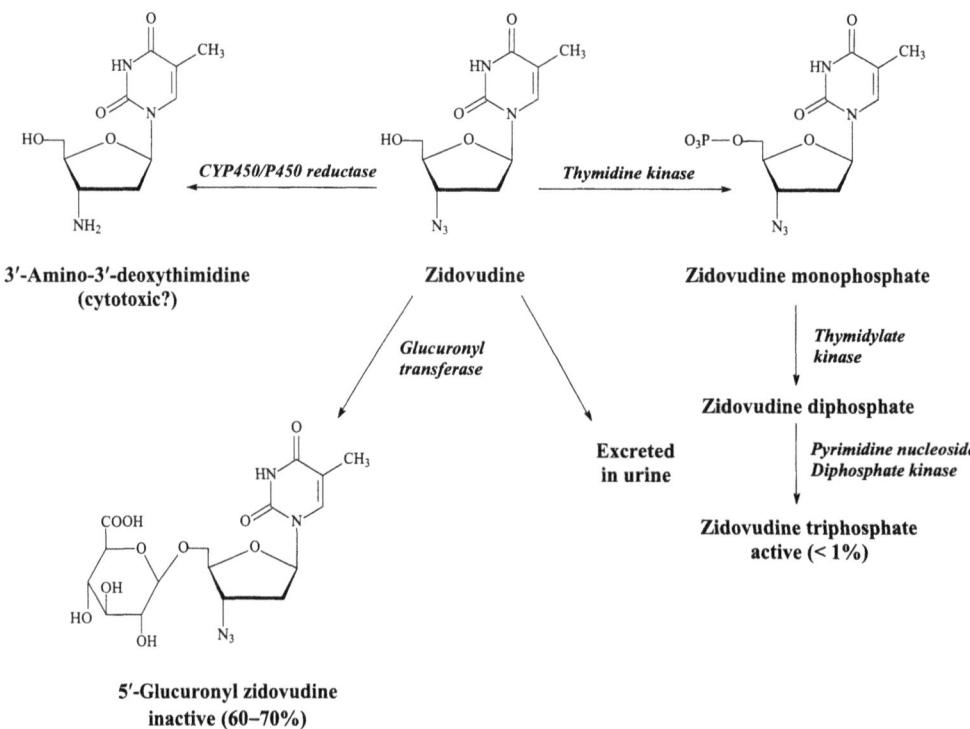

From Veal & Back (1995)

A second pathway involves the action of various hepatic CYP450 oxidases and reductases, resulting in the production of a toxic metabolite, 3'-amino-3'-deoxythymidine (Stagg et al., 1992; Acosta et al., 1996). This metabolite is formed to varying extents in different tissues and represents about 2% of the total dose in the urine. It has a longer plasma half-life than either zidovudine or 3'-azido-3'-deoxy-5'-O-α-D-glucopyranosyl-thymidine (Stagg et al., 1992). In one study (Hoetelmans et al., 1997) of samples from 23 patients, the amount of 3'-amino-3'-deoxythymidine in cerebrospinal fluid was about 1.8% that of zidovudine, and similar ratios were found in plasma.

The metabolic pathway responsible for the antiviral activity is phosphorylation (Figure 1). The mono-, di- and triphosphates of zidovudine are formed rapidly through the action of thymidine kinase, thymidylate kinase and pyrimidine nucleoside diphosphate kinase, respectively (Stretcher, 1995; Veal & Back, 1995; Acosta et al., 1996; Hoetelmans et al., 1996; Peter & Gambertoglio, 1998). Since zidovudine is a good substrate for thymidine kinase, with 60% of the maximal velocity (V_{max}) of thymidine, zidovudine monophosphate accumulates and typically comprises about 90% of the total intracellular zidovudine phosphates in healthy individuals (Hoetelmans et al., 1996; Peter & Gambertoglio, 1998). Zidovudine diphosphate and zidovudine triphosphate are present in equal proportions of ~5% (Peter & Gambertoglio, 1998). There is evidence (Stretcher, 1995; Acosta et al., 1996; Peter & Gambertoglio, 1996) that this balance is shifted in HIV-positive patients with CD4 counts between 300 and 500/mm^3, in whom zidovudine monophosphate constitutes about 74% of the total phosphates and zidovudine diphosphate and zidovudine triphosphate each account for about 13%. The difference may be due to the viral infection, since short-term and long-term exposure to zidovudine produced similar results (Peter & Gambertoglio, 1996). In patients, the zidovudine monophosphorylation pathway saturates after each dose of 100 mg or more, suggesting that monophosphorylation is largely independent of current clinical doses. Conversion to di- and triphosphates is more closely related to individual phosphorylation capacity (Stretcher, 1995). Zidovudine triphosphate is eventually incorporated into DNA, resulting in the termination of replication (Morse et al, 1993; Veal & Back, 1995; Peter & Gambertoglio, 1998). The antiviral activity of the drug is thought to result from direct inhibition of viral reverse transcriptase and truncation of proviral DNA replication (Peter & Gambertoglio, 1998). Although critical to the mechanism of antiviral activity, zidovudine phosphorylation is responsible for only a small fraction (~1%) of the total disposition of the drug.

After a woman received zidovudine intravenously by continuous infusion (0.12 mg/kg bw per h) 2 h before delivery, her blood contained 0.28 µg/mL and the blood of her newborn contained 0.27–0.51 µg/mL 6–48 h after birth. 3′-Azido-3′-deoxy-5′-O-α-D-glucopyranosyl-thymidine was present at a concentration of 1.12 µg/mL in the mother and 1.1–2.31 µg/mL in the infant (Chavanet et al., 1989).

O'Sullivan et al. (1993) studied the pharmacokinetics of zidovudine in eight near-term pregnant women given zidovudine orally at about 154 mg/kg bw per day before delivery. The mean body clearance rate was 26 ± 10 mL/min per kg bw and the half-time for elimination was 1.3 ± 0.2 h. The half-time for elimination in amniotic fluid was 13 ± 0.58 h, which was 10 times longer than in the mother.

4.1.2 *Experimental systems*

The absorption, distribution, metabolism and excretion of zidovudine have been determined in mice (Trang et al., 1993; Manouilov et al., 1995; Chow et al., 1997, 1998), rats (de Miranda et al., 1990) and rhesus monkeys (Boudinot et al., 1990; Cretton et al., 1991). The basic metabolic pathways of glucuronidation, phosphorylation and reduction to 3′-amino-3′-deoxythymidine are similar in all these species, but the bioavailability and pharmacokinetics vary. Absorption, distribution and elimination are more rapid in rodents than in humans, and the bioavailability is greater in rats and mice than in primates. Non-human primates appear to be excellent human surrogates because the pharmacokinetics of zidovudine, including clearance and steady-state volume of distribution, is virtually identical to that in humans.

In female B6C3F$_1$ mice given doses of 15, 30 and 60 mg/kg bw zidovudine by gavage, the maximum serum concentrations of 9, 18 and 40 µg/mL, respectively, were reached at 15–22 min (Trang et al., 1993). The half-time for elimination was 16–22 min. The absolute bioavailability was estimated to be 86%. The disposition of zidovudine followed a one-compartment open model, with first-order absorption and elimination after oral dosing and first-order elimination after intravenous injection. The pharmacokinetics of zidovudine in mice was not dependent on the route of administration.

Concentrations of zidovudine were determined in plasma and lymph nodes of female NIH Swiss mice given 50 mg/kg bw zidovudine intravenously, intraperitoneally or orally (Manouilov et al., 1995). The maximum serum concentrations of zidovudine were obtained after about 5 min with all routes, and the half-time for removal was 23–46 min. The absolute bioavailability was 49% after oral administration and 100% after administration by the other two routes. The concentrations of zidovudine in the neck, axillary and mesenteric lymph nodes reached about 30% of those in serum.

Female C57BL/6 mice, with and without retroviral infection, were given a single subcutaneous dose of 25 mg/kg bw [^{3}H]zidovudine, and tissues were examined after 30, 60 and 90 min for concentrations of zidovudine and zidovudine triphosphate (Chow et al., 1997). Healthy and infected animals showed a similar pattern of distribution in 10 organs, the highest concentrations being found in kidney and muscle and the lowest in thymus, lymph nodes and brain. In uninfected mice, the highest concentrations of zidovudine monophosphate were observed in the bone marrow, kidney and spleen and the lowest in thymus, lymph nodes and brain, although infected mice had relatively high concentrations of zidovudine triphosphate in lymph nodes. In similarly designed studies (Chow et al., 1998), mice were given subcutaneous injections of 25 mg/kg bw zidovudine twice daily for eight weeks. The profiles of zidovudine and zidovudine monophosphate were generally similar to those observed in the single-dose experiments; however, after multiple injections, zidovudine triphosphate accumulated preferentially in the spleen and bone marrow owing to the high cell density in those organs.

The tissue disposition and metabolism of zidovudine were studied in rats given a single dose of 10 mg/kg bw [^{3}H]zidovudine by gavage (de Miranda et al., 1990). The drug was absorbed and distributed rapidly in all tissues, with peak concentrations occurring by 15 min. The concentrations of zidovudine and its metabolites (zidovudine equivalents) in most tissues were similar to or higher than those in plasma, but very low concentrations were observed in brain, suggesting slow cerebrospinal fluid uptake. The disappearance of radiolabel from blood and plasma was biphasic. Urinary (78%) and faecal (21%) excretion of the drug was complete by 24 h. In urine, 88% of radiolabel was associated with unchanged drug and the remainder with five metabolites. 3'-Azido-3'-deoxy-5'-O-α-D-glucopyranosyl-thymidine and 3'-amino-3'-deoxythymidine were detected in both plasma and urine, and 7% of the radioactive dose was excreted, primarily as 3'-azido-3'-deoxy-5'-O-α-D-glucopyranosyl-thymidine, in the bile. The major faecal metabolite (> 70%) was 3'-amino-3'-deoxythymidine.

Rhesus monkeys received oral doses of 60 or 200 mg/kg bw zidovudine and an intravenous dose of 60 mg/kg bw. The bioavailability was 92% after the lower oral dose and about 50% after the higher dose, and the plasma half-time was 30–45 min at the lower dose and 80–120 min at the higher dose. Diffusion of zidovudine into cerebrospinal fluid was much slower than that into plasma, and the peak concentration in cerebrospinal fluid was 5–21% of that in plasma (Boudinet *et al.*, 1990).

After administration of 33.3 mg/kg bw zidovudine to rhesus monkeys by subcutaneous injection, the maximum concentrations of zidovudine, 3'-azido-3'-deoxy-5'-*O*-α-D-glucopyranosyl-thymidine and 3'-amino-3'-deoxythymidine in plasma were found at 45 min, with half-times of 1 h for zidovudine and the glucuronide and 1.6 h for 3'-amino-3'-deoxythymidine. In the urine, about 27% of the total dose was excreted as zidovudine, 60% as 3'-azido-3'-deoxy-5'-*O*-α-D-glucopyranosyl-thymidine and 1.8% as either 3'-azido-3'-deoxy-5'-*O*-α-D-glucopyranosyl-thymidine or 3'-amino-3'-deoxythimidine within the first 24 h. The average peak concentrations of zidovudine in the cerebrospinal fluid were 30% of those observed in plasma, but were highly variable between monkeys, and very little 3'-azido-3'-deoxy-5'-*O*-α-D-glucopyranosyl-thymidine was recovered from the cerebrospinal fluid (Cretton *et al.*, 1991).

Perfused human placentas were used to show that zidovudine readily crosses the human placenta and that the passage is bidirectional, with no evidence of active or carrier-mediated transport. No evidence for glucuronide conjugation of zidovudine by the placenta was reported (Schenker *et al.*, 1990).

Zidovudine added at a concentration of 3.8 mmol/L to a human placental perfusion on three separate occasions during 14 h reduced the concentration of human chorionic gonadotropin by 75% (Boal *et al.*, 1997). When human placental tissue and human trophoblast cells (Jar) were exposed to zidovudine at a concentration of 7.6 mmol/L for 48 h in culture and placental lobular tissue was perfused with 3.8 mmol/L zidovudine for 14 h, no zidovudine monophosphate was detected in any sample, and zidovudine inhibited cell proliferation by 72% in the Jar cells (Plessinger *et al.*, 1997). [The Working Group noted that the concentrations used were 1000 times the plasma concentrations found normally after therapy.]

Zidovudine readily crosses the placenta of pregnant non-human primates, probably by passive diffusion (Lopez-Anaya *et al.*, 1990). Zidovudine, zidovudine monophosphate and 3'-azido-3'-deoxy-5'-*O*-α-D-glucopyranosyl-thymidine glucuronide were detected in most fetal tissues after administration to pregnant rhesus monkeys (Patterson *et al.*, 1997). After exposure of pregnant pigtailed macaques to zidovudine, the fetal:maternal plasma concentration ratio of zidovudine was 0.76 (Tuntland *et al.*, 1998). Zidovudine administered to a baboon in late pregnancy resulted in a fetal:maternal plasma concentration ratio of 0.84, and the concentration of 3'-azido-3'-deoxy-5'-*O*-α-D-glucopyranosyl-thymidine in the fetus was seven times that of the mother (Garland *et al.*, 1996; Stark *et al.*, 1997; Garland *et al.*, 1998).

4.2 Toxic effects

4.2.1 Humans

Zidovudine has a broad spectrum of toxicity, some of which may be difficult to distinguish from that due to the presence of the HIV virus in patients receiving anti-retroviral therapy (Styrt et al., 1996). Toxic effects caused only by the drug have been elucidated in uninfected individuals accidentally exposed to body fluids from HIV-infected patients, such as health-care workers given prophylactic zidovudine therapy, and in cases in which toxicity has resolved after discontinutation of therapy. In one study involving 674 health-care workers (Ippolito et al., 1997), 49% reported at least one adverse effect and 20% had discontinued treatment because of side-effects. Nausea was reported by 243 individuals, and others reported vomiting, gastric pain, asthenia and headache. Ten individuals had anaemia and seven had transient increases in the activity of liver enzymes. All of these effects were reversible when the drug was discontinued. This pattern of toxicity is similar in African–American, Hispanic and white HIV-positive patients (Jacobson et al., 1996).

(a) Haematotoxicity

Pancytopenia and bone-marrow aplasia are the dose-limiting toxic effects for zidovudine (Gill et al., 1987; Moore et al., 1996; Styrt et al., 1996). In early trials, doses of 1200 mg/day were not uncommon, and Moore et al. (1991b), who studied 886 patients with AIDS, reported that serious anaemia and neutropenia occurred in 30% and 37% of patients, respectively, who were given this dose. In the same study, 70% of patients had had to interrupt dosing at least once, and increased haematocrit was observed after dosing cessation in 52% of patients. In later trials at lower doses, the absolute rates of anaemia and neutropenia were considerably decreased: Ippolito et al. (1997) reported 10 cases of anaemia in 674 HIV-negative health-care workers, and Vella et al. (1994) reported that 23 of 936 patients with asymptomatic HIV infection had neutropenia. A related haematotoxic effect, macrocytosis with decreasing haemoglobin concentrations, was also observed in several studies (Mathé et al., 1996; Styrt et al., 1996; Vella et al., 1994). Vella et al. (1994) reported that 18 of 936 patients had a ≥ 25% decrease in haemoglobin concentration. A survey by the Spontaneous Reporting System of the US Food and Drug Administration (Styrt et al., 1996) included some 2000 case reports of toxicity due to zidovudine and confirmed the profile of haematotoxicity previously described in clinical trials.

(b) Hepatotoxicity

Transiently increased liver transaminase activities that returned to normal after discontinuation of the drug were reported in seven of 674 health-care workers (Ippolito et al., 1997) and in 63 of 936 HIV-positive patients (Vella et al., 1994). Hepatic toxicity appears to be a more frequent consequence of long-term (3–12 months) exposure to zidovudine, and increases in liver enzyme activity have been accompanied by hepatomegaly with macrovesicular steatosis and frequently fatal lactic acidosis (Freiman *et al.*, 1993; Olano *et al.*, 1995; Acosta & Grimsley, 1999; Chariot *et al.*, 1999).

(c)   *Myopathy and neurotoxicity*

Long-term use of zidovudine (2–12 months) has been associated with skeletal muscle and cardiomyopathy in adult patients with AIDS (Mhiri *et al.*, 1991; Peters *et al.*, 1993; Dalakas *et al.*, 1994; Cupler *et al.*, 1995). Skeletal muscle myopathy has been observed in up to 27% of patients with a clinical presentation including fatigue, myalgia, muscle weakness, wasting, elevated serum creatine kinase activity and decreased carnitine concentration. In skeletal muscle biopsy samples, accumulation of lipid in muscle fibres, accumulation of mitochondria in the subsarcolemmal space (ragged red fibres) and morphologically abnormal mitochondria have been observed (Mhiri *et al.*, 1991; Dalakas *et al.*, 1994). In addition, long-term treatment with zidovudine has been associated with dilated cardiomyopathy in adult AIDS patients. Congestive heart failure, left ventricular dilatation, reduced ejection fractions (7–26%) and morphologically abnormal mitochondria have been demonstrated after prolonged (two years or more) use (Lewis, 1998). In one study (Barbaro *et al.*, 1998), abnormal echocardiograms were observed in 76 of 962 HIV-positive patients. The clinical, morphological and biochemical manifestations of cardiac and skeletal muscle myopathy improved when zidovudine use was terminated (Mhiri *et al.*, 1991; Lewis, 1998).

Analysis of neuromuscular function in a multicentre trial of patients receiving 600 mg/day zidovudine showed that 225 of 2467 patients had ≥ grade 2 peripheral neuropathy or distal symmetrical neuropathy. Of these cases, about 20% were considered to be related to treatment with zidovudine. Patients (7%) receiving zidovudine alone reported muscle weakness and ache, while 37% had difficulty in performing a series of tasks (Simpson *et al.*, 1998).

4.2.2   *Experimental systems*

(a)   *Haematotoxicity*

Most of the studies of the toxicity of zidovudine in animal models were performed in mice and, as in humans, the most frequently cited effect after either short-term or long-term dosing involved the haematopoietic system (Cronkite & Bullis, 1990; Bogliolo *et al.*, 1991; Thompson *et al.*, 1991; Scheding *et al.*, 1994; Omar *et al.*, 1996; Inoue *et al.*, 1997; Rao *et al.*, 1998). Also as in humans, the effects were typically reversible within days to weeks after discontinuation of the drug. In one study (Du *et al.*, 1992), normal bone marrow samples were obtained from patients undergoing hip replacement surgery and from mice, and the cells were exposed in culture to 0.1, 1.0, 10 or 100 μmol/L zidovudine. Continuous exposure caused greater inhibition of cell growth than a 1-h exposure, and the mouse cells were slightly more sensitive than the human cells to the toxic effects of zidovudine.

The effects of acute administration were examined by Scheding et al. (1994) in female B6C3F$_1$ mice given 30, 60, 90, 120 or 240 mg/kg bw zidovudine by bolus intravenous injection or by a 24-h intravenous infusion. The animals given bolus doses showed no toxicity, but those given the 24-h infusion had significantly decreased numbers of bone-marrow erythroid progenitor cells. Similar results were obtained by Bogliolo et al. (1991), who gave an intravenous dose of 240 mg/kg bw per day to mice for five days. The numbers of bone-marrow myeloid and erythroid progenitors reached the lowest point at five days and had returned to normal within two to five days after exposure. Exposure of mice to 500 mg/kg bw zidovudine for 7–14 days produced thymic involution, with a decreased percentage of CD4 and CD8 cells and a decrease in the ability of T cells to respond to foreign antigens (McKallip et al., 1995).

Long-term exposure to zidovudine results in more extensive haematopoeitic effects. For example, when 0.75 mg/mL zidovudine in drinking-water was administered to mice on days 84–687 of age, the primary toxic effects were thrombocytopenia and myelodysplasia (Inoue et al., 1997). In CBA/Ca mice given 1.0 mg/mL zidovudine in the drinking-water for seven weeks, neutropenia and lymphopenia, which did not resolve, and macrocytic anaemia and changes in bone-marrow cellularity were seen which returned to normal after discontinuation of treatment (Cronkite & Bullis, 1990). In other studies, doses of 25–1000 mg/kg bw zidovudine given to B6C3F$_1$ mice by gavage daily for 13 weeks caused bone-marrow depression and macrocytic anaemia, both of which were reversible when the drug was discontinued (Thompson et al., 1991; Rao et al., 1998).

Cats infected with feline leukaemia virus were given 7.5, 15, 30 or 60 mg/kg bw zidovudine per day for 32–34 days (Haschek et al., 1990). The 60- and 30-mg doses produced anaemia by days 4 and 13, respectively, and decreased packed red cell volume, bone-marrow hypercellularity and splenic extramedullary haematopoiesis were seen, similar to the effects in humans.

Ayers et al. (1996b) studied the toxic effects of zidovudine in CD rats, beagle dogs and cynomolgus monkeys given large single doses and lower doses over longer periods. In rats given 225–250 mg/kg bw zidovudine twice daily and monkeys given 17.5–150 mg/kg bw twice daily for 3–12 months, macrocytic, normochromic anaemia was observed. After 12 months of dosing, the erythrocyte counts were decreased in rats and those of leukocytes were slightly decreased in monkeys. In dogs given 62.5–250 mg/kg bw zidovudine for 14 days, cell replication was inhibited in bone marrow, gastrointestinal epithelium and lymphoid tissue.

(b) Myopathy

Functional, morphological and biochemical changes, similar to the cardiac and skeletal muscle myopathy seen in HIV-positive individuals given long-term zidovudine treatment, have been observed in rats exposed to zidovudine (Lamperth et al., 1991; Pindado et al., 1994; McCurdy & Kennedy, 1996; Masini et al., 1999). The animal models are particularly valuable because they clearly demonstrate that the drug alone can induce muscle myopathy associated with mitochondrial damage (see Section 4.5), independently of the effects of the HIV virus. Lamperth et al. (1991) compared human muscle cultured with zidovudine for three weeks with muscle tissue from rats given 17–51 mg/kg bw zidovudine per day for three months. In the rats, zidovudine was preferentially concentrated in heart and skeletal muscle. In both species, the mitochondria were enlarged with disorganized or absent cristae and abnormal functioning of oxidative phosphorylation. Complexes I and II were observed. In a study (Pindado et al., 1994) in which rats were given 1–2 mg/mL zidovudine in the drinking-water for 30, 60 or 120 days, the cardiac muscle mitochondria were increased in size and showed disrupted cristae. McCurdy and Kennedy (1996) found decreased amounts of mitochondrial DNA and a diminished response to electrical stimulation in skeletal muscle of rats given 1 mg/mL zidovudine in the drinking-water for 35 days. They concluded that zidovudine treatment induces changes in mitochondria that result in diminished contractile capacity of skeletal muscle. Masini et al. (1999) demonstrated depleted concentrations of mitochondrial DNA in skeletal muscle of rats given 1 mg/mL zidovudine in the drinking-water (about 40 mg/kg bw zidovudine per day) for 90 days.

4.3 Reproductive and prenatal effects

4.3.1 *Humans*

Studies of the efficacy of zidovudine in reducing maternal–infant transmission of HIV have included information on the reproductive and prenatal effects of this drug.

In a review of the medical records of 104 HIV-infected women who were treated with zidovudine at various times during pregnancy at one clinic in India, there were eight spontaneous first-trimester abortions, eight therapeutic terminations and eight cases of fetal abnormality, of which two occurred in women treated during the first trimester (Kumar et al., 1994). No specific abnormality could reasonably be attributed to the therapy.

White et al. (1997) used the files of an international Antiviral Pregnancy Register, set up in the USA in 1989 to monitor the safety of prenatal exposure to antiretroviral agents, to evaluate birth outcomes for 198 of 249 women who had been treated during pregnancy with zidovudine and for whom the pregnancy outcome was known by the authors. The outcomes included nine (4.5%) induced abortions, two (1.0%) spontaneous abortions and seven (3.7%; 95% CI, 1.6–7.8%) birth defects of which one occurred among the subgroup of 73 women who were exposed during the first trimester. The prevalence of birth defects among the zidovudine-treated pregnant women did not exceed the rate of 3–4% which is estimated to occur in the general population of the USA.

In a retrospective cohort study, Sperling et al. (1992) reported on 43 women with AIDS who had been treated at 17 different institutions in the USA, where they received doses of zidovudine ranging from 300 to 1200 mg per day during part of or all of pregnancy. All 45 newborns, including two sets of twins, were born alive. No increased risk for premature births, intrauterine growth retardation or newborn asphyxia was found, and 41 of the 45 infants were born at term. Among the 12 newborns who had been exposed to zidovudine during the first trimester, no malformations were reported.

In a randomized, placebo-controlled trial, Connor *et al.* (1994) included 477 HIV-infected pregnant women from various treatment centres in France and the USA in 1991–93. The women were randomly assigned to receive either zidovudine or placebo. During the study period, 409 gave birth to 415 liveborn infants. There were eight fetal or neonatal deaths, five in the group receiving zidovudine and three in the group given the placebo. None of these deaths was considered by the authors to be attributable to the drug. Seven infants died beyond the neonatal period, six (two in the group given zidovudine) from HIV infection and one (in the group given zidovudine) due to trauma.

In order to determine the safety of zidovudine administered during pregnancy, Sperling *et al.* (1998) reanalysed the findings of a randomized placebo-controlled trial in which HIV-infected women between 14 and 34 weeks' gestation with CD4 cell counts > 200/μL and no maternal indications for antiretroviral therapy were enrolled from 55 treatment centres in France and the USA. During the inclusion period of 1991–93, 424 eligible women were randomized to either zidovudine or placebo, and the women were followed through six months *post partum*, while their infants were followed through 18 months of age. Five women given zidovudine and two given placebo had either a spontaneous abortion or a stillbirth. Among the infants born live to women receiving zidovudine, 19 (9%) had major structural abnormalities and 28 (13%) had minor structural abnormalities, while among the infants born live to women given placebo the equivalent figures were 17 (8%) and 35 (17%).

Lorenzi *et al.* (1998) reported on a small prospective study conducted in Switzerland of 33 HIV-infected women who had received combined antiretroviral therapy including zidovudine during pregnancy in 1996–98. Among the 33 liveborn neonates, one (3.0%) case of congenital malformation was found.

In the French National Epidemiological Network, records have been kept of 1754 children of women seropositive for HIV-1 who were treated during pregnancy with zidovudine (500 mg per day) or with zidovudine and lamivudine (300 mg per day) for a mean prenatal exposure of 17.2 weeks (range, 0–40 weeks). After birth, the children of these women were given daily doses of 8 mg/kg bw zidovudine and/or 4 mg/kg bw lamivudine for an average of 5.2 weeks (range, 2–6 weeks). Two of the HIV-negative children, who had received both zidovudine and lamivudine transplacentally, died at approximately one year of age with symptoms of mitochondrial disorders, including seizures, brain lesions identified by nuclear magnetic resonance, persistent lactic acidosis and abnormal mitochondrial oxidative phosphorylation (respiratory chain) function in skeletal muscle, lymphocytes and liver. Six other HIV-negative children between the ages of seven months and 4.4 years, two of whom had received zidovudine and lamivudine and four of whom had received zidovudine alone, had various combinations of brain lesions, seizures and persistent lactic acidosis. All of these children had abnormal mitochondrial oxidative phosphorylation, and three had no other clinical symptoms (Blanche et al., 1999).

Culnane et al. (1999) reported on the Pediatric AIDS Clinical Trial Group Protocol 076, a multicentre, randomized, double-blind, placebo-controlled trial in which zidovudine was used to prevent perinatal HIV-1 transmission. The median age of 234 uninfected children born to 2330 HIV-infected women at the time of the follow-up visit was 4.2 years (range, 3.2–5.6 years). There were no significant differences between children exposed to zidovudine (122) and those who received placebo (112) with respect to weight, height, head circumference or cognitive development. No deaths or malignancies were reported.

4.3.2 *Experimental systems*

Bone-marrow aspirates from women of child-bearing age, bone marrow and liver from seven mid-trimester abortuses and umbilical cord blood from seven term infants were treated *in vitro* with zidovudine at a concentration of 0.1, 1.0, 10, 100 or 500 μmol/L. Erythroid progenitor cells from all fetal and neonatal sources were more sensitive to zidovudine than those from the bone marrow of adult women (Shah et al., 1996).

Aliquots of 16–20 fertilized mouse (FVB/N) oocytes at the one-cell stage were isolated and treated with zidovudine at a concentration of 0, 0.1, 1.0 or 10 μg/mL. Exposure to the two higher doses was reported to reduce blastocyst formation (Toltzis et al., 1991). This study was replicated with two-cell embryos in the same laboratory, with the same result (Toltzis et al., 1994).

Male and female embryos collected from pregnant Wistar rats on day 9.5 of gestation were cultured for 48 h with 0, 50, 500, 1000 or 3000 μmol/L zidovudine. At the highest concentration, zidovudine was reported to produce a 40% incidence of abnormal embryos (Klug et al., 1991).

In a 14-week study of reproductive toxicity in 10 $B6C3F_1$ mice dosed by gavage with 0, 100, 800 or 2000 mg/kg bw zidovudine, no treatment-related effects were found on spermatid or epididymal spermatozoal parameters in males or oestrone cycle characteristics in females (National Toxicology Program, 1999).

The toxicity of zidovudine was evaluated in groups of 10 adult male Swiss (CD-1) mice treated by gavage with 200 or 400 mg/kg bw zidovudine or with vehicle for 20–21 days and 20 adult female mice given the same doses for either 28–32 days or on days 6–15 of gestation. Zidovudine treatment at both doses caused decreased sperm motility and reduced the number of pregnant mice per group. In pregnant dams, the average numbers of corpora lutea and implantations per litter were not affected by treatment, but the number of live fetuses per litter was decreased and the average number of early and/or late deaths increased. The mean fetal body weight per litter was reduced by treatment with either dose (National Institute of Environmental Health Sciences, 1998).

In a separate study of the same design, zidovudine at doses of 100, 200 or 400 mg/kg bw given to pregnant mice decreased body-weight gain, reportedly due to reduced litter sizes, increased the number of resorptions and reduced the fetal weights per litter. No statistically significant increase in the number of litters or fetuses with gross external alterations was reported, and no statistically significant effect on sperm motility was observed (National Institute of Environmental Health Sciences, 1999).

Pregnant transgenic mice carrying the Moloney murine leukaemia virus in the germ line were treated with zidovudine dissolved in the drinking-water at a concentration of 0.1, 0.2, 0.4 or 0.6 mg/mL. Dosing began on either gestational day 10 or 19 and was continued throughout lactation and weaning. After weaning, the offspring received zidovudine directly in their drinking-water. No results were given for the group receiving 0.6 mg/mL zidovudine, but at the other doses, only mild macrocytic anaemia was reported. No gross teratological effects and no effect on litter size were reported. Histopathological analyses of the offspring revealed no specific sequelae (Sharpe et al., 1988). [The Working Group noted that the methods for collection of reproductive and histopathological data were not described and no individual or mean data were shown for these developmental toxicological end-points.].

Mature, female C3H/He mice were treated with 0, 0.25, 0.50 or 2.5 mg/mL zidovudine in the drinking-water at eight weeks of age and were mated after eight weeks of therapy. Dosing was continued throughout gestation. Two of the three untreated mice but none of the nine treated animals produced offspring. Mature female C3H/He mice (20 per group) were either untreated or treated with 0.25 mg/mL zidovudine in the drinking-water beginning at six weeks of age and were mated after six weeks of treatment. Dosing was continued up to days 12–17 of gestation. Treatment with zidovudine was reported to reduce the occurrence of pregnancy and the number of fetuses per litter and to increase the number of resorptions. No physical anomalies were noted on gross examination of surgically removed fetuses at 12–17 days of gestation (Toltzis et al., 1991). [The Working Group noted that the gestational days of exposure and age at sacrifice were not clear, having an apparent range of 12–17 days.]

Groups of 6–10 pregnant CD-1 mice were treated with zidovudine at 0, 0.1 or 0.5 mg/mL in the drinking-water on days 1–13 of gestation. Fetuses, examined at day 13 of gestation, were reported to be smaller, with fewer fetuses per litter and decreased colony-forming ability of erythroid progenitor cells collected from fetal hepatic tissue (Gogu et al., 1992).

Groups of 7–12 pregnant Swiss-derived CD-1 mice were given 0, 0.2, 0.4 and 2.0 mg/mL zidovudine in the drinking-water from day 10 of gestation to delivery. The body weights (day 16) and water intake (days 12–14 and 14–16) of the dams at the highest dose were significantly decreased. Only two of 12 dams at this dose had viable litters, and the pups in these litters were lighter, smaller and less active than controls. Maternal cannibalization may have accounted for some of the pup deaths. The serum concentrations of zidovudine in treated dams were 0.87 µg/mL at 0.2 mg/mL, 1.4 µg/mL at 0.4 mg/mL and 1.7 µg/mL at 2.0 mg/mL. Behavioural analysis of the pups of dams given 0.2 or 0.4 mg/mL and comparison with controls revealed reduced pup weight gain (males and females combined), delayed appearance of the pole-grasping reflex (males at 0.4 mg/mL only) and slight but significant impairment during acquisition sessions of the passive avoidance test (at 0.2 and 0.4 mg/mL). The dose of 0.4 mg/mL appeared to reduce the sex differences in two sexually dimorphic aspects of the social behaviour repertoire (Calamandrei et al., 1999).

Groups of six male Wistar rats, 40 days old, were treated with 0, 0.1 or 1.0 mg/mL zidovudine (approximately equivalent to 15 and 150 mg/kg bw per day) in the drinking-water for four weeks. Body-weight gain was similar in control and treated animals, but ventral prostate weight, seminal vesicle weight and serum testosterone concentrations were decreased and serum luteinizing hormone and prolactin concentrations were increased as compared with controls (Sikka et al., 1991).

Groups of 20 pregnant Wistar rats were treated with water or 100 mg/kg bw zidovudine orally three times at 5-h intervals (total dose, 300 mg/kg bw) on day 10 of gestation. No adverse effects were reported on maternal body weight, food consumption, reproductive capacity or haematological parameters. No effects of zidovudine on the survival or growth of offspring and no treatment-related gross histopathological lesions were reported in the weanling rats. The mean concentration of zidovudine in day-10 embryonal homogenates, collected 30 min after the third dose, was 21 µg/g tissue (Greene et al., 1990).

Groups of 35 male and female Sprague-Dawley CD rats were treated twice daily by gavage with zidovudine in 0.5% methylcellulose at a dose of 0, 25, 75 or 225 mg/kg bw. Starting at seven weeks of age, F_0 generation males were dosed for 85 days before mating and afterwards, for a total of 175 days. F_0 females were treated daily for 26 days before mating and throughout gestation and lactation. No consistent adverse effects were reported in the males or in the offspring of untreated females. Early embryo mortality was increased and the number of live fetuses per litter was decreased at 75 and 225 mg/kg bw zidovudine. Fetal body weight was decreased at the highest dose (Greene et al., 1996).

Groups of 12 mature female CD rats were treated twice daily by gavage with zidovudine in 0.5% methylcellulose at a dose of 225 mg/kg bw 26 days before mating through postnatal day 15; 26 days before mating through to day 10 of gestation; 26 days before mating until pregnancy was confirmed or from day 1 of gestation through postnatal day 15. Zidovudine-induced embryotoxicity was limited to early embryos, and no gross or histological changes were reported in the offspring (Greene et al., 1996).

Groups of 21–24 pregnant CD rats were treated orally twice daily with zidovudine at a dose of 0, 62.5, 125 or 250 mg/kg bw on days 6–15 of gestation. No toxic effects were reported in dams or their offspring (Greene et al., 1996).

Groups of 30 pregnant CD rats were treated twice daily by gavage with zidovudine in 0.5% methylcellulose at a dose of 0, 25, 75 or 225 mg/kg bw from day 17 of gestation through delivery until postnatal day 21. No consistent or dose-related effects on growth, development (including behaviour) or reproductive performance were reported (Greene *et al.*, 1996).

Sixteen pregnant VAF Sprague-Dawley rats were treated by gavage with 150 mg/kg bw per day zidovudine for 22 days from day 1 of gestation. A control group of 14 rats received water. On day 22 of gestation, no gross structural malformations were found in the 12 litters examined (six per group). Treatment reduced the litter size and increased the weights of both male and female offspring. On postnatal days 21–22, the pups were injected subcutaneously with amphetamines (0.25–1.0 mg/kg bw) and their behaviour was observed. The locomotion response to amphetamines was increased only in female pups given zidovudine (Applewhite-Black *et al.*, 1998).

Pregnant Sprague-Dawley rats were given zidovudine by gavage in water at a dose of 0, 50, 100 or 150 mg/kg bw on days 19–22 of gestation, and individual offspring were treated by gavage on postnatal days 2–20 at the same doses. Behaviour after intraperitoneal injection of amphetamines (0.25, 0.50, 0.75 or 1.0 mg/kg bw) was assessed on postnatal day 21. The authors concluded that perinatal exposure to zidovudine altered one aspect of behaviour—locomotion—the threshold for this effect depending on sex. Because no effects were seen on litter size or on maternal or pup weight gain, they concluded that zidovudine alters neurodevelopmental processes without producing overt toxicity (Busidan & Dow-Edwards, 1999a). In a follow-up study of 12–15 litters per group, behaviour after an intraperitoneal injection of amphetamine (0.1, 0.5, 1.0 or 2.0 mg/kg bw) was assessed on postnatal days 59–65. Treatment did not alter open-field behaviour (Busidan & Dow-Edwards, 1999b).

Pregnant New Zealand white rabbits were treated orally twice daily at a 6-h interval with zidovudine in 0.5% methylcellulose at a dose of 0, 37.5, 75 or 250 mg/kg bw on days 6–18 of gestation. Twenty-two rabbits per group were killed on day 29. Dams given 250 mg/kg bw were reported to have reduced weight gain during days 6–18 of gestation and decreased haemoglobin concentration, haematocrit and red blood cell count. The effects on fetuses included increased numbers of resorptions and decreased weights at 250 mg/kg bw. No teratogenic effects were reported. At 250 mg/kg bw, the mean peak concentration of zidovudine in maternal plasma was 92.7 µg/mL (Greene *et al.*, 1996).

Female pigtail monkeys (*Macaca nemestrina*) were given zidovudine at a dose of 1.5 mg/kg bw or vehicle every 4 h via a gastric catheter for at least 10 days before conception and throughout pregnancy. Nine of the zidovudine-treated monkeys became pregnant and carried to term, as did seven control monkeys. The treated mothers developed asymptomatic macrocytic anaemia and showed decreased total leukocyte counts. The zidovudine-exposed infants were mildly anaemic at birth and showed deficits in growth, rooting and snouting reflexes and in the ability to fixate and follow near stimuli visually. These deficits disappeared over time after birth (Ha *et al.*, 1994, 1998).

4.4 Genetic and related effects

4.4.1 *Humans*

There are few published data of the effects of zidovudine on the genome of zidovudine-treated patients. The drug has not been reported to be mutagenic. Shafik *et al.* (1991) reported high levels of clastogenicity, but a later study with more reliable methods failed to find a similar effect (Witt *et al.*, 1999, abstract). Shafik *et al.* (1991) assessed the frequency of chromosomal aberrations in HIV-infected patients who were non-smokers and who had received zidovudine at 1200 mg/day for four weeks to seven months. One hundred metaphases from first-division cells from each culture of peripheral lymphocytes were scored for aberrations, mainly of the chromatid type. The frequencies of breaks in the zidovudine-treated and non-HIV-infected control groups were 8.3 ± 2.0 and 0.5 ± 0.3 per 100 cells, respectively. Witt *et al.* (1999, abstract) evaluated the frequency of chromosomal aberrations in two healthy men occupationally exposed to HIV and in 22 HIV-positive men who had not previously received antiviral drugs, after treatment with zidovudine and other dideoxynucleosides according to standard protocols. The mitotic index and frequency of chromosomal aberrations were measured in peripheral lymphocytes collected before initiation of drug therapy and at approximately four and 12 weeks during treatment. No significant treatment-related changes in mitotic index or in the percentage of aberrant cells were observed.

Olivero *et al.* (1999) quantified the zidovudine incorporated into peripheral blood leukocyte DNA from 24 of 28 HIV-positive non-pregnant adults receiving 600 mg zidovudine per day and in peripheral blood leukocyte DNA from eight of 12 pregnant women who had received zidovudine for periods varying from the last three weeks to the whole nine months of pregnancy. The values varied from 22 to 544 molecules of zidovudine/10^6 nucleotides. Of a group of 22 infants exposed to zidovudine *in utero*, including children of the 12 women mentioned above, 15 had measurable values for incorporation of zidovudine into DNA in cord blood leukocytes, varying from 22 to 452 molecules of zidovudine/10^6 nucleotides. The results show that the amounts of zidovudine incorporated into human DNA are similar in adults and in infants exposed *in utero*.

4.4.2 *Experimental systems*

These studies are summarized in Table 1.

(a)   In vitro

Testing of zidovudine in prokaryotic systems *in vitro* is limited to a few studies performed by three groups. Zidovudine induced reverse mutation in only one strain of *Salmonella typhimurium* and produced marginal or no differential toxicity in *Escherichia coli* and *Bacillus subtilis*. Mamber *et al.* (1990) assessed the ability of zidovudine and representative dideoxynucleosides to induce two SOS functions, cell filamentation

Table 1. Genetic and related effects of zidovudine

Test system	Result[a] Without exogenous metabolic system	Result[a] With exogenous metabolic system	Dose[b] (LED/HID)	Reference
Escherichia coli BR513 (*uvrB envA lacZ::lambda*), prophage induction, SOS repair (spot and liquid suspension tests)	+	NT	0.064	Mamber et al. (1990)
Escherichia coli PQ37 (*uvrA rfa lacZ::sulA*), cell filamentation, SOS repair (spot and liquid suspension tests)	+	NT	0.5	Mamber et al. (1990)
Escherichia coli CM871 (*uvrA recA lexA*), differential toxicity (vs *Escherichia coli* WP2)	(+)	NT	1000	Mamber et al. (1990)
Bacillus subtilis M45 *rec* strain, differential toxicity	–	NT	NR	Mamber et al. (1990)
Salmonella typhimurium TA100, TA1535, TA1537, TA1538, TA88, reverse mutation	–	–	10 μg/plate	Ayers et al. (1996a)
Salmonella typhimurium TA100, TA104, TA 1535, TA98, TA97, reverse mutation	–	–	1–3 μg/plate	National Toxicology Program (1999)
Salmonella typhimurium TA 102, reverse mutation	(+)	(+)	0.3 μg/plate	National Toxicology Program (1999)
Bacillus subtilis H17, gene mutation	–	NT	NR	Mamber et al. (1990)
Gene mutation, Chinese hamster ovary cells *in vitro*, *Hprt* locus	–	NT	10 000	Grdina et al. (1992)
Gene mutation, mouse lymphoma L5178Y cells, *Tk* locus, 4-h treatment *in vitro*	(+)[c]	(+)	1000	Ayers et al. (1996a)
Gene mutation, mouse lymphoma L5178Y cells, *Tk* locus, 24-h treatment *in vitro*	+	NT	25	Ayers et al. (1996a)
Sister chromatid exchange, Chinese hamster cells *in vitro*	+	NT	500	González Cid & Larripa (1994)
Sister chromatid exchange, Chinese hamster cells *in vitro*	+	+	8.3	National Toxicology Program (1999)
Chromosomal aberrations, Chinese hamster cells *in vitro*	+	NT	1000	González Cid & Larripa (1994)

Table 1 (contd)

Test system	Result[a] Without exogenous metabolic system	Result[a] With exogenous metabolic system	Dose[b] (LED/HID)	Reference
Chromosomal aberrations, Chinese hamster cells in vitro	–	–	2500	National Toxicology Program (1999)
Cell transformation, BALB/c 3T3 mouse cells	+	NT	0.5	Ayers et al. (1996a)
Gene mutation, human HepG2 cells in vitro, HPRT locus	+	NT	100	Grdina et al. (1992)
Gene mutation, human TK6 lymphoblastoid cells in vitro, TK locus	+	NT	9 × 3 d	Meng et al. (2000a)
Gene mutation, human TK6 lymphoblastoid cells in vitro, HPRT locus	+	NT	80 × 3 d	Sussman et al. (1999)
Sister chromatid exchange, human lymphocytes in vitro	+	NT	50	González Cid & Larripa (1994)
Micronucleus formation, human lymphocytes in vitro	+	NT	500	González Cid & Larripa (1994)
Chromosomal aberrations, human lymphocytes in vitro	+	NT	100	González Cid & Larripa (1994)
Chromosomal aberrations, human lymphocytes in vitro	+	NT	3	Ayers et al. (1996a)
Chromosomal aberrations, H9 human lymphocytic cells in vitro	+	NT	6.7 × 7 mo	Agarwal & Olivero (1997)
Irreversible telomere shortening, mouse brain and liver cells in utero	+		25 mg/d, d 12–18 of gestation	Olivero et al. (1997)
Irreversible telomere shortening, Erythrocebus patas cells in utero (various organs)	–		10 mg/d, 5 d/wk; last 9.5–10 wk of gestation	Olivero et al. (1997)

Table 1 (contd)

Test system	Result[a]		Dose[b] (LED/HID)	Reference
	Without exogenous metabolic system	With exogenous metabolic system		
Micronucleus formation, mouse peripheral blood lymphocytes and bone-marrow cells in vivo	+		100 po × 4 wk	Oleson & Getman (1990); Ayers et al. (1996a)
Micronucleus formation, mouse peripheral blood lymphocytes and bone-marrow cells in vivo	+		NR iv × 4 d	Oleson & Getman (1990); Ayers et al. (1996a)
Micronucleus formation, B6C3F₁ mouse bone-marrow cells in vivo	+		200 po × 3	Phillips et al. (1991)
Micronucleus formation, B6C3F₁ mouse bone-marrow cells in vivo	+		100 po × 13 wk	Phillips et al. (1991)
Micronucleus formation, Swiss Webster mouse bone-marrow cells in vivo	−		14.4 ip × 1	Motimaya et al. (1994a)
Micronucleus formation, Swiss Webster mouse bone-marrow cells in vivo	−		28.6 ip × 1	Motimaya et al. (1994b)
Micronucleus formation, BALB/c mouse bone-marrow cells in vivo	+		17 ip × 5; 2 wk	Dertinger et al. (1996)
Micronucleus formation, rat bone-marrow cells in vivo	+		500 po × 7	Oleson & Getman (1990); Ayers et al. (1996a)
Chromosomal aberrations, mouse bone-marrow cells in vivo	+		33 po (drinking-water) × 4 wk	Olivero et al. (1994a)
Chromosomal aberrations, rat bone-marrow cells in vivo	−		300 iv × 1	Ayers et al. (1996a)

ZIDOVUDINE

Table 1 (contd)

Test system	Result[a] Without exogenous metabolic system	Result[a] With exogenous metabolic system	Dose[b] (LED/HID)	Reference
Binding (covalent) to telomeric and Z-DNA, Chinese hamster ovary cells *in vitro*	+		214	Olivero & Poirier (1993); Gomez et al. (1995); Parra et al. (1997)
Binding (covalent) to DNA, Chinese hamster ovary cells *in vitro*	+		5.3	Olivero et al. (1994b)
Binding (covalent) to DNA, mouse NIH 3T3 cells *in vitro*	+		5.3	Olivero et al. (1994b)
Binding (covalent) to DNA, CCRF/CEM human lymphoid cells *in vitro*	+		0.27	Avramis et al. (1989)
Binding (covalent) to DNA, human bone-marrow cells *in vitro*	+		2.7	Sommadossi et al. (1989)
Binding (covalent) to DNA, K562 human leukaemic cells *in vitro*	+		2.7	Vazquez-Padua et al. (1990)
Binding (covalent) to DNA, HL60 human leukaemic cells *in vitro*	+		5.3	Olivero et al. (1994b)
Binding (covalent) to DNA, HCT-8 human colon cancer cells *in vitro*	+		5.3	Darnowski & Goulette (1994)
Binding (covalent) to DNA, H9 human lymphocytic cells *in vitro*	+		6.7 × 7 mo	Agarwal & Olivero (1997)
Binding (covalent) to DNA, TK6 human lymphoblastoid cells *in vitro*	+		80 × 3 d	Sussman et al. (1999)
Binding (covalent) to DNA, TK6 human lymphoblastoid cells *in vitro*	+		9 × 3 d	Meng et al. (2000b)
Binding (covalent) to DNA, mouse vaginal epithelial cells *in vivo*	+		33 po (drinking-water) × 4 wk	Olivero et al. (1994a)
Binding (covalent) to nuclear and mitochondrial DNA, mouse kidney, liver, lung and skin cells *in utero*	+		25 mg/d; d 12–18 of gestation	Olivero et al. (1997)

Table 1 (contd)

Test system	Result[a]		Dose[b] (LED/HID)	Reference
	Without exogenous metabolic system	With exogenous metabolic system		
Binding (covalent) to nuclear and mitochondrial DNA, *Erythrocebus patas* cells *in utero* (brain, heart, kidney, liver, lungs, placenta)	+		10 mg/d, 5 d/wk; last 9.5–10 wk of gestation	Olivero *et al.* (1997)

[a] +, positive; (+), weak positive; –, negative; NT, not tested
[b] LED, lowest effective dose; HID, highest ineffective dose; in-vitro tests, µg/mL; in-vivo tests, mg/kg bw per day; NR, not reported; po, oral; iv, intravenous; ip, intraperitoneal; mo, month; d, day; wk, week
[c] Positive at 4000–5000 µg/mL only

and prophage lambda, in *E. coli*. Zidovudine was the most potent inducer of the SOS response, with a minimal active concentration that was 100-fold lower than those of the dideoxypurine nucleosides. These results indicate that zidovudine and dideoxynucleosides do not cause DNA lesions that are removed by the excision repair (*uvr*A) or error-free postreplication repair (*rec*A) processes. Rather, in acting as DNA chain terminators, they may generate an SOS-inducing response leading to inhibition of DNA replication.

The results of studies in animal cells *in vitro* have generally indicated mutagenic effects of zidovudine. In several tests with high doses of zidovudine that are not clinically relevant, it did not induce mutations at the hypoxanthine-guanine phosphoribosyl (*Hprt*) locus but significantly increased the frequencies of sister chromatid exchange and chromosomal aberrations in cultured Chinese hamster ovary cells. Zidovudine was also mutagenic at the thymidine kinase (*Tk*) locus of mouse lymphoma cells, and it caused cell transformation in 3T3 mouse cells.

The results of tests for gene mutation and clastogenicity in zidovudine-exposed human cells have been consistently positive, both at high doses and at low doses approximating the plasma concentrations in treated patients. Zidovudine induced mutations at the *HPRT* locus of HepG2 cells at high doses, but addition of a cytoprotective agent concomitantly or after zidovudine was effective in reducing the mutagenic effects. Sussman *et al.* (1999) investigated the relationships between incorporation of zidovudine into DNA [see (c) below], mutant frequency and the spectrum of deletion mutations in *HPRT* of human lymphoblastoid TK6 cells exposed to a concentration 10–20 times higher than the peak plasma concentrations in adult patients given a dose of 200 mg zidovudine. Treatment of TK6 cells with zidovudine significantly increased the *HPRT* mutant frequency, and molecular analyses showed that the differences between the control and treated groups was due mainly to an increase (by 16–37%) in the frequency of total gene deletion mutations. These results indicate that the primary mechanism of zidovudine-induced mutagenicity in TK6 cells is production of large deletions as a result of incorporation into DNA and subsequent chain termination. The mutational spectra also suggested that zidovudine induces point mutations, either directly by some unknown mechanism or indirectly by damaging genes that affect the frequency of endogenous mutational events. This hypothesis is supported by the finding of distinctive point mutations in Ha-*ras* in skin tumours from mice exposed *in utero* to zidovudine.

Sussman *et al.* (1999) also exposed TK6 cells to a minor metabolite of zidovudine, 3'-amino-3'-deoxythymidine, to evaluate its relative cytotoxic and mutagenic potency. 3'-Amino-3'-deoxythymidine was more cytotoxic than zidovudine at equimolar doses, and the amino metabolite did not produce a mutagenic response in TK6 cells. 3'-Amino-3'-deoxythymidine thus appears to contribute little to the mutagenic potency of zidovudine *in vivo* as only small amounts are formed in humans and relatively small amounts are incorporated into DNA after zidovudine treatment of human cells (Darnowski & Goulette, 1994; Acosta *et al.*, 1996).

Meng et al. (2000a) evaluated the relationships between incorporation of zidovudine into DNA, mutant frequency and loss of heterozygosity at the *TK* locus of TK6 cells exposed to zidovudine at concentrations down to the peak plasma levels found in some patients. The *TK* mutant frequencies increased in a time-dependent manner in treated cells and appeared to approach a plateau after 6 days of exposure. The frequencies were significantly increased over the background value at all doses, including that which corresponded to a clinically relevant concentration. Southern blot analyses indicated that 84% of the zidovudine-induced *TK* mutants had loss of heterozygosity due to large deletions, consistent with the known mechanism of action of zidovudine as a DNA chain terminator.

The fact that TK6 cells are heterozygous at the *TK* locus and hemizygous at the *HPRT* locus can affect both the magnitude and the nature of the mutagenic response to chemically induced lesions at these two reporter genes (Meng et al., 2000b). Many mutagenic mechanisms that involve homologous interaction, such as gene conversion and mitotic recombination, cannot occur at the X-linked *HPRT* locus. In addition, multi-locus deletions are likely to be lethal to the *HPRT* gene, because these gross deletions may span the adjacent genes essential for cell survival. Therefore, if the primary mechanism of mutation induction by a chemical implicates homologous interaction or a large deletion, the mutagenicity of that agent will be significantly underestimated in the *HPRT* assay; indeed, the average zidovudine-induced *TK* mutant frequency was significantly greater than the average zidovudine-induced *HPRT* mutant frequency in the same cell samples. Awareness of these differences is important because *HPRT*, but not *TK*, mutant frequencies can be measured in zidovudine-treated patients (Meng et al., 2000b).

The potential role of large-scale DNA damage in zidovudine-induced mutagenicity is supported by the finding of increased frequencies of sister chromatid exchange, micronuclei and chromosomal aberrations in zidovudine-exposed human cells *in vitro*. Agarwal and Olivero (1997) reported that seven months' exposure of human lymphocytic H_9 cells in culture to concentrations of zidovudine equivalent to the peak plasma concentrations of this drug in some patients significantly increased the frequency of chromosomal aberrations, the most dramatic increases being observed in the number of breaks and fragments. These two aberrations are consistent with integration of zidovudine into DNA and prevention of chain elongation.

Gomez et al. (1998) sought to determine if long-term exposure of human cells to zidovudine *in vitro* results in telomere shortening and if this shortening is reversible. They cultured HeLa cells with zidovudine and found that, as the passage number increased, the length of the telomere decreased markedly. This phenomenon correlated with incorporation of zidovudine into the telomere by telomerase and subsequent chain termination. The shortened telomeric repeats did not elongate after being cultured without zidovudine for additional passages, but no evidence of cell senescence was detected.

(b) *In vivo*

Studies of the mutagenicity of zidovudine in animals *in vivo* are limited to assays for micronuclei and chromosomal aberrations in rodents; the results of seven of 10 studies were positive. In the only study of micronucleus formation in which negative results were obtained, Motimaya *et al.* (1994a,b) reported no effect in mice given single intraperitoneal doses of 14.3–28.6 mg/kg bw. Although the doses used approximated the recommended daily dose for a person of average (70 kg) weight, Shelby (1994) pointed out that zidovudine therapy in patients involves long-term treatment. The finding raised questions about the clastogenic potential of zidovudine at clinically relevant doses as well as the sensitivity of the micronucleus assays used: either low doses of zidovudine do not induce micronuclei in mice or the genotoxic effects at these doses are too small to be detected in the tests as performed (Shelby, 1994). Dertinger *et al.* (1996) addressed these issues by scoring micronuclei with high throughput flow cytometry after intraperitoneal administration of zidovudine at 0 or 17 mg/kg bw to groups of five female and five male mice on five days a week for two weeks. The modest yet highly significant clastogenic effect observed in both sexes was below the limit of detection of conventional micronucleus assays which rely on microscopic inspection to score the rare micronucleated cell population. This study strongly suggested that low, clinically relevant concentrations of zidovudine are clastogenic.

Olivero *et al.* (1997) reported that transplacental exposure of mice to zidovudine at 25 mg/day by gavage during the last third of gestation resulted in shorter chromosomal telomeres in the liver and brain of most newborn mice. This effect was not observed in offspring of *Erythrocebus patas* monkeys given 20% of the human equivalent dose of zidovudine during the last half of gestation.

(c) *DNA incorporation of zidovudine*

The direct effects of zidovudine on DNA include incorporation into host cell nuclear and/or mitochondrial DNA and/or inhibition of nuclear or mitochondrial DNA polymerases. The first phenomenon results in termination of the DNA chain, and both phenomena lead to a reduction of DNA synthesis, with resultant effects on cell growth and viability. Thus, techniques have been devised to determine the amount of zidovudine incorporated, to elucidate the conditions under which such incorporation occurs and to define the generalized toxic and specific mutagenic consequences of such incorporation. The observed toxic and mutagenic effects of zidovudine may also be related to indirect interaction with host cell DNA through zidovudine-mediated alterations in deoxynucleotide pools, inhibition of DNA anabolic enzymes and interference with DNA repair processes. Only a brief review of the experimental evidence for incorporation of zidovudine into DNA as it relates to possible mutagenic and tumorigenic outcomes is given here.

Numerous studies have demonstrated that zidovudine is incorporated into the nuclear DNA of a variety of cell types (e.g. ovary cells, fibroblasts, lymphoblastoid/

lymphocytic cells, leukaemic cells, colon cancer epithelium and vaginal epithelium) *in vitro* and *in vivo* and in whole tissues in several species (e.g. hamsters, mice, monkeys and humans). As mentioned earlier, zidovudine is preferentially incorporated into the telomeric regions of some cell types (Olivero & Poirier, 1993; Gomez *et al.*, 1995; Parra *et al.*, 1997).

In most of the studies referred to in Table 1, mutagenicity and DNA incorporation were not conducted in the same samples, precluding a direct evaluation of the relationship between the two. In the study of Meng *et al.* (2000a) of the relationship between duration of exposure and concentration, incorporation of zidovudine into genomic DNA and mutagenic responses at the *HPRT* and *TK* loci of TK6 cells exposed in culture to concentrations down to the peak plasma concentrations in some patients, they found a significant correlation between incorporation of zidovudine into DNA and *HPRT* and *TK* mutant frequencies in relation to both duration and dose, strongly indicating that incorporation of zidovudine into nuclear DNA has a direct role in its mutagenicity.

In the study of Sussman *et al.* (1999), described above, of the relationships between duration of exposure, incorporation of zidovudine into genomic DNA and the mutagenic response at the *HPRT* locus of TK6 cells exposed in culture, although the concentration of zidovudine in the medium was 10–20 times higher than the peak plasma concentrations in some adult patients, the amount of zidovudine incorporated into DNA was comparable to those found after exposure of CD-1 mice, *E. patas* and *Macaca mulatta* monkeys and human infants to zidovudine *in utero*. Furthermore, exposure of TK6 cells to the equivalent of peak plasma concentrations of zidovudine for three days led to the incorporation of much smaller amounts of zidovudine than in cells from monkey and human infants exposed to clinical doses of zidovudine *in utero* (Meng *et al.*, 2000a). Comparisons of the amounts of zidovudine incorporated into DNA with duration and dose are presented in Table 2.

It is noteworthy that short-term exposure (three days) of human cells in culture to moderately high concentrations of zidovudine, short-term transplacental exposure of mice to high concentrations and long-term transplacental exposure of monkeys and humans to clinical doses of zidovudine had nearly the same effect in terms of incorporation into DNA. Exposure of human cells in culture to zidovudine can be correlated directly with a significant mutagenic response, and the exposure of mice led to increased incidences of transplacentally induced cancers and inactivation of Ha-*ras* oncogene in skin tumours. These results indicate that the dose and plasma concentrations of zidovudine do not account by themselves for its mutagenic and carcinogenic effects. Rather, the duration of exposure and other yet to be determined factors (such as species and inter-individual genetic variations in enzymes involved in anabolism of zidovudine and repair of zidovudine-induced DNA damage) must participate in zidovudine-mediated mutagenesis and carcinogenesis.

Table 2. Relationships between exposure to zidovudine, incorporation into DNA and mutagenic or carcinogenic effects

Sample source	Cell or tissue type	Dose of zidovudine or exposure	Molecules of zidovudine per 10^6 nucleotides	Mutagenic or carcinogenic response	Reference
Pregnant women	Peripheral blood lymphocytes	600 mg/day orally during last three weeks up to nine months of pregnancy	25–215	Unknown	Olivero et al. (1999)
Newborns	Cord blood lymphocytes	Transplacental via their mothers' therapy	22–452	Unknown	Olivero et al. (1999)
Monkey fetuses (*Macaca mulatta*)	Brain, heart, liver, lung, skeletal muscle, placenta, testis	In pregnant monkeys: 8 mg/kg bw intravenously 4 h before hysterectomy	29–1944	Unknown	Poirier et al. (2000)
Monkey fetuses (*Erythrocebas patas*)	Brain, heart, kidney, liver, lung, placenta	In pregnant monkeys: 10 mg/day orally five days per week, last 9.5–10 weeks of gestation	7–246	Unknown	Olivero et al. (1997)
CD-1 mouse fetuses	Brain, kidneys, liver, lung, skin	In pregnant mice: 25 mg/day by gavage last seven days of gestation	7–101	Tumours of liver, lung and reproductive system	Olivero et al. (1997)

Table 2 (contd)

Sample source	Cell or tissue type	Dose of zidovudine or exposure	Molecules of zidovudine per 10^6 nucleotides	Mutagenic or carcinogenic response	Reference
Human cells	TK6 lymphoblastoid cells	In culture: 33 μmol/L for three days		Significantly mutagenic at *TK* locus	Meng *et al.* (2000b)
		100 μmol/L for three days		Significantly mutagenic at *TK* and *HPRT* loci	
		33 μmol/L plus 33 μmol/L for three days		Synergistic mutagenic effects at *TK* and *HPRT* loci	
		100 μmol/L plus 100 μmol/L for three days		Synergistic mutagenic effects at *TK* and *HPRT* loci	
Human cells	TK6 lymphoblastoid cells	In culture: 300 μmol/L for three to six days	102 ± 15	Significantly mutagenic at *TK* locus	Sussman *et al.* (1999)

(*d*) *Genotoxicity of zidovudine in combinations*

In theory, a combination of two nucleoside analogues of two different bases could have at least an additive genotoxic effect in host cells. Meng *et al.* (2000b) tested two components of the frequently used clinical combination therapies, zidovudine and didanosine, by measuring the incorporation of zidovudine into nuclear DNA and the mutagenic responses at *HPRT* and *TK* in TK6 cells exposed to either drug alone and in combination at doses down to the peak plasma concentrations found in some patients. Didanosine was more cytotoxic than zidovudine, and didanosine alone was less mutagenic than zidovudine alone at both genes. An unexpected and striking finding was that equimolar combinations of zidovudine and didanosine not only significantly increased the *HPRT* and *TK* mutant frequencies at all doses, but the induced mutant frequencies at both loci were three to four times greater than the additive values obtained after exposure to zidovudine or didanosine alone. In addition, the amounts of zidovudine incorporated into DNA of cells exposed to zidovudine plus didanosine were 1.8 and 2.4 times greater than those in cells exposed to analogous concentrations of zidovudine alone. These results indicate that the mutagenic potentiation in human cells exposed to zidovudine plus didanosine is partly due to enhanced incorporation of zidovudine into cellular DNA. Further investigations are needed to determine if other clinically relevant combinations of antiretroviral agents have synergistic genotoxic effects in cell culture, in animal models and in human populations.

4.5 Mechanistic considerations

The toxicological and mutagenic consequences of exposure to zidovudine and the carcinogenic effects of this agent in rodents arise primarily as a result of its incorporation into host cell DNA and the concomitant termination of DNA replication. There is overwhelming evidence that zidovudine is incorporated into host cell nuclear and mitochondrial DNA in multiple systems, including cultured cells, animal models and humans. Incorporation values of about 7–500 molecules/10^6 nucleotides (approximately 10 000–100 000 zidovudine molecules/cell) have been obtained in adults and transplacentally exposed mice, monkeys (*E. patas* and *M. mulatta*) and humans given the drug alone or in therapeutic combinations (Table 2).

In human cells exposed to zidovudine, the amounts of zidovudine incorporated into cellular DNA correlated significantly with the frequencies of mutations induced in two target genes, strongly indicating that its incorporation into host cell DNA results in the observed mutagenicity. Consistent with the demonstrated chain termination, the potential for induction of large DNA deletions is supported by the consistent finding of clastogenicity (sister chromatid exchange, micronuclei and chromosomal aberrations) in human cells *in vitro* and in rodent cells *in vivo* after exposure to both high and low, clinically relevant doses. In addition, molecular analyses of mutations in zidovudine-exposed human cells have confirmed that the mutagenic response is mainly, but not exclusively, due to the production of large deletions leading to loss of heterozygosity in autosomal cells.

The mutational spectra also suggest that zidovudine produces point mutations, either directly by some unknown mechanism or indirectly through inhibition of DNA polymerases, alterations in nucleotide pools, inhibition of DNA anabolic enzymes and/or interference with DNA repair processes. The presence of distinct activating point mutations in Ha-*ras* of zidovudine-induced mouse skin tumours suggests that multiple mechanisms, which include point mutations and clastogenic events, with concomitant loss of heterozygosity, are all likely to be involved in the process of zidovudine-induced tumour formation.

Although the phenomenon is not directly related to carcinogenesis, it is worth noting that zidovudine is also incorporated into mitochondrial DNA and inhibits mitochondrial DNA polymerases, with resultant effects on cell growth and viability. The amounts incorporated into mitochondrial DNA are similar to those in nuclear DNA, resulting in 1–10 molecules of zidovudine per mitochondrion.

5. Summary of Data Reported and Evaluation

5.1 Exposure data

Zidovudine (AZT) is a nucleoside analogue that has been used in the treatment and prevention of HIV infection in adults and children since the mid-1980s. Zidovudine is in widespread use in combination regimens with other antiretroviral agents. It is currently indicated in the treatment of HIV-positive pregnant women and to prevent mother-to-infant transmission.

5.2 Human carcinogenicity data

No difference in the incidence of non-Hodgkin lymphoma relative to that in the general population was seen before and after introduction of zidovudine therapy.

In a large case–control study from the USA of HIV-infected patients, no association was found between the incidence of non-Hodgkin lymphoma and therapeutic use of zidovudine.

A large cohort study from the USA with limited length of follow-up suggested a linear increase in the cumulative risk for non-Hodgkin lymphoma over time among adult patients with AIDS, but this was not related to treatment with zidovudine. A number of other cohort studies were available which also involved limited length of follow-up and few subjects. No data were available on the risks for types of cancers other than non-Hodgkin lymphoma.

None of the studies provided information on the risk for cancer associated with use of zidovudine for more than three years.

5.3 Animal carcinogenicity data

Zidovudine was tested for carcinogenicity in mice and rats by oral administration, in mice by intravaginal administration and in mice by transplacental and by transplacental and postnatal exposure. Zidovudine was also administered with 12-O-tetradecanoylphorbol 13-acetate (TPA) in a transplacental experiment in mice and in combination with α-interferon in mice.

Administration of zidovudine by gavage induced vaginal squamous-cell carcinomas in two studies in mice. A low incidence of vaginal tumours was observed in rats treated with the highest dose. Administration of zidovudine to mice by the intravaginal route resulted in an increased incidence of vaginal squamous-cell carcinomas. Combined administration of zidovudine with α-interferon also induced vaginal tumours in mice. Vaginal squamous-cell tumours are very rare in untreated animals.

Transplacental administration to mice resulted in an increased incidence and multiplicity of lung and liver tumours and in an increased incidence of female reproductive tract tumours in one study, whereas no increased tumour incidence was associated with treatment in another study at a lower dose. After transplacental and postnatal administration of zidovudine to mice, an increased incidence of vaginal squamous-cell carcinomas was seen. Zidovudine given transplacentally followed by postnatal topical application of TPA to mice resulted in an increased incidence and multiplicity of skin tumours (mostly papillomas).

5.4 Other relevant data

The pharmacokinetics of zidovudine in humans shows large inter- and intra-individual variation. The achievement of maximum plasma concentrations and removal from plasma of the parent compound are rapid except in patients with compromised renal function. The pharmacokinetics in nonhuman primates is virtually identical to that in humans. The absorption, distribution and elimination of zidovudine in rodents are more rapid than in humans, and its bioavailability is higher in rats and mice than in primates. Zidovudine is metabolized by three pathways: glucuronidation, which accounts for up to three-quarters of the human urinary product; mixed-function oxidase-mediated reactions, giving 3'-amino-3'-deoxythymidine, a minor urinary metabolite; and phosphorylation, which is fundamental to the antiviral activity of zidovudine but accounts for only about 1% of its total disposition. Unchanged zidovudine constitutes up to one-fifth of the human urinary products. In rats and mice, unchanged drug accounts for up to 90% of the urinary recovery, which represents about 80% of the dose; the remaining urinary products consist of five metabolites, which have been identified.

The serious adverse effects of treatment with zidovudine, reported in a small proportion of people, include haematotoxicity (anaemia, neutropenia), hepatotoxicity and cardiac and skeletal myopathy (due to mitochondrial effects). Similar toxic effects are found in treated mice.

Zidovudine crosses the placenta by bidirectional passive diffusion, and the drug and its monophosphate and monoglucuronide metabolites were observed in fetal tissue. Studies of children up to 4.2 years of age who had been exposed *in utero* and for up to six weeks after birth to zidovudine provided no evidence for an increased incidence of structural developmental abnormalities or cognitive or immune dysfunction. Studies in mice, rats and rabbits given zidovudine transplacentally showed no increase in the frequency of malformations, but some studies showed increased numbers of fetal resorptions and decreased fetal weights after oral administration of zidovudine at doses of 200–500 mg/kg bw per day during gestation. Studies in monkeys and rats indicated that the behavioural alterations in offspring exposed to zidovudine *in utero* were generally reversible.

Zidovudine is incorporated into nuclear and mitochondrial DNA in mammalian cells in culture, in experimental animals and in humans. It appears to cause mutations primarily by inducing large deletions, consistent with its action as a DNA chain terminator. It produces clastogenic effects in cultured human cells and in mice exposed to either high or clinically relevant concentrations. Analyses of mutations induced in human cells in culture and in skin tumours from transplacentally treated mice showed that exposure to zidovudine also causes point mutations.

5.5 Evaluation

There is *inadequate evidence* in humans for the carcinogenicity of zidovudine.

There is *sufficient evidence* in experimental animals for the carcinogenicity of zidovudine.

Overall evaluation

Zidovudine is *possibly carcinogenic to humans (Group 2B)*.

6. References

Acosta, B.S. & Grimsley, E.W. (1999) Zidovudine-associated type B lactic acidosis and hepatic steatosis in an HIV-infected patient. *South. med. J.*, **92**, 421–423

Acosta, E.P., Page, L.M. & Fletcher, C.V. (1996) Clinical pharmacokinetics of zidovudine. An update. *Clin. Pharmacokinet.*, **30**, 251–262

Agarwal, R.P. & Olivero, O.A. (1997) Genotoxicity and mitochondrial damage in human lymphocytic cells chronically exposed to 3'-azido-2',3'-dideoxythymidine. *Mutat. Res.*, **390**, 223–231

American Hospital Formulary Service (1997) *AHFS Drug Information® 97*, Bethesda, MD, American Society of Health-System Pharmacists, pp. 538–557

Applewhite-Black L.E., Dow-Edwards, D.L. & Minkoff, H.L. (1998) Neurobehavioral and pregnancy effects of prenatal zidovudine exposure in Sprague-Dawley rats: Preliminary findings. *Neurotoxicol. Teratol.*, **20**, 251–258

Avramis, V.I., Markson, W., Jackson, R.L. & Gomperts, E. (1989) Biochemical pharmacology of zidovudine in human T-lymphoblastoid cells (CEM). *AIDS*, **3**, 417–422

Ayers, K.M., Clive, D., Tucker, W.E., Hajian, G. & de Miranda, P. (1996a) Nonclinical toxicology studies with zidovudine: Genetic toxicity tests and carcinogenicity bioassays in mice and rats. *Fundam. appl. Toxicol.*, **32**, 148–158

Ayers, K.M., Tucker, W.E., Jr, Hajian, G. & de Miranda, P. (1996b) Nonclinical toxicology studies with zidovudine: Acute, subacute, and chronic toxicity in rodents, dogs, and monkeys. *Fundam. appl. Toxicol.*, **32**, 129–139

Ayers, K.M., Torrey, C.E. & Reynolds, D.J. (1997) A transplacental carcinogenicity bioassay in CD-1 mice with zidovudine. *Fundam. appl. Toxicol.*, **38**, 195–198

Bacellar, H., Munoz, A., Miller, E.N., Cohen, B.A., Besley, D., Selnes, O.A., Becker, J.T. & McArthur, J.C. (1994) Temporal trends in the incidence of HIV-1-related neurologic diseases: Multicenter AIDS cohort study, 1985–1992. *Neurology*, **44**, 1892–1900

Baldeweg, T., Riccio, M., Gruzelier, J., Hawkins, D., Burgess, A., Irving, G., Stygall, J., Catt, S. & Catalan, J. (1995) Neurophysiological evaluation of zidovudine in asymptomatic HIV-1 infection: A longitudinal placebo-controlled study. *J. neurol. Sci.*, **132**, 162–169

Barbaro, G., Di Lorenzo, G., Grisorio, B. & Barbarini, G. (1998) Incidence of dilated cardiomyopathy and detection of HIV in myocardial cells of HIV-positive patients. *New Engl. J. Med.*, **339**, 1093–1099

Barry, M., Mulcahy, F., Merry, C., Gibbons, S. & Back, D. (1999) Pharmacokinetics and potential interactions amongst antiretroviral agents used to treat patients with HIV infection. *Clin. Pharmacokinet.*, **36**, 289–304

Blanche, S., Tardieu, M., Rustin, P., Slama, A., Barrett, B., Firtion, G., Ciraru-Vigneron, N., Lacroix, C., Rouzioux, C., Mandelbrot, L., Desguerre, I., Rötig, A., Mayaux, M.-J. & Delfraissy, J.-F. (1999) Persistent mitochondrial dysfunction and perinatal exposure to antiretroviral nucleoside analogues. *Lancet*, **354**, 1084–1089

Boal, J.H., Plessinger, M.A., van den Reydt, C. & Miller, R.K. (1997) Pharmacokinetic and toxicity studies of AZT (zidovudine) following perfusion of human term placenta for 14 hours. *Toxicol. appl. Pharmacol.*, **143**, 13–21

Bogliolo, G., Lerza, R., Mencoboni, M., Flego, G., Gasparini, L. & Pannacciulli, I. (1991) Hematoxic effects on mice of combined administration of azidothymidine and acyclovir. *Exp. Hematol.*, **19**, 838–841

Boudinot, F.D., Schinazi, R.F., Gallo, J.M., McClure, H.M., Anderson, D.C., Doshi, K.J., Kambhampathi, P.C. & Chu, C.K. (1990) 3'-Azido-2',3'-dideoxyuridine (AzddU): Comparative pharmacokinetics with 3'-azido-3'-deoxythymidine (AZT) in monkeys. *AIDS Res. hum. Retroviruses*, **6**, 219–228

British Medical Association/Royal Pharmaceutical Society of Great Britain (1998) *British National Formulary*, No. 36, London, pp. 278–279

British Pharmacopoeia Commission (1996) *British Pharmacopoeia 1993, Addendum 1996*, London, Her Majesty's Stationery Office, pp. 1846–1847

Budavari, S., ed. (1996) *The Merck Index*, 12th Ed., Whitehouse Station, NJ, Merck & Co., p. 1732

Busidan, Y. & Dow-Edwards, D.L. (1999a) Neurobehavioral effects of perinatal AZT exposure in Sprague-Dawley weanling rats. *Pharmacol. Biochem. Behav.*, **354**, 1–7

Busidan, Y. & Dow-Edwards, D.L. (1999b) Neurobehavioral effects of perinatal AZT exposure in Sprague-Dawley adult rats. *Neurotoxicol. Teratol.*, **21**, 359–363

Calamandrei, G., Venerosi, A., Branchi, I., Chiarotti, F., Verdina, A., Bucci, F. & Alleva, E. (1999) Effects of prenatal AZT on mouse neurobehavioral development and passive avoidance learning. *Neurotoxicol. Teratol.*, **21**, 29–40

Canadian Pharmaceutical Association (1997) *CPS Compendium of Pharmaceuticals and Specialties*, 32nd Ed., Ottawa, pp. 115, 1074–1076, 1357–1361

Centers for Disease Control and Prevention (1998a) Public health service task force recommendations for the use of antiretroviral drugs in pregnant women infected with HIV-1 for maternal health and for reducing perinatal HIV-1 transmission in the United States. *Morb. Mortal. wkly Rep.*, **47**, 1–26

Centers for Disease Control and Prevention (1998b) Public health service guidelines for the management of health-care worker exposures to HIV and recommendations for postexposure prophylaxis. *Morb. Mortal. wkly Rep.*, **47**, 1–28

Chariot, P., Drogou, I., de Lacroix-Szmania, I., Eliezer-Vanerot, M.-C., Chazaud, B., Lombès, A., Schaeffer, A. & Zafrani, E.S. (1999) Zidovudine-induced mitochondrial disorder with massive liver steatosis, myopathy, lactic acidosis, and mitochondrial DNA depletion. *J. Hepatol.*, **30**, 156–160

Chavanet, P., Diquet, B., Waldner, A. & Portier, H. (1989) Prenatal pharmacokinetics of zidovudine. *New Engl. J. Med.*, **321**, 1548–1549

Chow, H.-H., Li, P., Brookshier, G. & Tang, Y. (1997) *In vivo* tissue disposition of 3′-azido-3′-deoxythymidine and its anabolites in control and retrovirus-infected mice. *Drug Metab. Dispos.*, **25**, 412–422

Chow, H.-H., Brookshier, G. & Li, P. (1998) Tissue disposition of zidovudine and its phosphorylated metabolites in zidovudine-treated healthy and retrovirus infected mice. *Pharm. Res.*, **15**, 139–144

Chu, C.K., Beach, J.W., Ullas, G.V. & Kosugi, Y. (1988) An efficient total synthesis of 3′-azido-3′-deoxythymidine (AZT) and 3′-azido-2′,3′-dideoxyuridine (AZDDU, CS-87) from D-mannitol. *Tetrahedron Lett.*, **29**, 5349–5352

CIS Information Services (1998) *Worldwide Bulk Drug Users Directory 1997/98 Edition*, Dallas, TX [CD-ROM]

Concorde Coordinating Committee (1994) Concorde: MRC/ANRS randomised double-blind controlled trial of immediate and deferred zidovudine in symptom-free HIV infection. *Lancet*, **343**, 871–881

Connor, E.M., Sperling, R.S., Gelber, R., Kiselev, P., Scott, G., O'Sullivan, M.J., VanDyke, R., Bey, M., Shearer, W., Jacobson, R.L., Jimenez, E., O'Neill, E., Bazin, B., Delfraissy, J.-F., Culnane, M., Coombs, R., Elkins, M., Moye, J., Stratton, P. & Basley, J. for the Pediatric AIDS Clinical Trials Group Protocol 076 Study Group (1994) Reduction of maternal–infant transmission of human immunodeficiency virus type I with zidovudine treatment. *New Engl. J. Med.*, **331**, 1173–1180

Coté, T.R. & Biggar, R.J. (1995) Does zidovudine cause non-Hodgkin's lymphoma? *AIDS*, **9**, 404–405

Council of Europe (1997) *European Pharmacopoeia*, 3rd Ed., Strasbourg, pp. 1739–1740

Cretton, E.M., Schinazi, R.F., McClure, H.M., Anderson, D.C. & Sommadossi, J.-P. (1991) Pharmacokinetics of 3'-azido-3'-deoxythymidine and its catabolites and interactions with probenecid in rhesus monkeys. *Antimicrob. Agents Chemother.*, **35**, 801–807

Cronkite, E.P. & Bullis, J. (1990) In vivo toxicity of 3'-azido-3'-deoxythymidine (AZT) on CBA/Ca mice. *Int. J. Cell Cloning*, **8**, 332–345

Culnane, M., Fowler, M., Lee, S.S., McSherry, G., Brady, M., O'Donnell, K., Mofenson, L., Gortmaker, S.L., Shapiro, D.E., Scott, G., Jimenez, E., Moore E.C., Diaz, C., Flynn, P.M., Cunningham, B. & Oleske, J. for the Pediatric AIDS Clinical Trials Group Protocol 219/076 Teams (1999) Lack of long-term effects of in utero exposure to zidovudine among uninfected children born to HIV-infected women. *J. Am. med. Assoc.*, **281**, 151–157

Cupler, E.J., Danon, M.J., Jay, C., Hench, K., Ropka, M. & Dalakas, M.C. (1995) Early features of zidovudine-associated myopathy: Histopathological findings and clinical correlations. *Acta neuropathol.*, **90**, 1–6

Dabis, F., Msellati, P., Meda, N., Welffens-Ekra, C., You, B., Manigart, O., Leroy, V., Simonon, A., Cartoux, M., Combe, P., Ouangré, A., Ramon, R., Ky-Zerbo, O., Montcho, C., Salamon, R., Rouzioux, C., Van de Perre, P. & Mande, L. for the DIATRAME Study Group (1999) 6-Month efficacy, tolerance, and acceptability of a short regimen of oral zidovudine to reduce vertical transmission of HIV in breastfed children in Côte d'Ivoire and Burkina Faso: A double-blind placebo-controlled multicentre trial. *Lancet*, **353**, 786–792

Dalakas, M.C., Leon-Monzon, M.E., Bernardini, I., Gahl, W.A. & Jay, C.A. (1994) Zidovudine-induced mitochondrial myopathy is associated with muscle carnitine deficiency and lipid storage. *Ann. Neurol.*, **35**, 482–487

Darnowski, J.W. & Goulette, F.A. (1994) 3'Azido-3'-deoxythymidine cytotoxicity and metabolism in the human colon tumor cell line HCT-8. *Biochem. Pharmacol.*, **48**, 1797–1805

Delta Coordinating Committee (1996) Delta: A randomised double-blind controlled trial comparing combinations of zidovudine plus didanosine or zalcitabine with zidovudine alone in HIV-infected individuals. *Lancet*, **348**, 283–291

Dertinger, S.D., Torous, D.K. & Tometsko, K.R. (1996) Induction of micronuclei by low doses of azidothymidine (AZT). *Mutat. Res.*, **368**, 301–307

Du, D.-L., Volpe, D.A., Grieshaber, C.K. & Murphy, M.J., Jr (1992) *In vitro* toxicity of 3'-azido-3'-deoxythymidine, carbovir and 2',3'-didehydro-2',3'-dideoxythymidine to human and murine haematopoietic progenitor cells. *Br. J. Haematol.*, **80**, 437–445

Dudley, M.N. (1995) Clinical pharmacokinetics of nucleoside antiretroviral agents. *J. infect. Dis.*, **171**, S99–S112

Editions du Vidal (1998) *Dictionnaire Vidal 1998*, 74th Ed., Paris, OVP, pp. 1566–1573

Fischl, M.A., Richman, D.D., Hansen, N., Collier, A.C., Carey, J.T., Para, M.F., Hardy, D., Dolin, R., Powderly, W.G., Allan, J.D., Wong, B., Merigan, T.C., McAuliffe, V.J., Hyslop, N.E., Rhame, F.S., Balfour, H.H., Jr, Spector, S.A., Volberding, P., Pettinelli, C., Andersen, J. & the AIDS Clinial Trials Group (1990) The safety and efficacy of zidovudine (AZT) in the treatment of subjects with mildly symptomatic human immunodeficiency virus type 1 (HIV) infection. *Ann. intern. Med.*, **112**, 727–737

Forseter, G., Joline, C. & Wormser, G.P. (1994) Tolerability, safety, and acceptability of zidovudine prophylaxis in health care workers. *Arch. intern. Med.*, **154**, 2745–2749

Freiman, J.P., Helfert, K.E., Hamrell, M.R. & Stein, D.S. (1993) Hepatomegaly with severe steatosis in HIV-seropositive patients. *AIDS*, **7**, 379–385

Gail, M.H., Rosenberg, P.S. & Goedert, J.J. (1990) Therapy may explain recent deficits in AIDS incidence. *J. acquir. Immune Defic. Syndr.*, **3**, 296–306

Gallicano, K., Sahai, J., Ormsby, E., Cameron, D.W., Pakuts, A. & McGilveray, I. (1993) Pharmacokinetics of zidovudine after the initial single dose and during chronic-dose therapy in HIV-infected patients. *Br. J. clin. Pharmacol.*, **36**, 128–131

Garcia, P.M., Kalish, L.A., Pitt, J., Minkoff, H., Quinn, T.C., Burchett, S.K., Kornegay, J., Jackson, B., Moye, J., Hanson, C., Zorrilla, C. & Lew, J.F. (1999) Maternal levels of plasma human immunodeficiency virus type 1 RNA and the risk of perinatal transmission. *New Engl. J. Med.*, **341**, 394–402

Garland, M., Szeto, H.H., Daniel, S.S., Tropper, P.J., Myers, M.M. & Stark, R.I. (1996) Zidovudine kinetics in the pregnant baboon. *J. acquir. immune Defic. Syndr. hum. Retrovirol.*, **11**, 117–127

Garland, M. Szeto, H.H., Daniel, S.S., Tropper, P.J., Myers, M.M. & Stark, R.I. (1998) Placental transfer and fetal metabolism of zidovudine in the baboon. *Pediatr. Res.*, **44**, 47–53

Gennaro, A.R. (1995) *Remington: The Science and Practice of Pharmacy*, 19th Ed., Easton, PA, Mack Publishing, Vol. II, p. 1336

Gill, P.S., Rarick, M., Brynes, R.K., Causey, D., Loureiro, C. & Levine, A.M. (1987) Azidothymidine associated with bone marrow failure in the acquired immunodeficiency syndrome (AIDS). *Ann. intern. Med.*, **107**, 502–505

Glinski, R.P., Khan, M.S. & Kalamas, R.L. (1973) Nucleotide synthesis. IV. Phosphorylated 3'-amino-3'-deoxythymidine and 5'-amino-5'-deoxythymidine and derivatives. *J. org. Chem.*, **38**, 4299–4305

Gogu, S.R., Beckman, B.S. & Agrawal, K.C. (1992) Amelioration of zidovudine-induced fetal toxicity in pregnant mice. *Antimicrob. Agents Chemother.*, **36**, 2370–2374

Gomez, D.E., Kassim, A. & Olivero, O.A. (1995) Preferential incorporation of 3'-azido-2',3'-dideoxythymidine (AZT) in telomeric sequences of CHO cells. *Int. J. Oncol.*, **7**, 1057–1060

Gomez, D.E., Tejera, A.M. & Olivero, O.A. (1998) Irreversible telomere shortening by 3'-azido-2',3'-dideoxythymidine (AZT) treatment. *Biochem. biophys. Res. Commun.*, **246**, 107–110

González Cid, M. & Larripa, I. (1994) Genotoxic activity of azidothymidine (AZT) in in vitro systems. *Mutat. Res.*, **321**, 113–118

Good, S.S., Koble, C.S., Crouch, R., Johnson, R.L., Rideout, J.L. & de Miranda, P. (1990) Isolation and characterization of an ether glucuronide of zidovudine, a major metabolite in monkeys and humans. *Drug Metab. Dispos.*, **18**, 321–326

Graham, N.M.H., Zeger, S.L., Park, L.P., Vermund, S.H., Detels, R., Rinaldo, C.R. & Phair, J.P. (1992) The effects on survival of early treatment of human immunodeficiency virus infection. *New Engl. J. Med.*, **326**, 1037–1042

Grdina, D.J., Dale, P. & Weichselbaum, R. (1992) Protection against AZT-induced mutagenesis at the HGPRT locus in a human cell line by WR-151326. *Int. J. Radiat. Oncol. Biol. Phys.*, **22**, 813–815

Greene, J.A., Ayers, K.M., de Miranda, P. & Tucker, W.E., Jr (1990) Postnatal survival in Wistar rats following oral dosage with zidovudine on gestation day 10. *Fundam. appl. Toxicol.*, **15**, 201–206

Greene, J.A., Ayers, K.M., Tucker, W.E., Jr & de Miranda, P. (1996) Nonclinical toxicology studies with zidovudine: Reproductive toxicity studies in rats and rabbits. *Fundam. appl. Toxicol.*, **32**, 140–147

Ha, J.C., Nosbisch, C., Conrad, S.H., Ruppenthal, G.C., Sackett, G.P., Abkowitz, J. & Unadkat, J.D. (1994) Fetal toxicity of zidovudine (azidothymidine) in *Macaca nemestrina*: Preliminary observations. *J. acquir. Immune Defic. Syndr.*, **7**, 154–157

Ha, J.C., Botisch, C., Abokowitz, J.L., Conrad, S.H., Mottet, N.K., Ruppenthal, G.C., Robinette, R,. Sackett, G.P. & Unadkat, J.D. (1998) Fetal, infant, and maternal toxicity of zidovudine (azidothymidine) administered throughout pregnancy in *Macaca nemestrina*. *J. acquir. Immune Defic. Syndr. hum. Retrovirol.*, **7**, 154–157

Hammer, S.M., Squires, K.E., Hughes, M.D., Grimes, J.M., Demeter, L.M., Currier, J.S., Eron, J.J., Jr, Feinberg, J.E., Balfour, H.H., Jr, Deyton, L.R., Chodakewitz, J.A. & Fischl, M.A. (1997) A controlled trial of two nucleoside analogues plus indinavir in persons with human immunodeficiency virus infection and CD4 cell counts of 200 per cubic millimeter or less. *New Engl. J. Med.*, **337**, 725–733

Hanson, I.C., Antonelli, T.A., Sperfling, R.S., Oleske, J.M., Cooper, E., Culnane, M., Fowler, M.G., Kalish, L.A., Lee, S.S., McSherry, G., Mofenson, L. & Shapiro, D.E. (1999) Lack of tumors in infants with perinatal HIV-1 exposure and fetal/neonatal exposure to zidovudine. *J. acquir. Immune Defic. Syndr. hum. Retrovirol.*, **20**, 463–467

Haschek, W.M., Weigel, R.M., Scherba, G., DeVera, M.C., Feinmehl, R., Solter, P., Tompkins, M.B. & Tompkins, W.A.E. (1990) Zidovudine toxicity to cats infected with feline leukemia virus. *Fundam. appl. Toxicol.*, **14**, 764–775

Henry, K., Erice, A., Tierney, C., Balfour, H.H., Jr, Fischl, M.A., Kmack, A., Liou, S.H., Kenton, A., Hirsch, M.S., Phair, J., Martinez, A. & Kahn, J.O. (1998) A randomized, controlled, double-blind study comparing the survival benefit of four different reverse transcriptase inhibitor therapies (three-drug, two-drug, and alternating drug) for the treatment of advanced AIDS. AIDS Clinical Trial Group 193A Study Team. *J. acquir. Immune Defic. Syndr. hum. Retrovirol.*, **19**, 339–349

Hirschel, B., Glauser, M., Chave, J.P. & Taüber, M. (1988) Zidovudine for the treatment of thrombocytopenia associated with human immunodeficiency virus (HIV). A prospective study. *Ann. intern. Med.*, **109**, 718–721

Hoetelmans, R.M.W., Burger, D.M., Meenhorst, P.L. & Beijnen, J.H. (1996) Pharmacokinetic individualisation of zidovudine therapy. Current state of pharmacokinetic–pharmacodynamic relationships. *Clin. Pharmacokinet.*, **30**, 314–327

Hoetelmans, R.M.W., Kraaijeveld, C.L., Meenhorst, P.L., Mulder, J.W., Burger, D.M., Koks, C.H.W. & Beijnen, J.H. (1997) Penetration of 3'-amino-3-deoxythymidine, a cytotoxic metabolite of zidovudine, into the cerebrospinal fluid of HIV-1-infected patients. *J. acquir. Immune Defic. Syndr. hum. Retrovirol.*, **15**, 131–136

Husson, R.N., Mueller, B.U., Farley, M., Woods, L., Kovacs, A., Goldsmith, J.C., Ono, J., Lewis, L.L., Balis, F.M., Brouwers, P., Avramis, V.I., Church, J.A., Butler, K.M., Rasheed, S., Jarosinski, P., Venzon, D. & Pizzo, P.A. (1994) Zidovudine and didanosine combination therapy in children with human immunodeficiency virus infection. *Pediatrics*, **93**, 316–322

Inoue, T., Cronkite, E.P., Hirabayashi, Y., Bullis, J.E., Jr, Mitsui, H. & Umemura, T. (1997) Lifetime treatment of mice with azidothymidine (AZT) produces myelodysplasia. *Leukemia*, **3**, 123–127

Ippolito, G., Puro, V. & the Italian Registry of Antiretroviral Prophylaxis (1997) Zidovudine toxicity in uninfected healthcare workers. *Am. J. Med.*, **102**, 58–62

Jacobson, M.A., Gundacker, H., Hughes, M., Fischl, M. & Volberding, P. (1996) Zidovudine side effects as reported by black, Hispanic, and white/non-Hispanic patients with early HIV disease: Combined analysis of two multicenter placebo-controlled trials. *J. acquir. Immune Defic. Syndr. hum. Retrovirol.*, **11**, 45–52

Kamali, F. (1993) Clinical pharmacology of zidovudine and other 2′,3′-dideoxynucleoside analogues. *Clin. Invest.*, **71**, 392–405

Katz, M.H. & Gerberding, J.L. (1997) Postexposure treatment of people exposed to the human immunodeficiency virus through sexual contact or injection-drug use. *New Engl. J. Med.*, **336**, 1097–1100

Klug, S., Lewandowski, C., Merker, H.-J., Stahlmann, R., Wildi, L. & Neubert, D. (1991) In vitro and in vivo studies on the prenatal toxicity of five virustatic nucleoside analogues in comparison to aciclovir. *Arch. Toxicol.*, **65**, 283–291

Kumar, R.M., Hughes, P.F. & Khurranna, A. (1994) Zidovudine use in pregnancy: A report on 104 cases and the occurrence of birth defects. *J. acquir. Immune Defic. Syndr.*, **7**, 1034–1039

Lamperth, L., Dalakas, M.C., Dagani, F., Anderson, J. & Ferrari, R. (1991) Abnormal skeletal and cardiac muscle mitochondria induced by zidovudine in human muscle *in vitro* and in an animal model. *Lab. Invest.*, **65**, 742–751

Larder, B.A. & Kemp, S.D. (1989) Multiple mutations in HIV-1 reverse transcriptase confer high-level resistance to zidovudine (AZT). *Science*, **246**, 1155–1158

Larder, B.A., Darby, G. & Richman, D.D. (1989) HIV with reduced sensitivity to zidovudine (AZT) isolated during prolonged therapy. *Science*, **243**, 1731–1734

Levine, A.M., Bernstein, L., Sullivan-Halley, J., Shibata, D., Bauch Mahterian, S. & Nathwani, B.N. (1995) Role of zidovudine antiretroviral therapy in the pathogenesis of acquired immunodeficiency syndrome-related lymphoma. *Blood*, **86**, 4612–4616

Lewis, W. (1998) Mitochondrial toxicity of antiretroviral nucleosides used in AIDS: Insights derived from toxic changes observed in tissues rich in mitochondria. In: Lipshultz, S.E., ed., *Cardiology in AIDS*, New York, Chapman & Hall, pp. 317–329

LINFO Läkemedelsinformation AB (1998) *FASS 1998 Läkemedel i Sverige*, Stockholm, pp. 1019–1021

Lopez-Anaya, A., Unadkat, J.D., Schumann, L.A. & Smith, A.L. (1990) Pharmacokinetics of zidovudine (azidothymidine). I. Transplacental transfer. *J. acquir. Immune Defic. Syndr.*, **3**, 959–964

Lorenzi, P., Spicher, V.M., Laubereau, B., Hirchel, B., Kind, C., Rudin, C., Irion, O., Kaiser, L., the Swiss HIV Cohort Study, the Swiss Collaborative HIV and Pregnancy Study, & the Swiss Neonatal HIV Study (1998) Antiretroviral therapies in pregnancy: Maternal, fetal and neonatal effects. *AIDS*, **12**, 241–247

Mamber, S.W., Brookshire, K.W. & Forenza, S. (1990) Induction of the SOS response in *Escherichia coli* by azidothymidine and dideoxynucleotides. *Antimicrob. Agents Chemother.*, **34**, 1237–1243

Manouilov, K.K., White, C.A., Boudinot, F.D., Fedorov, I.I. & Chu, C.K. (1995) Lymphatic distribution of 3′-azido-3′-deoxythymidine and 3′-azido-2′,3′-dideoxyuridine in mice. *Drug Metab. Dispos.*, **23**, 655–658

Masini, A., Scotti, C., Calligaro, A., Cazzalini, O., Stivala, L.A., Bianchi, L., Giovannini, F., Ceccarelli, D., Muscatello, U., Tomasi, A. & Vannini, V. (1999) Zidovudine-induced experimental myopathy: Dual mechanism of mitochondrial damage. *J. neurol. Sci.*, **166**, 131–140

Mathé, G., Pontiggia, P., Orbach-Arbouys, S., Triana, K., Ambetima, N., Morette, C., Hallard, M. & Blanquet, D. (1996) AIDS therapy with two, three or four agent combinations, applied in short sequences, differing from each other by drug rotation. I. First of two parts: a phase I trial equivalent, concerning five virostatics: AZT, ddI, ddC, acriflavine and an ellipticine analogue. *Biomed. Pharmacother.*, **50**, 220–227

McCurdy, D.T., III & Kennedy, J.M. (1996) Skeletal muscle mitochondria from AZT-treated rats have a diminished response to chronic electrical stimulation. *J. appl. Physiol.*, **81**, 326–334

McKallip, R.J., Nagarkatti, M. & Nagarkatti, P.S. (1995) Immunotoxicity of AZT: Inhibitory effect on thymocyte differentiation and peripheral T cell responsiveness to gp120 of human immunodeficiency virus. *Toxicol. appl. Pharmacol.*, **131**, 53–62

Meng, Q., Su, T., Olivero, O.A., Poirier, M.C., Shi, X., Ding, X. & Walker, V.E. (2000a) Relationships between DNA incorporation, mutant frequency, and loss of heterozygosity at the *TK* locus in human lymphoblastoid cells exposed to 3′-azido-3′-deoxythymidine. *Toxicol. Sci.*, **54**, 322–329

Meng, Q., Olivero, O.A., Shi, X., Walker, D.W., Antiochos, B., Poirier, M.C. & Walker, V.E. (2000b) Enhanced DNA incorporation of AZT and synergistic effects of AZT and DDI in inducing *HPRT* and *TK* mutations in human cells (abstract). *Environ. mol. Mutag.*, **35** (Suppl. 31), 43

Mentré, F., Escolano, S., Diquet, B., Golmard, J.-L. & Mallet, A. (1993) Clinical pharmacokinetics of zidovudine: Inter and intraindividual variability and relationship to long term efficacy and toxicity. *Eur. J. clin. Pharmacol.*, **45**, 397–407

Mhiri, C., Baudrimont, M., Bonne, G., Geny, C., Degoul, F., Marsac, C., Roullet, E. & Gherardi, R. (1991) Zidovudine myopathy: A distinctive disorder associated with mitochondrial function. *Ann. Neurol.*, **29**, 606–614

de Miranda, P., Burnette, T.C. & Good, S.S. (1990) Tissue distribution and metabolic disposition of zidovudine in rats. *Drug Metab. Dispos.*, **18**, 315–320

Mofenson, L.M., Lambert, J.S., Stiehm, E.R., Bethel, J., Meyer, W.A., III, Whitehouse, J., Moye, J., Jr, Reichelderfer, P., Harris, D.R., Fowler, M.G., Mathieson, B.J. & Nemo, G.J. for the Pediatric AIDS Clinical Trials Group Study 185 Team (1999) Risk factors for perinatal transmission of human immunodeficiency virus type 1 in women treated with zidovudine. *New Engl. J. Med.*, **341**, 385–393

Montaner, J.S., Reiss, P., Cooper, D., Vella, S., Harris, M., Conway, B., Wainberg, M.A., Smith, D., Robinson, P., Hall, D., Myers, M. & Lange, J.M. (1998) A randomized, double-blind trial comparing combinations of nevirapine, didanosine, and zidovudine for HIV-infected patients: The INCAS Trial. Italy, The Netherlands, Canada and Australia Study. *J. Am. med. Assoc.*, **279**, 930–937

Moore, R.D., Kessler, H., Richman, D.D., Flexner, C. & Chaisson, R.E. (1991a) Non-Hodgkin's lymphoma in patients with advanced HIV infection treated with zidovudine. *J. Am. med. Assoc.*, **265**, 2208–2211

Moore, R.D., Creagh-Kirk, T., Keruly, J., Link, G., Wang, M.-C., Richman, D., Chaisson, R.E. & Zidovudine Epidemiology Study Group (1991b) Long-term safety and efficacy of zidovudine in patients with advanced human immunodeficiency virus disease. *Arch. intern. Med.*, **151**, 981–986

Moore, R.D., Fortgang, I., Keruly, J. & Chaisson, R.E. (1996) Adverse events from drug therapy for human immunodeficiency virus disease. *Am. J. Med.*, **101**, 34–40

Morse, G.D., Shelton, M.J. & O'Donnell, A.M. (1993) Comparative pharmacokinetics of antiviral nucleoside analogues. *Clin. Pharmacokinet.*, **24**, 101–123

Motimaya, A.M., Subramanya, K.S., Curry, P.T. & Kitchin, R.M. (1994a) Evaluation of the genotoxic potential of selected anti-AIDS treatment drugs at clinical doses in vivo in mice. *Toxicol. Lett.*, **70**, 171–183

Motimaya, A.M., Subramanya, K.S., Curry, P.T. & Kitchin, R.M. (1994b) Lack of induction of micronuclei by azidothymidine (AZT) in vivo in mouse bone marrow cells. *Environ. mol. Mutag.*, **23**, 74–76

Muñoz, A., Schrager, L.K., Bacellar, H., Speizer, I., Vermund, S.H., Detels, R., Saah, A.J., Kingsley, L.A., Seminara, D. & Phair, J.P. (1993) Trends in the incidence of outcomes defining acquired immunodeficiency (AIDS) in the multicenter AIDS cohort study: 1985–1991. *Am. J. Epidemiol.*, **137**, 423–438

National Cancer Institute (1989) *Infrared, Ultraviolet, ^{1}H-Nuclear Magnetic Resonance and Mass Spectrum of AZT* (NSC#602, 670, Lot No. AJ-A1.0 and AJ-A1-1), Bethesda, MD, National Institutes of Health

National Institute of Environmental Health Sciences (1998) *NIEHS Technical Report on the Reproductive, Developmental, and General Toxicity Study of 3'-Azido-3'-deoxythymidine (AZT), Trimethoprim (TMP/Sulfamethoxazole (SMX), and Folinic Acid Combinations Administered by Gavage to Swiss (CD-1®) Mice* (NIEHS AIDS Therapeutics Toxicity Report No. 2; NIH Publ. No. 99-3940), Research Triangle Park, NC

National Institute of Environmental Health Sciences (1999) *NIEHS Technical Report on the Reproductive, Developmental, and General Toxicity Study of 3'-Azido-3'-deoxythymidine (AZT) and Isoniazid Combinations (CAS Nos. 30516-87-1 and 54-85-3) Administered by Gavage to Swiss (CD-1®) Mice* (NIEHS AIDS Therapeutics Toxicity Report No. 3; NIH Publ. No. 99-3941), Research Triangle Park, NC

National Toxicology Program (1999) *Toxicology and Carcinogenesis Studies of AZT (CAS No. 30516-87-1) and AZT/α-Interferon A/D in B6C3F$_1$ Mice (Gavage Studies)* (NTP TR 469; NIH Publication No. 99-3959), Research Triangle Park, NC

Olano, J.P., Borucki, M.J., Wen, J.W. & Haque, A.K. (1995) Massive hepatic steatosis and lactic acidosis in a patient with AIDS who was receiving zidovudine. *Clin. infect. Dis.*, **21**, 973–976

Oleson, F.B. & Getman, S.M. (1990) Multiple-dose erythrocyte micronucleus assays in mice and rats with azidothymidine (AZT) (Abstract). *Environ. mol. Mutag.*, **15** (Suppl. 17), 46

Olivero, O.A. & Poirier, M.C. (1993) Preferential incorporation of 3'-azido-2',3'-dideoxythymidine into telomeric DNA and Z-DNA-containing regions of Chinese hamster ovary cells. *Mol. Carcinog.*, **8**, 81–88

Olivero, O., Beland, F.A., Fullerton, N.F. & Poirier, M.C. (1994a) Vaginal epithelial DNA damage and expression of preneoplastic markers in mice during chronic dosing with tumorigenic levels of 3'-azido-2',3'-dideoxythymidine. *Cancer Res.*, **54**, 6235–6242

Olivero, O., Beland, F.A. & Poirier, M.C. (1994b) Immunofluorescent localization and quantitation of 3'-azido-2',3'-dideoxythymidine (AZT) incorporated into chromosomal DNA of human, hamster and mouse cell lines. *Int. J. Oncol.*, **4**, 49–54

Olivero, O.A., Anderson, L.M., Diwan, B.A., Haines, D.C., Harbaugh, S.W., Moskal, T.J., Jones, A.B., Rice, J.M., Riggs, C.W., Logsdon, D., Yuspa, S.H. & Poirier, M.C. (1997) Transplacental effects of 3'-azido-2',3'-dideoxythymidine (AZT): Tumorigenicity in mice and genotoxicity in mice and monkeys. *J. natl Cancer Inst.*, **89**, 1602–1608

Olivero, O.A., Shearer, G.M., Chougnet, C.A., Kovacs, A.A.S., Landay, A.L., Baker, R., Stek, A.M., Khoury, M.M., Proia, L.A., Kessler, H.A., Sha, B.E., Tarone, R.E. & Poirier, M.C. (1999) Incorporation of zidovudine into leukocyte DNA of HIV-1-positive adults and pregnant women, and cord blood from infants exposed *in utero*. *AIDS*, **13**, 919–925

Omar, R.F., Gourde, P., Desormeaux, A., Tremblay, M., Beauchamp, D. & Bergeron, M.G. (1996) In vivo toxicity of foscarnet and zidovudine given alone or in combination. *Toxicol. appl. Pharmacol.*, **139**, 324–332

O'Sullivan, M.J,. Boyer, P.J., Scott, G.B., Parks, W.P., Weller, S., Blum, M.R., Balsley, J. & Bryson, Y.J. for the Zidovudine Collaborative Working Group (1993) The pharmacokinetics and safety of zidovudine in the third trimester of pregnancy for women infected with human immunodeficiency virus and their infants: Phase I acquired immunodeficiency syndrome clinical trials group study (protocol 0820). *Am. J. Obstet. Gynecol.*, **168**, 1510–1516

Parra, I., Flores, C., Adrian, D. & Windle, B. (1997) AZT induces high frequency, rapid amplification of centromeric DNA. *Cytogenet. Cell Genet.*, **76**, 128–133

Patterson, T.A., Binienda, Z.K., Lipe, G.W., Gillam, M.P., Slikker, W., Jr & Sandberg, J.A. (1997) Transplacental pharmacokinetics and fetal distribution of azidothyidine, its glucuronide, and phosphorylated metabolites and late-term rhesus macaqeues after maternal infusion. *Drug. Metab. Dispos.*, **25**, 453–459

Peter, K. & Gambertoglio, J.G. (1996) Zidovudine phosphorylation after short-term and long-term therapy with zidovudine in patients infected with the human immunodeficiency virus. *Clin. Pharmacol. Ther.*, **60**, 168–176

Peter, K. & Gambertoglio, J.G. (1998) Intracellular phosphorylation of zidovudine (ZDV) and other nucleoside reverse transcriptase inhibitors (RTI) used for human immunodeficiency virus (HIV) infection. *Pharm. Res.*, **15**, 819–825

Peters, B.S., Winer, J., Landon, D.N., Stotter, A. & Pinching, A.J. (1993) Mitochondrial myopathy associated with chronic zidovudine therapy in AIDS. *Q. J. Med.*, **86**, 5–15

Phillips, M.D., Nascimbeni, B., Tice, R.R. & Shelby, M.D. (1991) Induction of micronuclei in mouse bone marrow cells: An evaluation of nucleoside analogues used in the treatment of AIDS. *Environ. mol. Mutag.*, **18**, 168–183

Pindado, M.T.C., Bravo, A.L., Martinez-Rodrigues, R., Talavera, A.P., Aguado, F.G., Contreras, M.R., Alvarez, M.J.P., Garcia, A.F. & Martin, M.J.A. (1994) Histochemical and ultrastructural changes induced by zidovudine in mitochondria of rat cardiac muscle. *Eur. J. Histochem.*, **38**, 311–318

Pizzo, P.A., Eddy, J., Falloon, J., Balis, F.M., Murphy, R.F., Moss, H., Wolters, P., Brouwers, P., Jarosinski, P., Rubin, M., Broder, S., Yarchoan, R., Brunetti, A., Maha, M., Nusinoff-Lehrman, S. & Poplack, D.G. (1988) Effect of continuous intravenous infusion of zidovudine (AZT) in children with symptomatic HIV infection. *New Engl. J. Med.*, **319**, 889–896

Plessinger, M.A., Boal, J.H., & Miller, R.K. (1997) Human placenta does not reduce AZT (zidovudine) to 3'-amino-3'-deoxythymidine. *Proc. Soc. exp. Biol. Med.*, **215**, 243–247

Pluda, J.M., Yarchoan, R., Jaffe, E.S., Feuerstein, I.M., Solomon, D., Steinberg, S.M., Wyvill, K.M., Raubitschek, A., Katz, D. & Broder, S. (1990) Development of non-Hodgkin lymphoma in a cohort of patients with severe human immunodeficinecy virus (HIV) infection on long-term antiretroviral therapy. *Ann. intern. Med.*, **113**, 276–282

Pluda, J.M., Venzon, D.J., Tosato, G., Lietzau, J., Wyvill, K., Nelson, D.L., Jaffe, E.S., Karp, J.E., Broder, S. & Yarchoan, R. (1993) Parameters affecting the development of non-Hodgkin's lymphoma in patients with severe human immunodeficiency virus infection receiving antiretroviral therapy. *J. clin. Oncol.*, **11**, 1099–1107

Poirier, M.C., Patterson, T.A., Slikker, W., Jr & Olivero, O.A. (2000) Incorporation of 3'-azido-3'-deoxythymidine (AZT) into fetal DNA, and fetal tissue distribution of drug, after infusion of pregnant late-term rhesus macaques with a human-equivalent AZT dose. *J. AIDS hum. Retrovirol.* (in press)

Portegies, P., de Gans, J., Lange, J.M.A., Derix, M.M.A., Speelman, H., Bakker, M., Danner, S.A. & Goudsmit, J. (1989) Declining incidence of AIDS dementia complex after introduction of zidovudine treatment. *Br. med. J.*, **299**, 819–821

Raffi, F., Reliquet, V., Auger, S., Besnier, J.M., Chennebault, J.M., Billaud, E., Michelet, C., Perre, P., Lafeuillade, A., May, T. & Billaudel, S. (1998) Efficacy and safety of stavudine and didanosine combination therapy in antiretroviral-experienced patients. *AIDS*, **12**, 1999–2005

Rao, G.N., Lindamood, C., III, Heath, J.E., Farnell, D.R. & Giles, H.D. (1998) Subchronic toxicity of human immunodeficiency virus and tuberculosis combination therapies in B6C3F1 mice. *Toxicol. Sci.*, **45**, 113–127

Rolinski, B., Bogner, J.R., Sadri, I., Wintergerst, U. & Goebel, F.D. (1997) Absorption and elimination kinetics of zidovudine in the cerebrospinal fluid in HIV-1-infected patients. *J. acquir. Immune Defic. Syndr. hum. Retrovirol.*, **15**, 192–197

Rote Liste Sekretariat (1998) *Rote Liste 1998*, Frankfurt, Rote Liste Service GmbH, pp. 10–449

Royal Pharmaceutical Society of Great Britain (1999) *Martindale, The Extra Pharmacopoeia*, 13th Ed., London, The Pharmaceutical Press [MicroMedex Online: Health Care Series]

Scheding, S., Media, J.E. & Nakeff, A. (1994) Acute toxic effects of 3'-azido-3'-deoxythymidine (AZT) on normal and regenerating murine hematopoiesis. *Exp. Hematol.*, **22**, 60–65

Schenker, S., Johnson, R.F., King, T.S., Schenken, R.S. & Henderson, G.I. (1990) Azidothymidine (zidovudine) transport by the human placenta. *Am. J. med. Sci.*, **299**, 16–20

Sethi, M.L. (1991) Zidovudine. In: Florey, K., ed., *Analytical Profiles of Drug Substances*, New York, Academic Press, Vol. 20, pp. 729–765

Shafer, R.W., Iversen, A.K.N., Winters, M.A., Aguiniga, E., Katzenstein, D.A., Merigan, T.C. & the AIDS Clinical Trials Group 143 Virology Team (1995) Drug resistance and heterogeneous long-term virologic responses of human immunodeficiency virus type 1–infected subjects to zidovudine and didanosine combination therapy. *J. infect. Dis.*, **172**, 70–78

Shaffer, N., Chuachoowong, R., Mock, P.A., Bhadrakom, C., Siriwasin, W., Young, N.L., Chotpitayasunondh, T., Chearskul, S., Roongpisuthipong, A., Chinayon, P., Karon, J., Mastro, T.D., Simonds, R.J. on behalf of the Bangkok Collaborative Perinatal HIV Transmission Study Group (1999) Short-course zidovudine for perinatal HIV-1 transmission in Bangkok, Thailand: A randomised controlled trial. *Lancet*, **353**, 773–780

Shafik, H.M., Nokta, M.A. & Pollard, R.B. (1991) Recombinant human interferon beta ser protects against zidovudine-induced genetic damage in AIDS patients. *Antiviral Res.*, **16**, 205–212

Shah, M.M., Li, Y. & Christensen, R.D. (1996) Effects of perinatal zidovudine on hematopoiesis: A comparison of effects on progenitors from human fetuses versus mothers. *AIDS*, **10**, 1239–1247

Sharpe, A.H., Hunter, J.J., Ruptrecht, R.M. & Jaenisch, R. (1988) Maternal transmission of retroviral disease: Transgenic mice as a rapid test system for evaluating perintal and transplacental antiretroviral therapy. *Proc. natl Acad. Sci. USA*, **85**, 9792–9796

Shelby, M.D. (1994) The cytogenetic effects of AZT (Letter to the Editor). *Environ. mol. Mutag.*, **24**, 148–149

Sikka, S.C., Gogu, S.R. & Agrawal, K.D. (1991) Effect of zidovudine (AZT) on reproductive and hematopoietic systems in the male rat. *Biochem. Pharmacol.*, **42**, 1293–1297

Simonds, R.J., Steketee, R., Nesheim, S., Matheson, P., Palumbo, P., Alger, L., Abrams, E.J., Orloff, S., Lindsay, M., Bardeguez, A.D., Vink, P., Byers, R. & Rogers, M. for the Perinatal AIDS Collaborative Transmission Studies (1998) Impact of zidovudine use on risk and risk factors for perinatal transmission of HIV. *AIDS*, **12**, 301–308

Simpson, M.V., Chin, C.D., Keilbaugh, S.A., Lin, T. & Prusoff, W.H. (1989) Studies on the inhibition of mitochondrial DNA replication by 3'-azido-3'-deoxythymidine and other dideoxynucleoside analogs which inhibit HIV-1 replication. *Biochem. Pharmacol.*, **38**, 1033–1036

Simpson, D.M., Katzenstein, D.A., Hughes, M.D., Hammer, S.M., Williamson, D.L., Jiang, Q., Pi, J.-T. & the AIDS Clinical Trials Group 175/801 Study Team (1998) Neuromuscular function in HIV infection: Analysis of a placebo-controlled combination antiretroviral trial. *AIDS*, **12**, 2425–2432

Sommadossi, J.-P., Carlisle, R. & Zhou, Z. (1989) Cellular pharmacology of 3'-azido-3'-deoxythymidine with evidence of incorporation into DNA of human bone marrow cells. *Mol. Pharmacol.*, **36**, 9–14

Sperling, R.S., Stratton, P., O'Sullivan, M.J., Boyer, P., Watts, D.H., Lambert, J.S., Hammill, H., Livingston, E.G., Gloeb, D.J., Minkoff, H. & Fox, H.E. (1992) A survey of zidovudine use in pregnant women with human immunodeficiency virus infection. *New Engl. J. Med.*, **326**, 857–861

Sperling, R.S., Shapiro, D.E., McSherry, G.D., Britto, P., Cunningham, B.E., Culnane, M., Coombs, R.W., Scott, G., Van Dyke, R.B., Shearer, W.T., Jimenez, E., Diaz, C., Harrison, D.D. & Delfraissy, J.-F. for the Pediatric AIDS Clinical Trials Group Protocol 076 Study Group (1998) Safety of the maternal–infant zidovudine regimen utilized in the Pediatric AIDS Clinical Trial Group 076 study. *AIDS*, **12**, 1805–1813

Stagg, M.P., Cretton, E.M., Kidd, L., Diasio, R.B. & Sommadossi, J.-P. (1992) Clinical pharmacokinetics of 3'-azido-3'-deoxythymidine (zidovudine) and catabolites with formation of a toxic catabolite, 3'-amino-3'-deoxythymidine. *Clin. Pharmacol. Ther.*, **51**, 668–676

Stark, R.I., Garland, M., Daniel, S.S., Leung, K., Myers, M.M. & Tropper, P.J. (1997) Fetal cardiorespiratory and neurobehavioral response to zidovudine (AZT) in the baboon. *J. Soc. gynecol. Invest.*, **4**, 183–190

Staszewski, S., Katlama, C., Harrer, T., Massip, P., Yeni, P., Cutrell, A., Tortell, S.M., Harrigan, R.P., Steel, H., Lanier, R.E. & Pearce, G. (1998) A dose-ranging study to evaluate the safety and efficacy of abacavir alone or in combination with zidovudine and lamivudine in antiretroviral treatment-naive subjects. *AIDS*, **12**, 197–202

Stretcher, B.N. (1995) Pharmacokinetic optimisation of antiretroviral therapy in patients with HIV infection. *Clin. Pharmacokinet.*, **29**, 46–65

Styrt, B.A., Paizza-Hepp, T.D. & Chikami, G.K. (1996) Clinical toxicity of antiretroviral nucleoside analogs. *Antiviral Res.*, **31**, 121–135

Sussman, H.E., Olivero, O.A., Meng, Q., Pietras, S.M., Poirier, M.C., O'Neill, J.P., Finette, B.A., Bauer, M.J. & Walker, V.E. (1999) Genotoxicity of 3′-azido-3′-deoxythymidine in the human lymphoblastoid cell line, TK6: Relationships between DNA incorporation, mutant frequency, and spectrum of deletion mutations in *HPRT*. *Mutat. Res.*, **429**, 249–259

Swiss Pharmaceutical Society, ed. (1999) *Index Nominum, International Drug Directory*, 16th Ed., Stuttgart, Medpharm Scientific Publishers [MicroMedex Online: Health Care Series]

Thomas, J., ed. (1998) *Australian Prescription Products Guide*, 27th Ed., Victoria, Australian Pharmaceutical Publishing, Vol. 1, pp. 2447–2452

Thompson, M.B., Dunnick, J.K., Sutphin, M.E., Giles, H.D., Irwin, R.D. & Prejean, J.D. (1991) Hematologic toxicity of AZT and ddC administered as single agents and in combination to rats and mice. *Fundam. appl. Toxicol.*, **17**, 159–176

Tokars, J.I., Marcus, R., Culver, D.H., Schable, C.A., McKibben, P.S., Bandea, C.I. & Bell, D.M. for the CDC Cooperative Needlestick Surveillance Group (1993) Surveillance of HIV infection and zidovudine use among health care workers after occupational exposure to HIV-infected blood. *Ann. intern. Med.*, **118**, 913–919

Toltzis, P., Marx, C.M., Kleinman, N., Levine, E.M. & Schmidt, E.V. (1991) Zidovudine-associated embryonic toxicity in mice. *J. infect. Dis.*, **163**, 1212–1218

Toltzis, P., Mourton, T. & Magnuson, T. (1994) Comparative embryonic cytotoxicity of antiretroviral nucleosides. *J. infect. Dis.*, **169**, 1100–1102

Trang, J.M., Prejean, J.D., James, R.H., Irwin, R.D., Goehl, T.J. & Page, J.G. (1993) Zidovudine bioavailability and linear pharmacokinetics in female B6C3F1 mice. *Drug Metab. Dispos.*, **21**, 189–193

Tuntland, T., Odinecs, A., Nosbisch, C. & Unadkat, J.D. (1998) *In vivo* maternal–fetal–amniotic fluid pharmacokinetics of zidovudine in the pigtailed macaque: Comparison of steady-state and single-dose regimens. *J. Pharmacol. exp. Ther.*, **285**, 54–62

US Pharmacopeial Convention (1998a) *USP Dispensing Information*, Vol. I, *Drug Information for the Health Care Professional*, 18th Ed., Rockville, MD, pp. 3005–3009

US Pharmacopeial Convention (1998b) *The 1995 US Pharmacopeia*, 23rd Rev./*The National Formulary*, 18th Rev., Supplement 9, Rockville, MD, pp. 4277–4280

Vazquez-Padua, M., Starnes, M.C. & Cheng, Y.-C. (1990) Incorporation of 3′-azido-3′-deoxythymidine into cellular DNA and its removal in a human leukemic cell line. *Cancer Commun.*, **2**, 55–62

Veal, G.J. & Back, D.J. (1995) Metabolism of zidovudine. *Gen. Pharmacol.*, **26**, 1469–1475

Vella, S., Giuliano, M., Dally, L.G., Agresti, M.G., Tomino, C., Floridia, M., Chiesi, A., Fragola, V., Moroni, M., Piazza, M., Scalise, G., Ortona, L., Aiuti, F., Lazzarin, A., Carosi, G.P., Bassetti, D., Guzzanti, E., Dianzani, F. & the Italian Zidovudine Evaluation Group (1994) Long-term follow-up of zidovudine therapy in asymptomatic HIV infection: Results of a multicenter cohort study. *J. AIDS*, **7**, 31–38

Venturi, G., Romano, L., Catucci, M., Riccio, M.L., De Milito, A., Gonnelli, A., Rubino, M., Valensin, P.E. & Zazzi, M. (1999) Genotypic resistance to zidovudine as a predictor of failure of subsequent therapy with human immunodeficiency virus type-1 nucleoside reverse-transcriptase inhibitors. *Eur. J. clin. Microbiol. infect. Dis.*, **18**, 274–282

Wade, N.A., Birkhead, G.S., Warren, B.L., Charbonneau, T.T., French, P.T., Wang, L., Baum, J.B., Tesoriero, J.M. & Savicki, R. (1998) Abbreviated regimens of zidovudine prophylaxis and perinatal transmission of the human immunodeficiency virus. *New Engl. J. Med.*, **339**, 1409–1414

White, A., Eldridge, R., Andrews, E. & the Antiretroviral Pregnancy Registry Advisory Committee (1997) Birth outcomes following zidovudine exposure in pregnant women: The Antiretroviral Pregnancy Registry. *Acta paediatr.*, **421** (Suppl.), 86–88

Wiktor, S.Z., Ekpini, E., Karon, J.M., Nkengasong, J., Maurice, C., Severin, S.T., Roels, T.H., Kouassi, M.K., Lackritz, E.M., Coulibaly, I.M. & Greenberg, A.E. (1999) Short-course oral zidovudine for prevention of mother-to-child transmission of HIV-1 in Abidjan, Côte d'Ivoire: A randomised trial. *Lancet*, **353**, 781–785

Witt, K.L., Robbins, W., Bishop, J.B., Libbus, B., Cohen, M., Hamilton, C.D. & Shelby, M.D. (1999) Frequency of chromosomal aberrations in lymphocytes of patients before and after initiation of anti-HIV drug therapy with dideoxynucleosides. *Environ. mol. Mutag.*, **33** (Suppl. 30), 68

Zhang, Z., Diwan, B.A., Anderson, L.M., Logsdon, D., Oliverio, O.A., Haines, D.C., Rice, J.M., Yuspa, S.H. & Poirier, M.C. (1998) Skin tumorigenesis and Ki-*ras* and Ha-*ras* mutations in tumors from adult mice exposed in utero to 3'-azido-2',3'-dideoxythymidine. *Mol. Carcinog.*, **23**, 45–51

Zhu, Z., Hitchcock, M.J.M. & Sommadossi, J.-P. (1991) Metabolism and DNA interaction of 2',3'-didehydro-2',3'-dideoxythymidine in human bone marrow cells. *Mol. Pharmacol.*, **40**, 838–845

ZALCITABINE

1. Exposure Data

1.1 Chemical and physical data

1.1.1 *Nomenclature*

Chem. Abstr. Serv. Reg. No.: 7481-89-2
Chem. Abstr. Name: 2′,3′-Dideoxycytidine
IUPAC Systematic Name: 2′,3′-Dideoxycytidine
Synonyms: ddC; DDC; dideoxycytidine

1.1.2 *Structural and molecular formulae and relative molecular mass*

$C_9H_{13}N_3O_3$ Relative molecular mass: 211.22

1.1.3 *Chemical and physical properties of the pure substance*

(a) *Description*: White to off-white crystalline powder (American Hospital Formulary Service, 1997)
(b) *Melting-point*: 215–217 °C (Budavari, 1996)
(c) *Solubility*: Soluble in water (76.4 mg/mL at 25 °C) (American Hospital Formulary Service, 1997); soluble in dimethylsulfoxide (90–100 mg/mL); slightly soluble in ethanol (5–7 mg/mL) and methanol (8–10 mg/mL); insoluble in acetonitrile, chloroform, butanol, ethyl acetate, and toluene (National Cancer Institute, 1992)
(d) *Optical rotation*: $[\alpha]_D^{25}$, +81° (c = 0.635 in water) (Budavari, 1996)

1.1.4 *Technical products and impurities*

Zalcitabine is available as a 0.375- and 0.75-mg tablet. The tablets may also contain croscarmellose sodium, iron oxides (synthetic brown, black, red and yellow), lactose, macrogol, magnesium stearate, methylhydroxypropylcellulose, microcrystalline cellulose, polyethylene glycol, polysorbate 80 and titanium dioxide (Gennaro, 1995; Canadian Pharmaceutical Association, 1997; British Medical Association/Royal Pharmaceutical Society of Great Britain, 1998; Editions du Vidal, 1998; Rote Liste Sekretariat, 1998; Thomas, 1998; US Pharmacopeial Convention, 1998).

Trade names for zalcitabine include ddC Martian, Hivid and HIVID Roche (Swiss Pharmaceutical Society, 1999).

1.1.5 *Analysis*

The *United States Pharmacopeia* specifies infrared absorption spectrophotometry with comparison to standards, liquid chromatography and thin-layer chromatography as the methods for identifying zalcitabine; liquid chromatography is used to assay its purity. In pharmaceutical preparations, zalcitabine is identified and assayed by liquid chromatography (US Pharmacopeial Convention, 1997).

1.2 Production

Several methods have been reported for the synthesis of zalcitabine (Horwitz *et al.*, 1967; Marumoto & Honjo, 1974; Lin *et al.*, 1987).

Information available in 1999 indicated that it was manufactured and/or formulated in 33 countries (CIS Information Services, 1998; Swiss Pharmaceutical Society, 1999).

1.3 Use

Zalcitabine was among the first drugs (in the early 1990s) approved for use against human immunodeficiency virus (HIV) infection (Devineni & Gallo, 1995) but has passed out of common use in the industrialized world. Although many studies were conducted on its use in various combinations, several large clinical trials (Bartlett *et al.*, 1996; Delta Coordinating Committee, 1996; Hammer *et al.*, 1996; Schooley *et al.*, 1996; Henry *et al.*, 1998) have clearly demonstrated that zalcitabine-containing regimens are less effective than other combinations of antiviral nucleoside analogues with which it has been compared. Although it has been used to treat HIV infections in adults and children, the agent is regarded as obsolete if other nucleoside reverse transcriptase inhibitors are available.

Zalcitabine also has two serious toxic effects: a relatively high frequency of dose- and duration-related peripheral neuropathy and an idiosyncratic syndrome of ulcerations in the mucous membranes of patients (Indorf & Pegram, 1992; Roche Laboratories, 1998).

Zalcitabine has cross-resistance with didanosine (Roche Laboratories, 1998), which is generally more effective.

1.4 Occurrence

Zalcitabine is not known to occur as a natural product. No data on occupational exposure were available to the Working Group.

1.5 Regulations and guidelines

Zalcitabine is listed in the *United States Pharmacopeia* (Swiss Pharmaceutical Society, 1999).

2. Studies of Cancer in Humans

In a multicentre trial in the USA, Abrams *et al.* (1994) randomly assigned 467 symptomatic HIV-infected patients with CD4 counts of ≤ 300 cells/µL plasma, who had previously received zidovudine, to treatment with either zalcitabine at 2.25 mg per day ($n = 237$) or didanosine at 500 mg per day ($n = 230$). The patients were recruited during 1990–91 and were followed up for a median of 1.3 years and a maximum of only 1.8 years. Six cases of non-Hodgkin lymphoma were seen in the zalcitabine-treated group and three in the didanosine-treated group. [The Working Group noted that rate ratios were not calculated, although the risk ratio for non-Hodgkin lymphoma in patients treated with zalcitabine compared with that in patients receiving didanosine was 1.9 (95% CI, 0.49–7.7), with no adjustment for differences in survival between the two groups.]

In an international randomized trial, the Delta Coordinating Committee (1996) allocated 3207 individuals with antibodies to HIV, symptoms of infection or a CD4 count of < 350 cells/µL plasma to treatment with either zidovudine at 600 mg per day ($n = 1055$), zidovudine plus didanosine at 400 mg per day ($n = 1080$) or zidovudine plus zalcitabine at 2.25 mg per day ($n = 1072$). The patients were followed up for a median of 2.5 years (range, 1.8–2.9), during which time 14 deaths due to cancer [not further specified] occurred; five of the deaths occurred in the group treated with zidovudine alone, five in the group treated with zidovudine plus didanosine and four in the group treated with zidovudine plus zalcitabine.

In the study of Pluda *et al.* (1990, 1993), described in the monograph on zidovudine, two of 18 patients receiving zalcitabine alternated with zidovudine developed a high-grade, B-cell non-Hodgkin lymphoma. [The Working Group noted that the risk is difficult to interpret in the absence of a suitable reference group consisting of AIDS patients with a similar degree of immunosuppression.]

[The Working Group noted that these trials were designed to compare the efficacy of drugs in the treatment of patients with various degrees of severity of immunosuppression. For the purposes of evaluating cancer risk, therefore, the numbers of participants were too small and the length of follow-up too short, cancer incidence may have been underascertained, and cancer rates could not be analysed adequately.]

3. Studies of Cancer in Experimental Animals

Oral administration

Mouse

Groups of 10 male and 10 female $B6C3F_1$ mice, six weeks of age, were treated with zalcitabine (purity, > 99%) in a 0.5% methylcellulose and water suspension by gavage twice a day 6 h apart at a dose of 0 (control), 500 or 1000 mg/kg bw per day for 13 weeks, at which time all surviving mice were killed. An additional group of 10 female mice received 1000 mg/kg bw per day for 13 weeks and were then maintained without further treatment for a one-month recovery period before termination. The unexpected finding of thymic lymphomas in one female that received the low dose and one female that received the high dose prompted the authors to conduct an additional study (Sanders *et al.*, 1995).

Groups of 70 female $B6C3F_1$ mice, six weeks of age, were treated with zalcitabine (purity, > 99%) in a 0.5% methylcellulose and water suspension by gavage twice a day 6 h apart at a dose of 0 (control), 500 or 1000 mg/kg bw per day for 13 weeks, after which 20 animals per group were killed and necropsied. The remaining 50 mice per group were held without treatment for an additional three months before termination (recovery group). Thymic lymphomas were found in 2/19 mice that received the low dose and were necropsied at the end of the 13-week exposure period, and in 3/50 and 15/50 mice at the low and high doses, respectively, that were necropsied during or at the end of the three-month recovery period. No thymic lymphomas were seen in control mice (Sanders *et al.*, 1995).

Groups of 50 male and 50 female $B6C3F_1$ mice, six weeks of age, were treated with zalcitabine (purity > 99%) in a 0.5% methylcellulose and water suspension by gavage twice a day 6 h apart at a dose of 0 (control), 500 or 1000 mg/kg bw per day for six months. An additional group at the high dose was treated for three months and killed six months after the start of the experiment (recovery group). There were no treatment-associated deaths among male mice, but marked treatment-associated and lymphoma-associated mortality was seen in female mice receiving the high dose and in the recovery group. By the end of the experiment, the mortality rates in female mice were 0% in controls, 0% at the low dose, 6% at the high dose and 12% in the recovery group. The incidences of thymic lymphoma were 0%, 14%, 20% and 12% in males and 0%, 2%, 44% and 39% in females in these groups [effective numbers not reported for either sex], respectively. The thymic lymphomas involved other lymphoid organs, such as spleen and lymph nodes. Thymic atrophy was the commonest non-neoplastic lesion in treated mice, the incidences being 0%, 2%, 18% and 0% in males in the control, low-dose, high-dose and recovery groups and 0%, 12%, 20% and 0% in females in these groups, respectively. The recovery group had a lower incidence of thymic atrophy than mice at the high dose, indicating that cessation of treatment resulted in reversal of thymic atrophy (Rao et al., 1996).

Groups of 50 male and 50 female NIH Swiss mice, six weeks of age, were treated with zalcitabine (purity > 99%) in a 0.5% methylcellulose and water suspension by gavage twice a day 6 h apart at a dose of 0 (control), 500 or 1000 mg/kg bw per day for six months. An additional group at the high dose (recovery group) was treated for three months. All animals were killed six months after the start of the experiment. A treatment-related increase in mortality rate was seen in both males and females, with rates of 2%, 10%, 24% and 4% in males in the control, low-dose, high-dose and recovery groups and 0%, 14%, 50% and 46% in females in these groups, respectively. The deaths were due to thymic lymphomas in the females, whereas the male mice died from toxic effects of zalcitabine, such as anaemia. The incidences of thymic lymphoma were 0%, 15%, 55% and 47% in males in the control, low-dose, high-dose and recovery groups and 0%, 44%, 87% and 90% [effective numbers not reported for either sex] for females in these groups, respectively. Thymic atrophy was the commonest non-neoplastic lesion in treated mice, with incidences of 4%, 19%, 26% and 6% in males in the control, low-dose, high-dose and recovery groups and 0%, 2%, 10% and 2% in females in these groups, respectively. Both males and females in the recovery group had a lower incidence of thymic atrophy than those given the high dose continuously, indicating that cessation of treatment resulted in reversal of thymic atrophy (Rao et al., 1996).

4. Other Data Relevant to an Evaluation of Carcinogenicity and its Mechanisms

4.1 Absorption, distribution, metabolism and excretion

4.1.1 *Humans*

The absorption, distribution, metabolism and excretion of zalcitabine in adults have been reviewed extensively (Broder, 1990; Yarchoan et al., 1990; Burger et al., 1995; Devineni & Gallo, 1995; Vanhove et al., 1997). Because of the toxicity of zalcitabine, the dose range that can be used is narrow, and the drug is typically given three times daily for a total of 1.0–1.5 mg. This dose range is much lower than the 400- and 600-mg daily doses of didanosine and zidovudine, respectively, but the antiviral potency of zalcitabine in cell cultures is much greater than that of these other drugs. Zalcitabine is well absorbed when administered orally, with a bioavailability of the order of 80% (Klecker *et al.*, 1988; Broder, 1990; Burger *et al.*, 1995). About 75% of an oral dose is excreted unchanged in the urine, and measurable levels have been found in plasma and cerebrospinal fluid. The peak concentration of zalcitabine in cerebrospinal fluid 2 h after dosing has been reported to be 14% of that in plasma (Klecker *et al.*, 1988; Burger *et al.*, 1995; Devineni & Gallo, 1995). Zalcitabine is transported across the cell membrane by nucleoside carrier-mediated and non-carrier-mediated mechanisms, and < 5% is bound to protein (Burger *et al.*, 1995; Devineni & Gallo, 1995).

Zalcitabine is metabolized along only one pathway (Figure 1). About 10% of the drug appears in the faeces and ~75% is excreted unchanged in the urine, suggesting that renal integrity is important for clearance (Klecker *et al.*, 1988; Broder, 1990; Burger *et al.*, 1995; Beach, 1998). Hepatic metabolites have not been observed (Burger *et al.*, 1995). The antiviral action of zalcitabine, like that of zidovudine and didanosine, is dependent on phosphorylation and incorporation into DNA (Broder, 1990). The first step is the formation of zalcitabine monophosphate by the enzyme 2'-deoxycytidine kinase, which is followed by formation of the diphosphate and triphosphate metabolites through the action of the cytosine monophosphate kinase and nucleotide diphosphate kinase enzymes, respectively (Broder, 1990; Burger *et al*, 1995). Like zidovudine and didanosine, zalcitabine targets the viral reverse transcriptase and is simultaneously incorporated into DNA, where replication is unable to proceed further owing to lack of a 3'-hydroxyl group (Broder, 1990). Although phosphorylation is critical for the antiviral activity, it accounts for only a small fraction (probably ~1%) of the total drug disposition.

The pharmacokinetics of zalcitabine has been extensively reviewed (Yarchoan *et al.*, 1990; Burger *et al*, 1995; Devineni & Gallo, 1995; Vanhove *et al.*, 1997). Like that of zidovudine and didanosine, the pharmacokinetics of zalcitabine appears to be linear over a broad dose range, and the maximum concentration in plasma is reached by 1–2 h in adults (5–8 ng/mL after a 0.5–0.75-mg tablet orally three times a day); the plasma half-time is reported to be 1–2.7 h (Klecker *et al.*, 1988; Broder, 1990; Gustavson *et al.*, 1990; Burger *et al.*, 1995; Devineni & Gallo, 1995; Vanhove *et al.*, 1997). Because a lower dose is given, the peak plasma concentration is only about 10% of those found with zidovudine and 20% of those found with didanosine (Yarchoan *et al.*, 1990). The mean rate of plasma clearance was 14–25 L/h, but it decreased with increasing age and weight (Yarchoan *et al.*, 1990; Vanhove *et al.*, 1997). Renal clearance is also closely linked to creatinine clearance and body weight (Burger *et al.*, 1995; Bazunga *et al.*, 1998). The pharmacokinetics appeared to be similar after an inital dose and during long-term dosing, and there were no significant interactions between zalcitabine and concomitantly administered zidovudine (Vanhove *et al.*, 1997).

Figure 1. Pathways of anabolic phosphorylation of zalcitabine (2′,3′-dideoxycytidine, ddCyd) and its normal counterpart, 2′-deoxycytidine (dCyd)

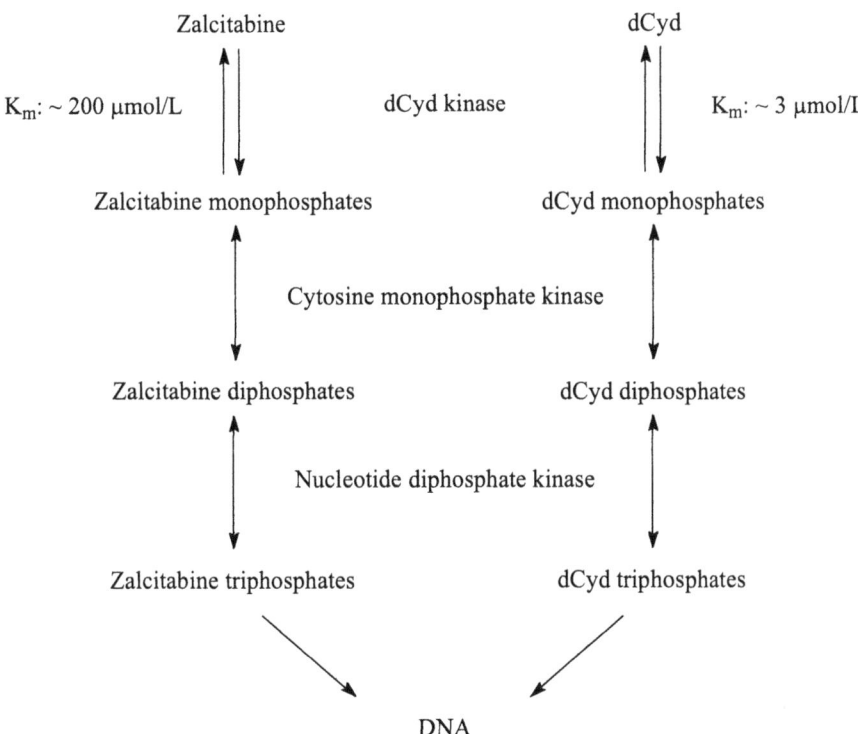

From Broder (1990)
The Michaelis constant for the first step of anabolic phosphorylation (mediated by 2′-deoxycytidine kinase) is shown for both the drug and the normal substrate.

4.1.2 Experimental systems

Pregnant rhesus monkeys (*Macaca mulatta*) that were near term (146 days) received radiolabelled zalcitabine as a bolus dose of 0.6 mg/kg bw via the radial vein. During a 3-h sampling of both the mother and the fetus, the fetal:maternal ratio of the integrated area under the curve of plasma concentration–time was 0.32 ± 0.02, and the fetal tissues were found to contain zalcitabine (0.05–0.8 µmol/L equivalents) and zalcitabine monophosphate (0.008–0.09 nmol/g) (Sandberg et al., 1995).

Four pregnant pigtailed macaques (*Macaca nemestrina*) that were near term (126 days) received an infusion of zalcitabine at a constant rate of 1.3 µg/min per kg bw through the femoral vein over 30 h. The authors concluded that passive transplacental transfer of zalcitabine occurred, with a fetal:maternal concentration ratio of 0.58 ± 0.06 (Tuntland et al., 1996).

The absorption, distribution, metabolism and excretion of zalcitabine have been reported in microswine (Swagler *et al.*, 1991), rats (Ibrahim & Boudinot, 1989, 1991), mice (Kelley *et al.*, 1987) and monkeys (Kelley *et al.*, 1987; Qian *et al.*, 1992). A review of data for several species (Devineni & Gallo, 1995) suggested that the pharmacokinetics in experimental animals and humans were essentially similar. Virtually no zalcitabine was found in cerebrospinal fluid (< 1%) in rats, dogs or monkeys. Approximately 50–80% of the drug was excreted unchanged in the urine, but urinary metabolites were detected only in monkeys. The half-time for drug elimination was similar in all species and averaged 1.4 h.

In four microswine given an intravenous bolus dose of 5 mg/kg bw zalcitabine (Swagler *et al.*, 1991), the rates of total and renal clearance were similar to those in humans, about 80% of the drug being excreted unchanged in the pigs and about 75% in humans (see section 4.1.1). The half-time for clearance of zalcitabine removal, 1.8 h in pigs, was also similar to that in humans (see section 4.1.1). Microswine are a good model for the pharmacokinetics of zalcitabine in humans but a less desirable model for the metabolism of zidovudine and didanosine, for which the clearance rates are significantly lower.

In rats, the pharmacokinetics of zalcitabine was stable over a dose range of 10–500 mg/kg bw. The half-time for removal of the drug from plasma and urine was 1–1.3 h. It bound to plasma proteins, and 50% of the original dose was excreted unchanged in the urine. Renal clearance exceeded the glomerular filtration rate, suggesting active renal tubular secretion (Ibrahim & Budinot, 1989, 1991). Zalcitabine accumulated preferentially in the liver and spleen of rats (Makabi-Panzu *et al.*, 1994). Interspecies scaling indicated that the concentrations in humans can be predicted from the pharmacokinetics in rats.

BDF_1 mice were given a single dose of 100 mg/kg bw zalcitabine orally or intravenously and continuous exposure to 47 mg/kg bw per day by Alzet pump. The plasma concentrations reached a maximum of about 15 μg/mL 45 min after oral dosing, and the half-time for plasma clearance was 67 min. About 80% of the drug was recovered unchanged in the urine after intravenous dosing, and about 60% of the drug was found in faeces after oral dosing. The phosphorylated metabolites constituted about 1–2% of the total dose. High concentrations of the drug were found in mouse kidney, pancreas and liver, and there was low penetration to the central nervous system (Kelley *et al.*, 1987).

In three rhesus monkeys given 100 mg/kg bw zalcitabine, recovery in the urine was about 75% by five days, as in humans, but only about 9% of the drug was excreted as dideoxyuridine, which is in contrast to the human metabolic pattern. Deamination of zalcitabine to dideoxyuridine does not appear to be a significant reaction in either mice or humans but is measurable in monkeys. The half-time for clearance from plasma was 1.8 h, and the concentration in cerebrospinal fluid was < 1% of the peak plasma level (Kelley *et al.*, 1987). When a much lower dose (5 mg/kg bw) of zalcitabine was given to three monkeys, 49–61% of the drug was excreted unchanged in the urine. The half-time for plasma clearance was 1.9 h, and the bioavailability was 61% (Qian *et al.*, 1992). The studies suggest that non-human primates are an appropriate model for studying the pharmacokinetics of zalcitabine in humans.

4.2 Toxic effects

4.2.1 *Humans*

Zalcitabine induces sensory peripheral neuropathy and a syndrome involving fever, rash and aphthous stomatitis, which are early toxic and dose-limiting effects (Yarchoan *et al.*, 1990; Burger *et al.*, 1995; Skowron, 1996; Beach, 1998). In some of the first clinical trials, peripheral neuropathy manifested as pain, numbness and weakness occurred in 70% of patients receiving doses of $\geq$ 4.5 mg per day but was reversible after discontinuation of the drug. At the lower doses used currently, the onset of neuropathy is more gradual and the symptoms resolve more rapidly (Skowron, 1996). For example, Fischl *et al.* (1995) studied 285 AIDS patients with CD4 counts of $\leq$ 300 cells/μL, who received 2.25 mg zalcitabine daily for 17 months (median time). Of these patients, 6% had neuropathy, 14% had anaemia or neutropenia, 6% had evidence of hepatic toxicity, 6% had stomatitis or rash and 3% had pancreatitis. Blum *et al.* (1996) reported that 34% of 79 HIV-infected individuals receiving zalcitabine at 2.25 mg/day developed neuropathy within a mean latency of 16 weeks (range, 1–51 weeks). Further reduction of the dose lessened the severity of symptoms but did not resolve the neuropathy.

In very highly compromised AIDS patients (median CD4 count, 59 cells/μL), toxic neuropathy was found in 27% of 51 patients receiving zalcitabine. The risk factors for peripheral neuropathy were low serum cobalamin and high alcohol consumption (Fichtenbaum *et al.*, 1995).

In contrast, two HIV-exposed health-care workers receiving prophylactic therapy that included zalcitabine and zidovudine had acute onset of rash, fever, nausea and increased activity of liver enzymes after three weeks of treatment. A liver biopsy specimen contained macrovesicular steatosis and lobular inflammation. These are known, but rare side-effects of zidovudine that may have been exacerbated by the presence of another nucleoside analogue drug, zalcitabine (Henry *et al.*, 1996).

Zalcitabine, like other anti-HIV nucleoside analogues, has been associated with a rare (1 in 10^5 to 1 in 10^6 patients) idiosyncratic syndrome of a progressive increase in the activity of liver enzymes in serum, fulminating hepatic steatosis and lactic acidosis. Failure to discontinue the drug can lead to death (US Food and Drug Administration Antiviral Advisory Committee, 1993).

4.2.2 *Experimental systems*

(a) *Haematotoxicity*

Although the haematotoxicity observed with zalcitabine is not as severe as that seen with zidovudine and is not the dose-limiting effect for zalcitabine, it is a feature of the toxic profile of zalcitabine (see section 4.2.1). It has been successfully modelled in mice, rats, dogs, rabbits and monkeys (Tsai *et al.*, 1989; Menconboni *et al.*, 1990; Luster *et al.*, 1991; Thompson *et al.*, 1991; Riley *et al.*, 1992; Taylor *et al.*, 1994).

Various classes of bone-marrow cells from mice given seven daily doses of 10 mg/kg bw zalcitabine were examined for 15 days after the initial exposure. By day 5, severe neutropenia was observed. The effect was greatest in committed progenitor cells of both erythroid and granulocyte–macrophage lineages and was reversible upon discontinuation of the drug (Menconboni *et al.*, 1990). Zalcitabine-induced regenerative macrocytic anaemia, but no immunosuppressive effects, were found when the drug was administered to mice for up to 94 days at a dose of 2000 mg/kg bw per day (Luster *et al.*, 1991). Similar results were observed by Thompson *et al.* (1991) with the same dose regimen, who found macrocytic anaemia and hypoplastic bone marrow in mice and rats, the effect being generally more severe in mice than in rats. The haematological effects were reversible upon discontinuation of treatment.

Rabbits treated daily for 13–18 weeks by intubation with 10–250 mg/kg bw zalcitabine per day showed persistent lymphopenia with decreased red and white blood cell counts, haematocrit and haemoglobin concentration. Most animals had non-regenerative macrocytic anaemia of bone-marrow origin and a progressive loss of lymphocytes until death (Riley *et al.*, 1992).

Pigtailed macaques were given zalcitabine at 15 or 30 mg/kg bw per day intravenously, either as a 24-h continuous infusion or a daily bolus dose for 10–12 days. All animals showed leukopenia, anaemia, lethargy and reduced appetite, and those given the bolus doses also had exfoliative dermatitis and peripheral neuropathy (Tsai *et al.*, 1989). In rhesus monkeys given lower doses (0.06–6.0 mg/kg bw per day) for up to 243 days, transient decreases in CD4 T and CD20 B cell counts were observed after 20 days of dosing, but few other haematological effects were found (Taylor *et al.*, 1994).

(b) *Neurotoxicity*

The neurotoxicity of zalcitabine in rabbits was modelled in a series of studies (Anderson *et al.*, 1991; Feldman *et al.*, 1992; Anderson *et al.*, 1994; Feldman & Anderson, 1994), which suggested that the underlying mechanism was mitochondrial damage (see section 4.5). New Zealand white rabbits were given zalcitabine at 0–250 mg/kg bw per day for 13–18 weeks. Rabbits at doses > 50 mg/kg bw per day developed hind-limb paresis and gait abnormalities and a 30–50% decrease in nerve conduction. Histological examination (Anderson *et al.*, 1991) revealed myelin splitting, demyelination and axonal loss in the sciatic nerve, but no alterations in the brain, spinal cord or retina. Electron microscopy showed demyelination of the sciatic nerve and ventral root, excess Schwann-cell basal lamina, abnormally shaped axons and the presence of lipid droplets (Feldman et al., 1992). In rabbits given 35 mg/kg bw zalcitabine per day for 24 weeks (Anderson et al., 1994), sciatic nerve analysis showed that by 16 weeks, there was evidence of prolonged F waves (a measure of proximal motor conduction, i.e. sciatic nerve function), myelin splitting, demyelination, remyelination, enlarged and damaged mitochondria in Schwann cells of sciatic and tibial nerves and dorsal root ganglia and a 30–50% decrease in myelin protein mRNA expression. The abnormal mitochondria were cup-shaped with tubular cristae (Feldman & Anderson, 1994).

4.3 Reproductive and prenatal effects

4.3.1 Humans

No data were available to the Working Group.

4.3.2 Experimental systems

C57BL/6N mice were given zalcitabine suspended in 0.5% methylcellulose by gavage twice a day on days 6–15 of gestation at a total daily dose of 0, 200, 400, 1000 or 2000 mg/kg bw. Maternal weight gain during the treatment period and gravid uterine weight were decreased at 2000 mg/kg bw per day, but weight gain corrected for gravid uterine weight was not affected. At this dose, the mean litter size was decreased, and the percentage of resorptions per litter was increased. The average fetal body weight per litter was decreased at 1000 and 2000 mg/kg bw per day. The number of fetuses with any malformation, the number of litters with one or more malformed fetuses and the percentage of malformed fetuses per litter were increased at the two higher doses. The malformations included open eyelids, micrognathia, kinked tail, clubbed paws, cleft palate, fused cervical arch, bent humerus and bent tibia (Lindström et al., 1990). [The Working Group noted the high doses used.]

The thymic lobes of fetal (day 17 of gestation) male and female Wistar rats were cultivated on membrane filters in 2 mL culture medium (RPMI 1640 plus 10% fetal calf serum), and zalcitabine was added to the cultures in water at final concentrations of 3, 10, 30, 100 and 300 µmol/L for seven days. The concentration of 10 µmol/L reduced the number of thymic cells on day 7, while 30 µmol/L reduced the percentages of $CD4^+/CD8^+$ and $CD4^+/CD8^-$ cells and increased that of $CD4^-/CD8^+$ cells. At 30 µmol/L, expression of the CD5 antigen was reduced, maturation of the thymocytes was inhibited, and the number of small thymocytes was reduced (Foerster et al., 1992).

4.4 Genetic and related effects

4.4.1 *Humans*

No data were available to the Working Group.

4.4.2 *Experimental systems*

These studies are summarized in Table 1.

Reports on the potential mutagenicity of zalcitabine are scarce. References such as *The Physician's Desk Reference* (Medical Economics Data Production, 1999) provide results but few or no details of the experimental conditions used in the assays. The manufacturer of the drug has yet to publish a detailed report equivalent to those available in the literature on aciclovir and zidovudine. Nevertheless, the limited genotoxicity data available indicate that zalcitabine is clastogenic at high doses.

Zalcitabine did not induce reverse mutation in *Salmonella typhimurium* [no information on doses or strains or the presence of exogenous metabolic activation] and did not induce gene mutation in unspecified tests in Chinese hamster lung and mouse lymphoma cells. It did not induce unscheduled DNA repair synthesis in rat hepatocytes under unspecified conditions. It induced cell transformation *in vitro* [cell type and experimental conditions not given] at doses ≥ 500 µg/mL (Medical Economics Data Production, 1999).

Mamber *et al.* (1990) conducted a series of assays primarily to characterize the ability of zalcitabine and other dideoxynucleosides to induce two SOS functions, cell filamentation and prophage lambda, in *Escherichia coli*. Induction of the SOS response was assessed by both agar spot methods and quantitative liquid suspension assays for β-galactosidase production in *E. coli* K-12 fusion strains BR513 and PQ37, respectively. Zalcitabine induced prophage lambda, but not *sulA*, in the liquid microsuspension assay at 1000 µg/mL. The combined results of tests for the induction of the SOS response in the nucleoside analogues evaluated in this volume indicate that the activity relationships can be ranked zidovudine > didanosine > zalcitabine. No effects of zalcitabine on DNA repair were observed in *E. coli* WP2 and CM871 *uvr*A *rec*A *lex*A or in the *Bacillus subtilis* H17 and M45 *rec*A, indicating that zalcitabine does not cause DNA lesions that require repair involving the excision repair (*uvr*A) or error-free postreplication repair (*rec*A) processes. Rather, zalcitabine, which acts as a DNA chain terminator, may generate an SOS-inducing response leading to inhibition of DNA replication.

Zalcitabine caused clastogenic effects in all studies performed *in vitro* and *in vivo*, except one. Human peripheral blood cells exposed to zalcitabine with and without exogenous metabolic activation showed increased frequencies of chromosomal aberrations at doses ≥ 1.5 µg/mL. Administration of oral doses of ≥ 500 mg/kg bw zalcitabine on three consecutive days to groups of five to seven male $B6C3F_1$ mice produced micronuclei. Zalcitabine was less potent than zidovudine in inducing micronuclei (Phillips

Table 1. Genetic and related effects of zalcitabine

Test system	Result[a] Without exogenous metabolic system	Result[a] With exogenous metabolic system	Dose[b] (LED/HID)	Reference
Escherichia coli BR513 (*uvrB envA lacZ::lambda*), prophage induction, SOS repair (spot and liquid suspension tests)	+	NT	1000	Mamber *et al.* (1990)
Escherichia coli PQ37 (*uvrA rfa lacZ::sulA*), cell filamentation, SOS repair (spot and liquid suspension tests)	–	NT	1000	Mamber *et al.* (1990)
Escherichia coli CM871 (*uvrA recA lexA*), differential toxicity (vs *Escherichia coli* WP2)	–	NT	1000	Mamber *et al.* (1990)
Bacillus subtilis M45 *rec* strain, differential toxicity	–	NT	NR	Mamber *et al.* (1990)
Salmonella typhimurium [strains not reported], reverse mutation	–	–	NR	Medical Economics Data Production (1999)
Bacillus subtilis H17, gene mutation	–	NT	NR	Mamber *et al.* (1990)
Unscheduled DNA synthesis, rat primary hepatocytes *in vitro*	–	NT	NR	Medical Economics Data Production (1999)
Gene mutation, Chinese hamster lung cells *in vitro*	–	NT	NR	Medical Economics Data Production (1999)
Gene mutation, mouse lymphoma cells *in vitro*	–	NT	NR	Medical Economics Data Production (1999)
Cell transformation [cells not specified]	+	NT	500	Medical Economics Data Production (1999)
Chromosomal aberrations, human lymphocytes *in vitro*	+	+	1.5	Medical Economics Data Production (1999)
Micronucleus formation, mouse cells *in vivo*	+		2500 po × 1	Medical Economics Data Production (1999)

Table 1 (contd)

Test system	Result[a]		Dose[b] (LED/HID)	Reference
	Without exogenous metabolic system	With exogenous metabolic system		
Micronucleus formation, mouse bone marrow *in vivo*	+		500 po × 3	Phillips *et al.* (1991)
Micronucleus formation, mouse bone marrow *in vivo*	–		0.12 ip × 1	Motimaya *et al.* (1994)

[a] +, positive; –, negative; NT, not tested
[b] LED, lowest effective dose; HID, highest ineffective dose; in-vitro tests, µg/mL; in-vivo tests, mg/kg bw per day; NR, not reported; po, orally; ip, intraperitoneally

et al., 1991), while single intraperitoneal injections of doses up to 0.12 mg/kg bw did not increase the frequency of micronucleated cells in groups of five female and five male Swiss Webster mice (Motimaya *et al.*, 1994). The highest dose used in the latter study was selected to represent the daily dose of a person of average body weight, whereas patient therapy with zalcitabine, in combination with other antiretroviral agents, involves long-term treatment. The question raised by this finding is whether this low dose of zalcitabine failed to induce micronuclei in the mice or whether the genotoxic effects at these exposure levels are too small to be detected in the tests as performed (Shelby, 1994) (see section 4.4.2 in the monograph on zidovudine for further discussion).

[The Working Group considered that a study should be conducted in which mice are exposed to clinically relevant doses of zalcitabine and the frequency of micronucleus formation is evaluated by flow cytometry, as has been done for zidovudine (see section 4.4.2 of the monograph on zidovudine).]

Zhuang *et al.* (1997, 1998) evaluated thymic lymphomas from mice exposed to zalcitabine or 1,3-butadiene for lesions, including homozygous deletions, hypermethylation and point mutations, in several genes critical for cancer. Southern blot analyses revealed homozygous deletions or rearrangements of $p16^{INK4a}$-β or $p15^{INK4b}$ genes in four of 16 tumours from zalcitabine-exposed mice. [The Working Group noted that the value of these studies is limited because spontaneous thymic lymphomas from untreated $B6C3F_1$ mice were not evaluated. Nevertheless, the occurrence of deletions in the tumours from zalcitabine-treated mice is consistent with the action of this drug as a chain terminator.]

4.5   Mechanistic considerations

On a molar basis, zalcitabine is a much more potent antiviral agent than zidovudine (Yarchoan *et al.*, 1989). In humans, the dose-limiting toxic effect, peripheral neuropathy, requires that the daily dose be limited to about 0.2% of that used for zidovudine and didanosine. The main mechanism of the antiviral activity and toxicity of zalcitabine and other 'dideoxy-type' nucleoside analogue drugs (see the monographs on zidovudine and didanosine, sections 4.5) is their phosphorylation and subsequent incorporation into DNA, which leads to inhibition of DNA replication due to lack of a free 3′-hydroxy group (Yarchoan *et al.*, 1990; Devineni & Gallo, 1995; Lewis & Dalakas, 1995) (see also section 4.2). These compounds can competitively inhibit binding of normal nucleotides to the nucleotide binding site of the reverse transcriptase and terminate replication once incorporation has occurred (Yarchoan *et al.*, 1989, 1990). By a similar mechanism, zalcitabine-triphosphate inhibits DNA polymerase β, involved in DNA repair, and DNA polymerase γ, the mitochondrial polymerase.

The inhibition of DNA polymerase γ by zalcitabine is considered to underlie its extensive mitochondrial toxicity and the depletion of mitochondrial DNA (Chen &

Cheng, 1992; Devineni & Gallo, 1995; Lewis & Dalakas, 1995; Benbrik *et al.*, 1997). Chen and Cheng (1992) showed that cells deficient in cytoplasmic deoxycytidine kinase, which were unable to phosphorylate zalcitabine, did not sustain mitochondrial damage or lose mitochondrial DNA. These investigators further demonstrated that zalcitabine, didanosine and zidovudine all induced loss of mitochondrial DNA and increased lactic acid production in the human lymphoblastoid cell line CEM (Chen *et al.*, 1991). In human muscle cells, the loss of mitochondrial DNA induced by either zalcitabine or zidovudine was accompanied by lipid droplet accumulation, lactate production and decreased activities of mitochondrial complexes II (succinate dehydrogenase) and IV (cytochrome *c* oxidase) (Benbrik *et al.*, 1997). The mitochondrial myopathy observed clinically after zidovudine therapy is not seen in patients receiving zalcitabine, perhaps because the doses are limited by the prevalence of peripheral neuropathy.

An association between zalcitabine and peripheral neuropathy was established in a rabbit model by Feldman and Anderson (1994), who observed that rabbits with zalcitabine-induced myelinopathy (section 4.2.2) had abnormal mitochondria in the Schwann cells of sciatic and tibial nerves but not in healthy nerves. The appearance of cup-shaped mitochondria with abnormal cristae coincided with the onset of physical symptoms. Further insight into the underlying mechanism was proposed by Lipman *et al.* (1993), who showed that the extent of zalcitabine phosphorylation is high in rabbits and humans, species which experience peripheral neuropathy, and low in rats and mice, which do not show this effect. Nucleoside phosphorylation and intracellular levels of phosphorylated metabolites play an important role in zalcitabine-related toxicity.

The doses at which zalcitabine induces thymic lymphomas in mice are about 1000-fold higher than the maximum doses tolerated by humans, non-human primates and rabbits.

Studies of the mutagenicity of zalcitabine are scarce; however, the available data indicate that it induces clastogenic effects *in vitro* and *in vivo* at high doses. Its clastogenicity is associated with its action as a DNA chain terminator. The potential importance of deletion mutations in zalcitabine-induced mutagenesis and carcinogenesis *in vivo* is supported by the high frequency of homozygous deletions in tumour suppressor genes in thymic lymphomas from zalcitabine-exposed $B6C3F_1$ mice. With regard to exposure, it is noteworthy that the maximum plasma concentration in mice dosed orally with 100 mg/kg bw is about 15 μg/mL, while the maximum concentration in humans receiving typical treatment with zalcitabine is 5–8 ng/mL (see section 4.1.1).

5. Summary of Data Reported and Evaluation

5.1 Exposure data

Zalcitabine is a nucleoside analogue that has been used to treat HIV infections in adults and children. The drug entered clinical use around 1990, but it is no longer in common use since several clinical studies showed it to be less active than other nucleoside analogues.

5.2 Human carcinogenicity data

The only data available were from two trials designed to assess the efficacy of zalcitabine in improving the degree of immunocompetence and survival of patients with HIV infection and one phase I trial of zalcitabine alternated with zidovudine. No conclusion could be drawn concerning carcinogenicity.

5.3 Animal carcinogenicity data

Zalcitabine was tested for carcinogenicity in four studies in mice by gavage. Treatment resulted in induction of thymic lymphomas in all studies.

5.4 Other relevant data

The human pharmacokinetics of orally administered zalcitabine appears to be linear over a broad dose range. Zalcitabine is about 80% bioavailable and is rapidly absorbed, distributed and eliminated in urine, mainly as the unchanged drug. Phosphorylation is essential to its antiviral activity but accounts for a very small fraction of its total disposition. Its pharmacokinetics in several species of experimental animals are similar to that in humans.

Side-effects observed in clinical trials and use include peripheral neuropathy, mucositis and, rarely, hepatotoxicity. Several of these effects, particularly neurotoxicity and hepatotoxicity, also occur in non-human primates, dogs, rabbits and rodents treated with zalcitabine.

No studies were available on the reproductive or prenatal effects of zalcitabine in humans. Developmental toxicity, with effects on litter size and fetal weight and malformations, was observed after oral administration of 1000 mg/kg bw per day zalcitabine to mice on days 6–15 of gestation. Studies of transplacental pharmacokinetics in monkeys indicated that zalcitabine crosses the placenta by passive diffusion; zalcitabine and zalcitabine monophosphate appear in fetal plasma and tissues after administration of zalcitabine to pregnant animals.

The limited data on genetic and related effects indicate that zalcitabine is primarily a clastogenic agent at high concentrations, consistent with its action as a DNA chain terminator.

5.5 Evaluation

There is *inadequate evidence* in humans for the carcinogenicity of zalcitabine.

There is *sufficient evidence* in experimental animals for the carcinogenicity of zalcitabine.

Overall evaluation

Zalcitabine is *possibly carcinogenic to humans (Group 2B)*.

6. References

Abrams, D.I., Goldman, A.I., Launer, C., Korvick, J.A., Neaton, J.D., Crane, L.R., Grodesky, M., Wakefield, S., Muth, K., Kornegay, S., Cohn, D.L., Harris, A., Luskin-Hawk, R., Markowitz, N., Sampson, J.H., Thompson, M., Deyton, L. & the Terry Beirn Community Programs for Clinical Research on AIDS (1994) A comparative trial of didanosine or zalcitabine after treatment with zidovudine in patients with human immunodeficiency virus infection. *New Engl. J. Med.*, **330**, 657–662

American Hospital Formulary Service (1997) *AHFS Drug Information® 97*, Bethesda, MD, American Society of Health-System Pharmacists, pp. 528–538

Anderson, T.D., Davidovich, A., Arceo, R., Brosnan, C., Arezzo, J. & Schaumburg, H. (1991) Peripheral neuropathy induced by 2′,3′-dideoxycytidine. A rabbit model of 2′,3′-dideoxycitidine neurotoxicity. *Lab. Invest.*, **66**, 63–74

Anderson, T.D., Davidovich, A., Feldman, D., Sprinkle, T.J., Arezzo, J., Brosnan, C., Calderon, R.O., Fossom, L.H., DeVries, J.T. & DeVries, G.H. (1994) Mitochondrial schwannopathy and peripheral myelinopathy in a rabbit model of dideoxycytidine neurotoxicity. *Lab. Invest.*, **70**, 724–739

Bartlett, J.A., Benoit, S.L., Johnson, V.A., Quinn, J.B., Sepulveda, G.E., Ehmann, W.C., Tsoukas, C., Fallon, M.A., Self, P.L. & Rubin, M. for the North American HIV Working Party (1996) Lamivudine plus zidovudine compared with zalcitabine plus zidovudine in patients with HIV infection. *Ann. intern. Med.*, **125**, 161–172

Bazunga, M., Tran, H.T., Kertland, H., Chow, M.S.S. & Massarella, J. (1998) The effects of renal impairment on the pharmacokinetics of zalcitabine. *J. clin. Pharmacol.*, **38**, 28–33

Beach, J.W. (1998) Chemotherapeutic agents for human immunodeficiency virus infection: Mechanism of action, pharmacokinetics, metabolism, and adverse reactions. *Clin. Ther.*, **20**, 2–25

Benbrik, E., Chariot, P., Bonavaud, S., Ammi-Saïd, M., Frisdal, E., Rey, C., Gherardi, R. & Barlovatz-Meimon, G. (1997) Cellular and mitochondrial toxicity of zidovudine (AZT), didanosine (ddI) and zalcitabine (ddC) on cultured human muscle cells. *J. neurol. Sci.*, **149**, 19–25

Blum, A.S., Dal Pan, G.J., Feinberg, J., Raines, C., Mayjo, K., Cornblath, D.R. & McArthur, J.C. (1996) Low-dose zalcitabine-related toxic neuropathy: Frequency, natural history, and risk factors. *Neurology*, **46**, 999–1003

British Medical Association/Royal Pharmaceutical Society of Great Britain (1998) *British National Formulary*, No. 36, London, p. 278

Broder, S. (1990) Pharmacodynamics of 2',3'-dideoxycytidine: An inhibitor of human immunodeficiency virus. *Am. J. Med.*, **88**, 2S–7S

Budavari, S., ed. (1996) *The Merck Index*, 12th Ed., Whitehouse Station, NJ, Merck & Co., p. 1730

Burger, D.M., Meenhorst, P.L. & Beijnen, J.H. (1995) Concise overview of the clinical pharmacokinetics of dideoxynucleoside antiretroviral agents. *Pharm. World Sci.*, **17**, 25–30

Canadian Pharmaceutical Association (1997) *CPS Compendium of Pharmaceuticals and Specialties*, 32nd Ed., Ottawa, pp. 667–671

Chen, C.-H. & Cheng, Y.-C. (1992) The role of cytoplasmic deoxycytidine kinase in the mitochondrial effects of the anti-human immunodeficiency virus compound, 2',3'-dideoxycytidine. *J. biol. Chem.*, **267**, 2856–2859

Chen, C.-H., Vazquez-Padua, M. & Cheng, Y.-C. (1991) Effect of anti-human immunodeficiency virus nucleoside analogs on mitochondrial DNA and its implication for delayed toxicity. *Mol. Pharmacol.*, **39**, 625–628

CIS Information Services (1998) *Worldwide Bulk Drug Users Directory 1997/98 Edition*, Dallas, TX [CD-ROM]

Delta Coordinating Committee (1996) Delta: A randomised double-blind controlled trial comparing combinations of zidovudine plus didanosine or zalcitabine with zidovudine alone in HIV-infected individuals. *Lancet*, **348**, 283–291

Devineni, D. & Gallo, J.M. (1995) Zalcitabine. Clinical pharmacokinetics and efficacy. *Clin. Pharmacokinet.*, **28**, 351–360

Editions du Vidal (1998) *Dictionnaire Vidal 1998*, 74th Ed., Paris, OVP, pp. 879–881

Feldman, D. & Anderson, T.D. (1994) Schwann cell mitochondrial alterations in peripheral nerves of rabbits treated with 2',3'-dideoxycytidine. *Acta neuropathol.*, **87**, 71–80

Feldman, D., Brosnan, C. & Anderson, T.D. (1992) Ultrastructure of peripheral neuropathy induced in rabbits by 2',3'-dideoxycytidine. *Lab. Invest.*, **66**, 75–85

Fichtenbaum, C.J., Clifford, D.B. & Powderly, W.G. (1995) Risk factors for dideoxynucleoside-induced toxic neuropathy in patients with the human immunodeficiency virus infection. *J. acquir. Immune Defic. Syndr.*, **10**, 169–174

Fischl, M.A., Stanley, K., Collier, A.C., Arduino, J.M., Stein, D.S., Feinberg, J.E., Allan, J.D., Goldsmith, J.C., Powderly, W.G. and the NIAID AIDS Clinical Trials Group (1995) Combination and monotherapy with zidovudine and zalcitabine in patients with advanced HIV disease. *Ann. intern. Med.*, **122**, 24–32

Foerster, M., Kastner, U. & Neubert, R. (1992) Effect of six virustatic nucleoside analogues on the development of fetal rat thymus in organ culture. *Arch. Toxicol.*, **66**, 688–699

Gennaro, A.R. (1995) *Remington: The Science and Practice of Pharmacy*, 19th Ed., Easton, PA, Mack Publishing, Vol. II, pp. 1335–1336

Gustavson, L.E., Fukuda, E.K., Rubio, F.A. & Dunton, A.W. (1990) A pilot study of the bioavailability and pharmacokinetics of 2′,3′-dideoxycytidine in patients with AIDS or AIDS-related complex. *J. aquir. Immune Defic. Syndr.*, **3**, 28–31

Hammer, S.M., Katzenstein, D.A., Hughes, M.D., Gundacker, H., Schooley, R.T., Haubrich, R.H., Henry, W.K., Lederman, M.M., Phair, J.P., Niu, M., Hirsch, M.S. & Merigan, T.C. for the AIDS Clinical Trials Group Study 175 Study Team (1996). A trial comparing nucleoside monotherapy with combination therapy in HIV-infected adults with CD4 cell counts from 200 to 500 per cubic millimeter. *New Engl. J. Med.*, **335**, 1081–1090

Henry, K., Acosta, E.P. & Jochimsen, E. (1996) Hepatotoxicity and rash associated with zidovudine and zalcitabine chemoprophylaxis (Letter to the Editor). *Ann. intern. Med.*, **124**, 855

Henry, K., Erice, A., Tierney, C., Balfour, H.H., Jr, Fischl, M.A., Kmack, A., Liou, S.H., Kenton, A., Hirsch, M.S., Phair, J., Martinez, A. & Kahn, J.O. for the AIDS Clinical Trial Group 193A Study Team (1998) A randomized, controlled, double-blind study comparing the survival benefit of four different reverse transcriptase inhibitor therapies (three-drug, two-drug, and alternating drug) for the treatment of advanced AIDS. *J. acquir. Immune Defic. Syndr. hum. Retrovirol.*, **19**, 339–349

Horwitz, J.P., Chua, J., Noel, M. & Donatti, J.T. (1967) Nucleosides. XI. 2′,3′-Dideoxycitidine. *J. org. Chem.*, **32**, 817–818

Ibrahim, S.S. & Boudinot, F.D. (1989) Pharmacokinetics of 2′,3′-dideoxycytidine in rats: Application to interspecies scale-up. *J. pharm. Pharmacol.*, **41**, 829–834

Ibrahim, S.S. & Boudinot, F.D. (1991) Pharmacokinetics of 2′,3′-dideoxycytidine after high-dose administration to rats. *J. pharm. Sci.*, **80**, 36–38

Indorf, A.S. & Pegram, P.S. (1992) Esophageal ulceration related to zalcitabine (ddC). *Ann. intern. Med.*, **117**, 133–134

Kelley, J.A., Litterst, C.L., Roth, J.S, Vistica, D.T., Poplack, D.G., Cooney, D.A., Nadkarni, M., Balis, F.M., Broder, S. & Johns, D.G. (1987) The disposition and metabolism of 2′,3′-dideoxycytidine, an *in vitro* inhibitor of human T-lymphotrophic virus type III infectivity, in mice and monkeys. *Drug Metab. Dispos.*, **15**, 595–601

Klecker, R.W., Jr, Collins, J.M., Yarchoan, R.C., Thomas, R., McAtee, N., Broder, S. & Myers, C.E. (1988) Pharmacokinetics of 2′,3′-dideoxycytidine in patients with AIDS and related disorders. *J. clin. Pharmacol.*, **28**, 837–842

Lewis, W. & Dalakas, M.C. (1995) Mitochondrial toxicity of antiviral drugs. *Nature Med.*, **1**, 417–422

Lin, T.S., Chen, M.S., McLaren, C., Gao, Y.S., Ghazzouli, I. & Prusoff, W.H. (1987) Synthesis and antiviral activity of various 3′-azido, 3′-amino, 2′,3′-unsaturated, and 2′,3′-dideoxy analogues of pyrimidine deoxyribonucleosides against retroviruses. *J. med. Chem.*, **30**, 440–444

Lindström, P., Harris, M., Hoberman, A.M., Dunnick, J.K. & Morrissey, R.E. (1990) Developmental toxicity of orally administered 2′,3′-dideoxycitidine in mice. *Teratology*, **42**, 131–136

Lipman, J.M., Reichert, J.A., Davidovich, A. & Anderson, T.D. (1993) Species differences in nucleotide pool levels of 2′,3′-dideoxycytidine: A possible explanation for species-specific toxicity. *Toxicol. appl. Pharmacol.*, **123**, 137–143

Luster, M.I., Rosenthal, G.J., Cao, W., Thompson, M.B., Munson, A.E., Prejean, J.D., Shopp, G., Fuchs, B.A., Germolec, D.R. & Tomaszewski, J.E. (1991) Experimental studies of the hematologic and immune system toxicity of nucleoside derivatives used against HIV infection. *Int. J. Immunopharmacol.*, **13**, 99–107

Makabi-Panzu, B., Lessard, C., Perron, S., Désormeaux, A., Tremblay, M., Poulin, L., Beauchamp, D. & Bergeron, M.G. (1994) Comparison of cellular accumulation, tissue distribution, and anti-HIV activity of free and liposomal 2′,3′-dideoxycytidine. *AIDS Res. hum. Retroviruses*, **10**, 1463–1470

Mamber, S.W., Brookshire, K.W. & Forenza, S. (1990) Induction of the SOS response in *Escherichia coli* by azidothymidine and dideoxynucleosides. *Antimicrob. Agents Chemother.*, **34**, 1237–1243

Marumoto, R. & Honjo, M. (1974) One-step halogenation at the 2′-position of uridine, and related reactions of cytidine and N^4-acetylcytidine. *Chem. pharm. Bull.*, **22**, 128–134

Medical Economics Data Production (1999) *PDR®: Physicians' Desk Reference*, 53rd Ed., Montvale, NJ, pp. 810–812

Menconi, M., Lerza, R., Bogliolo, G., Flego, G., Gasparini, L. & Pannacciulli, I. (1990) Dideoxycytidine toxicity on mouse hemopoietic progenitors. *In Vivo*, **4**, 171–174

Motimaya, A.M., Subramanya, K.S., Curry, P.T. & Kitchin, R.M. (1994) Evaluation of the genotoxic potential of selected anti-AIDS treatment drugs at clinical doses in vivo in mice. *Toxicol. Lett.*, **70**, 171–183

National Cancer Institute (1992) *NCI Investigational Drugs—Chemical Information—1992* (NIH Publication No. 92-2654), Bethesda, MD, National Institutes of Health, pp. 80–82

Phillips, M.D., Nascimbeni, B., Tice, R.R. & Shelby, M.D. (1991) Induction of micronuclei in mouse bone marrow cells: An evaluation of nucleoside analogues used in the treatment of AIDS. *Environ. mol. Mutag.*, **18**, 168–183

Pluda, J.M., Yarchoan, R., Jaffe, E.S., Feuerstein, I.M., Solomon, D., Steinberg, S.M., Wyvill, K.M., Raubitschek, A., Katz, D. & Broder, S. (1990) Development of non-Hodgkin's lymphoma in a cohort of patients with severe human immunodeficinecy virus (HIV) infection on long-term antiretroviral therapy. *Ann. intern. Med.*, **113**, 276–282

Pluda, J.M., Venzon, D.J., Tosato, G., Lietzau, J., Wyvill, K., Nelson, D.L., Jaffe, E.S., Karp, J.E., Broder, S. & Yarchoan, R. (1993) Parameters affecting the development of non-Hodgkin's lymphoma in patients with severe human immunodeficiency virus infection receiving antiretroviral therapy. *J. clin. Oncol.*, **11**, 1099–1107

Qian, M., Swagler, A.R., Fong, K.-L., Crysler, C.S., Mehta, M. & Gallo, J.M. (1992) Pharmacokinetic evaluation of drug interactions with anti-human immunodeficiency virus drugs. V. Effect of soluble CD4 on 2′,3′-dideoxycytidine kinetics in monkeys. *Drug Metab. Dispos.*, **20**, 396–401

Rao, G.N., Collins, B.J., Giles, H.D., Heath, J.E., Foley, J.F., May, R.D. & Buckley, L.A. (1996) Carcinogenicity of 2′,3′-dideoxycytidine in mice. *Cancer Res.*, **56**, 4666–4672

Riley, J.H., Davidovich, A., Lipman, J.M., Arceo, R. & Anderson, T.D. (1992) Hematological effects of 2′,3′-dideoxycytidine in rabbits. *Toxicol. Pathol.*, **20**, 367–375

Roche Laboratories (1998) *Hivid® (Zalcitabine) Tablets*, Nutley, NJ, pp. 1–11

Rote Liste Sekretariat (1998) *Rote Liste 1998*, Frankfurt, Rote Liste Service GmbH, pp. 10-448–10-449

Sandberg, J.A., Bintenda, Z., Lipe, G., Rose, L.M., Parker, W.B., Ali, S.F. & Slikker, W., Jr (1995) Placental transfer and fetal disposition of 2′,3′-dideoxycytidine and 2′,3′-dideoxyinosine in the rhesus monkey. *Drug Metab. Dispos.*, **23**, 881–884

Sanders, V.M., Elwell, M.R., Heath, J.E., Collins, B.J., Dunnick, J.K., Rao, G.N., Prejean, D., Lindamood, C. & Irwin, R.D. (1995) Induction of thymic lymphoma in mice administered the dideoxynucleoside ddC. *Fundam. appl. Toxicol.*, **27**, 263–269

Schooley, R.T., Ramirez-Ronda, C., Lange, J.M.A., Cooper, D.A., Lavelle, J., Lefkowitz, L., Moore, M., Larder, B.A., St Clair, M., Mulder, J.W., McKinnis, R., Pennington, K.N., Harrigan, P.R., Kinghorn, I., Steel, H., Rooney, J.F. & the Wellcome Resistance Study Collaborative Group (1996) Virologic and immunologic benefits of initial combination therapy with zidovudine and zalcitabine or didanosine compared with zidovudine monotherapy. *J. infect. Dis.*, **173**, 1354–1366

Shelby, M.D. (1994) The cytogenetic effects of AZT. *Environ. mol. Mutag.*, **24**, 148–149

Skowron, G. (1996) ddc (Zalcitabine). In: Mills, J., Volberding, P.A. & Corey, L., eds, *Antiviral Chemotherapy*, New York, Plenum Press, Vol. 4, pp. 257–269

Swagler, A.R., Qian, M. & Gallo, J.M. (1991) Pharmacokinetics of anti-HIV nucleosides in microswine. *J. pharm. Pharmacol.*, **43**, 823–826

Swiss Pharmaceutical Society, ed. (1999) *Index Nominum, International Drug Directory*, 16th Ed., Stuttgart, Medpharm Scientific Publishers [MicroMedex Online: Health Care Series]

Taylor, L.V.D., Binienda, Z., Schmued, L. & Slikker, W., Jr (1994) The effect of dideoxycytidine on lymphocyte subpopulations in nonhuman primates. *Fundam. appl. Toxicol.*, **23**, 434–438

Thomas, J., ed. (1998) *Australian Prescription Products Guide*, 27th Ed., Victoria, Australian Pharmaceutical Publishing, Vol. 1, pp. 1377–1384

Thompson, M.B., Dunnick, J.K., Sutphin, M.E., Giles, H.D., Irwin, R.D. & Prejean, J.D. (1991) Hematologic toxicity of AZT and ddC administered as single agents and in combination to rats and mice. *Fundam. appl. Toxicol.*, **17**, 159–176

Tsai, C.-C., Follis, K.E., Yarnall, M. & Blakley, G.A. (1989) Toxicity and efficacy of 2′,3′-dideoxycytidine in clinical trials of pigtailed macaques infected with simian retrovirus type 2. *Antimicrob. Agents Chemother.*, **33**, 1908–1914

Tuntland, T., Nosbisch, C., Baughman, W.L., Massarella, J. & Unadkat, J.D. (1996) Mechanism and rate of placental transfer of zalcitabine (2′,3′-dideoxycytidine) in *Macaca nemestrina*. *Am. J. Obstet. Gynecol.*, **174**, 856–863

US Food & Drug Administration Antiviral Drugs Advisory Committee (1993) *Mitochondrial Damage Associated with Nucleoside Analogues*, Rockville, MD

US Pharmacopeial Convention (1997) *The 1995 US Pharmacopeia*, 23rd Rev./*The National Formulary*, 18th Rev., Supplement 7, Rockville, MD, pp. 3949–3950

US Pharmacopeial Convention (1998) *USP Dispensing Information*, Vol. I, *Drug Information for the Health Care Professional*, 18th Ed., Rockville, MD, pp. 3002–3004

Vanhove, G.F., Kastrissios, H., Gries, J.-M., Verotta, D., Park, K., Collier, A.C., Squires, K., Sheiner, L.B. & Blaschke, T.F. (1997) Pharmacokinetics of saquinavir, zidovudine, and zalcitabine in combination therapy. *Antimicrob. Agents Chemother.*, **41**, 2428–2432

Yarchoan, R., Mitsuya, H., Myers, C.E. & Broder, S. (1989) Clinical pharmacology of 3′-azido-2′,3′-dideoxythymidine (zidovudine) and related dideoxynucleosides. *New Engl. J. Med.*, **321**, 726–738

Yarchoan, R., Pluda, J.M., Perno, C.F., Mitsuya, H., Thomas, R.V., Wyvill, K.M. & Broder, S. (1990) Initial clinical experience with dideoxynucleosides as single agents and in combination therapy. *Ann. N.Y. Acad. Sci.*, **616**, 328–343

Zhuang, S.-M., Cochran, C., Goudrow, T., Wiseman, R.W. & Söderkvist, P. (1997) Genetic alterations of *p53* and *ras* genes in 1,3-butadiene- and 2′,3′-dideoxycytidine-induced lymphomas. *Cancer Res.*, **57**, 2710–2714

Zhuang, S.-M., Shipput, A., Haugen-Srano, A., Wiseman, R.W. & Söderquist, P. (1998) Inactivations of p15^{INK4a}-α, P16^{INK4a}-β, and p15^{INK4b} genes in 2′,3′-dideoxycytidine- and 1,3-butadiene-induced murine lymphomas. *Oncogene*, **16**, 803–808

DIDANOSINE

1. Exposure Data

1.1 Chemical and physical data

1.1.1 Nomenclature

Chem. Abstr. Serv. Reg. No.: 69655-05-6
Chem. Abstr. Name: 2′,3′-Dideoxyinosine
IUPAC Systematic Name: 2′,3′-Dideoxyinosine
Synonyms: ddI; DDI; dideoxyinosine

1.1.2 Structural and molecular formulae and relative molecular mass

$C_{10}H_{12}N_4O_3$ Relative molecular mass: 236.23

1.1.3 Chemical and physical properties of the pure substance

(a) *Description*: White, nonhygroscopic crystalline powder (American Hospital Formulary Service, 1997)
(b) *Melting-point*: 160–163 °C (Budavari, 1996)
(c) *Spectroscopy data*: Infrared, ultraviolet, nuclear magnetic resonance (proton and ^{13}C) and mass spectral data have been reported (Nassar *et al.*, 1993).
(d) *Solubility*: Soluble in water (27.3 mg/mL at 25 °C and pH 6.2); soluble in dimethylsulfoxide; slightly soluble in ethanol and methanol; insoluble in chloroform (National Cancer Institute, 1992; Nassar *et al.*, 1993; American Hospital Formulary Service, 1997)

(e) *Stability*: Stable at neutral or slightly alkaline pH, but unstable at acidic pH. At pH less than 3, complete hydrolysis to hypoxanthine and 2',3'-dideoxyribose occurs in less than 2 min at 27 °C (American Hospital Formulary Service, 1997)

(f) *Dissociation constant*: pK_a, 9.13 (American Hospital Formulary Service, 1997)

(g) *Optical rotation*: $[\alpha]_D^{20}$, –25.7 ± 2° (National Cancer Institute, 1992)

1.1.4 *Technical products and impurities*

Didanosine is available as a 25-, 50-, 100- and 150-mg chewable, dispersible buffered tablet, a 100-, 167-, 250- and 375-mg buffered powder for oral solution and a 2- and 4-g unbuffered paediatric powder for oral solution. The tablets may also contain aspartame, calcium carbonate, dihydroxyaluminium sodium carbonate, flavours (mandarin orange, wintergreen), magnesium hydroxide, magnesium stearate, microcrystalline cellulose, phenylalanine, polyplasdone, silicon dioxide, sodium citrate, sorbitol and sucrose. The buffered powder for oral solution is buffered with a citrate–phosphate buffer (composed of dibasic sodium phosphate, sodium citrate and citric acid) and sucrose (Gennaro, 1995; American Hospital Formulary Service, 1997; Canadian Pharmaceutical Association, 1997; Bristol-Myers Squibb Co., 1998; British Medical Association/Royal Pharmaceutical Society of Great Britain, 1998; Editions du Vidal, 1998; LINFO Läkemedelsinformation AB, 1998; Rote Liste Sekretariat, 1998; Thomas, 1998; US Pharmacopeial Convention, 1998).

Trade names for didanosine include DDI Filaxis, Megavir, Ronvir and Videx (Swiss Pharmaceutical Society, 1999).

1.1.5 *Analysis*

Several reverse-phase high-performance liquid chromatography (HPLC) methods have been reported for the determination of didanosine and its impurities or degradates in bulk drug substance or formulations. HPLC procedures also have been developed for the analysis of didanosine and its major metabolite, hypoxanthine, in biological fluids, including plasma, urine and cerebrospinal fluid (Nassar *et al.*, 1993).

1.2 Production

2',3'-Dideoxynucleosides are typically synthesized from 2'-deoxynucleosides by Barton-type deoxygenation reactions or from intact nucleosides by several steps involving deoxygenation reactions to 2',3'-unsaturated deoxynucleosides, which are then hydrogenated. Approaches through ketonucleosides and a photoreductive process have also been described (Nassar *et al.*, 1993).

Selective benzoylation of the 5′-hydroxyl group of 2′-deoxyinosine is achieved by dropwise addition of a pyridine solution of benzoyl chloride to 2′-deoxyinosine suspended in pyridine. The 5′-*O*-benzoyl-2′-deoxyinosine formed is then treated in one portion with 1,1′-thiocarbonyldiimidazole to form the thioimidazolide. Deoxygenation at the 3′ position of the thioimidazolide gives 5′-*O*-benzoyl-2′,3′-dideoxyinosine. Removal of the benzoate group by treatment with anhydrous methanol saturated with anhydrous ammonia at 0 °C yields didanosine in 90% yield (Nassar *et al.*, 1993).

Didanosine has also been prepared enzymatically by deamination of 2′,3′-dideoxyadenosine with adenosine deaminase at room temperature. Recrystallization from methanol gave an 85% yield (Nassar *et al.*, 1993).

Information available in 1999 indicated that didanosine was manufactured and/or formulated in 26 countries (CIS Information Services, 1998; Swiss Pharmaceutical Society, 1999).

1.3   Use

Didanosine is a nucleoside analogue and a highly potent nucleoside reverse transcriptase inhibitor, which has been used in the treatment of human immunodeficiency virus (HIV) infections since 1990 (Lambert *et al.*, 1990). It is among the most durable agents in this class (i.e. viral resistance develops most slowly) (Kahn *et al.*, 1992; Spruance *et al.*, 1994; Dolin *et al.*, 1995; Hammer *et al.*, 1996; Englund *et al.*, 1997), although resistance does eventually develop (Kozal *et al.*, 1994). It has been extensively studied both as a single therapy and in combinations, especially with zidovudine (see monograph, this volume) and didehydrodideoxythymidine (stavudine) (Montaner *et al.*, 1998; Raffi *et al.*, 1998); combinations are more effective than monotherapy (McKinney *et al.*, 1998).

The major drawback of the agent in its current formulation is that its acid lability requires administration on an empty stomach with a substantial quantity of antacid, which can lead to gastrointestinal intolerance (Pike & Nicaise, 1993; American Hospital Formulary Service, 1997). An enteric coated form, which still must be taken on an empty stomach but does not contain antacids, is being developed.

The rare development of pancreatitis (which can be severe) and peripheral neuropathy limited use of this agent in initial therapy in the past (Pike & Nicaise, 1993). It is currently being prescribed for once-daily administration (Cooley *et al.*, 1990), and in combination with hydroxyurea to potentiate its antiviral effect (see the monograph on hydroxyurea, this volume).

Like most nucleoside analogues, didanosine is excreted primarily in the kidney, and the dose should probably be modified for patients with renal dysfunction (Singlas *et al.*, 1992; Knupp *et al.*, 1996).

1.4 Occurrence

Didanosine is not known to occur as a natural product. No data on occupational exposure were available to the Working Group.

1.5 Regulations and guidelines

Didanosine is not listed in any international pharmacopoeias.

2. Studies of Cancer in Humans

Pluda *et al.* (1993) examined the records of 61 patients with AIDS or severe AIDS-related complex (defined as having either oral candidiasis, oral hairy leukoplakia or weight loss of > 10% of total body weight) who were entered into a phase I study of didanosine and 2′,3′-dideoxyadenosine during 1988–89. 2′,3′-Dideoxyadenosine is rapidly converted to didanosine after its administration. All patients had fewer than 350 CD4 cells/µL plasma at the time of entry. They were treated and followed for a maximum of 3.7 years, during which time four (6.6%) developed a non-Hodgkin lymphoma, all of which were characterized as high-grade B-cell tumours. The estimated cumulative risk of all 61 patients of developing non-Hodgkin lymphoma by 24 months of therapy was 6.2% (95% confidence interval [CI], 2.1–17%, Kaplan-Meier method), increasing to 9.5% (3.6–23%) by 36 months. [The Working Group noted that the cumulative risks are difficult to interpret in the absence of a suitable reference group consisting of AIDS patients with a similar degree of immunosuppression.]

In a multicentre trial in the USA, Abrams *et al.* (1994) randomly assigned 467 symptomatic HIV-infected patients with CD4 counts of ≤ 300 cells/µL plasma who had previously received zidovudine to treatment with either didanosine at 500 mg per day ($n = 230$) or zalcitabine at 2.25 mg per day ($n = 237$). The patients were recruited during 1990–91 and were treated and followed up for a median of 1.3 years and a maximum of 1.8 years. Three cases of non-Hodgkin lymphoma was seen in the didanosine-treated group and six in the zalcitabine-treated group. [The Working Group noted that rate ratios were not calculated, although the risk ratio for non-Hodgkin lymphoma in patients treated with didanosine compared with that in the patients receiving zalcitabine was 0.5 (95% CI, 0.13–2.0), with no adjustment for differences in survival between the two groups.]

In an international randomized trial, the Delta Coordinating Committee (1996) allocated 3207 individuals with antibodies to HIV, symptoms of infection or a CD4 count of 350 cells/µL plasma to treatment with either zidovudine at 600 mg per day ($n = 1055$), zidovudine plus didanosine at 400 mg per day ($n = 1080$) or zidovudine plus zalcitabine at 2.25 mg per day ($n = 1072$). The patients were treated and followed up for a median of 2.5 years (range, 1.8–2.9), during which time 14 deaths due to cancer [not further specified] occurred; five of the deaths occurred in the group treated with zidovudine alone, five in the group treated with zidovudine plus didanosine and four in the group treated with zalcitabine.

[The Working Group noted that these trials were designed to compare the efficacy of drugs in the treatment of patients with various degrees of severity of immunosuppression. For the purposes of evaluating cancer risk, therefore, the numbers of participants were too small and the length of follow-up too short, cancer incidence may have been underascertained, and cancer rates could not be analysed adequately.]

3. Studies of Cancer in Experimental Animals

No data were available to the Working Group.

4. Other Data Relevant to an Evaluation of Carcinogenicity and its Mechanisms

4.1 Absorption, distribution, metabolism and excretion

4.1.1 *Humans*

The pharmacokinetics of didanosine has been reviewed and summarized extensively (Hartman *et al.*, 1990; Yarchoan *et al.*, 1990a; Knupp *et al.*, 1991; Faulds & Brogden, 1992; Perry & Balfour, 1996; Beach, 1998). The pharmacokinetics is linear over a broad dose range (0.4–16.5 mg/kg bw) and is similar after a single initial oral dose and after weeks of oral dosing (Knupp *et al.*, 1991). Drug disposition can be slowed significantly, however, in patients with compromised renal function (Burger *et al.*, 1995; Perry & Balfour, 1996). The peak concentration in plasma ranges between 2.2 and 11.8 μmol/L (0.52–2.8 mg/L) for doses between 125 and 375 mg and is reached after 30–60 min (Hartman *et al.*, 1990; Burger *et al.*, 1995; Perry & Balfour, 1996). The half-time for removal of the drug from plasma is approximately 1 h (Hartman *et al.*, 1990; Knupp *et al.*, 1991; Faulds & Brogden, 1992; Perry & Balfour, 1996). The total body clearance rate after oral administration has been reported to be 20–60 L/h, and the renal clearance is somewhat slower, about 20–30 L/h (Hartman *et al.*, 1990; Knupp *et al.*, 1991; Faulds & Brogden, 1992; Perry & Balfour, 1996; Beach, 1998). The pharmacokinetics of didanosine is not significantly altered when it is administered with zidovudine (Morse *et al.*, 1995; Sahai *et al.*, 1995).

A single oral dose of 375 mg didanosine was administered to two pregnant women (length of amenorrhoea, 21 and 24 weeks). Maternal blood was collected by venepuncture, and amniotic fluid and fetal blood samples were taken 65 and 78 min after treatment. Didanosine crossed the placenta, with fetal:maternal ratios of 0.14 and 0.19 (Pons et al., 1991).

Single, isolated portions (cotyledons) of fresh, full-term human placenta were perfused from both the fetal and the maternal side with Krebs-Ringer buffer (closed or open system). The transfer of didanosine (3–30 μmol/L) across the placenta was reported to be passive, with equal transfer in both directions. Little or no placental metabolism of didanosine was reported (Dalton & Au, 1993; Henderson et al., 1994).

Single, isolated cotyledons of fresh, full-term placenta were perfused from both the fetal and the maternal side with Earle's buffered salt solution with added glucose, amino acids and serum albumin (concentration of didanosine, 1–500 μmol/L). Neither perfusate was recirculated. HPLC of the maternal outflow indicated that 25% of the didanosine was metabolized, whereas about 50% of that in the fetal perfusate was metabolized. No didanosine triphosphate was detected in the placenta (Dancis et al., 1993).

The absorption, distribution, metabolism and excretion of didanosine in adults with and without HIV infection have been reviewed extensively (Yarchoan et al., 1990a; Faulds & Brogden, 1992; Burger et al., 1995; Perry & Balfour, 1996; Beach, 1998). Most of these studies and the use of the drug in clinical practice involve oral dosing at 400 mg/day, although intravenous dosing was documented in a number of studies (Perry & Balfour, 1996). Oral dosing poses specific problems because the drug is acid-labile and its bioavailability decreases in the presence of food (Hartman et al., 1991). When didanosine is given with antacid at doses of 0.8–10.2 mg/kg bw per day to fasting patients, its bioavailability is 35–40% (Yarchoan et al., 1990a; Hartman et al., 1991; Knupp et al., 1991; Perry & Balfour, 1996), and its entry into cells is thought to occur by passive diffusion (Faulds & Brogden, 1992). Didanosine is poorly bound to plasma proteins ($\leq 5\%$) (Burger et al., 1995; Perry & Balfour, 1996) and is apparently less widely distributed than zidovudine because it is less lipophilic (Perry & Balfour, 1996). It is, however, distributed to plasma and cerebrospinal fluid, the concentrations in the latter typically being much lower than those in plasma (Hartman et al., 1990; Yarchoan et al., 1990a; Perry & Balfour, 1996; Beach, 1998).

Didanosine is metabolized along two pathways (Figure 1). A quantitatively minor pathway that is responsible for the antiretroviral activity of the drug involves phosphorylation and reversible amination of didanosine monophosphate to dideoxyadenosine monophosphate through the action of adenylosuccinate synthetase and adenylosuccinate lyase (Yarchoan et al., 1990a; Back et al., 1992; Faulds & Brogden, 1992). The dideoxyadenosine monophosphate is further phosphorylated to the triphosphate (ddATP) by purine nucleoside monophosphate kinase and purine nucleoside diphosphate kinase. The intracellular half-time of ddATP is 12–24 h, suggesting that less frequent dosing may be required than with zidovudine or zalcitabine (Yarchoan et al., 1990a). In addition to inhibiting the viral reverse transcriptase, ddATP becomes incorporated into DNA and terminates the replicating DNA chain in both cellular and viral DNA (Faulds & Brogden, 1992). Although dideoxyadenosine phosphorylation is

Figure 1. Metabolic pathways of didanosine

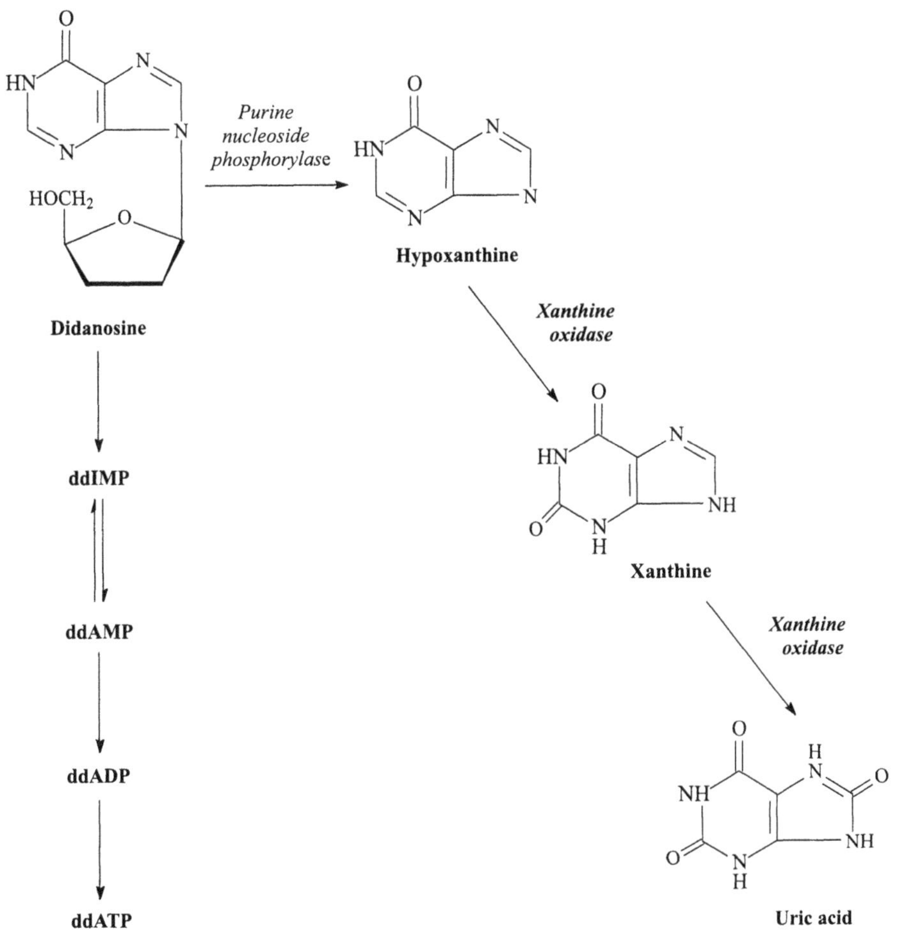

From Back et al. (1992)
ddIMP, didanosine 5'-monophosphate; ddAMP, 2',3'-dideoxyadenosine 5'-monophosphate; ddADP, 2'3'-dideoxyadenosine 5'-diphosphate; ddATP, 2'3'-dideoxyadenoxine 5'-triphosphate

critical to the mechanism of antiviral activity, it is responsible for only a small fraction of the total drug disposition. Approximately 40% of the total dose is recovered as unchanged drug in the urine, about 50% as hypoxanthine and about 4% as uric acid (Yarchoan et al., 1990a; Faulds & Brogden, 1992; Burger et al., 1995; Perry & Balfour, 1996; Beach, 1998), while non-renal clearance occurs via metabolism and/or biliary excretion (Back et al., 1992; Burger et al., 1995). The major metabolic pathway (Figure 1) involves metabolism to uric acid through purine nucleotide phosphorylase, which produces hypoxanthine. This compound either re-enters the purine nucleotide pools or is further metabolized to xanthine and uric acid through the action of xanthine oxidase (Hartman et al., 1990; Back et al., 1992; Burger et al., 1995).

4.1.2 *Experimental systems*

The pharmacokinetics of didanosine in monkeys is somewhat similar to that in humans (Qian *et al.*, 1991; Ravasco *et al.*, 1992; Hawkins *et al.*, 1995). The time to maximum plasma concentration was 30 min (Ravasco *et al.*, 1992), and the half-time for removal of the drug from plasma varied between 1.2 and 1.8 h (Qian *et al.*, 1991; Ravasco *et al.*, 1992; Hawkins *et al.*, 1995). The plasma clearance rate ranged from 9.6 to 16.7 mL/min per kg bw (Qian *et al.*, 1991; Ravasco *et al.*, 1992; Hawkins *et al.*, 1995), while the renal clearance was reported to be 2 mL/min per kg bw (Ravasco *et al.*, 1992). The proportion of the drug excreted unchanged in the urine was reported to be either 19% (Qian *et al.*, 1991) or 74% (Ravasco *et al.*, 1992). There is evidence of extensive distribution in the body, although the concentration in cerebrospinal fluid was 4.8% of that observed in plasma (Hawkins *et al.*, 1995).

In rats, didanosine is distributed to the plasma, kidney, brain, cerebrospinal fluid and intestine after oral or intravenous dosing at 40–200 mg/kg bw (Hoesterey *et al.*, 1991; Wientjes & Au, 1992a,b; Bramer *et al.*, 1993; Hasegawa *et al.*, 1996). Bioavailability of 14–33% has been reported after oral and rectal administration (Wientjes & Au, 1992a,b; Bramer *et al.*, 1993; Hasegawa *et al.*, 1996); intestinal absorption was reduced by digestive tract acidity (Hasegawa *et al.*, 1996). The rate of clearance of the drug from plasma was 66–115 mL/min per kg bw, while the renal clearance rate in the same rats was 18–33 mL/min per kg bw (Wientjes & Au, 1992a,b). The time from dosing to maximum plasma concentration was reported to be 8–35 min (Hoesterey *et al.*, 1991; Wientjes & Au, 1992a; Bramer *et al*, 1993), and the half-time for removal from plasma was 24–38 min (Hoesterey *et al.*, 1991; Wientjes & Au, 1992a,b). Unchanged drug in the urine accounted for 4% of the total dose after several hours (Wientjes & Au, 1992a) and 18% in a 24-h urine collection (Bramer *et al.*, 1993). The clearance rates appear to slow with increasing dose, and the biphasic decline in plasma concentrations after dosing was suggestive of a slow equilibrium with tissue. The concentrations of drug in the brain and cerebrospinal fluid reached 5% and 2%, respectively, of those in plasma (Hoesterey *et al.*, 1991). Clearance of didanosine from the brain and cerebral spinal fluid is retarded by probenecid (Hoesterey *et al*, 1991). The pharmacokinetics does not change in the presence of zidovudine (Wientjes & Au, 1992b).

In dogs, didanosine given orally or intravenously at doses of 20–500 mg/kg bw was metabolized rapidly, and 46–51% of the dose was recovered in urine; the other 50% was unaccounted for. The rate of clearance from plasma was 23 mL/min per kg bw, and the half-time for removal was 30–60 min (Kaul *et al.*, 1991; Wientjes *et al.*, 1991). The concentrations in cerebrospinal fluid were 3–11% of those in plasma (Wientjes *et al.*, 1991).

Three pregnant rhesus monkeys (*Macaca mulatta*) that were near term (146 days) received radiolabelled didanosine as a bolus dose of 2.0 mg/kg bw into the radial vein. During a 3-h sampling period of both the mothers and the fetuses, the fetal:maternal ratio of the integrated area under the curve of plasma concentration–time was 0.33 ± 0.08 at 3 h, and fetal tissues contained 0.2–4 μmol/L didanosine (Sandberg *et al.*, 1995)

4.2 Toxic effects

4.2.1 *Humans*

Didanosine is toxic primarily to the nervous system, inducing peripheral neuropathy and headache; the gastrointestinal system, inducing pancreatitis and hepatitis; and the haematological system, inducing leukopenia (Yarchoan *et al.*, 1990a,b; Pike & Nicaise, 1993; Beach, 1998). In an early study (Rozencweig *et al.*, 1990) of 92 patients treated with didanosine, 12 experienced neuropathy, nine had liver enzyme abnormalities, four had myelosuppression, three had pancreatitis, and two had skin rash. Later studies suggested that didanosine has a weaker association with peripheral neuropathy than was suggested in phase I clinical trials (Kelleher *et al.*, 1999). Peripheral neuropathy has been observed mainly at high doses and in individuals treated for at least four months. The effect has been demonstrated in 12–34% of didanosine-treated patients, and is reversible upon withdrawal of the drug (Rozencweig *et al.*, 1990; Yarchoan *et al.*, 1990b; Simpson & Tagliati, 1995; Kelleher *et al.*, 1999).

Acute pancreatitis was reported by Maxson *et al.* (1992) in 12 of 51 patients during about eight months of follow-up after the start of didanosine therapy. In a second study (Seidlin *et al.*, 1992), seven of 44 patients developed pancreatitis lasting from one to seven weeks and varying in severity from mild to life-threatening. Among 7806 zidovudine-resistant patients participating in the Didanosine Expanded Access Program, 5% reported pancreatitis (Pike & Nicaise, 1993). In all of the studies, the symptoms correlated with cumulative treatment and typically subsided after discontinuation of therapy.

Like zidovudine and zalcitabine, didanosine occasionally caused a rare (1 in 10^5 to 1 in 10^6 patients) idiosyncratic syndrome consisting of increased liver enzyme activity, hepatic steatosis, fulminant hepatitis and severe lactic acidosis after long-term (more than three months) treatment; this syndrome can be fatal (Lai *et al.*, 1991; Bissuel *et al.*, 1994; Hu & French, 1997). Other miscellaneous and rare human toxic effects include acute, reversible thrombocytopenia (Lor & Liu, 1993), retinal toxicity (Cobo *et al.*, 1996), nephrotoxicity (Crowther *et al.*, 1993) and widespread cutaneous eruption, possibly associated with malignancies and infections (Just *et al.*, 1997).

4.2.2 *Experimental systems*

Most of the studies of the toxicity of didanosine in animal models have addressed immune competence (Phillips & Munson, 1997; Phillips *et al.*, 1997), neurotoxicity (Warner *et al.*, 1995; Schmued *et al.*, 1996) and pancreatic toxicity (Grady *et al.*, 1992; Nordback *et al.*, 1992).

In B6C3F$_1$ mice given didanosine by gastric intubation at 100, 250, 500 or 1000 mg/kg bw per day for 14, 28 or 180 days, virtually no toxic effects were seen in specific organs, with the exception of spleen and thymus (Phillips & Munson, 1997; Phillips *et al.*, 1997). Cell-mediated (T cell) immunity was moderately suppressed at 250 mg/kg bw for > 14 days, and suppression of humoral (B cell) immune response was observed at 100 mg/kg bw given for > 28 days.

In order to investigate the mechanism of didanosine-induced neuropathy, rats were dosed orally twice daily with 41.5 or 415 mg/kg bw didanosine in a phosphate buffer vehicle. Myelin splitting and intramyelin oedema were observed in the sciatic nerves of treated animals in a dose-related fashion (Schmued *et al.*, 1996). In rabbits given 750 or 1500 mg/kg bw didanosine per day for 6 or 16 weeks, no evidence of peripheral neuropathy was found (Warner *et al.*, 1995).

Attempts to model the effects of didanosine in the human pancreas have been unsuccessful. Grady *et al.* (1992) gave male Wistar rats didanosine at 100 or 1400 mg/kg bw per day for about one month and found no alterations in pancreatic morphology, lysozymal cathepsin B activity or amylase secretion. Nordback *et al.* (1992) perfused the pancreas of dogs with 500 μmol/L didanosine for 4 h and found that the oxygen consumption and protein secretion decreased, but these changes did not mimic the typical response seen in human pancreatitis.

4.3 Reproductive and prenatal effects

4.3.1 *Humans*

No data were available to the Working Group.

4.3.2 *Experimental systems*

Groups of 5–15 pregnant CD1 mice were given didanosine subcutaneously at 10, 30, 100 or 300 mg/kg bw per day throughout gestation. No changes in the numbers of resorptions or pups per litter or in external embryo morphology were reported in animals examined on gestational day 11. The pups of treated dams were born live, developed at a normal rate and had a normal lifespan (Sieh *et al.*, 1992).

Human embryonic or fetal cells (6–11 weeks of development) exposed to didanosine at 10 mmol/L were reported to contain less protein than control cells [data not shown as mean ± SD]. Cells prepared from 11-day CD1 mouse embryos were treated in culture with didanosine at concentrations of 1 μmol/L to 10 mmol/L. Concentrations > 5 mmol/L decreased the protein content. No selective cytotoxicity was seen in neuronal, cardiac or skeletal muscle or cartilage cells (Sieh *et al.*, 1992).

4.4 Genetic and related effects

4.4.1 *Humans*

No data were available to the Working Group.

4.4.2 *Experimental systems*

Reports on the potential mutagenicity of didanosine are sparse. References such as *The Physician's Desk Reference* (Medical Economics Data Production, 1999) provide results but few or no details of the experimental conditions used in the assays. The manufacturer of the drug has yet to publish a detailed report equivalent to those available in the literature on aciclovir and zidovudine. Mutagenicity was seen *in vitro* and *in vivo* only with high doses of didanosine (Table 1).

Didanosine did not induce reverse mutation in *Salmonella typhimurium* with or without exogenous metabolic activation [no information on doses or strains] and did not induce differential toxicity in *Escherichia coli* or *Bacillus subtilis*.

Didanosine marginally increased the number of revertants in *E. coli* WP2 *uvr*A. Mamber *et al.* (1990) assessed the ability of didanosine to induce two SOS functions, cell filamentation and prophage lambda, in *E. coli*. The combined results of tests for the induction of the SOS response in the nucleoside analogues evaluated in this volume indicate that the activity relationships can be ranked zidovudine > didanosine > zalcitabine. The results indicate that didanosine does not cause DNA damage that requires repair involving the excision repair (*uvr*A) or error-free postreplication repair (*rec*A) processes. Rather, didanosine, which acts as a DNA chain terminator, may generate an SOS-inducing response leading to inhibition of DNA replication. Didanosine caused clastogenic effects in Chinese hamster ovary cells and human lymphocytes.

Studies of the mutagenicity of didanosine in animals *in vivo* are limited to assays for micronucleus formation in rodents. Phillips *et al.* (1991) administered didanosine to mice by gavage for three days or 13 weeks (five days per week) and found no increase in micronuclei even at extremely high doses. As didanosine can be inactivated by the low pH of the stomach, it was subsequently administered by intraperitoneal injection for three consecutive days. A significant clastogenic response was found in peripheral blood at the low and high doses.

Concomitant exposure of human lymphoblastoid TK6 cells to equimolar concentrations of didanosine and zidovudine potentiated the mutagenic responses at both the *HPRT* and *TK* loci. Over a range of concentrations, the induced mutant frequencies at the two loci were three to four times greater than the values obtained after exposure to didanosine or zidovudine alone. In addition, the levels of DNA incorporation of zidovudine in cells exposed to the combination of drugs was about twofold greater than those measured in cells exposed to analogous concentrations of zidovudine alone (Meng *et al.*, 2000) (see section 4.4.2 in the monograph on zidovudine).

Table 1. Genetic and related effects of didanosine

Test system	Result[a] Without exogenous metabolic system	Result[a] With exogenous metabolic system	Dose[b] (LED/HID)	Reference
Salmonella typhimurium [strains not reported], reverse mutation	–	–	NR	Medical Economics Data Production (1999)
Escherichia coli BR513 (*uvrB envA lacZ::lambda*), prophage induction, SOS repair (spot and liquid suspension tests)	+	NT	50	Mamber *et al.* (1990)
Escherichia coli PQ37 (*uvrA rfa lacZ::sulA*), cell filamentation, SOS repair (spot and liquid suspension tests)	+	NT	[X]	Mamber *et al.* (1990)
Escherichia coli WP2 *uvrA*, reverse mutation	(+)	(+)	NR	Medical Economics Data Production (1999)
Escherichia coli CM871 (*uvrA recA lexA*), differential toxicity (vs *Escherichia coli* WP2)	–	NT	1000	Mamber *et al.* (1990)
Bacillus subtilis M45 *rec* strain, differential toxicity	–	NT	NR	Mamber *et al.* (1990)
Bacillus subtilis H17, gene mutation	–	NT	NR	Mamber *et al.* (1990)
Gene mutation, mouse lymphoma L5178Y cells, *Tk* locus *in vitro*	(+)	(+)	2000	Medical Economics Data Production (1999)
Chromosomal aberrations, Chinese hamster cells *in vitro*	+	NT	500	Medical Economics Data Production (1999)
Cell transformation, BALB/c 3T3 mouse cells	+	NT	3000	Medical Economics Data Production (1999)
Chromosomal aberrations, human lymphocytes *in vitro*	+	NT	500	Medical Economics Data Production (1999)
Micronucleus formation, mouse cells *in vivo*	–		NR	Medical Economics Data Production (1999)
Micronucleus formation, mouse bone-marrow cells *in vivo*	–		3000 po × 3	Phillips *et al.* (1991)
Micronucleus formation, mouse peripheral blood cells *in vivo*	–		1000 po × 5; 13 wk	Phillips *et al.* (1991)

Table 1 (contd)

Test system	Result[a]		Dose[b] (LED/HID)	Reference
	Without exogenous metabolic system	With exogenous metabolic system		
Micronucleus formation, mouse peripheral blood cells *in vivo*	+		200 ip × 5; 13 wk	Phillips *et al.* (1991)
Micronucleus formation, mouse bone-marrow cells *in vivo*	–		108 ip × 1	Motimaya *et al.* (1994)
Micronucleus formation, rat cells *in vivo*	–		NR	Medical Economics Data Production (1999)

[a] +, positive; (+), weak positive; –, negative; NT, not tested
[b] LED, lowest effective dose; HID, highest ineffective dose; in-vitro tests, µg/mL; in-vivo tests, mg/kg bw per day; NR, not reported; po, orally; ip, intraperitoneally; wk, week; [X] indicated in figure but not clearly specified

4.5 Mechanistic considerations

The main mechanism of the toxicity and antiviral efficacy of didanosine appears to be related to its phosphorylation and subsequent incorporation into DNA (Brinkman et al., 1998; Peter & Gambertoglio, 1998). The monophosphate is converted to dideoxy-adenosine monophosphate, which is further phosphorylated before incorporation into DNA (Yarchoan et al., 1990a). Once incorporated, the absence of a 3′-hydroxy group on the ribose of the dideoxyadenosine molecule prevents extension of the replicating DNA chain (Brinkman et al., 1998). The antiviral activity of dideoxyadenosine triphosphate is thought to result both from direct inhibition of the viral reverse transcriptase and from truncation of proviral DNA replication (Yarchoan et al., 1990a; Brinkman et al., 1998; Peter & Gambertoglio, 1998).

Like other nucleoside analogue drugs, didanosine, which is converted to dideoxy-adenosine, can become incorporated into mitochondrial DNA and truncate its replication (Chen et al., 1991), impairing the oxidative phosphorylation capacity of the cell and depleting mitochondrial DNA (Youssef & Badr, 1992; Lewis & Dalakas, 1995; Benbrik et al., 1997; Brinkman et al., 1998).

The few available studies on the mutagenicity of didanosine show that it produces primarily clastogenic effects at high doses. This activity is consistent with its action as a DNA chain terminator.

5. Summary of Data Reported and Evaluation

5.1 Exposure data

Didanosine is a nucleoside analogue which has been used since approximately 1990 in the treatment of HIV infection in adults and children. It is in widespread use in combination regimens with other antiretroviral agents, and potentiation of the antiviral effect of didanosine by hydroxyurea is being investigated.

5.2 Human carcinogenicity data

The only data available were from three trials designed to assess the efficacy of didanosine in improving the degree of immunocompetence and survival of patients with HIV infection, and no conclusion could be drawn about carcinogenicity.

5.3 Animal carcinogenicity data

No data were available to the Working Group.

5.4 Other relevant data

The human pharmacokinetics of orally administered didanosine is linear over a broad range of doses. Didanosine is about 40% bioavailable. It is rapidly absorbed, distributed and eliminated. About half of the human urinary metabolites are represented by hypoxanthine, and 40% is unchanged drug. Phosphorylation is a minor pathway but is essential for the antiviral activity of the drug.

The toxic effects of didanosine in humans include peripheral neuropathy, pancreatitis, hepatitis and leukopenia.

No relevant studies of the reproductive and prenatal effects of didanosine in humans were available. Didanosine crosses the placenta of women and monkeys by bidirectional, passive diffusion. Didanosine but not didanosine triphosphate was observed in placental and fetal tissues.

Little information was available on the genetic and related effects of didanosine. Didanosine was mutagenic *in vitro* and *in vivo* only at high doses. Treatment of human cells in culture significantly increased the mutant frequencies after short-term exposure to concentrations 10–20-fold greater than the peak plasma concentrations found in some patients. In the same studies, didanosine was more cytotoxic and less mutagenic than zidovudine.

5.5 Evaluation

There is *inadequate evidence* in humans for the carcinogenicity of didanosine.

There is *inadequate evidence* in experimental animals for the carcinogenicity of didanosine.

Overall evaluation

Didanosine is *not classifiable as to its carcinogenicity to humans (Group 3)*.

6. References

Abrams, D.I., Goldman, A.I., Launer, C., Korvick, J.A., Neaton, J.D., Crane, L.R., Grodesky, M., Wakefield, S., Muth, K., Kornegay, S., Cohn, D.L., Harris, A., Luskin-Hawk, R., Markowitz, N., Sampson, J.H., Thompson, M., Deyton, L. & the Terry Beirn Community Programs for Clinical Research on AIDS (1994) A comparative trial of didanosine or zalcitabine after treatment with zidovudine in patients with human immunodeficiency virus infection. *New Engl. J. Med.*, **330**, 657–662

American Hospital Formulary Service (1997) *AHFS Drug Information® 97*, Bethesda, MD, American Society of Health-System Pharmacists, pp. 456–465

Back, D.J., Ormesher, S., Tjia, J.F. & Macleod, R. (1992) Metabolism of 2′,3′-dideoxyinosine (ddI) in human blood. *Br. J. clin. Pharmacol.*, **33**, 319–322

Beach, J.W. (1998) Chemotherapeutic agents for human immunodeficiency virus infection: Mechanism of action, pharmacokinetics, metabolism, and adverse reactions. *Clin. Ther.*, **20**, 2–25

Benbrik, E., Chariot, P., Bonavaud, S., Ammi-Saïd, M., Frisdal, E., Rey, C., Gherardi, R. & Barlovatz-Meimon, G. (1997) Cellular and mitochondrial toxicity of zidovudine (AZT), didanosine (ddI) and zalcitabine (ddC) on cultured human muscle cells. *J. neurol. Sci.*, **149**, 19–25

Bissuel, F., Bruneel, F., Habersetzer, F., Chassard, D., Cotte, L., Chevallier, M., Bernuau, J., Lucet, J.-C. & Trepo, C. (1994) Fulminant hepatitis with severe lactic acidosis in HIV-infected patients on didanosine therapy. *J. intern. Med.*, **235**, 367–372

Bramer, S.L., Wientjes, M.G. & Au, J.L.-S. (1993) Absorption of 2′,3′-dideoxyinosine from lower gastrointestinal tract in rats and kinetic evidence of different absorption rates in colon and rectum. *Pharm. Res.*, **10**, 763–770

Brinkman, K., ter Hofstede, H.J.M., Burger, D.M., Smeitink, J.A.M. & Koopmans, P.P. (1998) Adverse effects of reverse transcriptase inhibitors: Mitochondrial toxicity as common pathway. *AIDS*, **12**, 1735–1744

Bristol-Myers Squibb Co. (1998) *Package Insert: Videx® (Didanosine)*, Princeton, NJ

British Medical Association/Royal Pharmaceutical Society of Great Britain (1998) *British National Formulary*, No. 36, London, p. 277

Budavari, S., ed. (1996) *The Merck Index*, 12th Ed., Whitehouse Station, NJ, Merck & Co., p. 524

Burger, D.M., Meenhorst, P.L. & Beijnen, J.H. (1995) Concise overview of the clinical pharmacokinetics of dideoxynucleoside antiretroviral agents. *Pharm. World Sci.*, **17**, 25–30

Canadian Pharmaceutical Association (1997) *CPS Compendium of Pharmaceuticals and Specialties*, 32nd Ed., Ottawa, pp. 1710–1713

Chen, C.-H., Vazquez-Padua, M. & Cheng, Y.-C. (1991) Effect of anti-human immunodeficiency virus nucleoside analogs on mitochondrial DNA and its implication for delayed toxicity. *Mol. Pharmacol.*, **39**, 625–628

CIS Information Services (1998) *Worldwide Bulk Drug Users Directory 1997/98 Edition*, Dallas, TX [CD-ROM]

Cobo, J., Ruiz, M.F., Figueroa, M.S., Antela, A., Quereda, C., Pérez-Elías, M.J., Corral, I. & Guerrero, A. (1996) Renal toxicity associated with didanosine in HIV-infected adults. *AIDS*, **10**, 1297–1299

Cooley, T.P., Kunches, L.M., Saunders, C.A., Ritter, J.K., Perkins, C.J., McLaren, C., McCaffrey, R.P. & Liebman, H.A. (1990) Once-daily administration of 2′,3′-dideoxyinosine (ddI) in patients with the acquired immunodeficiency syndrome or AIDS-related complex. *New Engl. J. Med.*, **322**, 1340–1345

Crowther, M.A., Callaghan, W., Hodsman, A.B. & Mackie, I.D. (1993) Dideoxyinosine-associated nephrotoxicity. *AIDS*, **7**, 131–132

Dalton, J.T. & Au, J.L.-S. (1993) 2′,3′-Dideoxyinosine is not metabolized in human placenta. *Drug Metab. Dispos.*, **21**, 544–546

Dancis, J., Lee, J.D., Mendoza, S. & Liebes, L. (1993) Transfer and metabolism of dideoxyinosine by the perfused human placenta. *J. acquir. Immune Defic. Syndr.*, **6**, 2–6

Delta Coordinating Committee (1996) Delta: A randomised double-blind controlled trial comparing combinations of zidovudine plus didanosine or zalcitabine with zidovudine alone in HIV-infected individuals. *Lancet*, **348**, 283–291

Dolin, R., Amato, D.A., Fischl, M.A., Pettinelli, C., Beltangady, M., Liou, S.-H., Brown, M.J., Cross, A.P., Hirsch, M.S., Hardy, W.D., Mildvan, D., Blair, D.C., Powderly, W.G., Para, M.F., Fife, K.H., Steigbigel, R.T., Smaldone, L. & the AIDS Clinical Trials Group (1995) Zidovudine compared with didanosine in patients with advanced HIV type 1 infection and little or no previous experience with zidovudine. *Arch. intern. Med.*, **155**, 961–974

Editions du Vidal (1998) *Dictionnaire Vidal 1998*, 74th Ed., Paris, OVP, pp. 1967–1970

Englund, J.A., Baker, C.J., Raskino, C., McKinney, R.E., Petrie, B., Fowler, M.G., Pearson, D., Gershon, A., McSherry, G.D., Abrams, E.J., Schliozberg, J. & Sullivan, J.L. (1997) Zidovudine, didanosine, or both as the initial treatment for symptomatic HIV-infected children. *New Engl. J. Med.*, **336**, 1704–1712

Faulds, D. & Brogden, R.N. (1992) Didanosine. A review of its antiviral activity, pharmacokinetic properties and therapeutic potential in human immunodeficiency virus infection. *Drugs*, **44**, 94–116

Gennaro, A.R. (1995) *Remington: The Science and Practice of Pharmacy*, 19th Ed., Easton, PA, Mack Publishing Co., Vol. II, p. 1333

Grady, T., Saluja, A.K., Steer, M.L., Lerch, M.M., Modlin, I.M. & Powers, R.E. (1992) *In vivo* and *in vitro* effects of azidothymidine analog dideoxyinosine on the exocrine pancreas of the rat. *J. Pharmacol. exp. Ther.*, **262**, 445–449

Hammer, S.M., Katzenstein, D.A., Hughes, M.D., Gundacker, H., Schooley, R.T., Haubrich, R.H., Henry, W.K., Lederman, M.M., Phair, J.P., Niu, M., Hirsch, M.S. & Merigan, T.C. for the AIDS Clinical Trials Group Study 175 Study Team (1996) A trial comparing nucleoside monotherapy with combination therapy in HIV-infected adults with CD4 cell countrs from 200 to 500 per cubic millimeter. *New Engl. J. Med.*, **335**, 1081–1090

Hartman, N.R., Yarchoan, R., Pluda, J.M., Thomas, R.V., Marczyk, K.S., Broder, S. & Johns, D.G. (1990) Pharmacokinetics of 2′,3′-dideoxyadenosine and 2′,3′-dideoxyinosine in patients with severe human immunodeficiency virus infection. *Clin. Pharmacol. Ther.*, **47**, 647–654

Hartman, N.R., Yarchoan, R., Pluda, J.M., Thomas, R.V., Wyvill, K.M., Flora, K.P., Broder, S. & Johns, D.G. (1991) Pharmacokinetics of 2′,3′-dideoxyinosine in patients with severe human immunodeficiency infection. II. The effects of different oral formulations and the presence of other medications. *Clin. Pharmacol. Ther.*, **50**, 278–285

Hasegawa, T., Juni, K., Saneyoshi, M. & Kawaguchi, T. (1996) Intestinal absorption and first-pass elimination of 2′,3′-dideoxynucleosides following oral administration in rats. *Biol. pharm. Bull.*, **19**, 599–603

Hawkins, M.E., Mitsuya, H., McCully, C.M., Godwin, K.S., Murakami, K., Poplack, D.G. & Balis, F.M. (1995) Pharmacokinetics of dideoxypurine nucleoside analogs in plasma and cerebrospinal fluid of rhesus monkeys. *Antimicrob. Agents Chemother.*, **39**, 1259–1264

Henderson, G.I., Perez, A.B., Yang, Y., Hamby, R.L., Schenden, R.S. & Schenker, S. (1994) Transfer of dideoxyinosine across the human isolated placenta. *Br. J. clin. Pharmacol.*, **38**, 237–242

Hoesterey, B.L., Galinsky. R.E. & Anderson, B.D. (1991) Dose dependence in the plasma pharmacokinetics and uptake kinetics of 2′,3′-dideoxyinosine into brain and cerebrospinal fluid of rats. *Drug Metab. Dispos.*, **19**, 907–912

Hu, B. & French, S.W. (1997) 2′,3′-Dideoxyinosine-induced Mallory bodies in patients with HIV. *Am. J. clin. Pathol.*, **108**, 280–283

Just, M., Carrascosa, J.M., Ribera, M., Bielsa, I. & Ferrándiz, C. (1997) Dideoxyinosine-associated Ofuji papuloerythroderma in an HIV-infected patient. *Dermatology*, **195**, 410–411

Kahn, J.O., Lagakos, S.W., Richman, D.D., Cross, A., Pettinelli, C., Liou, S.-H., Brown, M., Volberding, P.A., Crumpacker, C.S., Beall, G., Sacks, H.S., Merigan, T.C., Beltangady, M., Smaldone, L., Dolin, R. & the NIAID AIDS Clinical Trials Group (1992) A controlled trial comparing continued zidovudine with didanosine in human immunodeficiency virus infection. *New Engl. J. Med.*, **327**, 581–587

Kaul, S., Knupp, C.A., Dandekar, K.A., Pittman, K.A. & Barbhaiya, R.H. (1991) Pharmacokinetics of 2′,3′-dideoxyinosine (BMY-40900), a new anti-human immunodeficiency virus agent, after administration of single intravenous doses to beagle dogs. *Antimicrob. Agents Chemother.*, **35**, 610–614

Kelleher, T., Cross, A. & Dunkle, L. (1999) Relation of peripheral neuropathy to HIV treatment in four randomized clinical trials including didanosine. *Clin. Ther.*, **21**, 1182–1192

Knupp, C.A., Shyu, W.C., Dolin, R., Valentine, F.T., McLaren, C., Martin, R.R., Pittman, K.A. & Barbhaiya, R.H. (1991) Pharmacokinetics of didanosine in patients with acquired immunodeficiency syndrome or acquired immunodeficiency syndrome- related complex. *Clin. Pharmacol. Ther.*, **49**, 523–535

Knupp, C.A., Hak, L.J., Coakley, D.F., Falk, R.J., Wagner, B.E., Raasch, R.H., van der Horst, C.M., Kaul, S., Barbhaiya, R.H. & Dukes, G.E. (1996) Disposition of didanosine in HIV-seropositive patients with normal renal function or chronic renal failure: Influence of hemodialysis and continuous ambulatory peritoneal dialysis. *Clin. Pharmacol. Ther.*, **60**, 535–542

Kozal, M.J., Kroodsma, K., Winters, M.A., Shafer, R.W., Efron, B., Katzenstein, D.A. & Merigan, T.C. (1994) Didanosine resistance in HIV-infected patients switched from zidovudine to didanosine monotherapy. *Ann. intern. Med.*, **121**, 263–268

Lai, K.K., Gang, D.L., Zawacki, J.K. & Cooley, T.P. (1991) Fulminant hepatic failure associated with 2′,3′-dideoxyinosine (ddI). *Ann. intern. Med.*, **115**, 283–284

Lambert, J.S., Seidlin, M., Reichman, R.C., Plank, C.S., Laverty, M., Morse, G.D., Knupp, C., McLaren, C., Pettinelli, C., Valentine, F.T. & Dolin, R. (1990) 2′,3′-Dideoxyinosine (ddI) in patients with the acquired immunodeficiency syndrome or AIDS-related complex. A phase I trial. *New Engl. J. Med.*, **322**, 1333–1340

Lewis, W. & Dalakas, M.C. (1995) Mitochondrial toxicity of antiviral drugs. *Nature Med.*, **1**, 417–422

LINFO Läkemedelsinformation AB (1998) *FASS 1998 Läkemedel i Sverige*, Stockholm, pp. 1243–1244

Lor, E. & Liu, Y.Q. (1993) Didanosine-associated eosinophilia with acute thrombocytopenia. *Ann. Pharmacother.*, **27**, 23–25

Mamber, S.W., Brookshire, K.W. & Forenza, S. (1990) Induction of the SOS response in *Escherichia coli* by azidothymidine and dideoxynucleotides. *Antimicrob. Agents Chemother.*, **34**, 1237–1243

Maxson, C.J., Greenfield, S.M. & Turner, J.L. (1992) Acute pancreatitis as a common complication of 2′,3′-dideoxyinosine therapy in the acquired immunodeficiency syndrome. *Am. J. Gastroenterol.*, **87**, 708–713

McKinney, R.E., Jr, Johnson, G.M., Stanley, K., Yong, F.H., Keller, A., O'Donnell, K.J., Brouwers, P., Mitchell, W.G., Yogev, R., Wara, D.W., Wiznia, A., Mofenson, L., McNamara, J. & Spector, S.A. (1998) A randomized study of combined zidovudine-lamivudine versus didanosine monotherapy in children with symptomatic therapy-naive HIV-1 infection. The Pediatric AIDS Clinical Trials Group Protocol 300 Study Team. *J. Pediatr.*, **133**, 500–508

Medical Economics Data Production (1999) *PDR®: Physicians' Desk Reference*, 53rd Ed., Montvale, NJ

Meng, Q., Olivero, O.A., Shi, X., Walker, D.W., Antiochos, B., Poirier, M.C. & Walker, V.E. (2000) Enhanced DNA incorporation of AZT and synergistic effects of AZT and DDI in inducing *HPRT* and *TK* mutations in human cells (abstract). *Environ. mol. Mutag.*, **35** (Suppl. 31), 43

Montaner, J.S.G., Reiss, P., Cooper, D., Vella, S., Harris, M., Conway, B., Wainberg, M.A., Smith, D., Robinson, P., Hall, D., Myers, M. & Lange, J.M.A. (1998) A randomized, double-blind trial comparing combinations of nevirapine, didanosine, and zidovudine for HIV-infected patients. The INCAS Trial. *J. Am. med. Assoc.*, **279**, 930–937

Morse, G.D., Shelton, M.J., Ho, M., Bartos, L., DeRemer, M. & Ragni, M. (1995) Pharmacokinetics of zidovudine and didanosine during combination therapy. *Antiviral Res.*, **27**, 419–424

Motimaya, A.M., Subramanya, K.S., Curry, P.T. & Kitchin, R.M. (1994) Evaluation of the genotoxic potential of selected anti-AIDS treatment drugs at clinical doses in vivo in mice. *Toxicol. Lett.*, **70**, 171–183

Nassar, M.N., Chen, T., Reff, M.J. & Agharkar, S.N. (1993) Didanosine. In: Brittain, H.G., ed., *Analytical Profiles of Drug Substances and Excipients*, New York, Academic Press, Vol. 22, pp. 185–227

National Cancer Institute (1992) *NCI Investigational Drugs—Chemical Information—1992* (NIH Publication No. 92-2654), Bethesda, MD, National Institutes of Health, pp. 83–85

Nordback, I.H., Olson, J.L., Chaisson, R.E. & Cameron, J.L. (1992) Acute effects of a nucleoside analog dideoxyinosine (DDI) on the pancreas. *J. surg. Res.*, **53**, 610–614

Perry, C.M. & Balfour, J.A. (1996) Didanosine. An update on its antiviral activity, pharmacokinetic properties and therapeutic efficacy in the management of HIV disease. *Drugs*, **52**, 928–962

Peter, K. & Gambertoglio, J.G. (1998) Intracellular phosphorylation of zidovudine (ZDV) and other nucleoside reverse transcriptase inhibitors (RTI) used for human immunodeficiency virus (HIV) infection. *Pharm. Res.*, **15**, 819–825

Phillips, K.E. & Munson, A.E. (1997) 2′,3′-Dideoxyinosine inhibits the humoral immune response in female B6C3F1 mice by targeting the B lymphocyte. *Toxicol. appl. Pharmacol.*, **145**, 260–267

Phillips, M.D., Nascimbeni, B., Tice, R.R. & Shelby, M.D. (1991) Induction of micronuclei in mouse bone marrow cells: An evaluation of nucleoside analogues used in the treatment of AIDS. *Environ. mol. Mutag.*, **18**, 168–183

Phillips, K.E., McCay, J.A., Brown, R.D., Musgrove, D.L., Meade, B.J., Butterworth, L.F., Wilson, S., White, K.L., Jr & Munson, A.E. (1997) Immunotoxicity of 2′,3′-dideoxyinosine in female B6C3F1 mice. *Drug chem. Toxicol.*, **20**, 189–228

Pike, I.M. & Nicaise, C. (1993) The didanosine Expanded Access Program: Safety analysis. *Clin. infect. Dis.*, **16** (Suppl. 1), S63–S68

Pluda, J.M., Venzon, D.J., Tosato, G., Lietzau, J., Wyvill, K., Nelson, D.L., Jaffe, E.S., Karp, J.E., Broder, S. & Yarchoan, R. (1993) Parameters affecting the development of non-Hodgkin lymphoma in patients with severe human immunodeficiency virus infection receiving antiretroviral therapy. *J. clin. Oncol.*, **11**, 1099–1107

Pons, J.C., Boubon, M.C., Tgaburet, A.M., Singlas, E., Chambrin, V., Frydman, R., Papiernik, E. & Delfraissy, J.F. (1991) Fetoplacental passage of 2′,3′-dideoxyinosine (Letter to the Editor). *Lancet*, **337**, 732

Qian, M., Finco, T.S., Swagler, A.R. & Gallo, J.M. (1991) Pharmacokinetics of 2′,3′-dideoxyinosine in monkeys. *Antimicrob. Agents Chemother.*, **35**, 1247–1249

Raffi, F., Reliquet, V., Auger, S., Besnier, J.-M., Chennebault, J.-M., Billaud, E., Michelet, C., Perre, P., Lafeuillade, A., May, T. & Billaudel, S. (1998) Efficacy and safety of stavudine and didanosine combination therapy in antiretroviral-experienced patients. *AIDS*, **12**, 1999–2005

Ravasco, R.J., Unadkat, J.D., Tsai, C.-C. & Nosbisch, C. (1992) Pharmacokinetics of dideoxyinosine in pigtailed macaques (*Macaca nemestrina*) after intravenous and subcutaneous administration. *J. acquir. Immune Defic. Syndr.*, **5**, 1016–1018

Rote Liste Sekretariat (1998) *Rote Liste 1998*, Frankfurt, Rote Liste Service GmbH, pp. 10–450

Rozencweig, M., McLaren, C., Beltangady, M., Ritter, J., Canetta, R., Schacter, L., Kelley, S., Nicaise, C., Smaldone, L., Dunkle, L., Barbhaiya, R., Knupp, C., Cross, A., Tsianco, M. & Martin, R.R. (1990) Overview of phase I trials of 2′,3′-dideoxyinosine (ddI) conducted on adult patients. *Rev. infect. Dis.*, **12**, S570–S575

Sahai, J., Gallicano, K., Garber, G., Pakuts, A. & Cameron, W. (1995) Pharmacokinetics of simultaneously administered zidovudine and didanosine in HIV-seropositive male patients. *J. acquir. Immune Defic. Syndr.*, **10**, 54–60

Sandberg, J.A., Binienda, Z., Lipe, G., Rose, L.M., Parker, W.B., Ali, S.F. & Slikker, W., Jr (1995) Placental transfer and fetal disposition of 2′,3′-dideoxycytidine and 2′,3′-dideoxyinosine in the rhesus monkey. *Drug Metab. Dispos.*, **23**, 881–884

Schmued, L.C., Albertson, C.M., Andrews, A., Sandberg, J.A., Nickols, J. & Slikker, W., Jr (1996) Evaluation of brain and nerve pathology in rats chronically dosed with ddI or isoniazid. *Neurotoxicol. Teratol.*, **18**, 555–563

Seidlin, M., Lambert, J.S., Dolin, R. & Valentine, F.T. (1992) Pancreatitis and pancreatic dysfunction in patients taking dideoxyinosine. *AIDS*, **6**, 831–835

Sieh, E., Coluzzi, M.L., Cusella de Angelis, M.G., Mezzogiorno, A., Foridia, M., Canipari, R., Cossu, G. & Vella, S. (1992) The effects of AZT and DDI on pre- and postimplantation mammalian embryos: An in vivo and in vitro study. *AIDS Res. hum. Retroviruses*, **8**, 639–649

Simpson, D.M. & Tagliati, M. (1995) Nucleoside analogue-associated peripheral neuropathy in human immunodeficiency virus infection. *J. acquir. Immune Defic. Syndr. hum. Retrovirol.*, **9**, 153–161

Singlas, E., Taburet, A.M., Lebas, F.B., de Curzon, O.P., Sobel, A., Chauveau, P., Viron, B., Al Khayat, R., Poignet, J.L., Mignon, F., Humbert, G. & Fillastre, J.P. (1992) Didanosine pharmacokinetics in patients with normal and impaired renal function: Influence of hemodialysis. *Antimicrob. Agents Chemother.*, **36**, 1519–1524

Spruance, S.L., Pavia, A.T., Peterson, D., Berry, A., Pollard, R., Patterson, T.F., Frank, I., Remick, S.C., Thompson, M., MacArthur, R.D., Morey, G.E., Jr, Ramirez-Ronda, C.H., Bernstein, B.M., Sweet, D.E., Crane, L., Peterson, E.A., Pachucki, C.T., Green, S.L., Brand, J., Rios, A., Dunkle, L.M., Cross, A., Brown, M.J., Ingraham, P., Gugliotti, R., Schindzielorz, A.H. & Smaldone, L. for the Bristol-Myers Squibb AI454-010 Study Group (1994) Didanosine compared with continuation of zidovudine in HIV-infected patients with signs of clinical deterioration while receiving zidovudine. A randomized double-blind clinical trial. *Ann. intern. Med.*, **120**, 360–368

Swiss Pharmaceutical Society, ed. (1999) *Index Nominum, International Drug Directory*, 16th Ed., Stuttgart, Medpharm Scientific Publishers [MicroMedex CD-ROM]

Thomas, J., ed. (1998) *Australian Prescription Products Guide*, 27th Ed., Victoria, Australian Pharmaceutical Publishing, Vol. 1, pp. 2907–2912

US Pharmacopeial Convention (1998) *USP Dispensing Information*, Vol. I, *Drug Information for the Health Care Professional*, 18th Ed., Rockville, MD, pp. 1178–1182

Warner, W.A., Bregman, C.L., Comereski, C.R., Arezzo, J.C., Davidson, T.J., Knupp, C.A., Kaul, S., Durham, S.K., Wasserman, A.J. & Frantz, J.D. (1995) Didanosine (ddI) and stavudine (d4T): Absence of peripheral neurotoxicity in rabbits. *Food chem. Toxicol.*, **33**, 1047–1050

Wientjes, M.G. & Au, J.L.-S. (1992a) Pharmacokinetics of oral 2′,3′-dideoxyinosine in rats. *Pharm. Res.*, **9**, 822–825

Wientjes, M.G. & Au, J.L.-S. (1992b) Lack of pharmacokinetic interaction between intravenous 2′,3′-dideoxyinosine and 3′-azido-3′-deoxythymidine in rats. *Antimicrob. Agents Chemother.*, **36**, 665–668

Wientjes, M.G., Placke, M.E., Chang, M.J.-W., Page, J.G., Kluwe, W.M. & Tomaszewski, J.E. (1991) Pharmacokinetics of 2′,3′-dideoxyadenosine in dogs. *Invest. new Drugs*, **9**, 159–168

Yarchoan, R., Pluda, J.M., Perno, C.F., Mitsuya, H., Thomas, R.V., Wyvill, K.M. & Broder, S. (1990a) Initial clinical experience with dideoxynucleosides as single agents and in combination therapy. *Ann. N.Y. Acad. Sci.*, **616**, 328–343

Yarchoan, R., Mitsuya, H., Pluda, J.M., Marczyk, K.S, Thomas, R.V., Hartman, N.R., Brouwers, P., Perno, C.-F., Allain, J.-P., Johns, D.G. & Broder, S. (1990b) The National Cancer Institute phase I study of 2′,3′-dideoxyinosine administration in adults with AIDS or AIDS-related complex: Analysis of activity and toxicity profiles. *Rev. infect. Dis.*, **12**, S522–S533

Youssef, J.A. & Badr, M.Z. (1992) Disruption of mitochondrial energetics and DNA synthesis by the anti-AIDS drug dideoxyinosine. *Toxicol. Lett.*, **60**, 197–202

DNA TOPOISOMERASE II INHIBITORS

ETOPOSIDE

1. Exposure Data

1.1 Chemical and physical data

1.1.1 *Nomenclature*

Etoposide

Chem. Abstr. Serv. Reg. No.: 33419-42-0
Chem. Abstr. Name: (5R,5aR,8aR,9S)-9-{[4,6-O-(1R)-Ethylidene-β-D-glucopyranosyl]oxy}-5,8,8a,9-tetrahydro-5-(4-hydroxy-3,5-dimethoxyphenyl)furo-[3′,4′:6,7]naphtho[2,3-d]-1,3-dioxol-6(5aH)-one
IUPAC Systematic Name: 4′-Demethylepipodophyllotoxin 9-(4,6-O-(R)-ethylidene-β-D-glucopyranoside)
Synonyms: 4′-Demethylepipodophyllotoxin 9-(4,6-O-ethylidene-β-D-glucopyranoside); 4′-demethylepipodophyllotoxin ethylidene-β-D-glucoside; (–)-etoposide; *trans*-etoposide; VP 16; VP 16-123; VP 16-213

Etoposide phosphate

Chem. Abstr. Serv. Reg. No.: 117091-64-2
Chem. Abstr. Name: (5R,5aR,8aR,9S)-5-[3,5-Dimethoxy-4-(phosphonooxy)phenyl]-9-{[4,6-O-(1R)-ethylidene-β-D-glucopyranosyl]oxy}-5,8,8a,9-tetrahydrofuro-[3′,4′:6,7]naphtho[2,3-d]-1,3-dioxol-6(5aH)-one
IUPAC Systematic Name: 4′-Demethylepipodophyllotoxin 9-(4,6-O-(R)-ethylidene-β-D-glucopyranoside), 4′-(dihydrogen phosphate)
Synonyms: {5R-[5α,5aβ,8aα,9β(R*)]}-5-[3,5-Dimethoxy-4-(phosphonooxy)-phenyl]-9-[(4,6-O-ethylidene-β-D-glucopyranosyl)oxy]-5,8,8a,9-tetrahydrofuro-[3′,4′:6,7]naphtho[2,3-d]-1,3-dioxol-6(5aH)-one; etoposide 4′-phosphate

1.1.2 Structural and molecular formulae and relative molecular mass

Etoposide

$C_{29}H_{32}O_{13}$ Relative molecular mass: 588.57

Etoposide phosphate

$C_{29}H_{33}O_{16}P$ Relative molecular mass: 668.55

1.1.3 *Chemical and physical properties of the pure substances*

Etoposide

(a) *Description*: White to yellow-brown crystalline powder (Gennaro, 1995; American Hospital Formulary Service, 1997)
(b) *Melting-point*: 236–251 °C (Budavari, 1996)
(c) *Spectroscopy data*: Infrared, ultraviolet, fluorescence emission, nuclear magnetic resonance (proton and ^{13}C) and mass spectral data have been reported (Holthuis *et al.*, 1989).
(d) *Solubility*: Sparingly soluble in water (approximately 0.03 mg/mL) and diethyl ether; slightly soluble in ethanol (approximately 0.76 mg/mL); very soluble in chloroform and methanol (Gennaro, 1995; American Hospital Formulary Service, 1997)
(e) *Optical rotation*: $[\alpha]_D^{20}$, –110.5° (c = 0.6 in chloroform) (Budavari, 1996)
(f) *Dissociation constant*: pK_a, 9.8 (Budavari, 1996)

Etoposide phosphate

(a) *Description*: White to off-white crystalline powder (American Hospital Formulary Service, 1997)
(b) *Solubility*: Very soluble in water (> 100 mg/mL); slightly soluble in ethanol (American Hospital Formulary Service, 1997)

1.1.4 *Technical products and impurities*

Etoposide is available as a 50- or 100-mg liquid-filled capsule and as a 20-mg/mL injection solution. The gelatin capsules may also contain citric acid, gelatin, glycerol, iron oxide, parabens (ethyl and propyl), polyethylene glycol 400, sorbitol and titanium dioxide. Etoposide concentrate for injection is a sterile, non-aqueous solution of the drug in a vehicle, which may be benzyl alcohol, citric acid, ethanol, polyethylene glycol 300 or polysorbate 80. The concentrate for injection is a clear, yellow solution and has a pH of 3–4.

Etoposide phosphate for injection is a sterile, non-pyrogenic, lyophilized powder containing sodium citrate and dextran 40; after reconstitution of the drug with water for injection to a concentration of 1 mg/mL, the solution has a pH of 2.9 (Gennaro, 1995; American Hospital Formulary Service, 1997; Canadian Pharmaceutical Association, 1997; British Medical Association/Royal Pharmaceutical Society of Great Britain, 1998; Editions du Vidal, 1998; Rote Liste Sekretariat, 1998; Thomas, 1998).

The following impurities are limited by the requirements of *The British Pharmacopoeia*: 4'-carbenzoxy ethylidene lignan P, picroethylidene lignan P, α-ethylidene lignan P, lignan P and 4'-demethylepipodophyllotoxin (British Pharmacopoeia Commission, 1994).

Trade names for etoposide include Abiposid, Cehaposid, Celltop, Citodox, Eposin, Etocris, Etomedac, Etopol, Etoposid Ebewe, Etoposid Pharmacia Upjohn, Etoposid Austropharm, Etoposida Filaxis, Etoposid, Etoposide Dakota, Etoposide Injection, Etoposide P&U, Etoposide Pierre Fabre, Etoposido Asofarma, Etoposido Dakota Farma, Etoposido Farmitalia, Etosid Euvaxon, Exitop, Kebedil, Labimion, Lastet, Optasid, Toposar, VePesid and Vépéside-Sandoz (Swiss Pharmaceutical Society, 1999).

Trade names for etoposide phosphate include Etopofos and Etopophos (Swiss Pharmaceutical Society, 1999).

1.1.5 *Analysis*

Several international pharmacopoeias specify infrared absorption spectrophotometry with comparison to standards and liquid chromatography as the methods for identifying etoposide; liquid chromatography is used to assay its purity. In pharmaceutical preparations, etoposide is identified by infrared absorption spectrophotometry and thin-layer chromatography; liquid chromatography is used to assay for etoposide content (British Pharmacopoeial Commission, 1994; US Pharmacopeial Convention, 1994; Council of Europe, 1997; US Pharmacopeial Convention, 1997).

Methods for the analysis of etoposide and its metabolites in plasma, serum and urine have included reversed-phase high-performance liquid chromatography with oxidative electrochemical detection, fluorescence detection and ultraviolet detection. The limit of detection of these methods is often < 100 ng/mL (Holthuis *et al.*, 1989).

1.2 Production

Etoposide is a semi-synthetic derivative of podophyllotoxin and was first synthesized in 1963. Podophyllotoxin is isolated from the dried roots and rhizomes of species of the genus *Podophyllin*, such as the may apple or American mandrake (*Podophyllin peltatum* L.) and *Podophyllin emodi* Wall (Holthuis *et al.*, 1989).

Etoposide can be synthesized from naturally occurring podophyllotoxin by first treating the podophyllotoxin with hydrogen bromide to produce 1-bromo-1-deoxyepipodophyllotoxin, which is demethylated to 1-bromo-4′-demethylepipodophyllotoxin. The bromine is replaced by a hydroxy group, resulting in 4′-demethylepipodophyllotoxin. After protection of the phenolic hydroxyl, the 4-hydroxy group is coupled with 2,3,4,6-tetra-O-acetyl-β-D-glucopyranose. The protecting group at the 4′-hydroxy is removed by hydrogenolysis and the acyl groups by hydrolysis, and the cyclic O-4,6 acetal is formed by reaction with acetaldehyde dimethyl acetal (Holthuis *et al.*, 1989).

Information available in 1999 indicated that etoposide was manufactured and/or formulated in 39 countries and etoposide phosphate in eight (CIS Information Services, 1998; Swiss Pharmaceutical Society, 1999).

1.3 Use

Podophyllotoxin is an extract of the roots and rhizomes of two plant species that have been used in folk medicine for several hundred years. It inhibits DNA topoisomerase II (Imbert, 1998). During early clinical trials for cancer chemotherapeutic use, podophyllotoxin proved to be too toxic and, in the 1960s, two epipodophyllotoxins were described, teniposide (see monograph, this volume) and etoposide (Keller-Juslén et al., 1971). The first clinical trial of etoposide was reported in 1971, and etoposide entered routine use after 1981 (Oliver et al., 1991). The drug was approved for use in the USA in 1983 (Imbert, 1998).

Etoposide is one of the most widely used cytotoxic drugs and has strong anti-tumour activity in cases of small-cell lung cancer, testicular cancer, lymphomas and a variety of childhood malignancies. It is one of the most active single agents in the treatment of small-cell lung cancer (Slevin et al., 1989a; Johnson et al., 1991), although it is commonly used in combination with cisplatin, often as part of alternating chemotherapy with the widely used cyclophosphamide–doxorubicin–vincristine regimen (Goodman et al., 1990; Roth et al., 1992).

For testicular germ-cell tumours, etoposide is used in combination with bleomycin and cisplatin. Durable complete responses were achieved in about 80% of patients with disseminated germ-cell tumours; in a randomized trial, the combination resulted in longer overall survival and less toxicity than the standard cisplatin–bleomycin–vinblastine regimen (Williams et al., 1987). Three or four cycles of etoposide with cisplatin and bleomycin are now generally regarded as the standard treatment for this disease (Nichols, 1992).

Etoposide is active as a single agent in non-Hodgkin lymphoma, with response rates of 17–40% in previously treated patients (O'Reilly et al., 1991). It has been investigated for use in combination with the widely used cyclophosphamide–doxorubicin–vincristine–prednisone regimen and in a number of new combinations.

Etoposide is less commonly used in a number of other tumour types, including non-small-cell lung cancer, breast, ovarian and gastric cancer, leukaemias, Kaposi sarcoma and in histiocytosis (Joel, 1996; Okada et al., 1998), typically as part of combination chemotherapy and often in patients in whom standard first-line treatments for these malignancies have failed.

The efficacy of etoposide is clearly schedule-dependent, longer exposures of three to five days being more active than a single dose (Slevin et al., 1989a). A typical intravenous dose is 375–500 mg/m^2 over three to five days days (90–120 mg/m^2 per day), repeated every three weeks. More prolonged dosing with etoposide has also been described.

Etoposide is available as intravenous and oral formulations. Owing to its poor solubility, a more water-soluble pro-drug, etoposide phosphate, was developed for clinical use. Once this drug enters the systemic circulation, the phosphate is rapidly and completely cleaved by circulating phosphatases. Early clinical trials showed that equimolar doses of etoposide and etoposide phosphate resulted in equivalent concentrations of etoposide in plasma (as measured by the area under the integrated plasma concentration–time curve) and equivalent biological effects (Schacter *et al.*, 1994; Kaul *et al.*, 1995).

1.4 Occurrence

Etoposide is not known to occur as a natural product. No data were available to the Working Group on occupational exposure.

1.5 Regulations and guidelines

Etoposide is listed in the British, Dutch, European, French, German, Swiss and US pharmacopoeias (Royal Pharmaceutical Society of Great Britain, 1999; Swiss Pharmaceutical Society, 1999).

2. Studies of Cancer in Humans

Several factors make it difficult to evaluate etoposide with respect to the incidence of second malignancies. First, most cancer patients are treated with combined treatment modalities (chemotherapy and radiotherapy), and multiple antineoplastic drugs are usually administered within combination chemotherapy regimens. The administration of possibly carcinogenic drugs other than etoposide was adjusted for in only a few studies. [The Working Group considered only studies in which etoposide was given to patients who did not receive treatments with alkylating agents (see IARC, 1987), with the exception of low doses of cyclophosphamide.] Secondly, first and second primary malignancies may have common risk factors. For example, there is now general agreement that the development of leukaemia in patients with mediastinal germ-cell cancer should be regarded as part of the natural history of the disease (Nichols *et al.*, 1990). In studies of the risk for treatment-related leukaemia, patients with mediastinal germ-cell cancer should therefore be excluded.

In studies in which patients were treated with etoposide and/or teniposide (see monograph, this volume), the authors used various conversion factors to derive an 'equivalent dose' of etoposide from that of teniposide. The conversions were based, however, on the therapeutic effects with regard to the possible leukaemogenic potency at a given dose rather than on metabolic considerations.

2.1 Case reports

Since the initial reports of treatment-related acute myeloid leukaemia after treatment of cancer patients with etoposide were published in the 1980s (e.g. Ratain *et al.*, 1986), more than 150 such reports have appeared. In all of these, however, the development of leukaemia followed the administration of etoposide in combination with other cytostatic drugs and/or irradiation. Since several cohort studies of patients with various malignancies have been conducted to estimate the risk for second malignancies after exposure to etoposide, this section includes only case reports of the specific group of patients with Langerhans cell histiocytosis and metastatic germ-cell tumours who received etoposide. Langerhans cell histiocytosis entails proliferation of connective tissue cells which originate in the bone marrow.

An eight-year-old Peruvian girl with Langerhans cell histiocytosis of the bone who had been treated according to an Italian protocol for this disease, consisting of etoposide at a dose of 200 mg/m^2 for three consecutive days every three weeks with 15 courses administered in one year for a cumulative dose of 8400 mg/m^2, was hospitalized for acute promyelocytic leukaemia 18 months after discontinuing therapy. Etoposide was the only cytotoxic agent that had been used before the onset of acute myeloid leukaemia. This patient was one of 26 treated only with an epipodophyllotoxin for Langerhans cell histiocytosis; their follow-up periods ranged between 11 and 44 months, with a median of 29.5 months (Haupt *et al.*, 1993).

In Japan, Horibe *et al.* (1993) reported two patients with secondary acute promyelocytic leukaemia after chemotherapy that included etoposide for the treatment of Langerhans cell histiocytosis. The first case was a four-year-old girl, in whom the disease was diagnosed in bone in July 1988. She initially received intravenous vinblastine and oral prednisolone, followed by etoposide injections alone at 200 mg/m^2 weekly, between June 1989 and January 1990. The total dose of etoposide administered was 6250 mg (9600 mg/m^2). In November 1990 (after 28 months), she developed acute promyelocytic leukaemia. The second case was in a five-month-old girl with Langerhans cell histiocytosis diagnosed in June 1987 who was treated with intravenous etoposide (100 mg/m^2 eight doses, two or three times a week), in addition to bolus vincristine, intravenous cyclophosphamide at doses unlikely to be leukaemogenic, intravenous methotrexate and oral prednisolone. The total doses of etoposide and cyclophosphamide administered were 1860 mg (4800 mg/m^2) and 4070 mg (10 800 mg/m^2), respectively. In June 1990 (after 36 months), acute promyelocytic leukaemia was diagnosed. Neither patient had undergone irradiation.

Oliver *et al.* (1991) reported in a letter to the editor that 115 patients in a series of 207 cases of metastatic germ-cell tumour (1978–90) in the United Kingdom were treated with low-dose etoposide combinations and that two cases of acute myeloid leukaemia occurred. The first patient, aged 34, developed acute myeloid leukaemia 63 months after treatment with bleomycin, cisplatin and etoposide. The cumulative etoposide dose was 710 mg/m^2. The other patient, aged 36, developed acute myelomonocytic leukaemia 27 months after radiotherapy and bleomycin, etoposide, vinblastine and cisplatin. The cumulative etoposide dose was 300 mg/m^2. There were also four non-haematological malignancies.

2.2 Cohort studies

In many of the cohort studies, the authors did not compare the observed number of secondary leukaemias with the number expected from rates for the general population; however, the expected number of cases of acute myeloid leukaemia in the general population can be approximated from a European standardized annual incidence rate of 3–4/100 000 (Parkin *et al.*, 1997), with little variation between the countries in which the studies were carried out. Thus, the observed cumulative incidences in most studies are clearly higher than the incidence in the general population.

2.2.1 *Langerhans cell histiocytosis*

The cohort studies of patients with Langerhans cell histiocytosis are summarized in Table 1.

An Austrian, Dutch, German, Swiss cohort was formed, consisting of 363 patients (223 boys, 140 girls) who were enrolled in trials for the treatment of newly diagnosed disseminated or relapsed Langerhans cell histiocytosis between 1983 (since use of etoposide began in these countries) and 1995 (Haupt *et al.*, 1997). The diagnoses were made between 1969 and 1992. The patients received various treatments, depending on the date of start. In 1983–91, the induction chemotherapy comprised prednisone, vinblastine and etoposide, and continuation treatment consisted of 46 weeks of therapy with 6-mercaptopurine and re-induction pulses of prednisone, vinblastine with/without etoposide, with/without methotrexate. The total cumulative dose of etoposide was 900 mg/m^2 for subjects who received the drug only in the induction phase and 2100 mg/m^2 for those given continuation treatment. In 1991–95, the patients were randomized into two groups, one receiving vinblastine and the other receiving etoposide (cumulative dose, 3600 mg/m^2). The median length of follow-up was 5.5 years. In this cohort, 123 patients had received etoposide alone or in combination with other drugs not known to be leukaemogenic, whereas 41 patients who had not responded adequately to these treatment protocols were subsequently given doxorubicin and/or cyclophosphamide in addition to etoposide. For subjects treated with etoposide, the total cumulative dose received ranged between 150 and 17 600 mg/m^2 (median, 2000 mg/m^2); only 14 patients were treated with doses exceeding 4000 mg/m^2. No cases of acute myeloid leukaemia were reported; however, the rate in the Saarland Cancer Registry in Germany indicated that only 0.005 cases were expected.

An Italian cohort (Haupt *et al.*, 1994, 1997) consisted of 241 patients (132 boys and 109 girls) who were treated between 1977 and 1995 for newly diagnosed or relapsed Langerhans cell histiocytosis. The median length of follow-up was 5.8 years. The expected number of cases of leukaemia was estimated from age- and sex-specific incidence rates derived from the Varese Cancer Registry in Italy. The standardized incidence ratio (SIR) of acute myeloid leukaemia for the extended Italian cohort (Haupt *et al.*, 1997) was 520 (95% CI, 168–1213). Eighty-two patients had received etoposide

Table 1. Cohort studies of the risk for secondary acute myeloid leukaemia (AML) after treatment of Langerhans cell histiocytosis with etoposide

Study population	Cumulative dose of etoposide (mg/m^2)	No. of patients	Additional chemotherapy or radiotherapy	No. of observed cases of secondary acute myeloid leukaemia	Median follow-up (years)	SIR for AML	Remarks
223 boys, 140 girls in Austria, Germany, Netherlands, Switzerland; cases diagnosed in 1969–92 (age not given)	150–17 600	123	None	0	Total group ($n = 363$; 342 alive): 5.5		Some patients received teniposide, and the cumulative dose of teniposide was transformed into equivalent etoposide dose assuming a 1:2 ratio. 14 (first cohort) patients received > 4000 mg/m^2.
	150–17 600	41	Alkylating, intercalating agents and/or radiotherapy	0			
	0	147	None	0			
	0	52	Alkylating, intercalating agents and/or radiotherapy	0			
132 boys, 109 girls in Italy; cases diagnosed in 1977–95; age, 22 days–19 years	100–30 000	82	None	4	Total group ($n = 241$): 5.8	1600 (440–4100)	All AML cases received cumulative etoposide doses > 4000 mg/m^2. The SIR for subjects exposed to high cumulative doses of etoposide is 1800 (570–4200). 70 patients received > 4000 mg/m^2.
	100–30 000	31	Alkylating, intercalating agents and/or radiotherapy	1			
	0	112	None	0			
	0	16	Alkylating, intercalating agents and/or radiotherapy	0			

From Haupt et al. (1997)
SIR, standardized incidence ratio

as a single agent or in combination with other drugs not known to be leukaemogenic, while 31 patients had received etoposide in combination with one or more agents with possible leukaemogenic activity (vincristine, prednisone, vinblastine, doxorubicin and cyclophosphamide); 128 patients were not treated with etoposide. The cumulative dose of etoposide ranged between 100 and 30 000 mg/m^2 (median, 5200 mg/m^2); 70 children received more than 4000 mg/m^2. Five cases of acute promyelocytic leukaemia were diagnosed, all in etoposide-treated patients (four girls, one boy; latency, 27–106 months). Four of the five patients had not been exposed to alkylating agents, intercalating agents or radiotherapy; the SIR for this group was 1600 (95% CI, 435–4096). The fifth case occurred in the group that had received both etoposide and alkylating agents, intercalating agents or radiotherapy (SIR, 776; 95% CI, 19–4325). All of the patients with acute promyelocytic leukaemia had received a cumulative dose of etoposide exceeding 4000 mg/m^2, and the SIR for this group was 1782 (95% CI, 574–4159). No cases of acute promyelocytic leukaemia were observed in patients who had not received etoposide.

[The Working Group noted that a possible explanation for the difference in the results of the multicentre and the Italian trials is the cumulative dose of etoposide given: The Italian patients received an average of 5200 mg/m^2 while those in the multicentre trial received 2000 mg/m^2. Moreover, when treated with etoposide, 62% of the Italian patients and 8.5% of those in the multicentre trial had received a cumulative dose of etoposide > 4000 mg/m^2. Other reasons for the difference in results cannot, however, be excluded. Both studies lacked sufficient power to detect a significant difference in leukaemia risk between patients with Langerhans cell histiocytosis treated with and without etoposide, although no cases of acute myeloid leukaemia were observed without etoposide treatment. The Working Group also noted that a small, unspecified proportion of patients in the Italian cohort were treated with teniposide (Haupt *et al.*, 1994).]

2.2.2 *Germ-cell tumours in men*

In the early years of platinum-based chemotherapy for testicular cancer, the large majority of patients received the cisplatin, vinblastine, bleomycin regimen. The absence of an increased risk for acute myeloid leukaemia after this regimen has now been documented in several large studies of the risk for second malignancies (Pedersen-Bjergaard *et al.*, 1991; Bokemeyer & Schmoll, 1993; van Leeuwen *et al.*, 1994; Bokemeyer & Schmoll, 1995; van Leeuwen, 1997). Further evidence for the absence of cases of acute myeloid leukaemia with myelodysplastic syndrome in patients treated with this regimen comes from several trials with long-term follow-up (Ozols *et al.*, 1988; Roth *et al.*, 1988).

The cohort studies of germ-cell tumours in men are summarized in Table 2.

Pedersen-Bjergaard *et al.* (1991) described four cases of acute myeloid leukaemia and one of myelodysplastic syndrome in a cohort of 212 patients in Denmark with

Table 2. Cohort studies of the risk for secondary acute myeloid leukaemia (AML) or myelodysplastic syndrome (MDS) after treatment of germ-cell tumours with etoposide-containing regimens

Reference	Study population receiving etoposide	Cumulative dose of etoposide (mg/m^2)	No. of patients	Additional chemotherapy or radiotherapy	No. of observed cases of second malignancies	Follow-up period (years)	Relative risk for AML or MDS (observed/expected)	Cumulative risk for AML or MDS (95% CI)	Remarks
Denmark									
Pedersen-Bjergaard et al. (1991)	212 men Diagnosed in 1979–89	1800–3600							
		1800–2000	130	Cisplatin, bleomycin	5	5.7	340 (92–860) (AML)	4.7% at 5.7 years (AML + MDS)	Etoposide-treated patients
					0				
		2000–3600	82		5 (4 AML, 1 MDS)			11% at 5.7 years	
Germany									
Bokemeyer & Schmoll (1993)	293 men Diagnosed in 1970–90	≤ 2000	221	Cisplatin, bleomycin, vinblastine, anthracyclines, dactinomycin, ifosfamide	3 (1 ALL + 2 solid)	Median, 5.1	2.3 (0.1–13)	1.0% at 5 years (0.0–2.2)	SMR for etoposide-treated patients
		> 2000	72		0				
Bokemeyer et al. (1995)	128 men Diagnosed in 1983–93	> 2000 Median cumulative dose:							Etoposide-treated patients
		3750	22	Cisplatin, bleomycin, ifosfamide	1 (AML)	4.5	30–35 (NS)	0.8% (0–2.3) at 4.5 years	
		3800	50	Cisplatin, bleomycin	1 (AML)	6.1			
		3800	41	Cisplatin, ifosfamide	0	5.2			
		5300	15	Carboplatin, ifosfamide, autologous stem-cell rescue	0	3.4			
					0	2.3			

Table 2 (contd)

Reference	Study population receiving etoposide	Cumulative dose of etoposide (mg/m^2)	No. of patients	Additional chemotherapy or radiotherapy	No. of observed cases of second malignancies	Follow-up period (years)	Relative risk for AML or MDS (observed/expected)	Cumulative risk for AML or MDS (95% CI)	Remarks
Germany + France									
Kollmannsberger et al. (1998)	302 men, 15–55 years old Diagnosed in 1986–96	2400–14 000			4	4.3 Median, 3.5	160 (44–411)	1.3% (0.4–3.4) at 4.3 years	SIR. Mediastinal germ-cell cancer patients were included. 161 patients were included in the trial after failing first-line therapy.
		First-line therapy 2400–6000	141	Cisplatin, ifosfamide, autologous stem-cell support	2 (AML)				
		2400–14 000	161	Cisplatin, cyclophosphamide, ifosfamide, carboplatin, autologous stem-cell support	2 (AML) (2 MDS in mediastinal germ-cell cancer patients)	4.8–5.6			
United Kingdom									
Boshoff et al. (1995)	679 men Diagnosed in 1979–92	500–5000		Vincristine, methotrexate, cisplatin, bleomycin, actinomycin D, cyclophosphamide, vinblastine, carboplatin	6 AML + 4 solid tumours	2 (n = 541) > 5 (n = 331) Median, 5.7	150 (55–326)	NR	Mediastinal germ cell-cancer patients included in patient population
		≤ 2000	636		4 (AML)				
		> 2000	25		2 (AML)				

Table 2 (contd)

Reference	Study population receiving etoposide	Cumulative dose of etoposide (mg/m^2)	No. of patients	Additional chemotherapy or radiotherapy	No. of observed cases of second malignancies	Follow-up period (years)	Relative risk for AML or MDS (observed/expected)	Cumulative risk for AML or MDS (95% CI)	Remarks
United States									
Bajorin et al. (1993) New York	340 men Diagnosed in 1982–90	800–5000		Cisplatin, cyclophosphamide	2 (AML) (1 after cyclophosphamide)	≥ 5	NR	< 1% at 5 years for 1 AML seen after etoposide only	Incidence
Nichols et al. (1993) Indiana	538 men Diagnosed in 1982–91	1500–2000		Cisplatin, bleomycin, ifosfamide	2 (AML)	Median, 4.9	66 (8–238)	NR	3 cases observed in another group (of unknown size) of patients treated with etoposide off clinical trial protocol; 2 patients received 2000 mg/m^2.

ALL, acute lymphoblastic leukaemia; AML, acute myeloid leukaemia; CI, confidence interval; MDS, myelodysplastic syndrome; NR, not reported; SIR, standardized incidence ratio; SMR, standardized morbidity ratio; NS, not significant mostly testicular germ-cell tumours who had been treated with bleomycin, etoposide and cisplatin, none of whom had mediastinal germ-cell tumours. Thirty-five patients, treated between 1979 and 1983, received cisplatin, vinblastine and bleomycin and, at relapse, bleomycin (15 mg/m^2 weekly), etoposide (120 mg/m^2 for five days) and cisplatin (20 mg/m^2 for five days). In the subgroup of 20 patients who had received a cumulative etoposide dose of > 2000 mg/m^2, two cases of acute myelomonocytic leukaemia occurred. The latent periods after etoposide treatment were 25 and 54 months, respectively. For the 177 patients treated after 1983 to 1989 with first-line bleomycin, etoposide and cisplatin, the doses were adjusted according to risk category: 115 patients received standard doses (100 mg/m^2 etoposide for five days (cumulative dose, 2000 mg/m^2), 20 mg/m^2 cisplatin for five days, 15 mg/m^2 bleomycin weekly). No cases of acute myeloid leukaemia were diagnosed. In 62 patients who received high-dose treatment consisting of etoposide (200 mg/m^2 for five days; cumulative dose, 3000 mg/m^2), cisplatin (40 mg/m^2 for five days) and bleomycin (15 mg/m^2 weekly), two cases of acute myeloblastic leukaemia (one in a patient with extragonal germ-cell tumour) and one case of myelodysplastic syndrome developed. The latencies after etoposide treatment were 15 and 29 months for acute myeloblastic leukaemia and 68 months for the case of myelodysplastic syndrome. The expected number of de-novo cases of acute myeloid leukaemia was estimated from the leukaemia incidence reported in the Danish Cancer Registry for 1973–77. In comparison with the risk of the general population, the relative risk for overt leukaemia was 336 (95% CI, 92–861). The mean cumulative risk (Kaplan–Meier method) for leukaemic complications was 4.7% (SE, 2.3) 5.7 years after the start of etoposide-containing chemotherapy. No leukaemias or dysplastic syndromes were observed among the 130 patients who had received ≤ 2000 mg/m^2 etoposide, whereas five cases were seen among the 82 patients who had received > 2000 mg/m^2 ($p = 0.004$). The cumulative risk for leukaemia among the 82 patients receiving high-dose etoposide (> 2000 mg/m^2) was 11% (SE, 5.0) 5.7 years after the start of chemotherapy. Although five cases of leukaemia and dysplastic syndrome were found in the 212 etoposide-treated patients, none was found in a previous cohort of 127 patients with germ-cell tumour treated with vinblastine and similar doses of cisplatin and bleomycin ($p = 0.08$).

Bokemeyer and Schmoll (1993) assessed the risk for secondary neoplasms after therapy for germ-cell tumours in 1025 patients treated between 1970 and 1990 in Germany. Patients followed-up for longer than 12 months were eligible (1018 patients; 394 had seminomatous germ-cell tumours). The median follow-up was 61 months, and the median age of the patients at diagnosis was 28.9 years. The chemotherapy regimens consisted mainly of cisplatin, bleomycin and either vinblastine or etoposide. A total of 293 patients received etoposide during their treatment: 221 patients received cumulative doses of ≤ 2000 mg/m^2; 72 patients received > 2000 mg/m^2. The cumulative incidence of second tumours after etoposide-containing therapy was 1.0% (95% CI, 0.0–2.2), while that after chemotherapy without etoposide was 0.8% (95% CI, 0.0–2.5) (not significant). The standardized morbidity ratio of second malignancy for patients treated with etoposide was 2.3 (95% CI, 0.1–13 (not significant)) when compared with the cancer incidence rate in the male German population (based on the Saarland Cancer Registry). Among the 221 patients who received ≤ 2000 mg/m^2 etoposide, three developed a secondary tumour: one carcinoid tumour, one rhabdomyosarcoma and one lymphoblastic leukaemia; the last patient had received four cycles of bleomycin, etoposide and cisplatin (cumulative dose of etoposide, 2000 mg/m^2), and the interval to second leukaemia was 16 months. In patients who received > 2000 mg/m^2 etoposide, no second malignancies occurred.

Bokemeyer *et al.* (1995) analysed the risk for leukaemia of long-term survivors of three treatment protocols of the German Testicular Cancer Study Group and of patients treated at Hannover University Medical School, all of whom had received cumulative doses of etoposide of > 2000 mg/m^2. All patients had non-seminomatous germ-cell tumours. The study was limited to those who had achieved complete remission or a stable partial response with no tumour markers after chemotherapy, with a minimum follow-up of 12 months. Patients with prior abdominal or mediastinal radiotherapy were excluded. The first cohort consisted of 22 patients who were treated between 1983 and 1989 with three or four cycles of bleomycin, etoposide and cisplatin as induction chemotherapy followed by cisplatin, etoposide and ifosfamide as salvage chemotherapy at relapse. The median cumulative dose of etoposide was 3750 mg/m^2. The second cohort was composed of 50 patients with metastatic testicular cancer who had been treated during 1984–88 with first-line chemotherapy consisting of a 'double-dose' of cisplatin, a 'double-dose' of etoposide and bleomycin (175 mg/m^2 cisplatin and 1000 mg/m^2 etoposide per cycle; four cycles). The median cumulative dose of etoposide was 3800 mg/m^2. The third cohort consisted of 41 patients who had been treated in a stepwise dose–escalation protocol with the cisplatin, etoposide and ifosfamide regimen as first-line therapy for 'advanced' germ-cell tumours. The patients were treated during 1989–92 with 150 mg/m^2 cisplatin and 8000 mg/m^2 ifosfamide plus either 750 mg/m^2 or 1000 g/m^2 etoposide per cycle for four consecutive cycles. The median total dose of etoposide given to these patients was 3800 mg/m^2. The fourth cohort consisted of 15 patients treated between 1990 and 1993 for relapsed testicular cancer with high doses of carboplatin, etoposide and ifosfamide followed by autologous stem-cell rescue. These patients had received primary chemotherapy that included etoposide and at least one regimen of salvage therapy with etoposide before the high-dose treatment, which resulted in a median cumulative dose of etoposide of 5300 mg/m^2. After a total median follow-up time of 4.5 years, one case of myelomonocytic leukaemia was diagnosed in the first cohort (after 6.1 years). The cumulative incidence of secondary leukaemia in the group of 128 patients after 4.5 years of median follow-up was 0.8% (95% CI, 0–2.34). When compared with the annual incidence of five cases of myeloid leukaemia per 100 000 persons in the general population, the relative risk for secondary leukaemia was increased approximately 30- to 35-fold, which is not statistically significant. [The Working Group noted that the power of this study was insufficient to detect an increased risk for leukaemia in the individual cohorts or to detect differences between low and high doses of etoposide-containing regimens. The Working Group also noted that there may have been overlap with the previous study.]

Kollmannsberger et al. (1998) examined the risk for acute myeloid leukaemia after high cumulative doses of etoposide (> 2000 mg/m^2) and stem-cell transplantation in patients with advanced or relapsed germ-cell tumours. The records of 302 patients (median age, 29 years) with germ-cell tumours (241 testicular, 33 retroperitoneal and 28 mediastinal) who were treated with high-dose chemotherapy in clinical trials in Germany and France between 1986 and 1996 were reviewed. Patients had to have had a minimal follow-up of 12 months. Of the three German trials, the first included first-line therapy with one cycle of standard-dose cisplatin 20 mg/m^2, etoposide 100 mg/m^2 and ifosfamide 1200 mg/m^2 daily for five days followed by three to four cycles of of the same treatment escalated over seven doses: the highest consisted of 20 mg/m^2 cisplatin, 300 mg/m^2 etoposide and 2400 mg/m^2 ifosfamide daily for five consecutive days every three weeks. In the second German trial, patients who relapsed after receiving cisplatin and etoposide-based chemotherapy received two cycles of a standard-dose cisplatin, etoposide and ifosfamide regimen followed by two cycles of 500 mg/m^2 carboplatin, 400 mg/m^2 etoposide and 2500 mg/m^2 cyclophosphamide. In the third German trial, patients who relapsed after initial therapy with cisplatin and etoposide received two cycles of standard-dose cisplatin, etoposide and ifosfamide followed by carboplatin, 300–400 mg/m^2 etoposide and ifosfamide. All the patients in France were treated with high-dose etoposide-containing chemotherapy including cisplatin, carboplatin and cyclophosphamide or ifosfamide, either as first-line consolidation therapy (patients with poor prognostic criteria) or as treatment for relapsed germ-cell tumour. All patients received either autologous bone marrow or autologous peripheral blood stem-cell support, and most patients also received granulocyte- or granulocyte–macrophage colony-stimulating factor after high-dose chemotherapy. The median cumulative dose of etoposide was 5000 mg/m^2 (range, 2400–14 000 mg/m^2). Six patients developed a secondary haematological malignancy (four acute myeloid leukaemias and two myelodysplastic syndromes). The two cases of myelodysplastic syndrome occurred in patients with a primary mediastinal germ-cell tumour and were excluded from the analysis. For the total group of 302 patients, the cumulative incidence of acute myeloid leukaemia was 1.3% (95% CI, 0.4–3.4%) at a median follow-up time of 4.3 years. The standardized incidence ratio in comparison with data from the Saarland Cancer Registry in Germany for 1989–93 was 160 (95% CI, 44–411). The latency from start of etoposide treatment was 24–58 months. Two of the malignancies were acute monoblastic leukaemia and two were acute myelomonocytic leukaemia; three were found in patients with testicular cancer as the primary tumour.

Boshoff et al. (1995) reported on the incidence of second cancer in 679 male patients (634 with testicular cancer) in the United Kingdom with advanced germ-cell cancer who had been treated with one of two etoposide-containing protocols. Between 1979 and 1992, 343 patients were treated with cisplatin, vincristine, methotrexate, bleomycin, actinomycin D, cyclophosphamide and etoposide, and 336 patients were treated with etoposide, platinum (cisplatin or carboplatin) and bleomycin with or without vinblastine. Patients who did not achieve complete remission or who died of germ-cell cancer were not excluded from the analysis. A total of 541 patients were followed-up for more than two years and 331 for more than five years. Six patients developed acute myeloid leukaemia, and four developed solid tumours. None of them had a primary mediastinal germ-cell tumour, and only one patient had received radiotherapy. The median interval between the onset of treatment and the development of leukaemia was 27 months. Four of six cases were acute myelomonocytic leukaemia, one was acute myeloid and the other acute myeloblastic leukaemia. The cumulative dose of etoposide in the cases of leukaemia ranged from 720 to 5000 mg/m^2. In the three cases treated with cisplatin, vincristine, methotrexate, bleomycin, actinomycin D, cyclophosphamide and etoposide, the relative risk for secondary leukaemia was 150 (95% CI, 55–326) ($p < 0.001$), on the basis of a comparison with data from the Office of Population Censuses and Surveys for England and Wales. Two of 25 patients who received total doses > 2000 mg/m^2 developed acute myeloid leukaemia, whereas four of 636 who received < 2000 mg/m^2 developed acute myeloid leukaemia ($p = 0.02$). Four patients developed solid tumours (excluding cancer of the contralateral testis). [The Working Group noted that the cumulative incidence in the patients given the low and high doses of etoposide was not properly compared; instead, the authors compared the frequency and also did not adjust for the doses of cyclophosphamide and actinomycin in the seven-agent regimen.]

In a study in New York, USA, Bajorin et al. (1993) investigated the risk for developing acute myeloid leukaemia of 503 patients with advanced germ-cell tumours who had been treated with etoposide-containing therapy according to a cancer centre protocol between 1982 and 1990; 340 patients with a minimum disease-free survival greater than one year were selected. Six patients with acute myeloid leukaemia were identified; however, four of them had a mediastinal germ-cell tumour. One patient aged 31 with testicular cancer had received cisplatin, etoposide (cumulative dose, 2000 mg/m^2), vinblastine, bleomycin, dactinomycin and cyclophosphamide as induction plus salvage therapy. After 56 months, he developed acute myeloblastic leukaemia. The second patient with testicular cancer, a man aged 35, had received induction therapy consisting of cisplatin, carboplatin and etoposide (cumulative dose, 1300 mg/m^2). After 26 months, he developed acute myeloblastic leukaemia. Thus, one of the 310 patients (291 treated with bleomycin, carboplastin and cisplatin) who had received only one etoposide-containing induction chemotherapy regimen subsequently developed acute myeloid leukaemia, giving a definite incidence [an approximate actuarial risk] of less than 1.0% at five years.

In a study in Indiana (USA) designed to estimate the risk for developing leukaemia of patients receiving conventional doses of etoposide, mostly with cisplatin and bleomycin, Nichols et al. (1993) reviewed the records of 538 previously untreated patients with (disseminated) germ-cell cancer entering clinical trials between 1982 and 1991, who were given conventional doses of etoposide (cumulative dose, 1500–2000 mg/m^2) in combination with cisplatin and either ifosfamide (190 cases) or bleomycin, in three or four cycles administered in short intravenous infusions of 100 mg/m^2 daily for five days. Of these patients, 337 had been followed-up for longer than two years. Five of the 538 patients developed a haematological malignancy. Three of the five developed acute leukaemia associated with a primary mediastinal germ-cell tumour and were excluded from the study. Two patients (0.37%) with a primary testicular cancer developed leukaemia: after the start of bleomycin, etoposide and cisplatin therapy (cumulative dose of etoposide for both, 2000 mg/m^2), one developed acute myelomonocytic leukaemia after 2.3 years and the other developed acute undifferentiated myeloid leukaemia after 2.0 years. The number of cases of leukaemia expected was estimated from the rates for white male US Navy personnel aged 17–34, who reflect the population of patients with testicular cancer entering clinical trials at Indiana University (Garland et al., 1990). The relative risk for developing leukaemia was 66 (95% CI, 8–238). [The Working Group calculated a cumulative incidence of < 1% at five years.] The authors also reported three cases of haematological abnormality (acute monoblastic leukaemia, acute myeloid leukaemia and refractory anaemia with excess blasts in transition (myelodysplastic syndrome)) in 'several hundred' patients who received a chemotherapy regimen containing etoposide, vinblastine, ifosfamide or cisplatin after failing to respond to primary chemotherapy involving treatment with total doses of etoposide of 2000 ($n = 2$) and 4400 ($n = 1$) mg/m^2.

[The Working Group calculated the relative risk for acute myeloid leukaemia or myelodysplastic syndrome in germ-cell tumour patients treated with etoposide-containing regimens with cisplatin and bleomycin and, in some cases, vinca alkaloids, from all of the studies reported above (see Table 3). Twelve cases of leukaemia or myelodysplastic syndrome (10 cases of acute myeloid leukaemia, one case of acute lymphoblastic leukaemia and one of myelodysplastic syndrome, were observed among 1720 patients with germ-cell tumours. On the basis of 8699 patient–years of follow-up and an annual incidence rate of 3–4 cases of acute myeloid leukaemia per 100 000 population (Parkin et al., 1997), the relative risk for acute myeloid leukaemia or myelodysplastic syndrome in the germ-cell tumour patients was significantly elevated by a factor of 40 (95% CI, 17–81).]

Since the background incidence of acute myeloid leukaemia in the population is low, this high relative risk translates to a rather low absolute risk. According to Bokemeyer and Schmoll (1995), the cumulative risk for acute myeloid leukaemia was only 0.58% (95% CI, 0.29–0.94%) after five years in 1868 published cases of patients treated with conventional etoposide-containing regimens (cumulative dose, ≤ 2000 mg/m^2), on the basis of the six cases reported by Boshoff et al. (1995), two by Nichols et al. (1993), two by Bajorin et al. (1993), one by Bokemeyer and Schmoll (1993) and none by Pedersen-Bjergaard et al. (1991).

Cohort studies of other types of cancer are summarized in Table 4 and are described below.

Table 3. Summary of studies in which 12 cases of leukaemia or myelodysplastic syndrome were found after treatment for germ-cell tumours with etoposide-containing regimens with cisplatin and bleomycin and, in some cases, vinca alkaloids

Reference	Cumulative dose of etoposide received	Type of malignancy	Agents other than etoposide	Number treated with this regimen	
				Patients	Person–years
Pedersen-Bjergaard et al. (1991)	7400 mg	AML	Cisplatin, bleomycin, vinblastine	212	[848]
	6075 mg	AML	Cisplatin, bleomycin, vinblastine, vincristine		
	4250 mg	AML	Cisplatin, bleomycin (X-ray)		
	7500 mg	MDS	Cisplatin, bleomycin (X-ray)		
	5250 mg	AML	Cisplatin, bleomycin		
Bokemeyer et al. (1995)	3800 mg	AML	Cisplatin, bleomycin	50	[225]
Bokemeyer & Schmoll (1993)	2000 mg/m^2	ALL	Cisplatin, bleomycin	293	[1465]
Bajorin et al. (1993)	1300 mg/m^2	AML	Cisplatin, carboplatin	291	[1455]
Nichols et al. (1993)	2000 mg/m^2	AML	Cisplatin, bleomycin	538[a]	[2690]
	2000 mg/m^2	AML	Cisplatin, bleomycin		
Boshoff et al. (1995)	720 mg/m^2	AML	Cisplatin, bleomycin, vinblastine	336	[2016]
	750 mg/m^2	AML	Cisplatin, bleomycin, vinblastine		
	1440 mg/m^2	AML	Carboplatin, bleomycin		
Total				1720	8699

AML, acute myeloid leukaemia; ALL, acute lymphoblastic leukaemia
[a] Patients treated with ifosfamide included

Table 4. Cohort studies of acute myeloid leukaemia (AML) or myelodysplastic syndrome (MDS) occurring after treatment with etoposide-containing regimens of cancers other than Langerhans cell histiocytosis and germ-cell tumours

Reference	Study population	Cumulative dose of etoposide (mg/m^2)	No. of patients	Additional chemotherapy or radiotherapy	No. of observed second malignancies	Follow-up period	Relative risk (observed/expected)	Cumulative risk (95 % CI)	Remarks
Acute lymphoblastic leukaemia in children									
Pui et al. (1991) (Tennessee, USA)	Diagnosed in 1979–88 < 19 years	No etoposide, no teniposide No etoposide, 600–4620 teniposide 9000 etoposide, 5100 teniposide	734 154 279 301	Prednisone, vincristine, asparaginase, methotrexate, mercaptopurine, cyclophosphamide, doxorubicin, cytarabine, cranial irradiation	21 (AML) 1 (AML) 7 (AML) 9 (AML) (+ 4 AML as second adverse effect)		NR	3.8% (2.3–6.1) at 6 years	Specific analysis for different schedules of drug administration
Winick et al. (1993) (Texas, USA)	Diagnosed in 1986–91 1–18 years	9900	203	Prednisone, vincristine, daunorubicin, asparaginase, methotrexate, mercaptopurine, leucovorin, cytarabine	10 (AML)		NR	5.9 % (SE 3.2%) at 4 years	The first 33 patients received teniposide instead of etoposide at half the dose.
Other types of childhood cancer									
Smith et al. (1993) (USA)	**Rhabdomyo-sarcoma** diagnosed around 1984	600–900	207	Dactinomycin, cisplatin, doxorubicin, cyclophosphamide (24 g/m^2)	4 (3 AML, 1 MDS)	Mean, 3.7 years	NR	3.2% (1.2–8.6) at 6 years	

Table 4 (contd)

Reference	Study population	Cumulative dose of etoposide (mg/m^2)	No. of patients	Additional chemotherapy or radiotherapy	No. of observed second malignancies	Follow-up period	Relative risk (observed/expected)	Cumulative risk (95 % CI)	Remarks
Other types of childhood cancer (contd)									
Smith et al. (1999) (USA)	**Various primary tumours** diagnosed in 1986–94; various ages	< 1500 (rhabdomyosarcoma, medulloblastoma)	451	Rhabdomyosarcoma: cyclophosphamide (25–35 g/m^2), ifosfamide	8 (4 AML, 4 MDS)	3 years	NR	2.1% (upper 95% CI bound, 3.7%) at 4 years	A 1:2 conversion was used to equate teniposide dose to etoposide dose. Each treatment stratum consists of patients with different primary tumours, ages, treatments.
		1500–3000 (neuroblastoma, germ-cell cancer, ALL)	1270	No cyclophosphamide	4 (2 AML, 2 MDS)			0.4% (upper 95% CI bound, 1.0%) at 4 years	
		> 3000 (rhabdomyosarcoma, Ewing sarcoma)	570	Cyclophosphamide (25–35 g/m^2), ifosfamide	5 (2 AML, 2 MDS, 1 T-cell ALL)			1.4% (upper 95% CI bound, 2.9%) at 4 years	
Heyn et al. (1994) (USA)	**Rhabdomyosarcoma** diagnosed in 1984–91; 0–21 years	643–3200	223	Cyclophosphamide, vincristine, dactinomycin, doxorubicin, cisplatin, radiotherapy	5 (4 AML, 1 MDS) + 1 osteogenic sarcoma	Median, 3.7 years	NR	Incidence of AML: 52/10 000 person–years	Preliminary results of low-dose study of Smith et al. (1999)

Table 4 (contd)

Reference	Study population	Cumulative dose of etoposide (mg/m²)	No. of patients	Additional chemotherapy or radiotherapy	No. of observed second malignancies	Follow-up period	Relative risk (observed/ expected)	Cumulative risk (95 % CI)	Remarks
Other types of childhood cancer (contd)									
Duffner et al. (1998) (USA)	**Brain tumours** diagnosed in 1986–90; < 3 years	Intravenous etoposide 6.5 mg/kg bw on 2 days per cycle	198	Vincristine, cyclophosphamide, cisplatin, irradiation		Median for 75 surviving children, 6.4 years	NR	Total group: Haematological and solid tumours: 11% (0–39%) (n = 198) at 8 years	No information on cumulative dose of etoposide
		≤ 2 years: 24 months etoposide	132		3 (2 MDS, 1 AML) + 1 sarcoma + 1 meningioma			19% (0–70%) at 8 years for children < 24 months at diagnosis;	
		2–3 years: 12 months etoposide	66					4.8% (0–38%) at 8 years for children 24–36 months at diagnosis	
Sugita et al. (1993) (Japan)	**Non-Hodgkin lymphoma** diagnosed in 1987–91 2–17 years; 28 boys, 10 girls	4200–5600	38	Prednisolone, vincristine, L-asparaginase, mercaptopurine, methotrexate, cranial irradiation, behenoyl cytarabine	5 AML + 3 haematological relapses	Median, 19 months (6–60 months)	NR	18% at 4 years	Short follow-up

Table 4 (contd)

Reference	Study population	Cumulative dose of etoposide (mg/m^2)	No. of patients	Additional chemotherapy or radiotherapy	No. of observed second malignancies	Follow-up period	Relative risk (observed/ expected)	Cumulative risk (95 % CI)	Remarks
Lung cancer									
Ratain et al. (1987) (USA)	Diagnosed in 1981–84 17 men, 7 women; median age, 56 (range, 38–69)	4382–7950	24	Cisplatin, vindesine, radiotherapy	4 (AML)		NR	15% (SE, 11%) at 2 years	3 patients (no AML cases) did not receive etoposide. Patients are 1-year survivors.
Breast cancer									
Yagita et al. (1998) (Japan)	Diagnosed in 1985–94; 24 women	< 2000 2000–5000 > 5000	7 10 7	Doxorubicin, vindesine, cyclophos-phamide, cisplatin	2 AML + 1 MDS	1–40 months	Total group 630 (130–1800)	$p < 0.01$	Short follow-up

ALL, acute lymphoblastic leukaemia; AML, acute myeloid leukaemia; CI, confidence interval; MDS, myelodysplastic syndrome; NR, not reported; SE, standard error. The expected number of cases of acute myeloid leukaemia in the general population can be approximated from a world standardized incidence rate of 4–5 per 100 000 persons (see text).

2.2.3 Acute lymphoblastic leukaemia in children

Pui *et al.* (1991) reported on the risk for acute myeloid leukaemia among 734 children (< 19 years old) in Tennessee, USA, in whom acute lymphoblastic leukaemia was diagnosed between 1979 and 1988. After having achieved complete remission, the patients received maintenance treatment with epipodophyllotoxins according to seven schedules (Table 5): 580 patients received teniposide (see monograph, this volume), and a substantial proportion of these (301) also received etoposide. In addition, most patients received methotrexate, mercaptopurine, prednisone, vincristine, asparaginase and cytarabine, and some patients received cyclophosphamide, doxorubicin and cranial irradiation. Acute myeloid leukaemia developed in 21 children (as a first adverse event in 17), with an overall cumulative risk of 3.8% (2.3–6.1%) at six years; one developed in a child not receiving etoposide or teniposide. The median interval between the diagnoses of acute lymphoblastic leukaemia and acute myeloid leukaemia was 40 months. Six of the cases were acute myelomonocytic leukaemia, eight were acute monoblastic leukaemia, three were acute myeloblastic leukaemia, one was acute megakaryoblastic leukaemia, one was acute myeloid leukaemia and two were acute undifferentiated leukaemia. In four patients, acute myeloid leukaemia developed after relapse had occurred, and these were not included in the statistical analyses. In the analysis of leukaemia risk, the doses of teniposide and etoposide were weighted equally, since the potency of teniposide *in vitro*—10 times that of etoposide—is offset *in vivo* by extensive protein binding, resulting in 10 times less unbound (active) drug (see section 4). The schedule of epipodophyllotoxin treatment appeared to be a crucial factor in determining the risk for acute myeloid leukaemia, as the strongest evidence was obtained by comparing two subgroups that differed only in their schedule of epipodophyllotoxin administration. The two groups were scheduled to receive the same cumulative doses of teniposide (5100 mg/m^2) and etoposide (9000 mg/m^2); among 84 patients in the first group (XI-HR3) who received epipodophyllotoxins weekly, the risk for acute myeloid leukaemia was clearly and significantly increased (12% at six years; 95% CI, 6.1–24%) as compared with the risk of the second subgroup of 148 patients (XI-HR2) who received the agents every other week (1.6% at six years; 95% CI, 0.4–6.1% [$p = 0.01$ by log-rank test for the difference between groups]. The multivariate analysis indicated that the frequency of epipodophyllotoxin administration was a much more important determinant of risk for acute myeloid leukaemia than cumulative dose. The frequency of treatment remained significant (relative risk, 6.7; 95% CI, 1.5–31; $p < 0.01$) after adjustment in a Cox model for all competing covariates, including cranial irradiation, cyclophosphamide and several factors characteristic of a poor prognosis for acute lymphoblastic leukaemia; however, since the total dose varied only slightly among the patients, its effects could not be assessed reliable. [The Working Group noted that the carcinogenic effects of etoposide could not be evaluated because all patients were treated with teniposide and none received etoposide alone, while patients treated with and without etoposide received teniposide at different schedules.]

Table 5. Risks for secondary acute myeloid leukaemia (AML) in children with acute lymphoblastic leukaemia treated with epipodophyllotoxins, according to regimen

Regimen	Prognosis	Planned cumulative dose (mg/m^2)		Epipodophyllotoxin schedule	No. of patients treated	No. of patients with AML	Six-year cumulative risk % (95% CI)
		Teniposide	Etoposide				
X-LR1	Low risk	0	0	None	154	1	1.0 (0.6–6.3)
X-LR2	Low risk	1350	0	Every other week	155	1	1.1 (0.1–7.1)
X-HR	High risk	4620	0	Twice weekly	85	6	12 (5.7–25)
XI-LR1	Low risk	600	0	Induction only	39	0	0
XI-LR2	Low risk	5100	9000	Every other week	69	0	0
XI-HR2	High risk	5100	9000	Every other week	148	2	1.6 (0.4–6.1)
XI-HR3	High risk	5100	9000	Weekly	84	7	12 (6.1–24)

From Pui et al. (1991)
CI, confidence interval

Winick et al. (1993) studied a cohort of 203 consecutive children aged 1–18 in Texas, USA, with early B-lineage acute lymphoblastic leukaemia diagnosed in 1986 and 1991, who received induction treatment and achieved complete remission. The induction and maintenance treatment consisted of prednisone, vincristine, daunorubicin, asparaginase, methotrexate, mercaptopurine, leucovorin, intravenous etoposide (300 mg/m^2) and cytarabine. The first 33 patients received teniposide instead of etoposide at half the dose. The planned cumulative dose of etoposide was 9900 mg/m^2. Only four patients received radiation therapy; none received alkylating agents. Ten children developed secondary acute myeloid leukaemia, two of which were of the myelomonocytic type and two of the monoblastic type; one developed myelodysplastic syndrome (consistent with chronic myelomonocytic leukaemia), and one had refractory anaemia with excess blasts in transformation. The interval between the diagnosis of acute lymphoblastic and acute myeloid leukaemia ranged from 23 to 68 months. The median dose of etoposide administered was 7900 mg/m^2 (range, 5100–9900 mg/m^2). One child with acute myeloid leukaemia had received teniposide instead of etoposide. The risk for secondary acute myeloid leukaemia at four years was 5.9% (SE, 3.2%), with risks for standard- and poor-risk patients of 6.3% (SE, 4.0%) and 4.7% (SE, 5.2%) respectively. [The Working Group noted that the patients treated with etoposide and teniposide were considered together as if they had received the same treatment, assuming equivalent leukaemogenic potencies. The Working Group also noted that it was not completely clear in these two studies whether the diagnosis of acute lymphoblastic leukaemia excluded primary mixed leukaemia and thus allowed differentiation of lymphoblastic from myeloid disease.]

2.2.4 *Other types of childhood cancer*

Smith et al. (1993) presented the first results of a monitoring plan for secondary acute myeloid leukaemia in clinical trials of the Cancer Therapy Evaluation Program of the National Cancer Institute in the USA. A total of 465 children [ages not given] with primary rhabdomyosarcoma (diagnosis around 1984) took part in this trial. The analysis was restricted to 207 children who had survived more than 36 weeks from entry into the protocol. They had received etoposide daily in combination with two courses of dactinomycin (cumulative dose of etoposide, 600 mg/m^2) or three courses of cisplatin (cumulative dose of etoposide, 900 mg/m^2), after they had been treated with induction regimens that included cyclophosphamide and doxorubicin. The mean duration of follow up was 3.7 years. Interim analyses of the risks for acute myeloid leukaemia and myelodysplastic syndrome were carried out when four cases had been observed. Two of the four cases had received etoposide (600 mg/m^2) and dactinomycin, and two had received etoposide (900 mg/m^2) and cisplatin. The three cases of acute myeloid leukaemia were of the myelomonocytic and monoblastic types and myelodysplastic syndrome progressing to acute myeloid leukaemia; the other case was myelodysplastic syndrome. The patients in the two treatment groups in which these four cases occurred had been treated for induction of remission with similar doses of doxorubicin (480 mg/m^2), cyclophosphamide (24 000 mg/m^2) and cisplatin (360 mg/m^2). The latency ranged from 2.0 to 3.3 years. The calculated cumulative six-year rate of development of acute myeloid leukaemia or myelodysplastic syndrome was 3.2% (95% CI, 1.2–8.6%). [The Working Group noted that the cumulative dose of cyclophosphamide was > 20 000 mg/m^2, which is known to be leukaemogenic (Curtis *et al.*, 1992).]

Smith *et al.* (1999) described the results of the second analysis of the monitoring plan, with results for the groups receiving low, moderate and higher cumulative doses of epipodophyllotoxins. Twelve trials were selected from a pool of approximately 100 in which etoposide or teniposide had been used. [The data from these trials do not appear to have been published elsewhere.] The 12 trials were selected on the basis of the length of accrual and the treatment of patient populations with significant numbers of survivors two to three years after treatment. Selection was made without knowledge of the number of secondary leukaemias that had occurred to date in the trials. The 12 trials (11 for patients with solid tumours and one for patients with acute lymphoblastic leukaemia) were divided into three strata according to the cumulative dose of etoposide: low (< 1500 mg/m^2), moderate (1500–3000 mg/m^2) and high (> 3000 mg/m^2). For trials in which teniposide was used, a 1:2 ratio was used to convert the dose of teniposide to that of etoposide. Patients treated with the low dose had primary rhabdomyosarcoma ($n = 222$) or medulloblastoma (advanced stage) ($n = 229$). The patients with rhabdomyosarcoma had also received cyclophosphamide or equivalent doses of ifosfamide (25 000–35 000 mg/m^2). Patients treated with the moderate dose had primary neuroblastoma ($n = 319$), germ-cell tumour (adult and paediatric) ($n = 700$) or acute lymphoblastic leukaemia (high risk) ($n = 251$). Patients given the higher dose had primary rhabdomyosarcoma ($n = 313$) or Ewing sarcoma ($n = 257$). They also received cyclophosphamide or equivalent doses of ifosfamide (25 000–35 000 mg/m^2). For each interim analysis (see Smith *et al.*, 1993), the total patient follow-up was calculated for all protocols within the treatment group, excluding the first 36 weeks of follow-up, since the incidence of leukaemia development during this period is extremely low, and the four-year and six-year cumulative incidence rates were estimated. The six-year actuarial risks for acute myeloid leukaemia or myelodysplastic syndrome were 3.3% (upper 95% CI bound, 5.9%) with the low cumulative dose of epipodophyllotoxin, 0.7% (upper 95% CI bound, 1.6%) with the moderate cumulative dose and 2.2% (upper 95% CI bound, 4.6%) with the high cumulative dose. The p values for homogeneity of the risks for secondary leukaemia across the cumulative dose strata were 0.012 (parametric test) and 0.011 (non-parametric test). Thus, the data provide no support for an effect of the cumulative dose of epipodophyllotoxins on leukaemogenic activity, at least not within the cumulative dose range encompassed by the monitoring plan. [The Working Group noted that the three treatment strata were compared as if the cumulative dose of epipodophyllotoxin were the only difference between them; however, the strata also differed with respect to the primary tumour (stratum with solid tumours versus stratum with solid and lymphoid tumours) and treatment (one stratum with high-dose epipodophyllotoxin and high-dose cyclophosphamide versus a stratum with no cyclophosphamide and a moderate dose of epipodophyllotoxin and a stratum with high-dose cyclophosphamide given to part (one trial) of the stratum with low dose epipodophyllotoxin). It is also not clear which patients received teniposide and which received etoposide.]

Between 1984 and 1991, 1062 patients with rhabdomyosarcoma (age, 0–21 years) entered a trial in the USA (Heyn et al., 1994). Of these, 223 patients received etoposide in combination with cyclophosphamide, vincristine, dactinomycin, doxorubicin and cisplatin, with a total dose of etoposide of 600–900 mg/m^2. All patients also received radiotherapy. The median follow-up time was 3.7 years. Four cases of acute myeloid leukaemia, one of myelodysplastic syndrome and one of osteogenic sarcoma were reported. The median time from the initiation of primary treatment to the diagnosis of leukaemia was 39 months. Three of four leukaemia patients had received etoposide in combination with doxorubicin, cyclophosphamide (13 000–21 900 mg/m^2), cisplatin and other agents and radiotherapy during their treatment. The cumulative doses of etoposide were 643, 765, 911 and 3197 mg/m^2. Two cases were myelomonocytic and two were monoblastic leukaemia. The incidence of acute myeloid leukaemia among patients who had received etoposide in combination with doxorubicin, cyclophosphamide, cisplatin and other agents and radiotherapy during their treatment was 52 per 10 000 person–years. When cyclophosphamide alone or cyclophosphamide plus doxorubicin but no etoposide was part of the regimen, the incidence was 7.6 per 10 000 person-years. The relative risk for acute myeloid leukaemia in a comparison of the etoposide-containing regimen and that without etoposide was thus 7.2 (95% CI, 0.8–65; $p = 0.06$). The patient who developed myelodysplastic syndrome after five years and seven months had received etoposide (840 mg/m^2) in combination with doxorubicin, cyclophosphamide (18 500 mg/m^2), cisplatin and other agents and radiotherapy during his treatment. [The Working Group noted that it is not clear whether the two treatment groups differed with respect to the doses of drugs other than etoposide or of radiation.]

Between 1986 and 1990, 198 children under three years of age with primary brain tumours were included in the study of Duffner et al. (1998) in the USA. Chemotherapy was started two to four weeks after surgery and consisted of vincristine, cyclophosphamide, cisplatinum and intravenous etoposide (6.5 mg/kg bw on days 3 and 4, every three months). Chemotherapy was planned for 24 months for children 0–23 months of age at diagnosis, and for 12 months for those 24–36 months of age. Irradiation therapy was started three to four weeks after the last cycle of chemotherapy. The median duration of follow-up for the 75 surviving children was 6.4 years. Five children developed a secondary malignancy. One developed a sarcoma, one a meningioma, and three developed haematological malignancies: two myelodysplastic syndromes with latencies of 7.7 and 4.8 years and an acute myeloid leukaemia with a latency of 2.8 years. The child with acute myeloid leukaemia had received a cumulative dose of etoposide of approximately 2400 mg/m^2. The actuarial risk for developing a second malignancy (solid or haematological) eight years after diagnosis was 11% (95% CI, 0–39). [The Working Group noted that the risk for secondary haematological malignancy was not analysed separately. The possibility that cyclophosphamide contributed to the risk for leukaemia could not be excluded, but the dose was lower than that considered to be leukaemogenic (Curtis *et al.*, 1992).]

Sugita *et al.* (1993) reported on 38 patients, 2–17 years old, in Japan who were treated for non-Hodgkin lymphoma diagnosed between 1987 and 1991 with a protocol that included etoposide (cumulative dose, 5600 mg/m^2). Etoposide (200 mg/m^2) and behenoyl cytarabine were given twice weekly before and after a conventional four-week induction course of prednisolone, vincristine and L-asparaginase. Maintenance therapy consisted of 6-mercaptopurine and methotrexate, administered for 2.5 years, with five two-week pulses of etoposide (200 mg/m^2) and behenoyl cytarabine given every 10 weeks during the first year. All received periodic infusions of methotrexate and prophylactic cranial irradiation. The median follow-up was 19 months. Five of eight patients with haematological relapses developed secondary acute myeloid leukaemia, with a cumulative risk at four years of 18.4% (Kaplan-Meier estimate). [Insufficient information was available to calculate the confidence interval.] Two cases occurred in patients while they were being treated with etoposide. One had been treated for relapse of non-Hodgkin lymphoma with higher doses of etoposide, cyclophosphamide, doxorubicin and also ifosfamide, vincristine, pirarubicin and mitoxantrone. The five patients with acute myeloid leukaemia had received a cumulative dose of etoposide of 4200–5600 mg/m^2; the latent period was 13–30 months. Four of the cases were acute monoblastic leukaemia and the other was acute myeloblastic leukaemia.

2.2.5 *Lung cancer*

Ratain *et al.* (1987) entered 119 patients with unresectable non-metastic lung cancer (histological type, other than small-cell) between 1981 and 1984 into a phase II trial of vindesine, etoposide (300 mg/m^2 intravenously) and cisplatin; etoposide (300 mg/m^2 intravenously) and cisplatin; or vindesine and cisplatin. The patients had had no prior chemotherapy. Twenty-four patients survived more than one year after initiation of therapy. Three of these had received vindesine and cisplatin, nine had received etoposide and cisplatin, and 12 had received vindesine, etoposide and cisplatin; 19 had received palliative radiotherapy (usually in the thorax). Four cases of acute myeloid leukaemia occurred (two acute monoblastic leukaemia, one acute myelomonocytic leukaemia). The rate of acute myeloid leukaemia was 0.30 per person–year (95% CI, 0.11–0.80), and the cumulative risk was 15% [95% CI, 2–45%] at two years. Two patients had received etoposide (7350 and 6240 mg/m^2) and cisplatin, and developed acute leukaemia 28 and 35 months after the start of therapy. The two others had received vindesine, etoposide (7950 and 4382 mg/m^2) and cisplatin, and developed acute myeloid leukaemia 19 and 13 months after the start of therapy, respectively. A comparison of the median cumulative dose of etoposide in the four patients with leukaemia (6795 mg/m^2) and the 20 patients without leukaemia (3025 mg/m^2) showed that those who eventually developed acute myeloid leukaemia had received significantly more etoposide than those who did not ($p < 0.01$). [The Working Group noted that three of the 24 one-year survivors who did not develop acute myeloid leukaemia had not received etoposide but were included in the calculation of cumulative risk.]

2.2.6 Breast cancer

A study in Japan (Yagita *et al.*, 1998) included 119 women who were treated for recurrent breast cancer between 1985 and 1994. Before recurrence, the patients had been treated with 5-fluorouracil, cyclophosphamide, doxorubicin, tamoxifen or radiation. All of the patients with recurrences were first treated with doxorubicin (or pirarubicin), vindesine and cyclophosphamide or cisplatin (or carboplatin). Twenty-four patients received etoposide (orally at 50 or 100 mg per day for five to seven days at four-week intervals); the cumulative doses were < 2000 mg for seven patients, 2000–5000 mg for 10 and > 5000 mg for seven. The length of follow-up from the start of etoposide treatment ranged from 1 to 40 months. The cumulative risk for acute myeloid leukaemia and myelodysplastic syndrome on the basis of three cases among the 119 patients was 9.1% (SE, 5.6%) 91–120 months after the operation. Two cases of acute myeloid leukaemia and one of myelodysplastic syndrome developed in the subgroup of 24 patients who had received etoposide orally, and no cases occurred in the group that did not receive etoposide ($p < 0.01$; Fisher's exact test). The latency from start of etoposide treatment was 31 months, 25 months and seven months, and the cumulative doses of etoposide were 1750 mg, 11 900 mg and 4550 mg, respectively. [The Working Group noted that one case of acute myeloid leukaemia occurred shortly (seven months) after the start of etoposide treatment. The comparison of etoposide-exposed patients with patients not treated with etoposide may not be valid, since the two groups were treated with different agents both initially and for recurrent breast cancer.]

3. Studies of Cancer in Experimental Animals

Oral administration

Mouse: Etoposide was tested in a neurofibromatosis type 1 (*Nf1*) transgenic knock-out mouse model of myeloid leukaemia. Approximately 10% of heterozygous *Nf1* mice (*Nf1*$^{+/-}$) spontaneously develop myeloid leukaemia at around 15 months of age. Groups of 31–46 *Nf1* wild-type (+/+) or *Nf1* heterozygous (+/–) mice, 6–10 weeks of age [sex unspecified], were treated with 0 or 100 mg/kg bw etoposide weekly for six weeks by gastric intubation and were observed for up to 18 months. Histological examination was limited to smears of peripheral blood and, in some cases, bone marrow and spleen. The incidences of leukaemia were 2/31 in controls and 8/46 in $Nf1^{+/+}$ and $Nf1^{+/-}$ mice compared with 0/26 in etoposide-treated $Nf1^{+/+}$ and 8/32 in $Nf1^{+/-}$ mice ($p = 0.20$). In contrast, the alkylating agent, cyclophosphamide, induced myeloid leukaemias in 0/5 $Nf1^{+/+}$ and 7/12 $Nf1^{+/-}$ treated mice (Mahgoub et al. (1999). [The Working Group noted that the model was applicable for alkylating agents.]

4. Other Data Relevant to an Evaluation of Carcinogenicity and its Mechanisms

4.1 Absorption, distribution, metabolism and excretion

4.1.1 *Humans*

Numerous studies and several reviews (Clark & Slevin, 1987; Fleming et al., 1989; Slevin, 1991) have reported the pharmacokinetics of etoposide after intravenous administration in humans. The pharmacokinetics of intravenously administered etoposide in children is similar to that in adults, with a total plasma clearance of 20–40 mL/min per m² in children and 15–35 mL/min per m² in adults, a distribution volume of 5–10 L/m² in children and 7–17 L/m² in adults and an elimination half-life of 3–7 h in children and 4–8 h in adults (Slevin, 1991). In most studies, a bi-exponential elimination is described, with a distribution half-life of about 1 h (Hande et al., 1984). The proportion of unchanged etoposide recovered in urine represented 20–40% of the dose, but more radiolabel was generally recovered in earlier studies with [³H]etoposide (Allen & Creaven, 1975) than with the more specific high-performance liquid chromatography or radioimmunoassay methods. Studies with high doses of etoposide (up to 3.5 g/m²) in which blood samples were collected longer than after standard dosing have shown tri-exponential elimination, with a terminal half-time of 18 h or longer, possibly reflecting release of etoposide from tissues (Holthuis et al., 1986; Mross et al., 1994). The area under the integrated time–concentration curve (AUC) was linear up to doses of 3 g/m² in one study (Holthuis et al., 1986). With standard doses of 100 mg/m² delivered over 1–2 h, the peak concentrations are 10–20 µg/mL (Clark et al., 1994).

The pharmacokinetics of orally administered etoposide has been summarized (Clark & Slevin, 1987; Fleming et al., 1989; Slevin, 1991). The bioavailability from an oral capsule is about 50%, but there is evidence that the bioavailability is dose-dependent, with decreasing absorption of doses > 200 mg (Harvey et al., 1986; Slevin et al., 1989b; Hande et al., 1993). In one study, the bioavailability of a 100-mg dose was 76%, while that of a 400-mg dose was 48% ($p < 0.01$) (Hande et al., 1993). This effect might be related to a concentration-dependent reduction in the solubility of etoposide in the stomach and small intestine (Joel et al., 1995a). The bioavailability of etoposide varies widely among and within patients (Harvey et al., 1985; Hande et al., 1993).

About 94% of a dose of etoposide is bound to protein in adult cancer patients with normal hepatic function (Liu et al., 1995; Joel et al., 1996; Liliemark et al., 1996; Nguyen et al., 1998) and 97.5% in children (Liliemark et al., 1996). The haematological toxicity of etoposide correlated better with the AUC for free compound than with that for total etoposide (Stewart et al., 1991; Joel et al., 1996). The AUC for intracellular etoposide in leukaemic cells from patients with acute myeloid leukaemia was ~10% that of the plasma AUC (Liliemark et al., 1993).

Little etoposide penetrates into other fluid spaces, almost certainly because of its extensive protein binding. The concentrations of etoposide in cerebrospinal fluid were only 1–2% of the plasma concentration after high doses (Hande et al., 1984; Postmus et al., 1984a; Holthuis et al., 1986), and none was detectable after a standard dose of etoposide (D'Incalci et al., 1982). Etoposide was detectable in brain tumours after standard doses (Stewart et al., 1984), at concentrations higher than in the cerebrospinal fluid immediately after administration of a high dose (400–800 mg/m^2 by infusion) (Hande et al., 1984), but the concentrations in tumours were generally lower in primary or metastasized intracerebral than in extracerebral tumours (Stewart et al., 1984). The concentration in saliva after a high dose was only 1.5% of the concurrent plasma concentration at several intervals (Holthuis et al., 1986). After administration of a high dose, the peak concentrations in ascites and pleural fluid were considerably lower than the peak plasma concentration, but at later times (> 10 h) the concentrations were higher than in plasma, suggesting slow clearance from these fluid compartments (Hande et al., 1984; Holthuis et al., 1986).

Because etoposide is excreted renally, clearance is reduced in patients with impaired renal function (Arbuck et al., 1986; D'Incalci et al., 1986; Pflüger et al., 1993; Joel et al., 1996). Changes in the pharmacokinetics of etoposide are more subtle in patients with impaired liver function. While the pharmacokinetics of total plasma etoposide may be unchanged, a reduction in protein binding has been reported in these patients, which is associated with decreased serum albumin and/or increased serum bilirubin (Stewart et al., 1989; Liu et al., 1995; Joel et al., 1996). This increase in free etoposide is associated with greater toxicity in this group of patients (Joel et al., 1996).

The fate of an intravenous dose of etoposide is still not clear. Generally, few or no etoposide metabolites have been detected in plasma. Etoposide is administered as the *trans*-lactone (ring furthest to the right, Figure 1), but *cis*-etoposide can also be detected in human urine (Holthuis et al., 1986). This might be a storage phenomenon, since isomerization sometimes occurs during freezing of plasma samples under slightly basic conditions (Rideout et al., 1984). The *cis* isomer accounts for < 1% of the dose (Holthuis et al., 1986; Holthuis, 1988). The catechol metabolite has also been reported in patients receiving 600 mg/m^2 etoposide, with an AUC of around 2.5% that of etoposide (Stremetzne et al., 1997). In patients given 90 mg/m^2 etoposide, the catechol metabolite represented 1.4–7.1% of the urinary etoposide and < 2% of the administered dose (Relling et al., 1994).

Figure 1. Possible metabolic conversions of etoposide

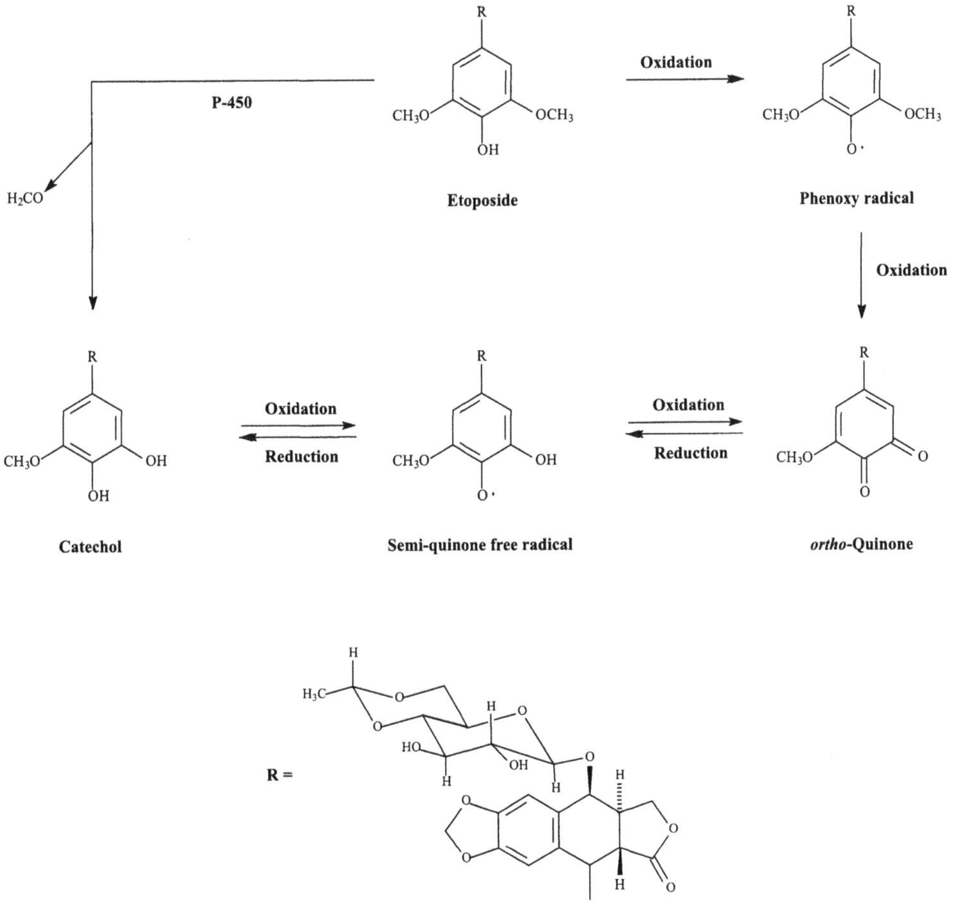

From Mans et al. (1990)
P-450, cytochrome P450 mixed-function oxidases

The major urinary metabolite of etoposide in humans is reported to be the glucuronide conjugate. Although urinary glucuronide and/or sulfate conjugates were reported to account for 5–22% of an intravenous dose of etoposide (D'Incalci et al., 1985), other studies suggest that the glucuronide predominates (Holthuis et al., 1986). Etoposide glucuronide in the urine of treated patients accounted for 8–17% of a dose of 0.5–3.5 g/m² etoposide (Holthuis et al., 1986) and 29% of a dose of 100–800 mg/m² etoposide (Hande et al., 1990), with no other metabolites other than etoposide glucuronide detected in the latter study. In patients with renal or liver impairment given somewhat lower doses of 70–150 mg/m², 3–17% of the dose was excreted in the urine within 72 h as etoposide glucuronide (D'Incalci et al., 1986).

The proposed hydroxy acid metabolite of etoposide, formed by opening of the lactone ring, has been detected in human urine, but only at low concentrations, accounting for 0.2–2.2% of the administered dose (Hande *et al.*, 1984; Holthuis *et al.*, 1986).

These findings are in broad agreement with those of early studies in which [^{3}H]etoposide was used, which indicated that 35–66% of the administered dose of radiolabel was recovered in the urine (Allen & Creaven, 1975).

Less than 4% of a dose was recovered in the bile after 48 h in patients with biliary drainage tubes (Arbuck *et al.*, 1986; D'Incalci *et al.*, 1986; Hande *et al.*, 1990). The faecal recovery of radiolabel after intravenous administration of [^{3}H]etoposide (130–290 mg/m^2) was variable, representing 0–16% of dose, but the collections were known to be incomplete because of faecal retention and other difficulties associated with the poor general condition of many of the patients (Creaven & Allen, 1975). In a study reported as an abstract in four patients with small-cell lung cancer given [^{14}C-glucopyranoside]etoposide, 56% of the radiolabel was recovered in urine and 44% in faeces over five days, for a total recovery of 100 ± 6% (Joel *et al.*, 1995b).

Studies in lung cancer patients have shown that the plasma concentrations associated with haematological toxicity are higher than those required for antitumour activity. The plasma concentration associated with antitumour activity may be different for different tumour types (Minami *et al.*, 1993; Clark *et al.*, 1994; Minami *et al.*, 1995; Joel *et al.*, 1998).

No differences in the pharmacokinetics of etoposide or in the AUC of etoposide catechol were seen in eight children who developed acute myeloid leukaemia after receiving etoposide as part of combination chemotherapy for acute lymphoblastic leukaemia, when compared with 23 children who did not develop secondary acute myeloid leukaemia (Relling *et al.*, 1998). These children were included in the study of Pui *et al.* (1991), described in section 2.2.3.

Felix *et al.* (1998) investigated the frequency of a cytochrome P450 CYP3A4 variant with an alteration in the 5' promoter region of the gene, in leukaemic cells with *MLL* translocations from 42 de-novo cases and 19 that followed epipodophyllotoxin treatment. A significantly decreased frequency of the CYP3A4 variant genotype was found in patients with leukaemia that occurred after treatment with epipodophyllotoxins. Possible changes in the pharmacokinetics related to the CYP3A4 variant were not investigated, but the wild type metabolizes epipodophyllotoxins to the catechol and quinone metabolites.

The pharmacokinetics of etoposide is influenced by concurrent administration of a number of other drugs: clearance may be increased by phenytoin (Mross *et al.*, 1994), strongly decreased by cisplatin, which is often given with etoposide, resulting in a 30% increase in the AUC for etoposide (Relling *et al.*, 1994), and decreased by up to 40% by ciclosporin, resulting in an increase in the AUC for etoposide of up to 80% (Lum *et al.*, 1992).

4.1.2 Experimental systems

Few published data on the pharmacokinetics of etoposide in non-human species are available, and many of the preliminary studies conducted before the early clinical trials have not been published in full.

Rhesus monkeys given [^{3}H]etoposide showed biphasic elimination, with a distribution phase half-time of about 1.3 h and a terminal elimination phase of 43 h, as reported in a review by Achterrath *et al.* (1982) that included unpublished reports. Sixty per cent of the dose was excreted renally within 60 h, and 30% faecally. Biphasic elimination was also observed in mice, with a distribution half-time of 1.5 min and an elimination half-time of 33 min. The clearance rate was 17 mL/kg bw per min, and the distribution volume was 820 mL/kg bw (Colombo *et al.*, 1986).

After intravenous infusion (5 min) of etoposide phosphate to beagle dogs at doses of 57–461 mg/m^2, a dose-proportional increase was seen in the maximal plasma concentration and AUC for etoposide. The total plasma clearance rate (342–435 mL/min per m^2) and the distribution volume (22–27 L/m^2) were not dose-dependent. The peak plasma concentration occurred at the end of the infusion of etoposide phosphate, indicating rapid conversion of the pro-drug to etoposide (Igwemezie *et al.*, 1995).

Thirty minutes after intravenous administration of etoposide to rats, the highest concentrations were found in the liver, kidneys and small intestine. By 24 h after the dose, the tissue concentrations were negligible (Achterrath *et al.*, 1982).

In leukaemic cells, the uptake appeared to be linear up to 5 min and reached a steady state by 20–30 min (Allen, 1978; Colombo *et al.*, 1986), with intracellular concentrations about twice those of the extracellular medium (Allen, 1978). After removal of the drug, an exponential efflux with a half-time of just 3 min was observed (Allen, 1978). At the same extracellular concentration, the intracellular concentrations of etoposide were 15–20 times lower than those of the closely related drug teniposide (Allen, 1978; Colombo *et al.*, 1986).

In rat liver homogenates, liver microsomes and in rats *in vivo*, etoposide was extensively metabolized to only one major metabolite, which was not formally identified (van Maanen *et al.*, 1982). In perfused isolated rat liver incubated with etoposide, the total recovery in bile was 60–85%, with roughly equal amounts of etoposide and two glucuronide metabolites (Colombo *et al.*, 1985; Hande *et al.*, 1988), confirmed as glucuronide species by liquid chromatography and mass spectrometry (Hande *et al.*, 1988). After intravenous injection of [^{3}H]etoposide to rabbits, the total urinary excretion of radiolabel was 30% after five days, with very little thereafter. A single glucuronide metabolite was identified in rabbit urine, which was present in larger amounts than etoposide. No hydroxy acid was identified in either species (Hande *et al.*, 1988).

A number of authors have reported the peroxidase-mediated oxidation of etoposide to a phenoxy radical, with further oxidation to the *ortho*-quinone, semi-quinone and catechol derivatives (Broggini *et al.*, 1985; van Maanen *et al.*, 1986; Haim *et al.*, 1987;

Kalyanaraman *et al.*, 1989). Cytochrome P450-mediated demethylation directly to the catechol has also been reported (van Maanen *et al.*, 1987; Relling *et al.*, 1992), which is catalysed mainly by the CYP3A4 isoform (Relling *et al.*, 1994). These reactive species bind to intracellular macromolecules, including DNA (Haim *et al.*, 1987). The *ortho*-quinone and catechol, but not etoposide itself, induced direct DNA damage, as measured by inactivation of single-stranded and double-stranded biologically active $\Phi \times 174$ [bacteriophage] DNA (van Maanen *et al.*, 1988). The *ortho*-quinone retains the DNA topoisomerase II inhibitory activity of etoposide (Gantchev & Hunting, 1998). It remains unclear how much these reactive metabolites contribute to the cytotoxic or mutagenic activity of etoposide.

4.2 Toxic effects

4.2.1 *Humans*

The toxicity of etoposide has been summarized (Fleming *et al.*, 1989; Hainsworth & Greco, 1995). The main, dose-limiting toxic effect is myelosuppression, manifest principally as leukopenia. After standard intravenous doses (375–500 mg/m² total dose) of etoposide administered alone over three to five days, 20–50% of previously untreated patients experienced moderate to severe leukopenia or neutropenia, typically occurring around day 10–12, with recovery by day 21. Nausea and vomiting are generally mild but may be more common after oral administration. Alopecia occurs in most patients. Mucositis can occur at standard doses, when it is generally mild, but at high doses (< 3500 mg/m²), mucositis can become dose-limiting (Postmus *et al.*, 1984b). Hypotension has been reported, which may be related to the duration of infusion.

Hypersensitivity reactions to etoposide have been reported but are uncommon (O'Dwyer & Weiss, 1984). In eight patients reported to the Investigational Drug Branch of the National Cancer Institute between January 1982 and May 1983, these reactions included flushing, respiratory problems, changes in blood pressure and abdominal pain, often occurring soon after the start of drug administration and generally resolving rapidly when the infusion was stopped. These reactions are less common with etoposide than with the related drug teniposide and have not been reported after oral administration, suggesting that other agents in the formulation may be at least partly responsible. The very low incidence of reported cases may reflect only serious hypersensitivity reactions (Weiss, 1992), as mild reactions were found in 51% of patients receiving etoposide as part of combination chemotherapy for Hodgkin disease (Hudson *et al.*, 1993) and 34% of children receiving etoposide as part of a multi-agent induction regime for leukaemia (Kellie *et al.*, 1991). Most patients can be successfully re-treated with etoposide after a premedication comprising antihistamine and/or corticosteroids (Hudson *et al.*, 1993).

Cardiotoxicity was reported in three of eight patients with pre-existing cardiac disease who received etoposide by infusion (Aisner *et al.*, 1982). Dose-related cutaneous toxicity has been reported, more commonly at doses > 2000 mg/m², but the symptoms can be controlled by corticosteroids (Murphy *et al.*, 1993).

4.2.2 *Experimental systems*

Much of the pre-clinical toxicology of etoposide has not been published in full, but summary data have been reported in reviews. The acute toxicity of the drug after intravenous dosing was investigated, with LD_{50} values of 118 mg/kg bw in mice, 68 mg/kg bw in rats and > 80 mg/kg bw in rabbits (Achterrath *et al.*, 1982). In a later study, the LD_{50} in mice after intraperitoneal administration was reported to be 108 mg/kg bw (Lee *et al.*, 1995).

Four-week studies of toxicity were conducted in rats treated intraperitoneally at 0.6–6.0 mg/kg bw per day and in monkeys treated intravenously at 0.4–3.6 mg/kg bw per day. At the highest doses, the main toxic effect was myelosuppression, with anaemia, leukopenia and thrombocytopenia, and some hepatotoxicity. Pathological changes were noted in the lung in rats, and mild enteritis was seen in dogs. After oral and intravenous administration at the same doses as in the previous studies, no additional toxicity was observed up to nine weeks (review of unpublished studies by Achterrath *et al.*, 1982).

Oral administration to rats and dogs at a dose of 0.5–5 mg/kg bw per day for five days a week for 26 weeks also resulted in myelosuppression as the major toxic effect in both species. No other effects were seen in the rats, while those in dogs included renal and hepatic impairment, electrocardiographic changes, decreased testis weight and disorders of spermatogenesis (review of unpublished studies by Achterrath *et al.*, 1982). These changes were largely reversible after four weeks without treatment.

After intraperitoneal administration of a clinical formulation or intrapleural administration of etoposide dissolved in dimethyl sulfoxide and Tween 80 diluted in Hank's buffer to rats and mice, delayed chronic pleuritis and peritonitis, with liver and spleen inflammation were reported. The vehicle had no effect when given alone (Stähelin, 1976).

After intravenous infusion of a single dose of 461 mg/m² etoposide phosphate to dogs over 5 min, all animals vomited, and leukopenia and thrombocytopenia were seen at this and lower doses (Igwemezie *et al.*, 1995).

Etoposide- and etoposide phosphate-induced sensory neuropathy has been reported in mice after single doses of 88 mg/kg bw and 100–150 mg/kg bw, respectively (Bregman *et al.*, 1994).

4.3   Reproductive and prenatal effects

4.3.1 *Humans*

Five case reports of treatment with etoposide during pregnancy were located. A woman was treated at 26 weeks of gestation with a combination of bleomycin, etoposide

(165 mg/day) and cisplatin on three consecutive days for an unknown primary cancer. Six days later, she developed neutropenia and septicaemia and had a spontaneous vaginal delivery. The female infant developed profound leukopenia with neutropenia three days later (10 days after in-utero exposure), which had resolved by day 13. At 10 days of age, the infant started to lose her hair, which was growing again when she was discharged at 12 weeks. At follow-up at one year, she was essentially normal (Raffles et al., 1989). A woman was treated for acute leukaemia at 25 and 30 weeks of gestation with cytarabine, daunorubicin and etoposide (400 mg/m^2 per day for three days). Her infant, delivered by caesarean section at 32 weeks because of fetal distress, had leukopenia with profound neutropenia, which was confirmed to be due to bone-marrow suppression by measurement of circulating haemopoietic progenitor cells. This condition responded to transfusion of packed cells and subcutaneous injections of granulocyte colony-stimulating factor, and the infant was well at follow-up at one year (Murray et al., 1994). Three women treated for acute leukaemia, ovarian cancer and non-Hodgkin lymphoma with multiple drug cycles including etoposide (100–125 mg/m^2 per day) in the third trimester had normal, healthy infants (Buller et al., 1992; Brunet et al., 1993; Rodriguez & Haggag, 1995). Etoposide was used to induce abortion in two cases of ectopic pregnancy. In one case, a woman with a cervical ectopic pregnancy of six weeks was given oral doses of etoposide of 200 mg/m^2 for five days. The pregnancy was terminated, but there was evidence of bone-marrow suppression in the mother and almost complete loss of hair (Segna et al., 1990). The second case, a tubal pregnancy of five weeks, was successfully terminated by two injections of 50 mg etoposide locally into the gestational sac, with no side-effects (Kusaka et al., 1994).

Ovarian function may be impaired by etoposide. In a study of 20 young and two older (> 50 years) women with gestational trophoblastic disease treated orally with etoposide and who had serial hormone assays, transient ovarian failure lasting two to four months was observed in five of the young women, and the two older women both had permanent ovarian failure. In the younger women, fertility was unaffected and six became pregnant within one year of therapy (Choo et al., 1985). In a similar study on 47 women treated with etoposide, ovulation ceased in about half of the patients but returned within four months after treatment in all of the patients under 40 years of age. In nine patients over 40 years of age, ovulation did not return within the follow-up period of 12 months. The effects on the ovary were not related to the dose of etoposide but were related to the age of the patient (Matsui et al., 1997). Etoposide was not found to have any long-term effect on fertility in 77 women treated for gestational trophoblastic tumours (Adewole et al., 1986).

Excretion of etoposide in breast milk was demonstrated in a woman with acute promyelocytic leukaemia receiving daily doses of 80 mg/m^2 [route not stated]. Peak concentrations of 0.6–0.8 μg/mL were measured immediately after dosing but had decreased to undetectable levels by 24 h (Azuno et al., 1995).

Reproductive capacity was assessed in 30 men with germ-cell tumours after treatment with cisplatin, etoposide and bleomycin. A single semen sample was obtained for analysis 24–78 months after initiation of therapy. The results are difficult to interpret, since most men with testis tumours are oligospermic before chemotherapy. Oligospermia ($< 40 \times 10^6$ total sperm) was diagnosed in 13 of the men, including six with azoospermia. Morphological abnormalities were common, and only one man had more than 50% normal sperm. Eight of the men subsequently fathered children, none of whom had birth defects (Stephenson et al., 1995).

Etoposide did not cause permanent damage to the germinal epithelium in 47 young men receiving it for Hodgkin disease (Gerres et al., 1998).

4.3.2 Experimental systems

Groups of 4–10 pregnant Swiss albino mice were given a single dose of etoposide at 1.0, 1.5 or 2.0 mg/kg bw intraperitoneally on day 6, 7 or 8 of gestation (vaginal plug, day 0), and the fetuses were removed and examined on day 17. No effect on maternal body-weight gain was seen in any group. In animals injected on day 6, no embryotoxicity was seen with 1.0 or 1.5 mg/kg bw, but 2.0 mg/kg bw increased the frequencies of intrauterine death, fetal malformations and reduced fetal body weight. Injection on day 7 caused dose-related embryolethality, fetal malformations and reduced fetal weight. Injection on day 8 caused no embryolethality and no effect on fetal body weight, but the frequency of fetal malformations was increased at doses of 1.0 and 2.0 mg/kg bw. The commonest malformations observed at the highest dose were hydrocephalus (12.2%) and open eyelids (16.7%) after injection on day 6, exencephaly and encephalocoele at frequencies of 13% and 10% on days 7 and 8 and axial skeletal defects at frequencies of 28% and 7.7% on days 7 and 8, respectively (Sieber et al., 1978).

The results of standard studies of reproductive toxicity with etoposide have been published. Groups of 30 male Crj:CD Sprague-Dawley rats were given etoposide at a dose of 1, 3 or 10 mg/kg bw orally by gavage for 64 days and 30 females for 15 days before mating, and treatment was continued during mating and, for females, until day 7 of gestation. The high dose suppressed body-weight gain during the first two weeks of treatment in the females only. In males at the highest dose, the weights of the testis, epididymides and thymus were reduced, and the organs appeared atrophic macroscopically; however, reproductive function was not significantly affected. Females at the high dose had decreased numbers of corpora lutea and implants and reduced litter size and an increased frequency of resorptions. Fetal body weight was significantly reduced and the number of malformed fetuses greater than in controls. The malformations observed included exencephaly, anury, cerebral atrophy, cerebral ventricular dilatation, anophthalmia and microphthalmia (Takahashi et al., 1986a).

Groups of 22–24 pregnant Crj:CD Sprague-Dawley rats were given etoposide at a dose of 1, 3 or 10 mg/kg bw orally by gavage from day 17 of gestation until day 20 post-partum. The high dose produced thymic atrophy in the dams but did not affect the duration of gestation or parturition. The mortality rate of pups was slightly increased during the first three days after birth, and their body-weight gain was transiently suppressed. Other aspects of postnatal physical, functional and behavioural development were unaffected. The reproductive function of the F_1 generation was normal, and the growth and development of the F_2 generation were normal. Long-term observation of the F_1 animals showed no delayed toxicity or carcinogenesis [details not given] (Takahashi et al., 1986b).

Groups of 20–22 male Crj:CD Sprague-Dawley rats were treated with etoposide at a dose of 0.05, 0.2 or 0.8 mg/kg bw intravenously for 61 days and females for 14 days before mating, and treatment was continued during mating and, for females, until day 7 of gestation. The high dose suppressed body-weight gain in animals of each sex. In males at the high dose, the weights of the testis and epididymides were reduced, and the organs appeared atrophic macroscopically; however, reproductive function was not significantly affected. The weight of the thymus was reduced at the intermediate and high doses. Females at the high dose had smaller litters and more resorptions than controls. Fetal body weight was significantly reduced, and the number of malformed fetuses was increased when compared with controls. The malformations observed included cerebral ventricular dilatation, anophthalmia and microphthalmia (Takahashi et al., 1986c).

Groups of 23–24 pregnant Crj:CD Sprague-Dawley rats were given etoposide intravenously at a dose of 0.05, 0.2 or 0.8 mg/kg bw from day 17 of gestation until day 20 *post-partum*. Animals at the intermediate and high doses had reduced body-weight gain and thymic atrophy, but the duration of gestation and parturition was not affected. Treatment had no effect on pup survival, but their body-weight gain was transiently suppressed. Other aspects of postnatal, physical, functional and behavioural development were unaffected, except for a slight delay in vaginal opening by 1.4 days in the group at the high dose. The reproductive function of the F_1 generation was normal, and the growth and development of the F_2 generation were normal (Takahashi et al., 1986d).

Day-10 rat embryos [strain not specified] cultured for 24 h *in vitro* were exposed for the first 3 h to etoposide at concentrations of 1.0–10 μmol/L. A dose-related increase in the incdence of malformations was observed at doses of 2.0 and 5.0 μmol/L, and at the latter concentration 100% of the embryos were malformed. The dose of 10 μmol/L was lethal to all embryos. The malformations observed consisted mainly of hypoplasia of the prosencephalon, microphthalmia and oedema of the rhombencephalon. Comparison of the concentrations necessary to produce 50% lethality and 50% malformations showed that amsacrine (see monograph, this volume) was 10 times and 20 times more potent, respectively, than etoposide. The authors suggested that the malformations were related to the inhibition of DNA topoisomerase II activity in the embryo, but presented no data to support the proposal (Mirkes & Zwelling, 1990).

Etoposide has been reported to cause degeneration of rat spermatogonia and early spermatocytes, the appearance of large multinucleated spermatids and nuclear and cytoplasmic changes in Sertoli cells. The stage-specific changes produced by etoposide were studied by following effects on DNA synthesis as measured by incorporation of

[³H]thymidine. Groups of three Sprague-Dawley rats, two to three months of age, were injected intraperitoneally with 5 or 10 mg/kg bw etoposide and killed 1, 3 or 18 days later. Premitotic DNA synthesis was inhibited by about 40–70% in spermatogonial stages II–V at both doses, when compared with controls. The effects on premeiotic DNA synthesis were less marked, with a maximum inhibition of about 40%. Markedly increased incorporation of thymidine was also observed at stage VII, at which no DNA synthesis normally occurs. The effects of etoposide were most marked after one and three days, but some effects were still present 18 days after treatment (Hakovirta *et al.*, 1993).

In adult Sprague-Dawley rats injected intraperitoneally with a single dose of 5 or 10 mg/kg bw etoposide, it was a powerful inducer of micronuclei in early spermatids, whereas the major cytotoxic action is on the early spermatogonial stages. Thus, the cytotoxicity is separate from genotoxicity (Lähdetie *et al.*, 1994).

In a study of teratogenicity, groups of 11–21 JW-NIBS rabbits were given 0.3, 1, 3 or 10 mg/kg bw etoposide orally by gavage on days 6–18 of gestation. The highest dose caused marked depression of body-weight gain and food intake throughout gestation, and only two animals were alive at the end of the study. Deaths were observed at 3 mg/kg bw per day, and only 16/21 animals in this group were alive at termination. Doses up to and including 3 mg/kg bw had no adverse effect on embryo or fetal development, fetal weight, ossification or the incidence of malformations (Takahashi *et al.*, 1986e).

Five groups of eight pregnant Japanese white rabbits (Kbl:JW) were given etoposide at a dose of 0, 0.25, 0.5, 1.0 or 2.0 mg/kg bw per day intravenously on days 7, 8 and 9 of gestation. The fetuses were removed for visceral and skeletal examination on day 28 of gestation. The body-weight gain of dams was depressed and liver damage was observed at the highest dose, but fetal survival and weight were unaffected and no gross malformations were observed. A low incidence (4/64, $p < 0.05$) of fetuses with rib and vertebral abnormalities was noted. Histological examination of the fetal telencephalon showed no increase in cell death (Nagao *et al.*, 1999).

4.4 Genetic and related effects

4.4.1 *Humans*

Evidence that etoposide causes genetic changes in humans derives from three lines of investigation. The first involves rather limited studies of DNA damage and mutations in patients undergoing treatment. The second involves cytogenetic analyses of cells from patients with leukaemias associated with this treatment. The third involves molecular characterization of the translocation break-points.

(a) *DNA damage and mutations in patients undergoing treatment with etoposide*

Osanto *et al.* (1991) examined the presence of micronuclei in binucleated peripheral blood lymphocytes of patients treated with etoposide-containing combination chemotherapy for testicular carcinoma. An increased frequency of micronuclei was found in these samples compared with those obtained from untreated cancer patients or healthy, age-matched controls at a mean interval of 4.6 years after cessation of chemotherapy. This indicates that DNA damage persists for a long time after treatment.

The analysis by Karnaoukhova *et al.* (1997) of *HPRT* gene mutation frequency and mutation spectra by a T-cell cloning assay in lymphocytes from 12 patients with small-cell lung cancer receiving chemotherapy with etoposide provides additional evidence that it is associated with genetic changes. The regimens included up to six cycles of two daily oral doses of 50 mg/kg bw over 10–14 days separated by two weeks of rest. The total doses ranged from 1.4 to 8.4 g, and follow-up was for 0.7–5.3 months from the start of treatment. There was considerable variation between patients, but no significant increase in *HPRT* gene mutation frequency was seen after treatment when compared with pre-treatment control values. The post-treatment mutation spectrum showed an increase in AT→TA transversions and a decrease in GC→TA transversions when compared with the pre-treatment spectrum. No gross rearrangements or deletions were detected.

(b) *Cytogenetic analyses of cells from patients with leukaemias associated with etoposide treatment*

The most direct evidence that etoposide causes genetic changes in humans *in vivo* derives from the finding in the 1980s of a distinct form of leukaemia characterized by chromosomal translocations at the time this agent was introduced into clinical usage. Taken together, these analyses suggest that etoposide is responsible for several non-random chromosomal translocations that are central to leukaemogenesis. It is also noteworthy that etoposide treatment of phytohaemagglutinin-stimulated human lymphocytes in culture is associated with an excess frequency of reciprocal translocations in addition to other abnormalities, which include dicentrics and, less often, unbalanced or complex rearrangements, deletions and inversions. Chromosomes 1, 11 and 17 are frequent targets of these abnormalities (Maraschin *et al.*, 1990; Pedersen-Bjergaard & Rowley, 1994).

Pedersen-Bjergaard *et al.* (1995) evaluated the cytogenetic characteristics in 137 cases of leukaemia and myelodysplastic syndrome after primary cancer treatment. The results of this analysis provide conclusive evidence that the kinds of aberrations associated with DNA topoisomerase II inhibitors are different from those observed with alkylating agents. Deletions or loss of chromosomes 5 and 7 were significantly associated with exposure to alkylating agents ($p = 0.002$), and balanced translocations to bands 11q23, 21q22 and 3q23 were seen with DNA topoisomerase II inhibitors ($p = 0.00005$).

Most of the translocations with which etoposide is associated in treated patients involve chromosome band 11q23, but this and other DNA topisomerase II inhibitors have also been associated with leukaemias with t(8;21), t(3;21), inv(16), t(15;17) or t(9;22) translocations (Ratain et al., 1987; Pui et al., 1990; Pedersen-Bjergaard & Philip, 1991; Pui et al., 1991; Detourmignies et al., 1992; Pedersen-Bjergaard, 1992; Hunger et al., 1993; Quesnel et al., 1993; Winick et al., 1993; Felix et al., 1995a; Nucifora & Rowley, 1995; Strissel Broeker et al., 1996; Pedersen-Bjergaard et al., 1997). These are also the common translocations in de-novo cases of leukaemia; however, while translocations of chromosome band 11q23 are present in most cases of acute lymphoblastic leukaemia in infants and cases of monoblastic leukaemia in infants and young children, they are found in only about 5% of acute leukaemias in adults. More recently, chromosome band 11p15 was recognized as a site of recurrent translocations in leukaemias that follow etoposide-containing therapy (Stark et al., 1994; Kobayashi et al., 1997).

(i) *Translocations involving band 11q23*

Etoposide has most often been used in combination chemotherapy. Ratain et al. (1987) described the occurrence of leukaemia, primarily with monoblastic features and translocations of chromosome band 11q23, in patients treated with etoposide in combination chemotherapy for non-small-cell carcinoma of the lung. A group of 119 patients with advanced non-small-cell lung cancer were treated with four different cisplatin-based regimens, one of which contained etoposide; four patients developed acute myeloid leukaemia 13, 19, 28 and 35 months after the start of treatment, respectively. All four had received etoposide and cisplatin with or without vindesine. Three of the leukaemias had monoblastic features; in one case there was a t(9;11)(p22;q23) translocation; in another there was t(9;11;18)(p22;q23;q12). The fourth case had a complex karyotype, with -5 and -7 abnormalities typical of alkylating agent-induced cases.

Several additional case reports and cohort studies have indicated that, while the 9p22 locus is commonly involved in translocations with band 11q23 (Pedersen-Bjergaard et al., 1991), chromosome band 11q23 can fuse with numerous other chromosomal loci. This was confirmed in studies of de-novo cases (Felix, 1998). For example, DeVore et al. (1989) and Nichols et al. (1993) reported cases of acute myeloid leukaemia with t(11;19)(q23;p13) after etoposide-containing chemotherapy of germ-cell tumours. Observations of cases of undifferentiated leukaemia and acute lymphoblastic leukaemia with t(4;11)(q21;q23) suggested additional heterogeneity in the partner chromosomes involved in translocations with band 11q23 (Hunger et al., 1992; Nichols et al., 1993).

When Pui et al. (1991) examined 21 cases of acute myeloid leukaemia that occurred as a second cancer in 734 children with acute lymphoblastic leukaemia who received maintenance therapy including teniposide with or without etoposide, a translocation of chromosome band 11q23 was found in 15 cases. The karyotype revealed t(9;11)(p21–p22;q23) in seven cases, but other chromosomal regions involved in translocations with band 11q23 in one case each were 21q22, Xq13, 12p13, 16p13, 19q13, 19p13, and 17q21. The translocation at band 11q23 was usually the only abnormality, but in five cases additional structural or numerical changes were detected. In one case the karyotype showed inv(11)(p15q23) and t(10;11)(p13;q13). Similarly, Winick et al. (1993) examined the occurrence of acute myeloid leukaemia as a second cancer in 205 children with B-lineage acute lymphoblastic leukaemia treated according to a protocol that included etoposide during central nervous system consolidation and continuation phases. Ten patients developed acute myeloid leukaemia. Translocation of chromosome band 11q23 occurred in eight of the 10 cases, with fusions to band 9p21 or 9p22 in three cases and fusions to band 17q25, 19p13.1, 16p13.3, 2q37 or 1q32 in one case each.

Heterogeneous translocations involving band 11q23 were also observed in cases of leukaemia after epipodophyllotoxin-containing treatment for paediatric solid tumours. In the series reported by Pui et al. (1990), 12 cases of leukaemia occurred in 3365 children, and cytogenetic analysis was available for eight cases. A translocation t(9;11)(p21;q23) was seen in two cases, one of which also contained t(4;11)(q26;p13). One case showed t(1;11)(p32;q23) and t(11;?)(p15;?). The treatment regimens were not described completely, but epipodophyllotoxins were used in two patients with translocations involving band 11q23. Laver et al. (1997) reported a case of myelodysplastic syndrome without excess blasts which showed t(11;16)(q23;p13.3) in a paediatric patient given etoposide-containing therapy for Ewing sarcoma. Karyotypic features in leukaemias were evaluated after more dose-intensive, repetitive administration of high-dose alkylating agents, anthracycline and etoposide for paediatric non-lymphoid solid tumours (Kushner et al., 1998a) and neuroblastoma (Kushner et al., 1998b), in which the incidence of leukaemia is high. Here, cytogenetic analysis revealed 5q and 7q deletions, consistent with alkylating agent-related leukaemia and myelodysplastic syndrome in some cases, and t(9;11)(p22;q23) translocation, more typical of leukaemias associated with DNA topoisomerase II inhibitors in others. One case that occurred 24 months after the start of neuroblastoma treatment showed del(7)(q22) and del(11)(q13q23), possibly reflecting the combined effects of an alkylating agent and an epipodophyllotoxin (Kushner et al., 1998b).

(ii) *Translocations t(8;21)(q22;q22) and t(3;21)(q26;q22)*

The t(8;21)(q22;q22) translocation is the hallmark of de-novo acute myeloid leukaemias of myeloblastic morphology, but this translocation is also observed after etoposide-containing therapy (Felix et al., 1995b). Two cases of acute myeloid leukaemia with t(8;21) were observed among 212 patients who received etoposide, cisplatin and bleomycin for germ-cell tumours (Pedersen-Bjergaard et al., 1991). Quesnel et al. (1993) identified the t(8;21) translocation in three cases of treatment-related leukaemia in which prior treatment had included an epipodophyllotoxin in combination with either an anthracycline or an alkylating agent, but it was not specified whether etoposide or teniposide was used. Translocation t(8;21) has been observed in cases of epipodophyllotoxin-related leukaemia occurring after paediatric solid tumours. In the paediatric patients with primary solid tumours reported by Pui *et al.* (1990), one leukaemia showed t(8;21)(q22;q22), with additional abnormalities of chromosome 17. One case showed t(8;21)(q22;q22) and del(16)(q22). Translocations t(3;21)(q26;q22) are uncommon variants in treatment-related acute myeloid leukaemia and treatment-related myelodysplastic syndrome (Nucifora & Rowley, 1995). Of five cases of leukaemia with t(3;21) after heterogeneous chemotherapy, one had been treated with etoposide (Rubin *et al.*, 1990).

(iii) *Abnormality inv(16)(p13q23)*

The chromosomal abnormality inv(16) is infrequent in treatment-related acute myeloid leukaemia associated with the monocytic subtype with eosinophilia (Quesnel *et al.*, 1993; Pedersen-Bjergaard & Rowley, 1994). Fenaux *et al.* (1989) described a case of acute monocytic leukaemia with eosinophilia in which the karyotype showed del(3)(q26), del(7)(q31), inv(16)(p13q23); the leukaemia had occurred after chemotherapy for Hodgkin disease with procarbazine, vincristine, prednisone and nitrogen mustard (MOPP) and for a germ-cell tumour with cisplatin, doxorubicin and etoposide in the same patient. Quesnel *et al.* (1993) identified the inv(16) in one case of treatment-related leukaemia in which prior treatment had included an epipodophyllotoxin in combination with an alkylating agent, but it was not specified whether etoposide or teniposide was used.

(iv) *Translocation t(15;17)*

Acute promyelocytic leukaemia with translocation t(15;17) occurs infrequently after treatment with etoposide and other DNA topoisomerase II-targeted anticancer drugs. Individual case reports indicate that t(15;17) is also a recurrent chromosomal alteration after etoposide-containing treatment for a variety of tumours (Raiker *et al.*, 1989; Detourmignies *et al.*, 1992; Lopez-Andreu *et al.*, 1994; Smith *et al.*, 1999). Etoposide has rarely been used as a single agent, except in some cases for the treatment of Langerhans cell histiocytosis (Haupt *et al.*, 1997). Haupt *et al.* (1997) observed five cases of leukaemia among 241 patients, 113 of whom had received etoposide as part of their treatment. Morphologically, the leukaemias were acute promyelocytic. Although t(15;17) is present in the vast majority of cases of acute promyelocytic leukaemia, the karyotypes in cases where etoposide was used a single agent revealed -6, -10, +mar, +ring in one case and del(20)(q11q13) in another. Cytogenetic analysis in one case in which etoposide was used with vinblastine and high-dose methylprednisolone did reveal the t(15;17), but in another case in which etoposide was used the t(15;17) was detectable only by molecular analysis.

(v) *Translocation t(9;22)*

A case of chronic myeloid leukaemia with t(9;22) and the *BCR/ABL* fusion gene was observed in an adult male 5.5 years after treatment of testicular cancer with a regimen that contained etoposide. Acute lymphoblastic leukaemia and acute myeloid leukaemia with t(9;22) may also occur after treatment with etoposide (Pedersen-Bjergaard et al., 1997).

(vi) *Translocations involving chromosome band 11p15*

Chromosome band 11p15 has emerged as another site of chromosomal abnormalities in leukaemias occurring after etoposide-containing treatment. At the cytogenetic level, abnormalities including add(11)(p15), inv(11)(p15q22), t(11;20)(p15;q11.2) and t(2;11)(q31;p15) have been reported (Stark et al., 1994; Felix et al., 1995b; Kobayashi et al., 1997; Raza-Egilmez et al., 1998), while additional cases with inv(11)(p15q22) and t(1;11)(q23;p15) after unspecified DNA topoisomerase II inhibitors have been observed (Arai et al., 1997; Nakamura et al., 1999).

(c) *Molecular characterization of the etoposide-related translocation break-points*

Molecular characterization of the translocation break-points in the leukaemias provides detailed insight about the genetic changes associated with etoposide treatment and clues to the mechanism whereby they occur. Cytogenetic studies revealed that translocations, especially those involving chromosome band 11q23, are hallmark features of leukaemias related to etoposide. In the early 1990s, several laboratories isolated the break-point region of the relevant gene at chromosome band 11q23 and named the gene *ALL-1*, *MLL*, *HTRX1* and *HRX* (Djabali et al., 1992; Gu et al., 1992; McCabe et al., 1992; Tkachuk et al., 1992), the last two designations for its homology to *Drosophila trithorax*. After the cloning of the *MLL* gene, several laboratories used Southern blot analysis to study leukaemias that had occurred in etoposide-treated patients and isolated the genomic break-points and the fusion transcripts.

Southern blot analyses of leukaemias with cytogenetic evidence of translocations involving band 11q23 and chromosomal loci, such as 9p22, 19p13, 3q25, 1p32, 4q21, 6q27, 5q13, 9q27, 16p13 or del(11)(q23), revealed that virtually all disrupted the same break-point cluster region between exons 5 and 11 of the *MLL* gene, which is also involved in de-novo leukaemias with translocations of chromosome band 11q23 (Felix et al., 1993; Gill Super et al., 1993; Domer et al., 1995; Felix et al., 1995b; Strissel Broeker et al., 1996). In addition, Southern blot analysis indicated that *MLL* gene rearrangements could be present even when the karyotype did not reveal the translocation (Felix et al., 1995b). Later, detailed mapping by Southern blot analysis suggested a biased distribution of the translocation break-points in treatment-related leukaemias in the 3′ break-point cluster region (Strissel Broeker et al., 1996). Low-affinity and high-affinity scaffold attachment regions were identified centromeric to and within the telomeric break-point cluster region, respectively, and sequence homologies to a putative in-vitro DNA topoisomerase II recognition sequence were observed proximal to and within the telomeric scaffold attachment region, leading Strissel Broeker et al. (1996) to suggest that chromatin structure may be important in determining the distribution of the break-points.

Domer et al. (1995) were the first to clone an *MLL* genomic translocation break-point in a case of leukaemia after etoposide-containing therapy when they isolated the der(11) breakpoint junction in a case of acute lymphoblastic leukaemia with a t(4;11). The *MLL* break-point was 3' in intron 8. The partner gene was *AF-4* at band 4q21. The *MLL* and *AF-4* break-points were both proximal to regions of homology to a putative in-vitro DNA topoisomerase II recognition site. The authors suggested a role for DNA topoisomerase II in the translocation process. Cloning of additional *MLL* genomic break-points and attempts to understand the translocation mechanism followed.

The cloning of *MLL* translocation break-points in leukaemias in etoposide-treated patients has led to further characterization of intronic regions of known genes fused with *MLL* (typically called 'partner genes'), because the break-points are in introns. It also led to the discovery of new partner genes. This line of investigation yields insights about regions of the genome affected by the drugs and provides some clues about the mechanism. Megonigal et al. (1997) cloned the *MLL* genomic break-point in a case of acute lymphoblastic leukaemia with t(4;11)(q21;q23) in a patient treated with etoposide. The der(11) *MLL* translocation break-point was in intron 6 in the 5' break-point cluster region. The sequence of the partner DNA was not homologous to known cDNA or genomic sequences of the *AF-4* gene at chromosome band 4q21, but reverse transcriptase polymerase chain reaction analysis showed that the t(4;11) was an *MLL-AF-4* fusion. The break-point in the *MLL* break-point cluster region was in an *Alu* repeat and there was an *Alu* repeat near the break-point in the partner DNA, suggesting that the repetitive sequences are important for this type of rearrangements. The break-point deviated from the predilection for 3' distribution in the break-point cluster region that was suggested in the adult cases (Strissel Broeker et al., 1996).

While the karyotypes imply considerable overlap in partner genes in treatment-related and de-novo leukaemias with *MLL* gene translocations, some partner genes were discovered in etoposide-related acute myeloid leukaemia or myelodysplastic syndrome. Examples include the cAMP response element-binding (CREB) protein gene (*CBP*) at chromosome band 16p13.3 (Rowley et al., 1997; Sobulo et al., 1997; Taki et al., 1997) and the gene encoding p300 at chromosome band 22q13 (Ida et al., 1997). Sobulo et al. (1997) isolated the der (16) genomic break-point of a t(11;16) translocation and localized the *MLL* break-point to position 1502 in intron 6, also in the 5' break-point cluster region. The *MLL* genomic break-point in the der(11) chromosome of the t(11;22) translocation involving p300 was at position 7206 in intron 9 in the 3' break-point cluster region (Ida et al., 1997), confirming heterogeneity in *MLL* genomic break-point distribution. The *CBP* gene also contains mutations in patients with Rubenstein-Taybi syndrome, indicating involvement of a common region of the genome in leukaemia and a constitutional disorder (Taki et al., 1997). Since the *CBP* gene product is a histone acetyltransferase, the t(11;16) potentially could lead to histone acetylation of genomic regions targeted by *MLL* AT hooks and transcriptional deregulation (Sobulo et al., 1997). p300 is a transcriptional co-activator with *CBP* (Ida et al., 1997).

Thus, like *MLL* break-points in leukaemia in infants, *MLL* translocation breakpoints in etoposide-related leukaemias are distributed in introns within the 8.3-kilobase break-point cluster region between *MLL* exons 5–11. Heterogeneous partner genes have been reported to be involved in the translocation. The *MLL* genomic break-point region involved in translocations has been studied in DNA topoisomerase II cleavage assays of naked DNA and after exposing human haematopoietic cells to etoposide in tissue culture. In an assay for DNA topoisomerase II cleavage *in vitro*, Lovett *et al.* (1999) reported (in an abstract) that multiple DNA topoisomerase II cleavage sites within the *MLL* break-point cluster region are enhanced not only by etoposide but also by its catechol and quinone metabolites. Aplan *et al.* (1996) and Stanulla *et al.* (1997a) observed site-specific cleavage *in vitro* within the 3' *MLL* break-point cluster region by Southern blot analysis after exposing human peripheral blood mononuclear cells to etoposide as well as to doxorubicin, catalytic DNA topoisomerase II inhibitors and other genotoxic and non-genotoxic stimuli of apoptosis. The site-specific cleavage was attributed to the higher-order chromatin fragmentation which occurs during apoptosis. Similar site-specific cleavage was identified within *AML1*, the gene at band 21q22 in the t(8;21) and t(3;21) translocations (Stanulla *et al.*, 1997b). Indeed, it later was proposed that DNA cleavage induced directly by DNA topoisomerase II or by the drug-induced apoptotic cellular response is responsible for the non-random chromosomal translocations leading to leukaemogenesis (Dassonneville & Bailly, 1998).

The *NUP98* gene at chromosome 11p15 is involved in at least six different chromosomal aberrations and, like *MLL*, appears to be a target gene in treatment-related myelodysplastic syndrome and acute myeloid leukaemia, with multiple translocation partners. The NUP98 gene product is a 98-kDa component of the nuclear pore complex which functions as a docking protein in nucleocytoplasmic transport (Radu *et al.*, 1995). The multiple FXFG repeats in the N-terminal portion of the protein are required for its docking function. The translocations t(7;11)(p15;p15), t(2;11)(q31;p15), t(1;11)(q23;p15) and t(4;11)(q21;p15) and the inversion inv (11)(p15q22) result in fusion transcripts that encode chimaeric oncoproteins fusing the FXFG region of NUP98 with HOXA9, HOXD13, PMX-1, all homeodomain-containing proteins, or with RAP1GDS1 or DDX-10, a putative RNA helicase, respectively (Nakamura *et al.*, 1996; Arai *et al.*, 1997; Raza-Egilmez *et al.*, 1998; Hussey *et al.*, 1999; Nakamura *et al.*, 1999). Most recently, the t(11;20)(p15;q11) was identified in two paediatric cases of treatment-related myelodysplastic syndrome after exposure to multi-agent chemotherapy in which etoposide was included. The t(11;20) translocation fuses *NUP98* with the *TOP1* gene (Ahuja *et al.*, 1999).

4.4.2 *Experimental systems*

General reviews on the mutagenicity of inhibitors of DNA topoisomerase II enzymes, including etoposide, have been published (Anderson & Berger, 1994; Ferguson & Baguley, 1994, 1996; Baguley & Ferguson, 1998; Ferguson, 1998).

Jackson et al. (1996) collated a genetic activity profile for this drug. The results are summarized in Table 6.

Etoposide gave mainly negative responses in a range of assays in prokaryotes and lower eukaryotes. Thus, in most studies, it did not cause significant increases in reverse mutation frequency as measured in *Salmonella typhimurium* strains TA1535, TA1537, TA1538, TA98 and TA100, *Escherichia coli* WP2 *uvrA*, *E. coli* K12 (forward and reverse mutation) and in other *E. coli* assays in the presence or absence of exogenous metabolic activation. Etoposide caused a slight (about twofold) increase in the frequency of revertant colonies in *S. typhimurium* TA102 and a clearly positive response in strain TA1978. It caused differential toxicity in *Bacillus subtilis* H17 rec^+ and M45 rec^-. Toxicity but not mutagenicity occurred at a dose of about 800 μg/plate, which is higher than those studied in mammalian cells. In *Saccharomyces cerevisiae* strain D5, etoposide did not induce either mitochondrial 'petite' mutations or mitotic recombination. It did not induce forward or reverse mutations in *Neurospora crassa*.

Etoposide is a potent inducer of DNA breakage in mammalian cells, both *in vitro* and *in vivo*. It caused protein-masked DNA double-strand breaks, DNA–protein cross-links and a small proportion of DNA single-strand breaks in various animal cells as well as in human cell lines at a concentration of about 1 μmol/L. At lower concentrations, the DNA strand breakage caused by etoposide was enhanced by various metal ions, but this may occur through a mechanism involving free-radical formation rather than DNA topoisomerase II. Etoposide induced highly specific DNA double-strand cleavage in a range of human leukaemic cell lines. In particular, breaks were seen at *MLL* sites that have been associated with translocations in human leukaemia. Single-strand breaks typically occur rapidly during exposure to the drug, reaching a maximum by 15 min, whereas double-strand breaks accumulate more slowly, reaching a plateau between 1–2 h after the start of exposure (Long et al., 1985). These DNA strand breaks are rapidly repaired when cells are placed in a drug-free medium, and 50% of the strand breaks are repaired within 60 min. All of the DNA strand breaks induced by etoposide were protein-associated (Kerrigan et al., 1987), suggesting that its cytotoxicity is dependent on DNA topoisomerase II inhibition. As with the related drug teniposide, single-strand DNA breaks are more common at low concentrations of etoposide, the number of double-strand breaks increasing with increasing concentration (Long et al., 1985). Cells from patients with ataxia telangiectasia show increased sensitivity to etoposide, accompanied by an increased frequency of chromosomal aberrations (Pandita & Hittelman, 1992). Treatment of human leukaemic T lymphoblasts with etoposide led to DNA breakage and also caused a nadir in cellular nucleotide pools 2–6 h after treatment. Etoposide has been suggested to inactivate DNA synthesis by inhibiting replicon cluster initiation (Suciu, 1990). In DNA from HeLa cells, DNA topoisomerase II enzymes were active in cleaving the telomere DNA repeat at a 5'-TTAGG*G3' site, and this reaction was strongly stimulated by etoposide but not by other DNA topoisomerase II poisons (Yoon et al., 1998).

Table 6. Genetic and related effects of etoposide

Test system	Result[a] Without exogenous metabolic system	Result[a] With exogenous metabolic system	Dose[b] (LED or HID)	Reference
Bacillus subtilis H17 and M45 *rec* strains, differential toxicity	+	NT	50 μg/disc	Nakanomyo *et al.* (1986)
Salmonella typhimurium TA100, TA1535, reverse mutation	–	–	1000 μg/plate	Nakanomyo *et al.* (1986)
Salmonella typhimurium TA100, reverse mutation	–	–	500 μg/plate	Gupta *et al.* (1987)
Salmonella typhimurium TA102, reverse mutation	(+)	(+)	600 μg/plate	Gupta *et al.* (1987)
Salmonella typhimurium TA1537, TA1538, reverse mutation	–	–	1000 μg/plate	Ashby *et al.* (1994)
Salmonella typhimurium TA98, TA1537, TA1538, reverse mutation	(+)	(+)	1000 μg/plate	Nakanomyo *et al.* (1986)
Salmonella typhimurium TA98, TA1538, reverse mutation	–	NT	2000 μg/plate	Matney *et al.* (1985)
Salmonella typhimurium TA98, reverse mutation	–	–	800 μg/plate	Gupta *et al.* (1987)
Salmonella typhimurium TA98, reverse mutation	(+)	(+)	50 μg/plate	Ashby *et al.* (1994)
Salmonella typhimuriumi TA1978, reverse mutation	+	NT	200 μg/plate	Matney *et al.* (1985)
Escherichia coli 343/113, forward mutation	–	NT	500 μg/plate	Gupta *et al.* (1987)
Escherichia coli WP2 *uvrA*, reverse mutation	–	–	4000 μg/plate	Nakanomyo *et al.* (1986)
Escherichia coli WP2S, WP44SNF, reverse mutation	–	NT	400 μg/plate	Gupta *et al.* (1987)
Saccharomyces cerevisiae D5, mitochondrial 'petite' mutation	–	NT	3000	Ferguson & Turner (1988a)
Saccharomyces cerevisiae D5, mitotic recombination	–	NT	900	Ferguson & Turner (1988b)
Neurospora crassa, forward mutation	–	NT	100	Gupta (1990)
Neurospora crassa, reverse mutation	–	NT	470 μg/plate	Gupta (1990)
Drosophila melanogaster, genetic crossing-over or recombination (white–ivory assay)	+		25 in feed	Ferreiro *et al.* (1997)
Drosophila melanogaster, somatic mutation (and recombination)	+		300 in feed	Frei & Würgler (1996)
Drosophila melanogaster, somatic mutation (and recombination)	+		600 in feed	Torres *et al.* (1998)
DNA single- and double-strand breaks, mouse leukaemia L1210 cells *in vitro*	+	NT	1.8	Wozniak & Ross (1983)

Table 6 (contd)

Test system	Result[a]		Dose[b] (LED or HID)	Reference
	Without exogenous metabolic system	With exogenous metabolic system		
DNA double-strand breaks, L1210 mouse leukaemia cells in vitro	+	NT	3	Ross et al. (1984)
DNA single-strand breaks (protein-associated) and DNA–protein cross-links, mouse leukaemia L1210 cells in vitro	+[c]	NT	9	Kerrigan et al. (1987)
DNA single- and double-strand breaks, mouse embryo fibroblast 3T3 cells in vitro	+	NT	12	Markovits et al. (1987)
DNA–protein cross-links, Chinese hamster ovary CHO-K1 cells and xrs-1 cells in vitro	+	NT	3	Jeggo et al. (1989)
DNA–protein cross-links, MCF-7 cells in vitro	+	NT	12	Nutter et al. (1991)
DNA strand breaks (single-cell gel electrophoresis assay), Chinese hamster lung V79-171b cells in vitro	+	NT	2	Olive & Banáth (1993)
DNA double-strand breaks (contour clamped, homogeneous electric field assay), Chinese hamster ovary AA8 cells in vitro	+	NT	3	Sestili et al. (1995)
DNA strand breaks (single-cell gel electrophoresis assay), Chinese hamster CHO-K1 cells in vitro	+	NT	0.12	Vigreux et al. (1998)
Recombination, Chinese hamster lung V79-SP5 cells in vitro	–	NT	0.6	Zhang & Jenssen (1994)
Mutation, Chinese hamster ovary cells, Hprt locus in vitro	+	NT	0.8	Singh & Gupta (1983a)
Mutation, Chinese hamster ovary CHO W-14 cells, Hprt locus in vitro	+	NT	0.4	Singh & Gupta (1983b)
Mutation, mouse lymphoma L5178Y cells, Tk locus in vitro	+	NT	0.005	Ashby et al. (1994)
Mutation, mouse L cells, Hprt locus in vitro	+	NT	0.4	Gupta et al. (1987)
Sister chromatid exchange, Chinese hamster ovary cells in vitro	+	NT	0.1	Singh & Gupta (1983a)
Sister chromatid exchange, Chinese hamster lung DC3F cells in vitro	+[d]	NT	12	Pommier et al. (1988)
Micronucleus formation, spermatids of Sprague-Dawley rats in vitro	+	NT	0.3	Sjöblom et al. (1994)
Micronucleus formation, mouse splenocytes in vitro	+	NT	0.06	Record et al. (1995)

Table 6 (contd)

Test system	Result[a] Without exogenous metabolic system	Result[a] With exogenous metabolic system	Dose[b] (LED or HID)	Reference
Micronucleus formation, Chinese hamster ovary CHO-K1 cells in vitro	+	NT	1.2[e]	Johnston et al. (1997)
Chromosomal aberrations, Chinese hamster lung DC3F cells in vitro	+[d]	NT	12	Pommier et al. (1988)
Chromosomal aberrations, Chinese hamster lung CHL cells in vitro	+	NT	0.15	Suzuki & Nakane (1994)
Chromosomal aberrations, Chinese hamster ovary CHO-K1 cells in vitro	+	NT	0.12	Vigreux et al. (1998)
Chromosomal aberrations, mouse lymphoma L5178Y cells in vitro	+	NT	0.02	Ashby et al. (1994)
Polyploidy, Chinese hamster ovary CHO cells in vitro	+	NT	24	Sumner (1995)
DNA single-strand breaks, human carcinoma A549 cell line in vitro	+	NT	0.12	Long et al. (1985)
DNA single- and double-strand breaks, SW1272 human lung carcinoma cells in vitro	+	NT	0.06	Long et al. (1986)
DNA single-strand breaks (protein-associated) and DNA–protein cross-links, human embryo fibroblast VA-13 and colon carcinoma HT-29 cells in vitro	+[c]	NT	15	Kerrigan et al. (1987)
DNA double-strand breaks, T-47D human breast cancer cells in vitro	+	NT	1.5	Epstein & Smith (1988)
DNA single-strand breaks, MCF-7 human breast cancer cells in vitro	+	NT	3	Sinha et al. (1988)
DNA strand breaks, human leukaemic T lymphoblasts in vitro	+	NT	12	Marks & Fox (1991)
DNA double-strand breaks (DNA unwinding assay), human promyelocytic leukaemia HL60 WT cells in vitro	+	NT	1.5	Sinha & Eliot (1991)
DNA single-strand breaks, primary acute myeloid leukaemia cells in vitro	+	NT	5	Chiron et al. (1992)
DNA strand breaks, Molt 4 human T lymphoblastoid cells and HL-60 promyelocytic leukaemia cells in vitro	+	NT	1	Shimizu et al. (1992)
DNA double-strand breaks, human ovarian A2780 cells in vitro	+[f]	NT	3	Noviello et al. (1994)
DNA double-strand breaks, human T lymphocytes in vitro	+	NT	0.6	Russo et al. (1994)

Table 6 (contd)

Test system	Result[a]		Dose[b] (LED or HID)	Reference
	Without exogenous metabolic system	With exogenous metabolic system		
DNA double-strand breaks, human lung carcinoma A549 cells in vitro	+	NT	1.2	Long et al. (1985)
DNA double-strand breaks (MLL BCR site-specific), human leukaemia cell lines in vitro	+	NT	0.6	Aplan et al. (1996)
DNA strand breaks (single-cell electrophoresis assay), human lymphocytes in vitro	+	NT	12	Lebailly et al. (1997)
DNA double-strand breaks within the AML-1 locus, various human leukaemia cell lines in vitro	+	NT	6	Stanulla et al. (1997b)
DNA double-strand breaks, human lung carcinoma A549 cell line in vitro	+	NT	60	Vock et al. (1998)
Mutation, human lymphoid CCRF-CEM, HPRT locus (deletion exons 2 and 3) in vitro	+	NT	0.15	Chen et al. (1996a)
Sister chromatid exchange, human lymphocytes in vitro	+	NT	0.025	Tominaga et al. (1986)
Sister chromatid exchange, human lymphocytes in vitro	+	NT	0.06	Ribas et al. (1996)
Sister chromatid exchange, human ovarian A2780 cells in vitro	+[f]	NT	12	Noviello et al. (1994)
Sister chromatid exchange, human lymphoblastoid cell lines derived from patients with ataxia telangiectasia, in vitro	+	NT	0.002	Fantini et al. (1998)
Micronucleus formation, neonatal human lymphocytes in vitro	+	NT	0.03	Slavotinek et al. (1993)
Chromosomal aberrations, human lymphocytes in vitro	+	NT	0.025	Tominaga et al. (1986)
Chromosomal aberrations, human lymphocytes in vitro	+	NT	50	Maraschin et al. (1990)
Chromosomal aberrations at the 1cen–1q12 region, human lymphocytes in vitro	+	NT	0.12	Rupa et al. (1997)
Chromosomal aberrations, human lymphoblastoid cell lines derived from patients with ataxia telangiectasia, in vitro	+	NT	0.18	Caporossi et al. (1993)
Chromosomal aberrations, human ovarian A2780 cells in vitro	+[f]	NT	12	Noviello et al. (1994)

Table 6 (contd)

Test system	Result[a]		Dose[b] (LED or HID)	Reference
	Without exogenous metabolic system	With exogenous metabolic system		
Chromosomal aberrations, human lymphoblastoid cell lines derived from patients with ataxia telangiectasia, *in vitro*	+	NT	0.02	Fantini *et al.* (1998)
Chromosomal aberrations, TK6 and WI-L2-NS human B-lymphoblast cells *in vitro*	+	NT	1	Greenwood *et al.* (1998)
Chromosomal aberrations, human lymphocytes *in vitro*	+	NT	30	Mosesso *et al.* (1998)
Fragmentation of centromeric DNA, spermatids of BALB/c mice *in vivo*	+		10 ip × 1	Kallio & Lähdetie (1996)
Mutation, primary spermatocytes in (101/R1 × C3H/R1)F$_1$ mice *in vivo*	+		75 ip × 1	Russell *et al.* (1998)
Sister chromatid exchange, bone-marrow cells of male Swiss mice *in vivo*	+		0.5 ip × 1	Agarwal *et al.* (1994)
Micronucleus formation, bone-marrow cells of CD-1 mice *in vivo*	+		0.75 ip × 1	Nakanomyo *et al.* (1986)
Micronucleus formation, spermatids of Han:NMRI mice *in vivo*	+		25 ip × 1	Kallio & Lähdetie (1993)
Micronucleus formation, bone-marrow cells of mice *in vivo*	+		0.1 po × 1	Ashby *et al.* (1994)
Micronucleus formation, bone-marrow cells of male CBA mice *in vivo*	+		1 po or ip × 1	Ashby & Tinwell (1995)
Micronucleus formation, spermatids of BALB/c mice *in vivo* (kinetochore-positive, indicative of aneuploidy)	+		20 ip × 1	Kallio & Lähdetie (1997)
Micronucleus formation, spermatids of Sprague-Dawley rats *in vivo*	+		5 ip × 1	Lähdetie *et al.* (1994)
Micronucleus formation, bone-marrow cells of male and female Fischer 344 rats *in vivo*	+		57 po × 14	Garriot *et al.* (1995)

Table 6 (contd)

Test system	Result[a]		Dose[b] (LED or HID)	Reference
	Without exogenous metabolic system	With exogenous metabolic system		
Chromosomal aberrations, bone-marrow cells of pregnant Swiss mice and embryonic tissue cells *in vivo*	+		1.5 ip × 1, day 6 of gestation	Sieber *et al.* (1978)
Chromosomal aberrations, bone-marrow cells of male Swiss mice *in vivo*	+		5 ip × 1	Agarwal *et al.* (1994)
Chromosomal aberrations, metaphase II oocytes, ICR mice *in vivo*	+		40 ip × 1	Mailhes *et al.* (1994)
Aneuploidy, metaphase II oocytes, ICR mice *in vivo*	+		40 ip × 1	Mailhes *et al.* (1994)

[a] +, positive; (+), weak positive; −, negative; NT, not tested
[b] LED, lowest effective dose; HID, highest ineffective dose; in-vitro tests, μg/mL; in-vivo tests, mg/kg bw per day; ip, intraperitoneal; po, oral
[c] Protein-free single-strand breaks were not induced.
[d] Negative in topoisomerase II inhibitor-resistant DC3F/9-OHE cells
[e] CHO-K1 repair-deficient cells (*xrs* 5) were more sensitive (LED, 0.12 μg/mL) than CHO-K1 cells.
[f] Negative in multi-drug resistant, A2780-DX3 cells

Etoposide was highly effective in causing chromosomal aberrations in cultured Chinese hamster cells, in other rodent cell lines and in human peripheral blood lymphocytes in tissue culture. It also induced micronucleus formation in neonatal lymphocytes grown *in vitro* and in mouse splenocytes in culture. Various human lymphoblastoid cell lines derived from patients with ataxia telangiectasia were hypersensitive to the induction of chromosomal aberrations by etoposide. The Chinese hamster cell line *xrs-1* was also hypersensitive to etoposide, with an elevated frequency of micronucleus induction; however, the two ionizing radiation-sensitive cell lines, *irs1* and *irs3*, appeared to be similar to the parental V79-4 cell line in terms of micronucleus induction. Etoposide caused both clastogenic and aneuploidogenic effects in all these cell lines (Hermine *et al.*, 1997). Fluorescence in-situ hybridization techniques revealed that etoposide caused almost equal numbers of dicentric and stable translocations in human peripheral blood lymphocytes in culture (Mosesso *et al.*, 1998). It induced micronuclei and/or chromosomal aberrations in the bone marrow of mice and rats.

Etoposide induced sister chromatid exchange in Chinese hamster lung cells and in human lymphocytes and other human cell lines *in vitro*. Sister chromatid exchange induction has also been seen in mouse bone-marrow cells *in vivo*. Etoposide induced mutation and somatic recombination in *Drosophila melanogaster* in the wing spot test. It also induced a positive response in the *Drosophila white–ivory* assay, probably again through recombinogenic events.

Somatic intrachromosomal recombination can result in inversions and deletions in DNA. pKZ1 mice have an *E. coli lacZ* transgene that is expressed only after a DNA inversion involving the transgene; the *E. coli* β-galactosidase protein, which is encoded by the *lacZ* gene, can then be detected in frozen tissue sections with a chromogenic substrate. These mice can therefore be used to detect somatic intrachromosomal recombination inversion events *in vivo* in various tissues. When these mice were given a single intraperitoneal injection of etoposide and spleen cells were examined three days later, significant induction of inversion events was found by histochemical staining of tissue sections (Sykes *et al.*, 1999).

Etoposide induced mutations at the *HPRT* locus in human leukaemic CCRF-CEM cells and at the *Hprt* locus in Chinese hamster ovary and mouse L cells. It induced primarily small colony mutants at the *Tk* locus in mouse lymphoma L5178Y cells. Small colony mutants in L5178Y cells are usually caused by chromosomal mutations (DeMarini *et al.*, 1987). Di Leonardo *et al.* (1993) showed an etoposide-induced increase in resistance to *N*-phosphonoacetyl-L-aspartate, an event that has been shown to result from gene amplification.

Whether cellular damage results in mutation or apoptosis depends on a number of factors (Ferguson & Baguley, 1994). Etoposide-induced apoptosis has been demonstrated in cultured retinoblastoma Y79 cells (Lauricella *et al.*, 1998), in mouse fibroblasts (Mizumoto *et al.*, 1994), in human leukaemia HL-60 and K562 cells (Ritke *et al.*, 1994) and in neurons cultured from the fetal rat central nervous system (Nakajima *et al.*, 1994). It caused a concentration-dependent induction of apoptosis in immature thymocytes from male Fischer 344 rats (Sun *et al.*, 1994a,b). Fritsche *et al.* (1993) showed that etoposide caused accumulation of p53 protein in a range of murine, simian and human cell lines. In mice, etoposide caused apoptosis through a *p53*-dependent pathway in immature thymocytes and also through a *p53*-independent pathway in a particular sub-population of these cells. The drug induced apoptosis at significantly lower levels and at later times in *p53* null as compared with *p53* wild-type mice (MacFarlane *et al.*, 1996).

Chen *et al.* (1996a) provided evidence that etoposide-induced deletions in the *HPRT* gene of human lymphoid CCRF-CEM cells occur through illegitimate V(D)J recombination. In human leukaemic CCRF-CEM cells, etoposide concentrations resulting in equal cytotoxicity (95%) after a 4-h exposure (2.5 µmol/L) and a 24-h exposure (0.5 µmol/L) caused significantly fewer recombinogenic events (as measured by VDJ recombinase-mediated deletions in exons 2 and 3 of the *HPRT* gene at day 6) with the more prolonged schedule (4.1×10^{-7} after 24 h versus 14.2×10^{-7} after 4 h) (Chen *et al.*, 1996b). These results indicate an improved therapeutic index with the prolonged schedule. Similar results were not seen in the myeloid cell lines KG-1A or K562, but Edwards *et al.* (1987) observed that CCRF-CEM cells are especially sensitive to etoposide, probably because of their high content of DNA topoisomerase II enzymes. Aratani *et al.* (1996) used gene transfer assays to study whether etoposide affects non-homologous (illegitimate) recombination and found that it stimulated integration of closed circular or linearized plasmids carrying the wild-type *Aprt* gene into *Aprt*-deficient Chinese hamster cells by non-homologous (illegitimate) recombination. It did not, however, significantly influence intrachromosomal recombination in SP5/V79 Chinese hamster cells (Zhang & Jenssen, 1994). Given their size, it is probable that etoposide-induced deletions and recombination events are mediated by a series of subunit exchanges between overlapping DNA topoisomerase II dimers at the bases of replicons or larger chromosomal structures such as replicon clusters or chromosome minibands.

A fluorescence in-situ hybridization procedure involving tandem DNA probes was used to show that etoposide caused hyperdiploidy of chromosome 1 and stimulated DNA breakage in the centromeric region of this chromosome. Polyploidy was also demonstrated by cytogenetic techniques in Chinese hamster ovary cells. Etoposide inhibited accurate chromosomal segregation in both HeLa and PtK2 cells (Downes *et al.*, 1991). It also retarded chromatid separation *in vitro* in a system derived from sperm nuclei in an extract of *Xenopus laevis* eggs. Etoposide induced differentiation of human HL-60 leukaemia cells (Gieseler *et al.*, 1993). It caused hypermethylation of DNA at CpG sites, resulting in altered patterns of distribution of 5-methylcytosine residues at these sites, thereby modifying gene expression (Nyce, 1989; Wachsman, 1997).

In general, events in mammalian cells *in vitro* occurred in the absence of exogenous metabolic activation. Nevertheless, etoposide is metabolized by human liver microsomes (Kawashiro *et al.*, 1998). Various metabolic species have been identified, but their mutagenic properties have not been studied.

Etoposide mutates not only somatic cells but also germ cells. It readily induced micronuclei associated with aneuploidy in stage 1 spermatids. Sjöblom *et al.* (1994)

showed that the drug increased the frequency of meiotic micronuclei in cultured rat seminiferous tubules. Hakovirta *et al.* (1993) found that it affected stage-specific DNA synthesis during rat spermatogenesis, inhibiting specific stages of premitotic DNA synthesis more effectively than premeiotic DNA synthesis. Russell *et al.* (1998) commented that etoposide is almost unique in causing peak mutagenicity in primary spermatocytes of mice. These effects are manifest as recessive mutations at specific loci and dominants at other loci. Deletion mutations occurred commonly, and these authors suggested that they had a recombinational origin.

Treatment of germ cells of male BALB/c mice with etoposide led to fragmentation of centromeric DNA. Lähdetie *et al.* (1994) found that the sensitivity of rats to etoposide was greatest in diplotene-diakinesis of primary spermatocytes, reduced in late pachytene and low in preleptotene stages, a very different pattern from that induced by DNA alkylating chemicals. These authors suggested that etoposide caused a failure of resolution of recombined chromosome arms, probably associated with cell cycle arrest and triggering of the apoptotic pathway. Etoposide also induced aneuploidy, polyploidy and M-phase cycle arrest when introduced during the meiotic M phase. Kallio and Lähdetie (1996) reported etoposide-induced DNA breakage at both the centromeric regions and chromatid arms of dyads. Additionally, many cells were arrested at late anaphase I, and the frequency of second divisions with a diploid chromosome number was significantly elevated. These authors also noted some unique effects in etoposide-treated germ cells, including minute micronuclei most of which contained only centromeric DNA. Chromosomal aberrations and aneuploidy were induced in metaphase II oocytes of ICR mice treated *in vivo* with etoposide.

Cytogenetic changes were measured in pregnant mice given a single intraperitoneal injection of 1.5 mg/kg bw etoposide on day 6, 7 or 8 of gestation and killed 48 h later. Injection on day 7 increased the frequency of embryonic cells with structural aberrations, one-third of which were stable, consisting of chromosomes with metacentric or submetacentric markers. Injection on day 6 or 8 increased the percentage of embryonic cells with numerical aberrations, most of which were hypoploidy (monosomy) (Sieber *et al.*, 1978).

4.5 Mechanistic considerations

Etoposide has two properties that are likely to lead to mutation.

1. It is an inhibitor of DNA topoisomerase II enzymes: Etoposide is a eukaryotic DNA topoisomerase II poison that has been shown to promote DNA cleavage, with a strong preference for C and to a lesser extent T at the −1 position (Capranico & Binashi, 1998). It does not inhibit bacterial topoisomerases and may not mutate bacterial cells by the same mechanism as mammalian cells. Unlike many other DNA topoisomerase II poisons, etoposide does not bind to DNA, either covalently or by intercalation. Instead, it appears to interact directly with the DNA topoisomerase II enzyme (Burden & Osheroff, 1998). Most of the mutational events found in mammalian cells, including point mutations, chromosomal deletions and exchanges, as well as aneuploidy, can be explained by this activity.

   2. It possesses readily oxidizable functions: Some of the etoposide-induced effects have been ascribed to the formation of free radicals by oxidation of its 4′-phenolic hydroxy group to a semiquinone free radical (Sakurai *et al.*, 1991). The hydroxy radical •OH may be responsible for the metal- and photo-induced DNA breakage produced by this compound; however, none of the mutations seen with etoposide is of the type usually associated with oxygen radicals.

The role of etoposide in the translocations associated with leukaemia is unknown. Two possibilities are plausible. The first is that etoposide itself causes the translocations, perhaps through a cytotoxic action. The planar ring structures of epipodophyllotoxins confer an ability to form stable, stacked complexes with DNA and DNA topoisomerase II. DNA topoisomerase II changes the topology of DNA by transiently cleaving and re-ligating both strands of the double helix (Ross *et al.*, 1988; Liu & Wang, 1991; Pommier *et al.*, 1991; Pommier, 1993). In the presence of epipodophyllotoxin, the rate of re-ligation is decreased, causing double-stranded breaks in DNA that are ultimately cytotoxic (Chen *et al.*, 1984; Long *et al.*, 1985; Epstein, 1988; Osheroff, 1989; Wang *et al.*, 1990; Osheroff *et al.*, 1991; Chen & Liu, 1994). In one model in which the drugs cause the translocations, the process involves drug-induced DNA topoisomerase II-mediated chromosomal breakage and formation of the translocations by further processing and resolution of the breakage through cellular mechanisms of DNA repair (Felix, 1998).

The second possibility for the role of etoposide in causing translocations is that it selects for cells that already have translocations. Indeed, *MLL* tandem duplications, a form of translocation, have been identified in peripheral blood and bone marrow of healthy adults (Schnittger *et al.*, 1998). Chemotherapy has profound effects on the kinetics of the marrow: it causes cell death, forcing many marrow stem cells to divide, which might select for the rare stem cells with a translocation (Knudson, 1992).

In favour of the first possibility is the specificity of the association between DNA topoisomerase II inhibitors, but not other forms of chemotherapy that cause cell death in the bone marrow, and leukaemias characterized by translocations.

5. Summary of Data Reported and Evaluation

5.1 Exposure data

Etoposide is a semi-synthetic podophyllotoxin derivative that has been used in cancer treatment since the early 1970s. This DNA topoisomerase II inhibitor is one of the most widely used and effective cytotoxic drugs in combination therapy, particularly in the treatment of lymphoma, small-cell lung cancer, testicular cancer, childhood malignancies and, to a lesser extent, a number of other cancers.

5.2 Human carcinogenicity data

One cohort study of patients with Langerhans cell histiocytosis and several cohort studies of patients with germ-cell tumours or lung cancer treated with etoposide-containing chemotherapy showed increased risks for acute myeloid leukaemia.

In the patients with Langerhans cell histiocytosis, a strongly increased risk for acute myeloid leukaemia of the promyelocytic type was found after treatment with etoposide alone; however, the possibility could not be ruled out that such patients have an inherently increased risk for acute promyelocytic leukaemia.

In several cohort studies of germ-cell tumours in men, treatment with etoposide, cisplatin and bleomycin was associated with an increased risk for acute myeloid leukaemia. On the basis of the combined data from six studies, the relative risk for acute myeloid leukaemia was 40 times greater than that of the general population; substantially higher relative risks have been found with high cumulative doses of etoposide. Although the other two agents (cisplatin and bleomycin) in etoposide-containing chemotherapy regimens for germ-cell tumours may have contributed to the positive association seen in the cohort studies, use of these agents in a similar regimen without etoposide has not been associated with acute myeloid leukaemia. As the background risk for acute myeloid leukaemia is low, the absolute risk for this disease in men treated for germ-cell tumours with etoposide-containing regimens is low. A strongly increased risk for acute myeloid leukaemia was also found in one cohort study of lung cancer patients treated with etoposide, cisplatin and vindesine. The possibility cannot be excluded that etoposide exerts its effects only in the presence of other cytotoxic agents.

Several other cohort studies reported strongly increased risks for acute myeloid leukaemia following treatment of various primary malignancies with etoposide-containing regimens that also included alkylating agents, or etoposide-containing regimens in combination with teniposide. In these studies, the possibility cannot be excluded that the excess leukaemia risk was partly or wholly due to the other agents.

5.3 Animal carcinogenicity data

Etoposide was tested in one experiment in wild-type and heterozygous neurofibromatosis type 1 gene ($Nf1$) knock-out mice. No increase in the incidence of leukaemia was observed.

5.4 Other relevant data

In humans, etoposide is eliminated biphasically, with an elimination half-time of 3–9 h. The pharmacokinetics of this compound is linear up to 3.5 mg/m^2 (typical single dose, 100 mg/m^2). Its bioavailability is around 50%, but this decreases with oral doses of > 200 mg. Etoposide is about 95% protein-bound in plasma. About 50% of an intravenous dose of etoposide is recovered in urine; up to 17% is excreted as a glucuronide metabolite and less than 2% as a catechol metabolite. Preliminary studies suggest that the remainder of the dose is excreted in the faeces. The catechol metabolite has also been detected in plasma at concentrations around 2.5% that of etoposide.

Biphasic elimination is seen in a number of animal species. In rhesus monkeys, 60% of a radiolabelled dose of etoposide was excreted in urine and 30% in faeces. Glucuronide metabolites have been reported in the urine of rabbits and rats. Oxidation of etoposide to quinone species and a catechol metabolite have been reported in cell systems, occurring either by peroxidase oxidation or cytochrome P450-mediated demethylation involving CYP3A4. These oxidation products have cytotoxic activity, but it is unclear how much they contribute to the activity of etoposide.

The major dose-limiting toxic effect of etoposide in humans is myelosuppression, manifest principally as leukopenia. Other toxic effects include nausea and vomiting, mucositis and alopecia. Cases of hypotension were reported in early trials in which short infusions were given, but this effect is rarely seen with infusions of longer than 30 min. Hypersensitivity reactions have been reported but are seen much less frequently than with teniposide. Cardiotoxicity and cutaneous toxicity have been reported but are rare.

Myelosuppression was the main toxic effect of intravenously administered etoposide in a number of the animal species studied. Other effects included changes in the lung in rats and renal and hepatic toxicity, electrocardiographic changes, decreased testis weight and disorders of spermatogenesis in rats and dogs. After intrapleural and intraperitoneal administration to mice and rats, delayed chronic pleuritis and peritonitis, with liver and spleen inflammation, were reported. Teratogenic effects especially on the central nervous system have been observed.

Etoposide does not bind to DNA by forming covalent bonds or through intercalation. The drug is orders of magnitude more toxic in mammalian than in microbial cells. The effects in mammals arise primarily because etoposide is a poison of DNA topoisomerase II enzymes. Etoposide also induces both aneuploidy and polyploidy. It enhances gene amplification and affects gene expression through hypermethylation of DNA. Treatment of cells with etoposide leads to an accumulation of protein-masked double-stranded DNA breaks and, with time, a variety of chromosomal aberrations. The predominant mutagenic effects detected involve the deletion and/or interchange of large DNA segments, especially balanced translocations. *In vitro*, etoposide and its catechol and quinone metabolites enhanced DNA topoisomerase II-mediated DNA strand breaks within the *MLL* gene which is implicated in leukaemia.

Etoposide-containing regimens have been associated with the development, after a short latency, of leukaemia which is characterized by chromosomal translocations. The translocations that are observed are the same as those found in de-novo cases of acute leukaemia; however, while translocations of the *MLL* gene at chromosome band 11q23 occur in only about 5% of cases of leukaemia in adults and are seen primarily in de-novo leukaemia in infants and young children, translocations of chromosome band 11q23 comprise the majority of the aberrations that follow leukaemias associated with administration of DNA topoisomerase II inhibitors. The translocations are considered to be primary events in leukaemogenesis. Etoposide is often used in combination chemotherapy with alkylating agents, which are themselves associated with leukaemia with specific chromosomal aberrations after a longer latency. These chromosomal aberrations are unbalanced chromosomal losses and deletions, especially monosomy 7, 7q and 5q deletions. Since the primary aberrations associated with alkylating agents are distinct from the balanced translocations with which DNA topoisomerase II inhibitors are associated, balanced translocations are specific events of epipodophyllotoxins that can be distinguished even when DNA topoisomerase II inhibitors are used in combination chemotherapy.

5.5 Evaluation

There is *limited evidence* in humans for the carcinogenicity of etoposide.

There is *sufficient evidence* in humans for the carcinogenicity of etoposide given in combination with cisplatin and bleomycin.

There is *inadequate evidence* in experimental animals for the carcinogenicity of etoposide.

Overall evaluation

Etoposide is *probably carcinogenic to humans (Group 2A)*.

In reaching this conclusion, the Working Group noted that etoposide causes distinctive cytogenetic lesions in leukaemic cells that can be readily distinguished from those induced by alkylating agents. The short latency of these leukaemias contrasts with that of leukaemia induced by alkylating agents. Potent protein-masked DNA breakage and clastogenic effects occur in human cells *in vitro* and in animal cells *in vivo*.

Etoposide in combination with cisplatin and bleomycin is *carcinogenic to humans (Group 1)*.

6. References

Achterrath, W., Niederle, N., Raettig, R. & Hilgard, P. (1982) Etoposide—Chemistry, preclinical and clinical pharmacology. *Cancer Treat. Rev.*, **9** (Suppl. A), 3–13

Adewole, L.F., Rustin, G.J., Newlands, E.S., Dent, J. & Bagshawe, K.D. (1986) Fertility in patients with gestational trophoblastic tumors treated with etoposide. *Eur. J. Cancer clin. Oncol.*, **22**, 1479–1482

Agarwal, K., Mukherjee, A. & Sen, S. (1994) Etoposide (VP-16): Cytogenetic studies in mice. *Environ. mol. Mutag.*, **23**, 190–193

Ahuja, H.G., Felix, C.A. & Aplan, P.D. (1999) The t(11;20)(p15;q11) chromosomal translocation associated with therapy-related myelodysplastic syndrome results in an NUP98-TOP1 fusion. *Blood*, **94**, 3258–3261

Aisner, J., Van Echo, D.A., Whitacre, C. & Wiernik, P.H. (1982) A phase I trial of continuous infusion VP16-213 (etoposide). *Cancer Chemother. Pharmacol.*, **7**, 157–160

Allen, L.M. (1978) Comparison of uptake and binding of two epipodophyllotoxin glucopyranosides, 4'-demethyl epipodophyllotoxin thenylidene-β-D-glucoside and 4'-demethyl epipodophyllotoxin ethylidene-β-D-glucoside, in the L1210 leukemia cell. *Cancer Res.*, **38**, 2549–2554

Allen, L.M. & Creaven, P.J. (1975) Comparison of the human pharmacokinetics of VM-26 and VP-16, two antineoplastic epipodophyllotoxin glucopyranoside derivatives. *Eur. J. Cancer*, **11**, 697–707

American Hospital Formulary Service (1997) *AHFS Drug Information® 97*, Bethesda, MD, American Society of Health-System Pharmacists, pp. 746–753

Anderson, R.D. & Berger, N.A. (1994) Mtuagenicity and carcinogenicity of topoisomerase-interactive agents. *Mutat. Res.*, **309**, 109–142

Aplan, P.D., Chervinsky, D.S., Stanulla, M. & Burhans, W.C. (1996) Site-specific DNA cleavage within the *MLL* breakpoint cluster region induced by topoisomerase II inhibitors. *Blood*, **87**, 2649–2658

Arai, Y., Hosoda, F., Kobayashi, H., Arai, K., Hayashi, Y., Kamada, N., Kaneko, Y. & Ohki, M. (1997) The inv(11)(p15q22) chromosome translocation of de novo and therapy-related myeloid malignancies results in fusion of the nucleoporin gene, *NUP98*, with the putative RNA helicase gene, *DDX10*. *Blood*, **89**, 3936–3944

Aratani, Y., Andoh, T. & Koyama, H. (1996) Effects of DNA topoisomerase inhibitors on non-homologous and homologous recombination in mammalian cells. *Mutat. Res.*, **362**, 181–191

Arbuck, S.G., Douglass, H.O., Crom, W.R., Goodwin, P., Silk, Y., Cooper, C. & Evans, W.E. (1986) Etoposide pharmacokinetics in patients with normal and abnormal organ function. *J. clin. Oncol.*, **4**, 1690–1695

Ashby, J. & Tinwell, H. (1995) Activity of etoposide in the mouse bone marrow micronucleus test: Independence of route of exposure. *Mutat. Res.*, **328**, 243–244

Ashby, J., Tinwell, H., Glover, P., Poorman-Allen, P., Krehl, R., Callander, R.D. & Clive, D. (1994) Potent clastogenicity of the human carcinogen etoposide to the mouse bone marrow and mouse lymphoma L5178Y cells: Comparison to Salmonella responses. *Environ. mol. Mutag.*, **24**, 51–60

Azuno, Y., Kaku, K., Fujita, N., Okubo, M., Kaneko, T. & Matsumoto, N. (1995) Mitoxantrone and etoposide in breast milk (Letter to the Editor). *Am. J. Hematol.*, **48**, 131–132

Baguley, B.C. & Ferguson, L.R. (1998) Mutagenic properties of topoisomerase-targeted drugs. *Biochim. biophys. Acta*, **1400**, 213–222

Bajorin, D.F., Motzer, R.J., Rodriguez, E., Murphy, B. & Bosl, G.J. (1993) Acute nonlymphocytic leukemia in germ cell tumor patients treated with etoposide-containing chemotherapy (Brief communication). *J. natl Cancer Inst.*, **85**, 60–62

Bokemeyer, C. & Schmoll, H.-J. (1993) Secondary neoplasms following treatment of malignant germ cell tumors. *J. clin. Oncol.*, **11**, 1703–1709

Bokemeyer, C. & Schmoll, H.-J. (1995) Treatment of testicular cancer and the development of secondary malignancies. *J. clin. Oncol.*, **13**, 283–292

Bokemeyer, C., Schmoll, H.-J., Kuczyk, M.A., Beyer, J. & Siegert, W. (1995) Risk of secondary leukemia following high cumulative doses of etoposide during chemotherapy for testicular cancer (Letter to the Editor). *J. natl Cancer Inst.*, **87**, 58–60

Boshoff, C., Begent, R.H.J., Oliver, R.T.D., Rustin, G.J., Newlands, E.S., Andrews, R., Skelton, M., Holden, L. & Ong, J. (1995) Secondary tumours following etoposide containing therapy for germ cell cancer. *Ann. Oncol.*, **6**, 35–40

Bregman, C.L., Buroker, R.A., Hirth, R.S., Crosswell, A.R. & Durham, S.K. (1994) Etoposide- and BMY-40481-induced sensory neuropathy in mice. *Toxicol. Pathol.*, **22**, 528–535

British Medical Association/Royal Pharmaceutical Society of Great Britain (1998) *British National Formulary*, No. 36, London, p. 375

British Pharmacopoeia Commission (1994) *British Pharmacopoeia 1993, Addendum 1994*, London, Her Majesty's Stationery Office, pp. 1326–1327

Broggini, M., Rossi, C., Benfenati, E., D'Incalci, M., Fanelli, R. & Gariboldi, P. (1985) Horse-radish peroxidase/hydrogen peroxide-catalyzed oxidation of VP16-213. Identification of a new metabolite. *Chem.-biol. Interactions*, **55**, 215–224

Brunet, S., Sureda, A., Mateu, R. & Domingo-Albás, A. (1993) [Full-term pregnancy in a patient diagnosed with acute leukemia treated with a protocol including VP-16 (Letter to the Editor).] *Med. clin. Barcelona*, **100**, 757–758 (in Spanish)

Budavari, S., ed. (1996) *The Merck Index*, 12th Ed., Whitehouse Station, NJ, Merck & Co., p. 659

Buller, R.E., Darrow, V., Manetta, A., Porto, M. & DiSaia, P.J. (1992) Conservative surgical management of dysgerminoma concomitant with pregnancy. *Obstet. Gynecol.*, **79**, 887–890

Burden, D.A. & Osheroff, N. (1998) Mechanism of action of eukaryotic topoisomerase II and drugs targeted to the enzyme. *Biochim. biophys. Acta*, **1400**, 139–154

Caldecott, K., Banks, G. & Jeggo, P. (1990) DNA double-strand break repair pathways and cellular tolerance to inhibitors of topoisomerase II. *Cancer Res.*, **50**, 5778–5783

Canadian Pharmaceutical Association (1997) *CPS Compendium of Pharmaceuticals and Specialties*, 32nd Ed., Ottawa, pp. 1697–1699

Caporossi, D., Porfirio, B., Nicoletti, B., Palitti, F., Degrassi, F., De Salvia, R. & Tanzarella, C. (1993) Hypersensitivity of lymphoblastoid lines derived from ataxia telangiectasia patients to the induction of chromosomal aberrations by etoposide (VP-16). *Mutat. Res.*, **290**, 265–272

Capranico, G. & Binaschi, M. (1998) DNA sequence selectivity of topoisomerases and topoisomerase poisons. *Biochim. biophys. Acta*, **1400**, 185–194

Chen, A.Y. & Liu, L.F. (1994) DNA topoisomerases: Essential enzymes and lethal targets. *Ann. Rev. Pharmacol. Toxicol.*, **84**, 191–218

Chen, G.L., Yang, L., Rowe, T.C., Halligan, B.D., Tewey, K.M. & Liu, L.F. (1984) Nonintercalative antitumor drugs interfere with the breakage–reunion reaction of mamalian DNA topoisomerase II. *J. biol. Chem.*, **259**, 13560–13566

Chen, C.-L., Fuscoe, J.C., Liu, Q. & Relling, M.V. (1996a) Etoposide causes illegitimate V(D)J recombination in human lymphoid leukemic cells. *Blood*, **88**, 2210–2218

Chen, C.-L., Fuscoe, J.C., Liu, Q., Pui, C.H., Mahmoud, H.H. & Relling, M.V. (1996b) Relationship between cytotoxicity and site-specific DNA recombination after in vitro exposure of leukemia cells to etoposide. *J. natl Cancer Inst.*, **88**, 1840–1847

Chiron, M., Demur, C., Pierson, V., Jaffrezou, J.-P., Muller, C., Saivin, S., Bordier, C., Bousquet, C., Dastugue, N. & Laurent, G. (1992) Sensitivity of fresh acute myeloid leukemia cells to etoposide: Relationship with cell growth characteristics and DNA single-strand breaks. *Blood*, **80**, 1307–1315

Choo, Y.C., Chan, S.Y.W., Wong, L.C. & Ma, H.K. (1985) Ovarian dysfunction in patients with gestational trophoblastic neoplasia treated with short intensive courses of etoposide (VP-16-213). *Cancer*, **55**, 2348–2352

CIS Information Services (1998) *Worldwide Bulk Drug Users Directory 1997/98 Edition*, Dallas, TX [CD-ROM]

Clark, P.I. & Slevin, M.L. (1987) The clinical pharmacology of etoposide and teniposide. *Clin. Pharmacokinet.*, **12**, 223–252

Clark, P.I., Slevin, M.L., Joel, S.P., Osborne, R.J., Talbot, D.I., Johnson, P.W.M., Reznek, R., Masud, T., Gregory, W. & Wrigley, P.F.M. (1994) A randomized trial of two etoposide schedules in small-cell lung cancer: The influence of pharmacokinetics on efficacy and toxicity. *J. clin. Oncol.*, **12**, 1427–1435

Colombo, T., D'Incalci, M., Donelli, M.G., Bartosek, I., Benfenati, E., Farina, P. & Guaitani, A. (1985) Metabolic studies of a podophyllotoxin derivative (VP16) in the isolated perfused liver. *Xenobiotica*, **15**, 343–350

Colombo, T., Broggini, M., Vaghi, M., Amato, G., Erba, E. & D'Incalci, M. (1986) Comparison between VP 16 and VM 26 in Lewis lung carcinoma of the mouse. *Eur. J. Cancer clin. Oncol.*, **22**, 173–179

Council of Europe (1997) *European Pharmacopoeia*, 3rd Ed., Strasbourg, pp. 833–835

Creaven, P.J. & Allen, L.M. (1975) EPEG, a new antineoplastic epipodophyllotoxin. *Clin. Pharmacol. Ther.*, **18**, 221–226

Curtis, R.E., Boice, J.D., Jr, Stovall, M., Bernstein, L., Greenberg, R.S., Flannery, J.T., Schwartz, A.G., Weyer, P., Moloney, W.C. & Hoover, R.N. (1992) Risks of leukemia after chemotherapy and radiation treatment for breast cancer. *New Engl. J. Med.*, **326**, 1745–1751

Dassonneville, L. & Bailly, C. (1998) [Chromosomal translocations and leukaemias induced by anticarcinogenic drugs that inhibit topoisomerase II.] *Bull. Cancer*, **85**, 254–261 (in French)

DeMarini, D.M., Brock, K.H., Doerr, C.L. & Moore, M.M. (1987) Mutagenicity and clastogenicity of teniposide (VM-26) in L5178Y/TK $^{+/-}$ - 3.7.2C mouse lymphoma cells. *Mutat. Res.*, **187**, 141–149

Detourmignies, L., Castaigne, S., Stoppa, A.M., Harousseau, J.L., Sadoun, A., Janvier, M., Demory, J.L., Sanz, M., Berger, R., Bauters, F., Chomienne, C. & Fenaux, P. (1992) Therapy-related acute promyelocytic leukemia: A report on 16 cases. *J. clin. Oncol.*, **10**, 1430–1435

DeVore, R., Whitlock, J., Hainsworth, J.D. & Johnson, D.H. (1989) Therapy-related acute non-lymphocytic leukemia with monocytic features and rearrangement of chromosome 11q. *Ann. intern. Med.*, **110**, 740–742

Di Leonardo, A., Cavolina, P. & Maddalena, A. (1993) DNA topoisomerase II inhibition and gene amplification in V79/B7 cells. *Mutat. Res.*, **301**, 177–182

D'Incalci, M., Farina, P., Sessa, C., Mangioni, C., Conter, V., Masera, G., Rocchetti, M., Pisoni, M.B., Piazza, E., Beer, M. & Cavalli, F. (1982) Pharmacokinetics of VP16-213 given by different administration methods. *Cancer Chemother. Pharmacol.*, **7**, 141–145

D'Incalci, M., Sessa, C., Rossi, C., Roviaro, G. & Mangioni, C. (1985) Pharmacokinetics of etoposide in gestochoriocarcinoma. *Cancer Treat. Rep.*, **69**, 69–72

D'Incalci, M., Rossi, C., Zucchetti, M., Urso, R., Cavalli, F., Mangioni, C., Willems, Y. & Sessa, C. (1986) Pharmacokinetics of etoposide in patients with abnormal renal and hepatic function. *Cancer Res.*, **46**, 2566–2571

Djabali, M., Selleri, L., Parry, P., Bower, M., Young, B.D. & Evans, G.A. (1992) A trithorax-like gene is interrupted by chromosome 11q23 translocations in acute leukaemias. *Nature Genet.*, **2**, 113-118

Domer, P.H., Head, D.R., Renganathan, N., Raimondi, S.C., Yang, E. & Atlas, M. (1995) Molecular analysis of 13 cases of MLL/11q23 secondary acute leukemia and identification of topoisomerase II consensus-binding sequences near the chromosomal breakpoint of a secondary leukemia with the t(4;11). *Leukemia*, **9**, 1305–1312

Downes, C.S., Mullinger, A.M. & Johnson, R.T. (1991) Inhibitors of DNA topoisomerase II prevent chromatid separation in mammalian cells but do not prevent exit from mitosis. *Proc. natl Acad. Sci. USA*, **88**, 8895–8899

Duffner, P.K., Krischer, J.P., Horowitz, M.E., Cohen, M.E., Burger, P.C., Friedman, H.S., Kun, L.E. & the Pediatric Oncology Group (1998) Second malignancies in young children with primary brain tumors following treatment with prolonged postoperative chemotherapy and delayed irradiation: A Pediatric Oncology Group study. *Ann. Neurol.*, **44**, 313–316

Editions du Vidal (1998) *Vidal 1998*, 74th Ed., Paris, OVP, pp. 672–674, 1953

Edwards, C.M., Glisson, B.S., King, C.K., Smallwood-Kentro, S. & Ross, W.E. (1987) Etoposide-induced DNA cleavage in human leukemia cells. *Cancer Chemother. Pharmacol.*, **20**, 162–168

Epstein, R.J. (1988) Topoisomerases in human disease. *Lancet*, **i**, 521–524

Fantini, C., Vernole, P., Tedeschi, B. & Caporossi, D. (1998) Sister chromatid exchanges and DNA topoisomerase II inhibitors: Effect of low concentrations of etoposide (VP-16) in ataxia telangiectasia lymphoblastoid cell lines. *Mutat. Res.*, **412**, 1–7

Felix, C.A. (1998) Secondary leukemias induced by topoisomerase-targeted drugs. *Biochim. biophys. Acta*, **1400**, 233–255

Felix, C.A., Winick, N.J., Negrini, M., Bowman, W.P., Croce, C.M. & Lange, B.J. (1993) Common region of *ALL*-1 gene disrupted in epipodophyllotoxin-related secondary acute myeloid leukemia. *Cancer Res.*, **53**, 2954–2956

Felix, C.A., Lange, B.J., Hosler, M.R., Fertala, J. & Bjornsti, M.-A. (1995a) Chromosome band 11q23 translocation breakpoints are DNA topoisomerase II cleavage sites. *Cancer Res.*, **55**, 4287–4292

Felix, C.A., Hosler, M.R., Winick, N.J., Masterson, M., Wilson, A.E. & Lange, B.J. (1995b) *ALL-1* gene rearrangements in DNA topoisomerase II inhibitor-related leukemia in children. *Blood*, **85**, 3250–3256

Felix, C.A., Walker, A.H., Lange, B.J., Williams, T.M., Winick, N.J., Cheung, N.K., Lovett, B.D., Nowell, P.C., Blair, I.A. & Rebbeck, T.R. (1998) Association of CYP3A4 genotype with treatment related leukemia. *Proc. natl Acad. Sci. USA*, **95**, 13176–13181

Fenaux, P., Lucidarme, D., Laï, J.L. & Bauters, F. (1989) Favorable cytogenetic abnormalities in secondary leukemia. *Cancer*, **63**, 2505–2508

Ferguson, L.R. (1998) Inhibitors of topoisomerase II enzymes: A unique group of environmental mutagens and carcinogens. *Mutat. Res.*, **400**, 271–278

Ferguson, L.R. & Baguley, B.C. (1994) Topoisomerase II enzymes and mutagenicity. *Environ. mol. Mutag.*, **24**, 245–267

Ferguson, L.R. & Baguley, B.C. (1996) Mutagenicity of anticancer drugs that inhibit topoisomerase enzymes. *Mutat. Res.*, **355**, 91–102

Ferguson, L.R. & Turner, P.M. (1988a) 'Petite' mutagenesis by anticancer drugs in *Saccharomyces cerevisiae*. *Eur. J. Cancer clin. Oncol.*, **24**, 591–596

Ferguson, L.R. & Turner, P.M. (1988b) Mitotic crossing-over by anticancer drugs in *Saccharomyces cerevisiae* strain D5. *Mutat. Res.*, **204**, 239–249

Ferreiro, J.A., Consuegra, S., Sierra, L.M. & Comendador, M.A. (1997) Is the *white-ivory* assay of *Drosophila melanogaster* a useful tool in genetic toxicology? *Environ. mol. Mutag.*, **29**, 406–417

Fleming, R.A., Miller, A.A. & Stewart, C.F. (1989) Etoposide: An update. *Clin. Pharm.*, **8**, 274–293

Frei, H. & Würgler, F.E. (1996) Induction of somatic mutation and recombination by four inhibitors of eukaryotic topoisomerases assayed in the wing spot test of *Drosophila melanogaster*. *Mutagenesis*, **11**, 315–325

Fritsche, M., Haessler, C. & Brandner, G. (1993) Induction of nuclear accumulation of the tumor-suppressor protein p53 by DNA-damaging agents. *Oncogene*, **8**, 307–318

Gantchev, T.G. & Hunting, D.J. (1998) The *ortho*-quinone metabolite of the anticancer drug etoposide (VP-16) is a potent inhibitor of the topoisomerase II/DNA cleavable complex. *Mol. Pharmacol.*, **53**, 422–428

Garland, F.C., Shaw, E., Gorham, E.D., Garland, C.F., White, M.R. & Sinsheimer, P.J. (1990) Incidence of leukemia in occupations with potential electromagnetic field exposure in United States navy personnel. *Am. J. Epidemiol.*, **132**, 293–303

Garriott, M.L., Brunny, J.D., Kindig, D.E., Parton, J.W. & Schwier, L.S. (1995) The in vivo rat micronucleus test: Integration with a 14-day study. *Mutat. Res.*, **342**, 71–76

Gennaro, A.R. (1995) *Remington: The Science and Practice of Pharmacy*, 19th Ed., Easton, PA, Mack Publishing, Vol. II, pp. 1249–1250

Gerres, L., Brämswig, J.H., Schlegel, W., Jürgens, H. & Schellong, G. (1998) The effects of etoposide on testicular function in boys treated for Hodgkin's disease. *Cancer*, **83**, 2217–2222

Gieseler, F., Boege, F., Clark, M. & Meyer, P. (1993) Correlation between the DNA-binding affinity of topoisomerase inhibiting drugs and their capacity to induce hematopoetic cell differentiation. *Toxicol. Lett.*, **67**, 331–340

Gill Super, H.J., McCabe, N.R., Thirman, M.J., Larson, R.A., Le Beau, M.M., Pedersen-Bjergaard, J., Philip, P., Diaz, M.O. & Rowley, J.D. (1993) Rearrangements of the *MLL* gene in therapy-related acute myeloid leukemia patients previously treated with agents targeting DNA-topoisomerase II. *Blood*, **82**, 3705–3711

Goodman, G.E., Crowley, J.J., Blasko, J.C., Livingston, R.B., Beck, T.M., Demattia, M.D. & Bukowski, R.M. (1990) Treatment of limited small-cell lung cancer with etoposide and cisplatin alternating with vincristine, doxorubicin, and cyclophosphamide versus concurrent etoposide, vincristine, doxorubicin, and cyclophosphamide and chest radiotherapy: A Southwest Oncology Group Study. *J. clin. Oncol.*, **8**, 39–47

Gu, Y., Nakamura, T., Alder, H., Prasad, R., Canaani, O., Cimino, G., Croce, C.M. & Canaani, E. (1992) The t(4;11) chromosome translocation of human acute leukemias fuses the *ALL*-1 gene, related to *Drosophila trithorax*, to the *AF-4* gene. *Cell*, **71**, 701–708

Gupta, R. (1990) Tests for the genotoxicity of m-AMSA, etoposide, teniposide and ellipticine in *Neurospora crassa*. *Mutat. Res.*, **240**, 47–58

Gupta, R.S., Bromke, A., Bryant, D.W., Gupta, R., Singh, B. & McCalla, D.R. (1987) Etoposide (VP16) and teniposide (VM26): Novel anticancer drugs, strongly mutagenic in mammalian but not prokaryotic test systems. *Mutagenesis*, **2**, 179–186

Haim, N., Nemec, J., Roman, J. & Sinha, B.K. (1987) Peroxidase-catalyzed metabolism of etoposide (VP-16-213) and covalent binding of reactive intermediates to cellular macromolecules. *Cancer Res.*, **47**, 5835–5840

Hainsworth, J.D. & Greco, F.A. (1995) Etoposide: Twenty years later. *Ann. Oncol.*, **6**, 325–341

Hakovirta, H., Parvinen, M. & Lähdetie, J. (1993) Effects of etoposide on stage-specific DNA synthesis during rat spermatogenesis. *Mutat. Res.*, **301**, 189–193

Hande, K.R., Wedlund, P.J., Noone, R.M., Wilkinson, G.R., Greco, F.A. & Wolff, S.N. (1984) Pharmacokinetics of high-dose etoposide (VP-16-213) administered to cancer patients. *Cancer Res.*, **44**, 379–382

Hande, K., Anthony, L., Hamilton, R., Bennett, R., Sweetman, B. & Branch, R. (1988) Identification of etoposide glucuronide as a major metabolite of etoposide in the rat and rabbit. *Cancer Res.*, **48**, 1829–1834

Hande, K.R., Wolff, S.N., Greco, F.A., Hainsworth, J.D., Reed, G. & Johnson, D.H. (1990) Etoposide kinetics in patients with obstructive jaundice. *J. clin. Oncol.*, **8**, 1101–1107

Hande, K.R., Krozely, M.G., Greco, F.A., Hainsworth, J.D. & Johnson, D.H. (1993) Bioavailability of low-dose oral etoposide. *J. clin. Oncol.*, **11**, 374–377

Harvey, V.J., Slevin, M.L., Joel, S.P., Smythe, M.M., Johnston, A. & Wrigley, P.F.M. (1985) Variable bioavailability following repeated oral doses of etoposide. *Eur. J. Cancer clin. Oncol.*, **21**, 1315–1319

Harvey, V.J., Slevin, M.L., Joel, S.P., Johnston, A. & Wrigley, P.F.M. (1986) The effect of dose on the bioavailability of oral etoposide. *Cancer Chemother. Pharmacol.*, **16**, 178–181

Haupt, R., Comelli, A., Rosanda, C., Sessarego, M. & De Bernardi, B. (1993) Acute myeloid leukemia after single-agent treatment with etoposide for Langerhans' cell histiocytosis of bone. *Am. J. pediatr. Hematol. Oncol.*, **15**, 255–257

Haupt, R., Fears, T.R., Rosso, P., Colella, R., Loiacono, G., de Terlizzi, M., Mancini, A., Comelli, A., Indolfi, P., Donfrancesco, A., Operamolla, P., Grazia, G., Ceci, A. & Tucker, M.A. (1994) Increased risk of secondary leukemia after single-agent treatment with etoposide for Langerhans' cell histiocytosis. *Pediatr. Hematol. Oncol.*, **11**, 499–507

Haupt, R., Fears, T.R., Heise, A., Gadner, H., Loiacono, G., De Terlizzi, M. & Tucker, M.A. (1997) Risk of secondary leukemia after treatment with etoposide (VP-16) for Langerhans' cell histiocytosis in Italian and Austrian–German populations. *Int. J. Cancer*, **71**, 9–13

Hermine, T., Jones, N.J. & Parry, J.M. (1997) Comparative induction of micronuclei in repair-deficient and -proficient Chinese hamster cell lines following clastogen or aneugen exposures. *Mutat. Res.*, **392**, 151–163

Heyn, R., Khan, F., Ensign, L.G., Donaldson, S.S., Ruymann, F., Smith, M.A., Vietti, T. & Maurer, H.M. (1994) Acute myeloid leukemia in patients treated for rhabdomyosarcoma with cyclophosphamide and low-dose etoposide on Intergroup Rhabdomyosarcoma Study III: An interim report. *Med. Pediatr. Oncol.*, **23**, 99–106

Holthuis, J.J.M. (1988) Etoposide and teniposide. Bioanalysis, metabolism and clinical pharmacokinetics. *Pharm. Weekbl. Sci.*, **10**, 101–116

Holthuis, J.J.M., Postmus, P.E., Van Oort, W.J., Hulshoff, B., Verleun, H., Sleijfer, D.T. & Mulder, N.H. (1986) Pharmacokinetics of high dose etoposide (VP 16-213). *Eur. J. Cancer clin. Oncol.*, **22**, 1149–1155

Holthuis, J.J.M., Kettenes-van den Bosch, J.J. & Bult, A. (1989) Etoposide. In: Florey, K., ed., *Analytical Profiles of Drug Substances*, New York, Academic Press, Vol. 18, pp. 121–151

Horibe, K., Matsushita, T., Numata, S.-I., Miyajima, Y., Katayama, I., Kitabayashi, T., Yanai, M., Sekiguchi, N. & Egi, S. (1993) Acute promyelocytic leukemia with t(15;17) abnormality after chemotherapy containing etoposide for Langerhans cell histiocytosis. *Cancer*, **72**, 3723–3726

Hudson, M.M., Weinstein, H.J., Donaldson, S.S., Greenwald, C., Kun, L., Tarbell, N.J., Humphrey, W.A., Rupp, C., Marina, N.M., Wilimas, J. & Link, M.P. (1993) Acute hypersensitivity reactions to etoposide in a VEPA regimen for Hodgkin's disease. *J. clin. Oncol.*, **11**, 1080–1084

Hunger, S.P., Sklar, J. & Link, M.P. (1992) Acute lymphoblastic leukemia occurring as a second malignant neoplasm in childhood: Report of three cases and review of the literature. *J. clin. Oncol.*, **10**, 156–163

Hunger, S.P., Tkachuk, D.C., Amylon, M.D., Link, M.P., Carroll, A.J., Welborn, J.L., Willman, C.L. & Cleary, M.L. (1993) *HRX* involvement in de novo and secondary leukemias with diverse chromosome 11q23 abnormalities. *Blood*, **81**, 3197–3203

Hussey, D.J., Nicola, M., Moore, S., Peters, G.B. & Dobrovic, A. (1999) The (4;11)(q21;p15) translocation fuses the *NUP98* and *RAP1GDS1* genes and is recurrent in T-cell acute lymphocytic leukemia. *Blood*, **94**, 2072–2079

IARC (1987) *IARC Monographs on the Evaluation of Carcinogenic Risks to Humans*, Suppl. 7, *Overall Evaluations of Carcinogenicity: An Updating of* IARC Monographs *Volumes 1–42*, Lyon, IARC*Press*

Ida, K., Kitabayashi, I., Taki, T., Taniwaki, M., Noro, K., Yamamoto, M., Ohki, M. & Hayashi, Y. (1997) Adenoviral E1A-associated protein p300 is involved in acute myeloid leukemia with t(11;22)(q23;q13). *Blood*, **90**, 4699–4704

Igwemezie, L.N., Kaul, S. & Barbhaiya, R.H. (1995) Assessment of toxicokinetics and toxicodynamics following intravenous administration of etoposide phosphate in beagle dogs. *Pharm. Res.*, **12**, 117–123

Imbert, T.F. (1998) Discovery of podophyllotoxins. *Biochimie*, **80**, 207–222

Jackson, M.A., Stack, H.F. & Waters, M.D. (1996) Genetic activity profiles of anticancer drugs. *Mutat. Res.*, **355**, 171–208

Jeggo, P.A., Caldecott, K., Pidsley, S. & Banks, G.R. (1989) Sensitivity of Chinese hamster ovary mutants defective in DNA double strand break repair to topoisomerase II inhibitors. *Cancer Res.*, **49**, 7057–7063

Joel, S. (1996) The clinical pharmacology of etoposide. *Cancer Treat. Rev.*, **22**, 179–221

Joel, S.P., Clark, P.I. & Slevin, M.L. (1995a) Stability of the i.v. and oral formulations of etoposide in solution. *Cancer Chemother. Pharmacol.*, **37**, 117–124

Joel, S.P., Hall, M., Gaver, R.C. & Slevin, M.L. (1995b) Complete recovery of radioactivity after administration of ^{14}C-etoposide in man (Abstract). *Proc. ann. Meet. Am. Soc. clin. Oncol.*, **14**, 1

Joel, S.P., Shah, R., Clark, P.I. & Slevin, M.L. (1996) Predicting etoposide toxicity: Relationship to organ function and protein binding. *J. clin. Oncol.*, **14**, 257–267

Joel, S., O'Byrne, K., Penson, R., Papamichael, D., Higgins, A., Robertshaw, H., Rudd, R., Talbot, D. & Slevin, M. (1998) A randomised, concentration-controlled, comparison of standard (5-day) vs. prolonged (15-day) infusions of etoposide phosphate in small-cell lung cancer. *Ann. Oncol.*, **9**, 1205–1211

Johnson, D.H., Hainsworth, J.D., Hande, K.R. & Greco, F.A. (1991) Current status of etoposide in the management of small cell lung cancer. *Cancer*, **67**, 231–244

Johnston, P.J., Stoppard, E. & Bryant, P.E. (1997) Induction and distribution of damage in CHO-K1 and the X-ray-sensitive hamster cell line *xrs5*, measured by the cytochalasin-B-cytokinesis block micronucleus assay. *Mutat. Res.*, **385**, 1–12

Kallio, M. & Lähdetie, J. (1993) Analysis of micronuclei induced in mouse early spermatids by mitomycin C, vinblastine sulfate or etoposide using fluorescence *in situ* hybridization. *Mutagenesis*, **8**, 561–567

Kallio, M. & Lähdetie, J. (1996) Fragmentation of centromeric DNA and prevention of homologous chromosome separation in male mouse meiosis *in vivo* by the topoisomerase II inhibitor etoposide. *Mutagenesis*, **11**, 435–443

Kallio, M. & Lähdetie, J. (1997) Effects of the DNA topoisomerase II inhibitor merbarone in male mouse meiotic divisions in vivo: Cell cycle arrest and induction of aneuploidy. *Environ. mol. Mutag.*, **29**, 16–27

Kalyanaraman, B., Nemec, J. & Sinha, B.K. (1989) Characterization of free radicals produced during oxidation of etoposide (VP-16) and its catechol and quinone derivatives. An ESR Study. *Biochemistry*, **28**, 4839–4846

Karnaoukhova, L., Moffat, J., Martins, H. & Glickman, B. (1997) Mutation frequency and spectrum in lymphocytes of small cell lung cancer patients receiving etoposide chemotherapy. *Cancer Res.*, **57**, 4393–4407

Kaul, S., Igwemezie, L.N., Stewart, D.J., Fields, S.Z., Kosty, M., Levithan, N., Bukowski, R., Gandara, D., Goss, G., O'Dwyer, P., Schacter, L.P. & Barbhaiya, R.H. (1995) Pharmacokinetics and bioequivalence of etoposide following intravenous administration of etoposide phosphate and etoposide in patients with solid tumors. *J. clin. Oncol.*, **13**, 2835–2841

Kawashiro, T., Yamashita, K., Zhao, X.-J., Koyama, E., Tani, M., Chiba, K. & Ishizaki, T. (1998) A study on the metabolism of etoposide and possible interactions with antitumor or supporting agents by human liver microsomes. *J. Pharmacol. exp. Ther.*, **286**, 1294–1300

Keller-Juslén, C., Kuhn, M., Stahelin, H. & von Wartburg, A. (1971) Synthesis and antimitotic activity of glycosidic lignan derivatives related to podophyllotoxin. *J. med. Chem.*, **14**, 936–940

Kellie, S.J., Crist, W.M., Pui, C.-H., Crone, M.E., Fairclough, D.L., Rodman, J.H. & Rivera, G.K. (1991) Hypersensitivity reactions to epipodophyllotoxins in children with acute lymphoblastic leukemia. *Cancer*, **67**, 1070–1075

Kerrigan, D., Pommier, Y. & Kohn, K.W. (1987) Protein-linked DNA strand breaks produced by etoposide and teniposide in mouse L1210 and human VA-13 and HT-29 cell lines: Relationship to cytotoxicity. *Natl Cancer Inst. Monogr.*, **4**, 117–121

Knudson, A.G. (1992) Stem cell regulation, tissue ontogeny and oncogenic events. *Sem. Cancer Biol.*, **3**, 99–106

Kobayashi, H., Arai, Y., Hosoda, F., Maseki, N., Hayashi, Y., Eguchi, H., Ohki, M. & Kaneko, Y. (1997) Inversion of chromosome 11, inv(11)(p15q22), as a recurring chromosomal aberration associated with de novo and secondary myeloid malignancies: Identification of a P1 clone spanning the 11q22 breakpoint. *Genes Chromosomes Cancer*, **19**, 150–155

Kollmannsberger, C., Beyer, J., Droz, J.-P., Harstrick, A., Hartmann, J.T., Biron, P., Fléchon, A., Schöffski, P., Kuczyk, M., Schmoll, H.-J., Kanz, L. & Bokemeyer, C. (1998) Secondary leukemia following high cumulative doses of etoposide in patients treated for advanced germ cell tumors. *J. clin. Oncol.*, **16**, 3386–3391

Kusaka, M., Tanaka, T. & Fujimoto, S. (1994) Local etoposide injection for treatment of tubal pregnancy with cardiac activity. *Int. J. Fertil. menopausal Stud.*, **39**, 11–13

Kushner, B.H., Heller, G., Cheung, N.K., Wollner, N., Kramer, K., Bajorin, D., Polyak, T. & Meyers, P.A. (1998a) High risk of leukemia after short-term dose-intensive chemotherapy in young patients with solid tumors. *J. clin. Oncol.*, **16**, 3016–3020

Kushner, B.H., Cheung, N.K., Kramer, K., Heller, G. & Jhanwar, S.C. (1998b) Neuroblastoma and treatment-related myelodysplasia/leukemia: The Memoral Sloan-Kettering experience and a literature review. *J. clin. Oncol.*, **16**, 3880–3889

Lähdetie, J., Keiski, A., Suutari, A. & Toppari, J. (1994) Etoposide (VP-16) is a potent inducer of micronuclei in male rat meiosis: Spermatid micronucleus test and DNA flow cytometry after etoposide treatment. *Environ. mol. Mutag.*, **24**, 192–202

Lauricella, M., Giuliano, M., Emanuele, S., Vento, R. & Tesoriere, G. (1998) Apoptotic effects of different drugs on cultured retinoblastoma Y79 cells. *Tumor Biol.*, **19**, 356–363

Laver, J.H., Yusuf, U., Cantu, E.S., Barredo, J.C., Holt, L.B. & Abboud, M.R. (1997) Transient therapy-related myelodysplastic syndrome associated with monosomy 7 and 11q23 translocation. *Leukemia*, **11**, 448–455

Lebailly, P., Vigreux, C., Godard, T., Sichel, F., Bar, E., LeTalaër, J.Y., Henry-Amar, M. & Gauduchon, P. (1997) Assessment of DNA damage induced in vitro by etoposide and two fungicides (carbendazim and chlorothalonil) in human lymphocytes with the comet assay. *Mutat. Res.*, **375**, 205–217

Lee, J.S., Takahashi, T., Hagiwara, A., Yoneyama, C., Itoh, M., Sasabe, T., Muranishi, S. & Tashima, S. (1995) Safety and efficacy of intraperitoneal injection of etoposide in oil suspension in mice with peritoneal carcinomatosis. *Cancer Chemother. Pharmacol.*, **36**, 211–216

van Leeuwen, F.E. (1997) Second cancers. In: DeVita, V.T., Jr, Hellman, S. & Rosenberg, S.A., eds, *Cancer. Principles & Practice of Oncology*, 5th Ed., New York, Lippincott-Raven, Vol. 2, pp. 2773–2796

van Leeuwen, F.E., Stiggelbout, A.M., Delamarre, J.F.M. & Somers, R. (1994) Second cancer risk following testicular cancer. *Adv. Biosci.*, **91**, 359–369

Liliemark, E.K., Liliemark, J., Pettersson, B., Gruber, A., Bjorkholm, M. & Peterson, C. (1993) In vivo accumulation of etoposide in peripheral leukemic cells in patients treated for acute myeloblastic leukemia; relation to plasma concentrations and protein binding. *Leuk. Lymphoma*, **10**, 323–328

Liliemark, E., Söderhäll, S., Sirzea, F., Gruber, A., Ösby, E., Björkholm, M., Zhou, R., Peterson, C. & Liliemark, J. (1996) Higher in vivo protein binding of etoposide in children compared with adult cancer patients. *Cancer Lett.*, **106**, 97–100

Liu, F.L. & Wang, J.C. (1991) Biochemistry of DNA topoisomerase and their poisons. In: Potmesil, M. & Kohn, K., eds, *DNA Topoisomerases in Cancer*, New York, Oxford University Press, pp. 13–22

Liu, B., Earl, H.M., Poole, C.J., Dunn, J. & Kerr, D.J. (1995) Etoposide protein binding in cancer patients. *Cancer Chemother. Pharmacol.*, **36**, 506–512

Long, B.H., Musial, S.T. & Brattain, M.G. (1985) Single- and double-strand DNA breakage and repair in human lung adenocarcinoma cells exposed to etoposide and teniposide. *Cancer Res.*, **45**, 3106–3112

Long, B.H., Musial, S.T. & Brattain, M.G. (1986) DNA breakage in human lung carcinoma cells and nuclei that are naturally sensitive or resistant to etoposide and teniposide. *Cancer Res.*, **46**, 3809–3816

Lopez-Andreu, J.A., Ferrís, J., Verdeguer, A., Esquembre, C., Senent, M.L. & Castel, V. (1994) Secondary acute promyelocytic leukemia in a child treated with epipodophyllotoxins. *Am. J. Pediatr. Hematol./Oncol.*, **16**, 384–386

Lovett, B.D., Blair, I.A., Pang, S., Burden, A., Megonigal, M.D., Rappaport, E.F., Bjornsti, M.-A., Lange, B.J., Osheroff, N. & Felix, C.A. (1999) Etoposide metabolites enhance DNA topoisomerase II cleavage proximal to leukemia-associated *MLL* translocation breakpoints (Abstract No. 4506). *Proc. Am. Assoc. Cancer Res.*, **40**, 683

Lum, B.L., Kaubisch, S., Yahanda, A.M., Adler, K.M., Jew, L., Ehsan, M.N., Brophy, N.A., Halsey, J., Gosland, M.P. & Sikic, B.I. (1992) Alteration of etoposide pharmacokinetics and pharmacodynamics by cyclosporine in a phase I trial to modulate multidrug resistance. *J. clin. Oncol.*, **10**, 1635–1642

van Maanen, J.M.S, van Oort, W.J. & Pinedo, H.M. (1982) *In vitro* and *in vivo* metabolism of VP 16-213 in the rat. *Eur. J. Cancer clin. Oncol.*, **18**, 885–890

van Maanen, J.M.S., De Ruiter, C., Kootstra, P.R., de Vries, J. & Pinedo, H.M. (1986) Free radical formation from the antineoplastic agent VP 16-213. *Free Radic. Res. Commun.*, **1**, 263–272

van Maanen, J.M.S., de Vries, J., Pappie, D., van den Akker, E., Lafleur, V.M., Retèl, J., van der Greef, J. & Pinedo, H.M. (1987) Cytochrome P-450-mediated *O*-demethylation: A route in the metabolic activation of etoposide (VP-16-213). *Cancer Res.*, **47**, 4658–4662

van Maanen, J.M.S., Lafleur, M.V., Mans, D.R., van den Akker, E., De Ruiter, C., Kootstra, P.R., Pappie, D., de-Vries, J., Retel, J. & Pinedo, H.M. (1988) Effects of the ortho-quinone and catechol of the antitumor drug VP-16-213 on the biological activity of single-stranded and double-stranded phi X174 DNA. *Biochem. Pharmacol.*, **37**, 3579–3589

MacFarlane, M., Jones, N.A., Dive, C. & Cohen, G.M. (1996) DNA-damaging agents induce both p53-dependent and p53-independent apoptosis in immature thymocytes. *Mol. Pharmacol.*, **50**, 900–911

Mahgoub, N., Taylor,, B.R., Le Beau, M.M., Gratiot, M., Carlson, K.M., Atwater, S.K., Jacks, T. & Shannon, K.M. (1999) Myeloid malignancies induced by alkylating agents in *Nf1* mice. *Blood*, **93**, 3617–3623

Mans, D.R.A., Retèl, J., van Maanen, J.M.S., Lafleur, M.V.M., van Schaik, M.A., Pinedo, H.M. & Lankelma, J. (1990) Role of the semi-quinone free radical of the anti-tumour agent etoposide (VP-16-213) in the inactivation of single- and double-stranded ΦX174 DNA. *Br. J. Cancer*, **62**, 54–60

Maraschin, J., Dutrillaux, B. & Aurias, A. (1990) Chromosome aberrations induced by etoposide (VP-16) are not random. *Int. J. Cancer*, **46**, 808–812

Markovits, J., Pommier, Y., Kerrigan, D., Covey, J.M., Tilchen, E.J. & Kohn, K.W. (1987) Topoisomerase II-mediated DNA breaks and cytotoxicity in relation to cell proliferation and the cell cycle in NIH 3T3 fibroblasts and L1210 leukemia cells. *Cancer Res.*, **47**, 2050–2055

Marks, D.I. & Fox, R.M. (1991) DNA damage, poly (ADP-ribosyl)ation and apoptotic cell death as a potential common pathway of cytotoxic drug action. *Biochem. Pharmacol.*, **42**, 1859–1867

Matney, T.S., Nguyen, T.V., Connor, T.H., Dana, W.J. & Theiss, J.C. (1985) Genotoxic classification of anticancer drugs. *Teratog. Carcinog. Mutag.*, **5**, 319–328

Matsui, H., Seki, K., Sekiya, S. & Takamizawa, H. (1997) Reproductive status in GTD treated with etoposide. *J. reprod. Med.*, **42**, 104–110

McCabe, N.R., Burnett, R.C., Gill, H.J., Thirman, M.J., Mbangkollo, D., Kipiniak, M., van Melle, E., Ziemin-van der Poel, S., Rowley, J.D. & Diaz, M.O. (1992) Cloning of cDNAs of the *MLL* gene that detect DNA rearrangements and altered RNA transcripts on human leukemic cells with 11q23 translocations. *Proc. natl Acad. Sci. USA*, **89**, 11794–11798

Megonigal, M.D., Rappaport, E.F., Jones, D.H., Kim, C.S., Nowell, P.C., Lange, B.J. & Felix, C.A. (1997) Panhandle PCR strategy to amplify *MLL* genomic breakpoints in treatment-related leukemias. *Proc. natl Acad. Sci. USA*, **94**, 11583–11588

Minami, H., Shimokata, K., Saka, H., Saito, H., Ando, Y., Senda, K., Nomura, F. & Sakai, S. (1993) Phase I clinical and pharmacokinetic study of a 14-day infusion of etoposide in patients with lung cancer. *J. clin. Oncol.*, **11**, 1602–1608

Minami, H., Ando, Y., Sakai, S. & Shimokata, K. (1995) Clinical and pharmacologic analysis of hyperfractionated daily oral etoposide. *J. clin. Oncol.*, **13**, 191–199

Mirkes, P.E. & Zwelling, L.A. (1990) Embryotoxicity of the intercalating agents m-AMSA and o-AMSA and the epipodophyllotoxin VP-15 in postimplantation rat embryos in vitro. *Teratology*, **41**, 679–688

Mizumoto, K., Rothman, R.J. & Farber, J.L. (1994) Programmed cell death (apoptosis) of mouse fibroblasts is induced by the topoisomerase II inhibitor etoposide. *Mol. Pharmacol.*, **46**, 890–895

Mosesso, P., Darroudi, F., van den Berg, M., Vermeulen, S., Palitti, F. & Natarajan, A.T. (1998) Induction of chromosomal aberrations (unstable and stable) by inhibitors of topoisomerase II, m-AMSA and VP16, using conventional Giemsa staining and chromosome painting techniques. *Mutagenesis*, **13**, 39–43

Mross, K., Bewermeier, P., Krüger, W., Stockschläder, M., Zander, A. & Hossfeld, D.K. (1994) Pharmacokinetics of undiluted or diluted high-dose etoposide with or without busulfan administered to patients with hematologic malignancies. *J. clin. Oncol.*, **12**, 1468–1474

Murphy, C.P., Harden, E.A. & Herzig, R.H. (1993) Dose-related cutaneous toxicities with etoposide. *Cancer*, **71**, 3153–3155

Murray, N.A, Acolet, D., Deane, M., Price, J. & Roberts, I.A.G. (1994) Fetal marrow suppression after maternal chemotherapy for leukaemia. *Arch. Dis. Child.*, **71**, F209–F210

Nagao, T., Yoshimura, S., Saito, Y. & Imai, K. (1999) Developmental toxicity of the topoisomerase inhibitor, etoposide, in rabbits after intravenous administration. *Teratog. Carcinog. Mutag.*, **19**, 233–241

Nakajima, M., Kashiwagi, K., Ohta, J., Furukawa, S., Hayashi, K., Kawashima, T. & Hayashi, Y. (1994) Etoposide induces programmed death in neurons cultured from the fetal rat central nervous system. *Brain Res.*, **641**, 350–352

Nakamura, T., Largaespada, D.A., Lee, M.P., Johnson, L.A., Ohyashiki, K., Toyama, K., Chen, S.G., Willman, C.L., Chen, I.-M., Feinberg, A.P., Jenkins, N.A., Copeland, N.G. & Shaughnessy, J.D., Jr (1996) Fusion of the nucleoporin gene *NUP98* to *HOXA9* by the chromosome translocation t(7;11)(p15;p15) in human myeloid leukaemia. *Nature Genet.*, **12**, 154–158

Nakamura, T., Yamazaki, Y., Hatano, Y. & Miura, I. (1999) *NUP98* is fused to *PMX1* homeobox gene in human acute myelogenous leukemia with chromosome translocation t(1;11)(q23;p15). *Blood*, **94**, 741–747

Nakanomyo, H., Hiraoka, M. & Shiraya, M. (1986) [Mutagenicity tests of etoposide and teniposide.] *J. toxicol. Sci.*, **11**, 301–310 (in Japanese)

Nguyen, L., Chatelut, E., Chevreau, C., Tranchand, B., Lochon, I., Bachaud, J.-M., Pujol, A., Houin, G., Bugat, R. & Canal, P. (1998) Population pharmacokinetics of total and unbound etoposide. *Cancer Chemother. Pharmacol.*, **41**, 125–132

Nichols, C.R. (1992) The role of etoposide therapy in germ cell cancer. *Semin. Oncol.*, **19**, 72–77

Nichols, C.R., Roth, B.J., Heerema, N., Griep, J. & Tricot, G. (1990) Hematologic neoplasia associated with primary mediastinal germ-cell tumors. *New Engl. J. Med.*, **322**, 1425–1429

Nichols, C.R., Breeden, E.S., Loehrer, P.J., Williams, S.D. & Einhorn, L.H. (1993) Secondary leukemia associated with a conventional dose of etoposide: Review of serial germ cell tumor protocols. *J. natl Cancer Inst.*, **85**, 36–40

Noviello, E., Aluigi, M.-G., Cimoli, G., Rovini, E., Mazzoni, A., Parodi, S., De Sessa, F. & Russo, P. (1994) Sister-chromatid exchanges, chromosomal aberrations and cytotoxicity produced by topoisomerase II-targeted drugs in sensitive (A2780) and resistant (A2780-DX3) human ovarian cancer cells: Correlations with the formation of DNA double-strand breaks. *Mutat. Res.*, **311**, 21–29

Nucifora, G. & Rowley, J.D. (1995) AML1 and the 8;21 and 3;21 translocations in acute and chronic myeloid leukemia. *Blood*, **86**, 1–14

Nutter, L.M., Ngo, E.O. & Abul-Hajj, Y.J. (1991) Characterization of DNA damage induced by 3,4-estrone-o-quinone in human cells. *J. biol. Chem.*, **266**, 16380–16386

Nyce, J. (1989) Drug-induced DNA hypermethylation and drug resistance in human tumors. *Cancer Res.*, **49**, 5829–5836

O'Dwyer, P.J. & Weiss, R.B. (1984) Hypersensitivity reactions induced by etoposide. *Cancer Treat. Rep.*, **68**, 959–961

Okada, T., Katano, H., Tsutsumi, H., Kumakawa, T., Sawabe, M., Arai, T., Mori, S. & Mori, M. (1998) Body-cavity-based lymphoma in an elderly AIDS-unrelated male. *Int. J. Hematol.*, **67**, 417–422

Olive, P.L. & Banáth, J.P. (1993) Detection of DNA double-strand breaks through the cell cycle after exposure to X-rays, bleomycin, etoposide and ^{125}IdUrd. *Int J. Radiat. Biol.*, **64**, 349–358

Oliver, R.T.D., Ong, J.Y.H., Raja, M.A., Sperandio, P., Gibbons, B. & Walker, M. (1991) Secondary pre-leukaemia and etoposide (Letter to the Editor). *Lancet*, **338**, 1269–1270

O'Reilly, S.E., Klimo, P. & Connors, J.M. (1991) The evolving role of etoposide in the management of lymphomas and Hodgkin's disease. *Cancer*, **67**, 271–280

Osanto, S., Thijssen, J.C., Woldering, V.M., van Rijn, J.L., Natarajan, A.T. & Tates, A.D. (1991) Increased frequency of chromosomal damage in peripheral blood lymphocytes up to nine years following curative chemotherapy of patients with testicular carcinoma. *Environ. mol. Mutag.*, **17**, 71–78

Osheroff, N. (1989) Effect of antineoplastic agents on the DNA cleavage/religation reaction of eukaryotic topoisomerase II: Inhibition of DNA religation by etoposide. *Biochemistry*, **28**, 6157–6160

Osheroff, N., Robinson, M.J. & Zechiedrich, E.L. (1991) Mechanism of the topoisomerase II mediated DNA cleavage–religation reaction: Inhibition of DNA religation by antineoplastic drugs. In: Potmesil, M. & Kohn, K., eds, *DNA Topoisomerases in Cancer*, New York, Oxford University Press, pp. 230–239

Ozols, R.F., Ihde, D.C., Linehan, W.M., Jacob, J., Ostchega, Y. & Young, R.C. (1988) A randomized trial of standard chemotherapy vs a high-dose chemotherapy regimen in the treatment of poor prognosis nonseminomatous germ-cell tumors. *J. clin. Oncol.*, **6**, 1031–1040

Pandita, T.K. & Hittelman, W.N. (1992) Initial chromosome damage but not DNA damage is greater in ataxia telangiectasia cells. *Radiat. Res.*, **130**, 94–103

Parkin, D.M., Whelan, S.L., Ferlay, J., Raymond, L. & Young, J., eds (1997) *Cancer Incidence in Five Continents (Volume VII)* (IARC Scientific Publications No. 143), Lyon, IARC*Press*

Pedersen-Bjergaard, J. (1992) Radiotherapy- and chemotherapy-induced myelodysplasia and acute myeloid leukemia. A review. *Leuk. Res.*, **16**, 61–65

Pedersen-Bjergaard, J. & Philip, P. (1991) Balanced translocations involving chromosome bands 11q23 and 21q22 are highly characteristic of myelodysplasia and leukemia following therapy with cytostatic agents targeting at DNA-topoisomerase II. *Blood*, **78**, 1147–1148

Pedersen-Bjergaard, J. & Rowley, J.D. (1994) The balanced and the unbalanced chromosome aberrations of acute myeloid leukemia may develop in different ways and may contribute differently to malignant transformation. *Blood*, **83**, 2780–2786

Pedersen-Bjergaard, J., Daugaard, G., Hansen, S.W., Philip, P., Larsen, S.O. & Rorth, M. (1991) Increased risk of myelodysplasia and leukaemia after etoposide, cisplatin, and bleomycin for germ-cell tumours. *Lancet*, **338**, 359–363

Pedersen-Bjergaard, J., Pedersen, M., Roulston, D. & Philip, P. (1995) Different genetic pathways in leukemogenesis for patients presenting with therapy-related myelodysplasia and therapy-related acute myeloid leukaemia. *Blood*, **86**, 3542–3552

Pedersen-Bjergaard, J., Brøndum-Nielsen, K., Karle, H. & Johansson, B. (1997) Chemotherapy-related—and late occurring—Philadelphia chromosome in AML, ALL and CML. Similar events related to treatment with DNA topoisomerase II inhibitors? *Leukemia*, **11**, 1571–1574

Pflüger, K.H., Hahn, M., Holz, J.-B., Schmidt, L., Köhl, P., Fritsch, H.-W., Jungclas, H. & Havemann, K. (1993) Pharmacokinetics of etoposide: Correlation of pharmacokinetic parameters with clinical conditions. *Cancer Chemother. Pharmacol.*, **31**, 350–356

Pommier, Y. (1993) DNA topoisomerase I and II in cancer chemotherapy: Update and perspectives. *Cancer Chemother. Pharmacol.*, **32**, 103–108

Pommier, Y., Kerrigan, D., Covey, J.M., Kao-Shan, C.-S. & Whang-Peng, J. (1988) Sister chromatid exchanges, chromosomal aberrations, and cytotoxicity produced by antitumor topoisomerase II inhibitors in sensitive (DC3F) and resistant (DC3F/9-OHE) Chinese hamster cells. *Cancer Res.*, **48**, 512–516

Pommier, Y., Capranico, G., Orr, A. & Kohn, K.W. (1991) Local base sequence preferences for DNA cleavage by mammalian topoisomerase II in the presence of amsacrine or teniposide. *Nucleic Acids Res.*, **19**, 5973–5980

Postmus, P.E., Holthuis, J.J., Haaxma-Reiche, H., Mulder, N.H., Vencken, L.M., van Oort, W.J., Sleijfer, D.T. & Sluiter, H.J. (1984a) Penetration of VP 16-213 into cerebrospinal fluid after high-dose intravenous administration. *J. clin. Oncol.*, **2**, 215–220

Postmus, P.E., Mulder, N.H., Sleijfer, D.T., Meinesz, A.F., Vriesendorp, R. & de Vries, E.G. (1984b) High-dose etoposide for refractory malignancies: A phase I study. *Cancer Treat. Rep.*, **68**, 1471–1474

Pui, C.-H., Hancock, M.L., Raimondi, S.C., Head, D.R., Thompson, E., Wilimas, J., Kun, L.E., Bowman, L.C., Crist, W.M. & Pratt, C.B. (1990) Myeloid neoplasia in children treated for solid tumours. *Lancet*, **336**, 417–421

Pui, C.-H., Ribeiro, R.C., Hancock, M.L., Rivera, G.K., Evans, W.E., Raimondi, S.C., Head, D.R., Behm, F.G., Mahmoud, M.H., Sandlund, J.T. & Crist, W.M. (1991) Acute myeloid leukemia in children treated with epipodophyllotoxins for acute lymphoblastic leukemia. *New Engl. J. Med.*, **325**, 1682–1687

Quesnel, B., Kantarjian, H., Pedersen-Bjergaard, J., Brault, P., Estey, E., Lai, J.L., Tilly, H., Stoppa, A.M., Archimbaud, E., Harousseau, J.L., Bauters, F. & Fenaux, P. (1993) Therapy-related acute myeloid leukemia with t(8;21), inv(16), and t(8;16): A report on 25 cases and review of the literature. *J. clin. Oncol.*, **11**, 2370–2379

Radu, A., Moore, M.S. & Blobel, G. (1995) The peptide repeat domain of nucleoporin Nup98 functions as a docking site in transport across the nuclear pore complex. *Cell*, **81**, 215–222

Raffles, A., Williams, J., Costeloe, K. & Clark, P. (1989) Transplacental effects of maternal cancer chemotherapy. Case report. *Br. J. Obstet. Gynaecol.*, **96**, 1099–1100

Raiker, A., Green, W., Shabaik, A. & Perlin, E. (1989) Acute promyelocytic leukemia following treatment of non-Hodgkin's lymphoma. *Cancer*, **63**, 1402–1406

Ratain, M.J., Bitran, J.D., Larson, R.A., Golomb, H.M., Skosey, C., Purl, S., Hoffman, P.C., LeBeau, M.M., Wade, J., Vardiman, J.W. & Daly, K. (1986) Increased risk of acute non-lymphocytic leukemia following cisplatin, etoposide, vindesine therapy for advanced non-small cell lung cancer (Abstract No. 607). *Proc. Am. Assoc. Cancer Res.*, **27**, 153

Ratain, M.J., Kaminer, L.S., Bitran, J.D., Larson, R.A., Le Beau, M.M., Skosey, C., Purl, S., Hoffman, P.C., Wade, J., Vardiman, J.W., Daly, K., Rowley, J.D. & Golomb, H.M. (1987) Acute nonlymphocytic leukemia following etoposide and cisplatin combination chemotherapy for advanced non-small-cell carcinoma of the lung. *Blood*, **70**, 1412–1417

Raza-Egilmez, S.Z., Jani-Sait, S.N., Grossi, M., Higgins, M.J., Shows, T.B. & Aplan, P.D. (1998) *NUP98-HOXD13* gene fusion in therapy-related acute myelogenous leukemia. *Cancer Res.*, **58**, 4269–4273

Record, I.R., Jannes, M., Dreosti, I.E. & King, R.A. (1995) Induction of micronucleus formation in mouse splenocytes by the soy isoflavone genistein *in vitro* but not *in vivo*. *Food chem. Toxicol.*, **33**, 919–922

Relling, M.V., Evans, R., Dass, C., Desiderio, D.M. & Nemec, J. (1992) Human cytochrome P450 metabolism of teniposide and etoposide. *J. Pharmacol. exp. Ther.*, **261**, 491–496

Relling, M.V., Nemec, J., Schuetz, E.G., Schuetz, J.D., Gonzalez, F.J. & Korzekwa, K.R. (1994) *O*-Demethylation of epipodophyllotoxins is catalyzed by human cytochrome P450 3A4. *Mol. Pharmacol.*, **45**, 352–358

Relling, M.V., Yanishevski, Y., Nemec, J., Evans, W.E., Boyett, J.M., Behm, F.G. & Pui, C.D. (1998) Etopsoside and antimetabolite pharmacology in patients who develop secondary acute myeloid leukemia. *Leukemia*, **12**, 346–352

Ribas, G., Xamena, N., Creus, A. & Marcos, R. (1996) Sister-chromatid exchanges (SCE) induction by inhibitors of DNA topoisomerases in cultured human lymphocytes. *Mutat. Res.*, **368**, 205–211

Rideout, J.M., Ayres, D.C., Lim, C.K. & Peters, T.J. (1984) Determination of etoposide (VP16-213) and teniposide (VM-20) in serum by high-performance liquid chromatography with electrochemical detection. *J. pharm. biomed. Anal.*, **2**, 125–128

Ritke, M.K., Rusnak, J.M., Lazo, J.S., Allan, W.P., Dive, C., Heer, S. & Yalowich, J.C. (1994) Differential induction of etoposide-mediated apoptosis in human leukemia HL-60 and K562 cells. *Mol. Pharmacol.*, **48**, 605–611

Rodriguez, J.M. & Haggag, M. (1995) VACOP-B chemotherapy for high grade non-Hodgkin's lymphoma in pregnancy. *Clin. Oncol.*, **7**, 319–320

Ross, W.E., Sullivan, D.M. & Chow, K.-C. (1988) Altered function of DNA topoisomerases as a basis for antineoplastic drug action. In: DeVita, V., Hellman, S. & Rosenberg, S., eds, *Important Advances in Oncology*, Philadelphia, PA, J.B. Lippincott, pp. 65–79

Rote Liste Sekretariat (1998) *Rote Liste 1998*, Frankfurt, Rote Liste Service GmbH, pp. 86-103–86-104, 86-118

Roth, B.J., Greist, A., Kubilis, P.S., Williams, S.D. & Einhorn, L.H. (1988) Cisplatin-based combination chemotherapy for disseminated germ cell tumors: Long-term follow-up. *J. clin. Oncol.*, **6**, 1239–1247

Roth, B.J., Johnson, D.H., Einhorn, L.H., Schacter, L.P., Cherng, N.C., Cohen, H.J., Crawford, J., Randolph, J.A., Goodlow, J.L. & Broun, G.O. (1992) Randomized study of cyclophosphamide, doxorubicin, and vincristine versus etoposide and cisplatin versus alternation of these two regimens in extensive small-cell lung cancer: A phase III trial of the Southeastern Cancer Study Group. *J. clin. Oncol.*, **10**, 282–291

Rowley, J.D., Reshmi, S., Sobulo, O., Musvee, T., Anastasi, J., Raimondi, S., Schneider, N.R., Barredo, J.C., Cantu, E.S., Schlegelberger, B., Behm, F., Doggett, N.A., Borrow, J. & Zeleznik-Le, N. (1997) All patients with the t(11;16)(q23;p13.3) that involves *MLL* and *CBP* have treatment-related hematologic disorders. *Blood*, **90**, 535–541

Royal Pharmaceutical Society of Great Britain (1999) *Martindale, The Extra Pharmacopoeia*, 13th Ed., London, The Pharmaceutical Press [MicroMedex Online: Health Care Series]

Rubin, C.M., Larson, R.A., Anastasi, J., Winter, J.N., Thangavelu, M., Vardiman, J.W., Rowley, J.D. & Le Beau, M.M. (1990) t(3;21)(q26;q22): A recurring chromosomal abnormality in therapy-related myelodysplastic syndrome and acute myeloid leukemia. *Blood*, **76**, 2594–2598

Rupa, D.S., Schuler, M. & Eastmond, D.A. (1997) Detection of hyperdiploidy and breakage affecting the 1cen-1q12 region of cultured interphase human lymphocytes treated with various genotoxic agents. *Environ. mol. Mutag.*, **29**, 161–167

Russell, L.B., Hunsicker, P.R., Johnson, D.K. & Shelby, M.D. (1998) Unlike other chemicals, etoposide (a topoisomerase-II inhibitor) produces peak mutagenicity in primary spermatocytes of the mouse. *Mutat. Res.*, **400**, 279–286

Russo, P., Cimoli, G., Valenti, M., De Sessa, F., Parodi, S. & Pommier, Y. (1994) Induction of DNA double-strand breaks by 8-methoxycaffeine: Cell cycle dependence and comparison with topoisomerase II inhibitors. *Carcinogenesis*, **15**, 2491–2496

Sakurai, H., Miki, T., Imakura, Y., Shibuya, M. & Lee, K.-H. (1991) Metal- and photo-induced cleavage of DNA by podophyllotoxin, etoposide, and their related compounds. *Mol. Pharmacol.*, **40**, 965–973

Schacter, L.P., Igwemezie, L.N., Seyedsadr, M., Morgenthien, E., Randolph, J., Albert, E. & Santabarbara, P. (1994) Clinical and pharmacokinetic overview of parenteral etoposide phosphate. *Cancer Chemother. Pharmacol.*, **34**, S58–S63

Schnittger, S., Wormann, B., Hiddemann, W. & Griesinger, F. (1998) Partial tandem duplications of the MLL gene are detectable in peripheral blood and bone marrow of nearly all healthy donors. *Blood*, **92**, 1728–1734

Segna, R.A., Mitchell, D.R. & Misas, J.E. (1990) Successful treatment of cervical pregnancy with oral etoposide. *Obstet. Gynecol.*, **76**, 945–947

Sestili, P., Cattabeni, F. & Cantoni, O. (1995) Simultaneous determination of DNA double strand breaks and DNA fragment size in cultured mammalian cells exposed to hydrogen peroxide/histidine or etoposide with CHEF electrophoresis. *Carcinogenesis*, **16**, 703–706

Shimizu, T., Kubota, M., Adachi, S., Sano, H., Kasai, Y., Hashimoto, H., Akiyama, Y. & Mikawa, H. (1992) Pre-treatment of a human T-lymphoblastoid cell line with L-asparaginase reduces etoposide-induced DNA strand breakage and cytoxicity. *Int. J. Cancer*, **50**, 644–648

Sieber, S.M., Whang-Peng, J., Botkin, C. & Knutsen, T. (1978) Teratogenic and cytogenetic effects of some plant-derived antitumor agents (vincristine, colchicine, maytansine, VP-16-213 and VM-26) in mice. *Teratology*, **18**, 31–47

Singh, B. & Gupta, R.S. (1983a) Mutagenic responses of thirteen anticancer drugs on mutation induction at multiple genetic loci and on sister chromatid exchanges in Chinese hamster ovary cells. *Cancer Res.*, **43**, 577–584

Singh, B. & Gupta, R.S. (1983b) Comparison of the mutagenic responses of 12 anticancer drugs at the hypoxanthine-guanine phosphoribosyl transferase and adenosine kinase loci in Chinese hamster ovary cells. *Environ. Mutag.*, **5**, 871–880

Sinha, B.K. & Eliot, H.M. (1991) Etoposide-induced DNA damage in human tumor cells: Requirement for cellular activating factors. *Biochim. biophys. Acta*, **1097**, 111–116

Sinha, B.K., Haim, N., Dusre, L., Kerrigan, D. & Pommier, Y. (1988) DNA strand breaks produced by etoposide (VP-16,213) in sensitive and resistant human breast tumor cells: Implications for the mechanism of action. *Cancer Res.*, **48**, 5096–5100

Sjöblom, T., Parvinen, M. & Lähdetie, J. (1994) Germ-cell mutagenicity of etoposide: Induction of meiotic micronuclei in cultured rat seminiferous tubules. *Mutat. Res.*, **323**, 41–45

Slavotinek, A., Perry, P.E. & Sumner, A.T. (1993) Micronuclei in neonatal lymphocytes treated with the topoisomerase II inhibitors amsacrine and etoposide. *Mutat. Res.*, **319**, 215–222

Slevin, M.L. (1991) The clinical pharmacology of etoposide. *Cancer*, **67**, 319–329

Slevin, M.L., Clark, P.I., Joel, S.P., Malik, S., Osborne, R.J., Gregory, W.M., Lowe, D.G., Reznek, R.H. & Wrigley, P.F. (1989a) A randomized trial to evaluate the effect of schedule on the activity of etoposide in small-cell lung cancer. *J. clin. Oncol.*, **7**, 1333–1340

Slevin, M.L., Joel, S.P., Whomsley, R., Devenport, K., Harvey, V.J., Osborne, R.J. & Wrigley, P.F.M. (1989b) The effect of dose on the bioavailability of oral etoposide: Confirmation of a clinically relevant observation. *Cancer Chemother. Pharmacol.*, **24**, 329–331

Smith, M.A., Rubinstein, L., Cazenave, L., Ungerleider, R.S., Maurer, H.M., Heyn, R., Khan, F.M. & Gehan, E. (1993) Report of the Cancer Therapy Evaluation Program monitoring plan for secondary acute myeloid leukemia following treatment with epipodophyllotoxins. *J. natl Cancer Inst.*, **85**, 554–558

Smith, M.A., Rubinstein, L., Anderson, J.R., Arthur, D., Catalano, P.J., Freidlin, B., Heyn, R., Khayat, A., Krailo, M., Land, V.J., Miser, J., Shuster, J. & Vena, D. (1999) Secondary leukemia or myelodysplastic syndrome after treatment with epipodophyllotoxins. *J. clin. Oncol.*, **17**, 569–577

Sobulo, O.M., Borrow, J., Tomek, R., Reshmi, S., Harden, A., Schlegelberger, B., Housman, D., Doggett, N.A., Rowley, J.D. & Zeleznik-Le, N.J. (1997) MLL is fused to CBP, a histone acetyltransferase, in therapy-related acute myeloid leukemia with a t(11;16)(q23;p13.3). *Proc. natl Acad. Sci. USA*, **94**, 8732–8737

Stähelin, H. (1976) Delayed toxicity of epipodophyllotoxin derivatives (VM 26 and VP 16-213), due to a local effect. *Eur. J. Cancer*, **12**, 925–931

Stanulla, M., Wang, J., Chervinsky, D.S., Thandla, S. & Aplan, P.D. (1997a) DNA cleavage within the *MLL* breakpoint cluster region is a specific event which occurs as part of high-order chromatin fragmentation during the initial stages of apoptosis. *Mol. cell. Biol.*, **17**, 4070–4079

Stanulla, M., Wang, J., Chervinsky, D.S. & Aplan, P.D. (1997b) Topoisomerase II inhibitors induce DNA double-strand breaks at a specific site within the *AML1* locus. *Leukemia*, **11**, 490–496

Stark, B., Jeison, M., Shohat, M., Goshen, Y., Vogel, R., Cohen, I.J., Yaniv, I., Kaplinsky, C. & Zaizov, R. (1994) Involvement of 11p15 and 3q21q26 in therapy-related myeloid leukemia (t-ML) in children. *Cancer Genet. Cytogenet.*, **75**, 11–22

Stephenson, W.T., Poirier, S.M., Rubin, L. & Einhorn, L.H. (1995) Evaluation of reproductive capacity in germ cell tumor patients following treatment with cisplatin etoposide, and bleomycin. *J. clin. Oncol.*, **13**, 2278–2280

Stewart, D.J., Richard, M.T., Hugenholtz, H., Dennery, J.M., Belanger, R., Gerin-Lajoie, J., Montpetit, V., Nundy, D., Prior, J. & Hopkins, H.S. (1984) Penetration of VP-16 (etoposide) into human intracerebral and extracerebral tumors. *J. Neuro-oncol.*, **2**, 133–139

Stewart, C.F., Pieper, J.A., Arbuck, S.G. & Evans, W.E. (1989) Altered protein binding of etoposide in patients with cancer. *Clin. Pharmacol. Ther.*, **45**, 49–55

Stewart, C.F., Arbuck, S.G., Fleming, R.A. & Evans, W.E. (1991) Relation of systemic exposure to unbound etoposide and hematologic toxicity. *Clin. Pharmacol. Ther.*, **50**, 385–393

Stremetzne, S., Jaehde, U., Kasper, R., Beyer, J., Siegert, W. & Schunack, W. (1997) Considerable plasma levels of a cytotoxic etoposide metabolite in patients undergoing high-dose chemotherapy. *Eur. J. Cancer*, **33**, 978–979

Strissel Broeker, P.L., Gill Super, H., Thirman, M.J., Pomykala, H., Yonebayashi, Y., Tanabe, S., Zeleznik-Le, N. & Rowley, J.D. (1996) Distribution of 11q23 breakpoints within the MLL breakpoint cluster region in de novo acute leukemia and in treatment-related acute myeloid leukemia: Correlation with scaffold attachment regions and topoisomerase II consensus binding sites. *Blood*, **87**, 1912–1922

Suciu, D. (1990) Inhibition of DNA synthesis and cytotoxic effects of some DNA topoisomerase II and gyrase inhibitors in Chinese hamster V79 cells. *Mutat. Res.*, **243**, 213–218

Sugita, K., Furukawa, T., Tsuchida, M., Okawa, Y., Nakazawa, S., Akatsuka, J., Ohira, M. & Nishimura, K. (1993) High frequency of etoposide (VP-16)-related secondary leukemia in children with non-Hodgkin's lymphoma. *Am. J. pediatr. Hematol. Oncol.*, **15**, 99–104

Sumner, A.T. (1995) Inhibitors of topoisomerase II delay progress through mitosis and induce a doubling of the DNA content in CHO cells. *Exp. Cell Res.*, **217**, 440–447

Sun, X.-M., Carthew, P., Dinsdale, D., Snowden, R.T. & Cohen, G.M. (1994a) The involvement of apoptosis in etoposide-induced thymic atrophy. *Toxicol. appl. Pharmacol.*, **128**, 78–85

Sun, X.-M., Snowden, R.T., Dinsdale, D., Ormerod, M.G. & Cohen, G.M. (1994b) Changes in nuclear chromatin precede internucleosomal DNA cleavage in the induction of apoptosis by etoposide. *Biochem. Pharmacol.*, **47**, 187–195

Suzuki, H. & Nakane, S. (1994) Differential induction of chromosomal aberrations by topoisomerase inhibitors in cultured Chinese hamster cells. *Biol. pharm. Bull.*, **17**, 222–226

Swiss Pharmaceutical Society, ed. (1999) *Index Nominum, International Drug Directory*, 16th Ed., Stuttgart, Medpharm Scientific Publishers [MicroMedex Online: Health Care Series]

Sykes, P.J., Hooker, A.M. & Morley, A.A. (1999) Inversion due to intrachromosomal recombination produced by carcinogens in a transgenic mouse model. *Mutat. Res.*, **427**, 1–9

Takahashi, N., Kai, S., Kohmura, H., Ishikawa, K., Kuroyanagi, K., Hamajima, Y, Ohta, S., Kadota, T., Kawano, S. & Ohtak, K. (1986a) [Reproduction studies of VP 16-213. I. Oral administration to rats prior to and in the early stages of pregnancy.] *J. toxicol. Sci.*, **11** (Suppl. 1), 177–194 (in Japanese)

Takahashi, N., Kai, S., Kohmura, H., Ishikawa, K., Kuroyanagi, K., Hamajima, Y, Ohta, S., Kadota, T., Kawano, S. & Ohta, K. (1986b) [Reproduction studies of VP 16-213. IV. Oral administration to rats during the perinatal and lactation periods.] *J. toxicol. Sci.*, **11** (Suppl. 1), 241–261 (in Japanese)

Takahashi, N., Kai, S., Kohmura, H., Ishikawa, K., Tanaka, T., Kuroyanagi, K., Hamajima, Y, Ohta, S., Kadota, T. & Kawano, S. (1986c) [Reproduction studies of VP 16-213 V. Intravenous administration to rats prior to and in the early stages of pregnancy.] *J. toxicol. Sci.*, **11** (Suppl. 1), 263–279 (in Japanese)

Takahashi, N., Kai, S., Kohmura, H., Ishikawa, K., Kuroyanagi, K., Hamajima, Y, Ohta, S., Kadota, T., Kawano, S. & Ohta, K. (1986d) [Reproduction studies of VP 16-213. VI. Intravenous administration to rats during the perinatal and lactation periods.] *J. toxicol. Sci.*, **11** (Suppl. 1), 281–300 (in Japanese)

Takahashi, N., Kai, S., Kohmura, H., Ishikawa, K., Kuroyanagi, K., Hamajima, Y, Ohta, S., Kadota, T., Kawano, S. & Ohta, K. (1986e) [Reproduction studies of VP 16-213. III. Oral administration to rabbits during the period of fetal organogenesis.] *J. toxicol. Sci.*, **11** (Suppl. 1), 227–239 (in Japanese)

Taki, T., Sako, M., Tsuchida, M. & Hayashi, Y. (1997) The t(11;16)(q23;p13) translocation in myelodysplastic syndrome fuses the *MLL* gene to the *CBP* gene. *Blood*, **89**, 3945–3950

Thomas, J., ed. (1998) *Australian Prescription Products Guide*, 27th Ed., Victoria, Australian Pharmaceutical Publishing, Vol. 1, pp. 2896–2899

Tkachuk, D., Kohler, S. & Cleary, M.L. (1992) Involvement of a homolog of *Drosophila trithorax* by 11q23 chromosomal translocations in acute leukemias. *Cell*, **71**, 691–700

Tominaga, K., Shinkai, T., Saijo, N., Nakajima, T., Ochi, H. & Suemasu, K. (1986) Cytogenetic effects of etoposide (VP-16) on human lymphocytes; with special reference to the relation between sister chromatid exchange and chromatid breakage. *Jpn. J. Cancer Res.*, **77**, 385–391

Torres, C., Creus, A. & Marcos, R. (1998) Genotoxic activity of four inhibitors of DNA topoisomerases in larval cells of *Drosophila melanogaster* as measured in the wing spot assay. *Mutat. Res.*, **413**, 191–203

US Pharmacopeial Convention (1994) *The 1995 US Pharmacopeia*, 23rd Rev./*The National Formulary*, 18th Rev., Rockville, MD, pp. 648–649

US Pharmacopeial Convention (1997) *The 1995 US Pharmacopeia*, 23rd Rev./*The National Formulary*, 18th Rev., Supplement 7, Rockville, MD, pp. 3889–3890

Vigreux, C., Poul, J.M., Deslandes, E., Lebailly, P., Godard, T., Sichel, F., Henry-Amar, M. & Gauduchon, P. (1998) DNA damaging effects of pesticides measured by the single cell gel electrophoresis assay (comet assay) and the chromosomal aberration test, in CHOK1 cells. *Mutat. Res.*, **419**, 79–90

Vock, E.H., Lutz, W.K., Hormes, P., Hoffmann, H.D. & Vamvakas, S. (1998) Discrimination between genotoxicity and cytotoxicity in the induction of DNA double-strand breaks in cells treated with etoposide, melphalan, cisplatin, potassium cyanide, Triton X-100, and γ-irradiation. *Mutat. Res.*, **413**, 83–94

Wachsman, J.T. (1997) DNA methylation and the association between genetic and epigenetic changes: Relation to carcinogenesis. *Mutat. Res.*, **375**, 1–8

Wang, J.C., Caron, P.R. & Kim, R.A. (1990) The role of DNA topoisomerases in recombination and genome stability: A double-edged sword? *Cell*, **62**, 403–406

Weiss, R.B. (1992) Hypersensitivity reactions. *Semin. Oncol.*, **19**, 458–477

Williams, S.D., Birch, R., Einhorn, L.H., Irwin, L., Greco, F.A. & Lochrer, P.J. (1987) Treatment of disseminated germ-cell tumours with cisplatin, bleomycin, and either vinblastine or etoposide. *New Engl. J. Med.*, **316**, 1435–1440

Winick, N., McKenna, R.W., Shuster, J.J., Schneider, N.R., Borowitz, M.J., Bowman, W.P., Jacaruso, D., Kamen, B.A. & Buchanan, G.R. (1993) Secondary acute myeloid leukemia in children with acute lymphoblastic leukemia treated with etoposide. *J. clin. Oncol.*, **11**, 209–217

Wozniak, A.J. & Ross, W.E. (1983) DNA damage as a basis for 4'-demethylepipodophyllotoxin-9-(4,6-O-ethylidene-beta-D-glucopyranoside) (etoposide) cytotoxicity. *Cancer Res.*, **43**, 120–124

Yagita, M., Ieki, Y., Onishi, R., Huang, C.-L., Adachi, M., Horiike, S., Konaka, Y., Taki, T. & Miyake, M. (1998) Therapy-related leukemia and myelodysplasia following oral administration of etoposide for recurrent breast cancer. *Int. J. Oncol.*, **13**, 91–96

Yoon, H.J., Choi, I.Y., Kang, M.R., Kim, S.S., Muller, M.T., Spitzner, J.R. & Chung, I.K. (1998) DNA topoisomerase II cleavage of telomeres in vitro and in vivo. *Biochim. biophys. Acta*, **1395**, 110–120

Zhang, L.-H. & Jenssen, D. (1994) Studies on intrachromosomal recombination in SP5/V79 Chinese hamster cells upon exposure to different agents related to carcinogenesis. *Carcinogenesis*, **15**, 2303–2310

TENIPOSIDE

1. Exposure Data

1.1 Chemical and physical data

1.1.1 Nomenclature

Chem. Abstr. Serv. Reg. No.: 29767-20-2
Chem. Abstr. Name: (5*R*,5a*R*,8a*R*,9*S*)-5,8,8a,9-Tetrahydro-5-(4-hydroxy-3,5-dimethoxyphenyl)-9-{[4,6-*O*-[(*R*)-2-thienylmethylene]-β-D-glucopyranosyl]oxy}-furo[3′,4′:6,7]naphtho[2,3-*d*]-1,3-dioxol-6(5a*H*)-one
IUPAC Systematic Name: 4′-Demethylepipodophyllotoxin, 9-(4,6-O-2-thenylidene-β-D-glucopyranoside)
Synonyms: Epipodophyllotoxin; EPT; teniposide VM-26; VM 26; 5,8,8a,9-tetrahydro-5-(4-hydroxy-3,5-dimethoxyphenyl)-9-{[4,6-*O*-(2-thienylmethylene)-β-D-glucopyranosyl]oxy}furo[3′,4′:6,7]naphtho[2,3-*d*]-1,3-dioxol-6(5a*H*)-one

1.1.2 Structural and molecular formulae and relative molecular mass

$C_{32}H_{32}O_{13}S$ Relative molecular mass: 656.67

1.1.3 Chemical and physical properties of the pure substance

(*a*) *Description*: White, crystalline solid (Gennaro, 1995; Budavari, 1996)

(b) *Melting-point*: 242–246 °C (Gennaro, 1995; Budavari, 1996)

(c) *Spectroscopy data*: Ultraviolet, infrared, fluorescence emission, nuclear magnetic resonance (proton and ^{13}C) and mass spectral data have been reported (Kettenes-van den Bosch *et al.*, 1990).

(d) *Solubility*: Insoluble in water and diethyl ether; slightly soluble in methanol; very soluble in acetone and dimethylformamide (Medical Economics Data Production, 1999)

(e) *Optical rotation*: $[\alpha]_D^{20}$, –107° (9:1, chloroform/methanol) (Budavari, 1996)

(f) *Dissociation constant*: pK_a, 10.13 (Budavari, 1996)

1.1.4 *Technical products and impurities*

Teniposide is available as a 10-mg/mL injection solution. It is poorly soluble, and the 50-mg intravenous preparation typically also contains benzyl alcohol (0.15 g), *N,N*-dimethylacetamide (0.3 g), polyethoxylated castor oil (2.5 g), maleic acid to a pH of 5.1 and absolute ethanol to 5 mL (Gennaro, 1995; American Hospital Formulary Service, 1997; Canadian Pharmaceutical Association, 1997; LINFO Läkemedelsinformation AB, 1998; Rote Liste Sekretariat, 1998; Thomas, 1998; Medical Economics Data Production, 1999).

Trade names for teniposide include Vehem, Vehem-Sandoz, Vumon and Vumon Parenteral (Royal Pharmaceutical Society of Great Britain, 1999; Swiss Pharmaceutical Society, 1999).

1.1.5 *Analysis*

Standard analytical methods have not been established for teniposide. The methods for the analysis of teniposide in various matrices include high-performance liquid chromatography, thin-layer and paper chromatography and radioimmunoassay (Kettenes-van den Bosch *et al.*, 1990).

1.2 Production

Teniposide is prepared from etoposide by reaction with 2-thiophene carboxaldehyde, with zinc chloride as the catalyst (Kettenes-van den Bosch *et al.*, 1990).

Information available in 1999 indicated that teniposide is manufactured and/or formulated in 24 countries (CIS Information Services, 1998; Royal Pharmaceutical Society of Great Britain; 1999; Swiss Pharmaceutical Society, 1999).

1.3 Use

Teniposide is a semi-synthetic derivative of podophyllotoxin, an extract of the roots and rhizomes of two plant species that have been used in folk medicine for several hundred years. It inhibits DNA topoisomerase II (Imbert, 1998). During early clinical trials for cancer chemotherapeutic use, podophyllotoxin itself proved to be too toxic, and, in the 1960s, two epipodophyllotoxins, teniposide and etoposide (see monograph, this volume), were described (Keller-Juslén et al., 1971). The first clinical trial of teniposide in cancer treatment was reported in 1967. Marketing of teniposide in several countries began in 1976 (Imbert, 1998).

Teniposide is used in the treatment of adult and childhood leukaemia, typically at doses of 30–50 mg/m^2 per day for five days or three doses of about 200 mg/m^2 over seven days. The drug is also used in the treatment of brain tumours in adults and neuroblastoma in children. Teniposide is active against a number of other tumour types, including small-cell and non-small-cell lung cancer, lymphomas and bladder cancer. It is used much less commonly than the related drug etoposide (Giaccone, 1992; Giaccone et al., 1992; Hirsch et al., 1994; Muggia, 1994; Rivera et al., 1994).

1.4 Occurrence

Teniposide is not known to occur as a natural product. No data on occupational exposure were available to the Working Group.

1.5 Regulations and guidelines

Teniposide is not listed in any international pharmacopoeias.

2. Studies of Cancer in Humans

This section summarizes only studies in which tepinoside was given without agents with known or suspected leukaemogenic properties. In studies in which patients were treated with both tepinoside and etoposide, the authors used various conversion factors to derive an 'equivalent dose' of etoposide from that of teniposide. The conversions were based, however, on the therapeutic effects rather than on metabolic considerations.

2.1 Cohort studies

Sixty-two children in Spain in whom acute lymphoblastic leukaemia was newly diagnosed between 1985 and 1988 were initially treated with teniposide (165 mg/m^2), cytarabine, vincristine, L-asparaginase and prednisone and subsequently with teniposide (165 mg/m^2), cytarabine, vincristine, cranial irradiation, mercaptopurine, methothrexate and prednisone (Verdeguer et al., 1992). Of 60 patients in whom complete remission was achieved, 14 suffered a bone-marrow relapse. During treatment, acute myeloid leukaemia developed in three of these patients (two cases of acute monoblastic leukaemia, one of acute myelomonocytic leukaemia). Thus, the frequency of conversion from acute lymphoblastic leukaemia to acute myeloid leukaemia was 3/60. The time from diagnosis to conversion was 17, 23 and 29 months. The authors noted that 45 children with non-T-cell acute lymphoblastic leukaemia were treated between 1981 and 1984 with a regimen that did not include teniposide and cytarabine, and no cases of acute myeloid leukaemia were observed at relapse. [The Working Group noted that it is difficult to establish the difference between lineage switch and mixed-lineage leukaemia. Tests for myeloid marker cells had not been performed at initial diagnosis in any of the three cases reported. No appropriate comparison of leukaemia risk between the two treatment groups was made.]

In the study of Pui *et al.* (1991), described in the monograph on etoposide, acute myeloid leukaemia developed in 20 out of 580 children treated with teniposide with or without etoposide for acute lymphoblastic leukaemia; one case was found in a patient treated with neither etoposide nor teniposide. The overall cumulative risk was 3.8% at six years. The median interval between the diagnoses of acute lymphoblastic leukaemia and acute myeloid leukaemia was 40 months. Six cases were acute myelomonocytic leukaemia, eight were acute monoblastic leukaemia, three were acute myeloblastic leukaemia, one was acute megakaryoblastic leukaemia, one was acute myeloid leukaemia and two were acute undifferentiated leukaemia. In four patients, acute myeloid leukaemia developed after relapse had occurred, and these were not included in the analysis. In the analysis of leukaemia risk, the doses of teniposide and etoposide were weighted equally since the potency of teniposide *in vitro*—10 times that of etoposide—is offset *in vitro* by extensive protein binding, resulting in 10 times less unbound active drug. The analyses indicated the importance of the schedule and frequency of epipodophyllotoxin treatment in determining the risk for acute myeloid leukaemia (see Table 1).

In a combined analysis of 12 trials in patients with various primary tumours who developed acute myeloid leukaemia after treatment with epipodophyllotoxins (Smith *et al.*, 1999), described in the monograph on etoposide, the six-year actuarial risks for acute myeloid leukaemia or myelodysplastic syndrome were 3.3% (upper 95% confidence bound, 5.9%) with the low cumulative dose of epipodophyllotoxin, 0.7% (upper 95% confidence bound, 1.6%) with the moderate cumulative dose and 2.2% (upper 95% confidence bound, 4.6%) with the high cumulative dose. The *p* values for homogeneity of the risk for leukaemia across the cumulative dose strata were 0.012 (with a parametric test) and 0.011 (with a non-parametric test). In one of the trials, 251 patients with primary acute lymphoblastic leukaemia received only teniposide as three courses of 165 mg/m^2 for two days, for a cumulative dose of 990 mg/m^2, corresponding to a moderate cumulative dose of epipodophyllotoxin. No cases of leukaemia were observed. Thus, the data provide no support for an effect of the cumulative dose of epipodophyllotoxins on leukaemogenic activity, at least not within the cumulative dose range encompassed by the monitoring plan. [The Working Group noted that the

Table 1. Risks for secondary acute myeloid leukaemia (AML) in children with acute lymphoblastic leukaemia treated with epipodophyllotoxins, according to regimen

Regimen	Prognosis	Planned cumulative dose (mg/m^2)		Epipodophyllotoxin schedule	No. of patients treated	No. of patients with AML	Six-year cumulative risk % (95% CI)
		Teniposide	Etoposide				
X-LR1	Low risk	0	0	None	154	1	1.0 (0.6–6.3)
X-LR2	Low risk	1350	0	Every other week	155	1	1.1 (0.1–7.1)
X-HR	High risk	4620	0	Twice weekly	85	6	12 (5.7–25)
XI-LR1	Low risk	600	0	Induction only	39	0	0
XI-LR2	Low risk	5100	9000	Every other week	69	0	0
XI-HR2	High risk	5100	9000	Every other week	148	2	1.6 (0.4–6.1)
XI-HR3	High risk	5100	9000	Weekly	84	7	12 (6.1–24)

From Pui et al. (1991)
CI, confidence interval

three treatment strata were compared as if the cumulative dose of epipodophyllotoxin were the only difference between them; however, the strata also differed with respect to the primary tumour (stratum with solid tumours versus stratum with solid and lymphoid tumours) and treatment; one stratum with high-dose epipodophyllotoxin and high-dose cyclophosphamide versus a stratum with no cyclophosphamide and a moderate dose of epipodophyllotoxin and a stratum with high-dose cyclophosphamide given to part (one trial) of the stratum with low-dose epipodophyllotoxin. It is also not clear which patients received teniposide and which received etoposide.]

Negligible risks for acute myeloid leukaemia were reported in two large series of children with acute lymphoblastic leukaemia who received treatments without epipodophyllotoxins (Neglia et al., 1991; Kreissman et al., 1992). The patients in these series received treatments similar to those in the study by Pui et al. (1991): most received cranial irradiation, all received methotrexate, 6-mercaptopurine, prednisone, vincristine and L-asparaginase, and a substantial proportion received cyclophosphamide and doxorubicin. Neglia et al. (1991) reported only two cases of acute myeloid leukaemia among 9720 children treated according to protocols of the US Children's Cancer Study Group between 1972 and 1988. The median follow-up was 4.7 years. Kreissman et al. (1992) reported two cases of acute myeloid leukaemia in 779 children treated for acute lymphoblastic leukaemia at the Dana Farber Cancer Institute, Boston, USA. The median follow-up time was 4.4 years. The estimated overall risk for secondary acute myeloid leukaemia was 0.61 per 1000 patient–years of follow-up, which was significantly lower ($p = 0.0008$) than the reported risk of 5.8 per 1000 patient–years for patients with acute lymphoblastic leukaemia in the study of Pui et al. (1989) who were treated with epipodophyllotoxins.

2.2 Case–control studies

Hawkins et al. (1992) reported the results of a case–control study of secondary leukaemia nested in a cohort of 16 422 children aged < 15 years who had survived at least one year after a diagnosis of a childhood neoplasm in the United Kingdom between 1962 and 1983. The mean follow-up period beyond one year of survival for the entire cohort was 7.7 years. Twenty-six cases of secondary leukaemia occurring after diagnosis of the initial childhood neoplasm between 1940 and 1983 were each matched with up to four controls for sex, histological type of first cancer and age at first diagnosis. In addition, the controls had to have survived free of any second primary neoplasm for at least as long as the interval between the first primary neoplasm and secondary leukaemia in the corresponding case. Ninety-six controls were selected. Of those patients receiving chemotherapy (69% of cases, 55% of controls), 77% had received alkylating agents, 51% antibiotics, 54% antimetabolites, 97% vinca alkaloids and 30% epipodophyllotoxins. Ten patients with leukaemia had received epipodophyllotoxins during their treatment: nine had received teniposide and one had received etoposide. Two methods were used to categorize the doses of epipodophyllotoxins and the other groups of agents: first, a ranking method based on the assumption that all drugs within an etiological group have equal leukaemogenic potency within the corresponding third of their respective dose distributions; secondly, an approach based on the simple assumption that all agents in a particular group have equal leukaemogenic potency for a specified amount of drug given per unit of surface area. Multivariate analysis of the relative risk for leukaemia (adjusted for active bone marrow radiation dose and exposure to alkylating agents) according to the total dose of epipodophyllotoxins estimated by either method showed evidence of a trend ($p = 0.012$ and $p = 0.006$) in the relative risk with dose of epipodophyllotoxins (see Table 2). [The Working Group noted that, even though multivariate analysis was conducted to adjust for confounding by leukaemogenic agents, interaction between epipodophyllotoxins and these agents could not be ruled out.]

Detailed information from the medical records of a cohort of 1939 patients treated for Hodgkin disease between 1966 and 1986 in the Netherlands (van Leeuwen et al., 1994) was obtained for 32 cases of acute myeloid leukaemia, 12 cases of myelodysplastic syndrome and 124 matched controls in whom leukaemia had not developed. The controls had to have survived without a second cancer for at least as long as the interval between the diagnosis of Hodgkin disease and leukaemia in the case patient. Controls were matched to the case patient on cancer centre, sex, date of birth and date of diagnosis of Hodgkin disease. In multivariate analyses, all of the relative risks were adjusted for mechlorethamine dose, lomustine, dacarbazine, cyclophosphamide given in combinations, teniposide, interaction between cyclophosphamide and teniposide, splenectomy and number of episodes of chemotherapy. In these analyses, treatment with teniposide (median dose, 300 mg; seven cases, six controls) did not increase the risk for leukaemia (relative risk, 0.9; 95% confidence interval, 0.12–7.0) over that of patients never treated with teniposide. Since only one case patient and two controls received teniposide without cyclophosphamide, however, the independent effect of teniposide on the risk for leukaemia could not be assessed reliably. Treatment with cyclophosphamide alone was not significantly associated with an increased risk for leukaemia. The combination of cyclophosphamide and teniposide, which had been used in six patients who developed leukaemia and four controls, was associated with a strongly increased relative risk (125 000; $p = 0.03$). Most of the patients who received this combination were treated alternately with procarbazine, vincristine, prednisone and nitrogen mustard (MOPP) (see IARC, 1987), cyclophosphamide, doxorubicin, teniposide and prednisone. [The Working Group noted that the increased relative risk was based on very small numbers.]

3. Studies of Cancer in Experimental Animals

No data were available to the Working Group.

Table 2. Risks for acute myeloid leukaemia in children treated for primary neoplasms with epipodophyllotoxins, in relation to dose

Dose of epipodophyllotoxin	No. of leukaemia cases	No. of controls[a]	Adjusted relative risk[b]
Total dose by third of distribution			
0	16	85	1
First	2	5	2.9
Second	4	4	8.4
Third	4	2	24
Total equivalent (mg/m^2)			$p = 0.012$
0	16	85	1
1–750	2	5	2.6
751–1200	3	4	6.6
≥ 1201	5	2	17
Total	26	96	$p = 0.006$

From Hawkins et al. (1992)
[a] Patients with childhood malignancies who did not develop leukaemia
[b] Adjusted for radiation dose to the active bone marrow and exposure to alkylating agents

4. Other Data Relevant to an Evaluation of Carcinogenicity and its Mechanisms

4.1 Absorption, distribution, metabolism and excretion

4.1.1 Humans

The pharmacokinetics of teniposide in humans has been summarized (Clark & Slevin, 1987). After intravenous administration of 50–200 mg/m^2, the disposition of the drug typically fitted a two-compartment model, with terminal elimination half-times of 6–10 h (Rossi et al., 1984; D'Incalci et al., 1985; Gigante et al., 1995). Tri-exponential decay has also been reported, with terminal half-times of 26 h after administration of [^{3}H]teniposide (Creaven & Allen, 1975), 20 h after a low intravenous dose of 30 mg/m^2 (Canal et al., 1985) and 48 h after doses of ≤ 1000 mg/m^2 (Holthuis et al., 1987). The distribution volume of teniposide in these studies was 8–30 L/m^2, indicating that the drug is distributed mainly in the extracellular fluid compartment, with a total plasma clearance rate of 7–17 mL/min per m^2 and a low renal clearance rate of 0.8–2.2 mL/min per m^2 (Clark & Slevin, 1987). The pharmacokinetics of teniposide was linear up to 1000 mg/m^2, the highest dose tested (Holthuis et al., 1987).

The pharmacokinetics of teniposide in children is similar to that in adults, with elimination half-times of 9–10.3 h and a total plasma clearance rate of 5–15 mL/min per m^2, but possibly with a smaller distribution volume of 3–10 L/m^2 (Evans et al., 1983; Sinkule et al., 1984; Rodman et al., 1987; Petros et al., 1991).

After intravenous infusion of 150 mg/m^2 over 24 h in adults, the peak plasma concentrations were 4–12 µg/mL (D'Incalci et al., 1985). In children receiving 450 mg/m^2 over 72 h, 10 of 11 values were between 4 and 13 µg/mL, and the remaining value was 30 µg/mL (Rodman et al., 1987).

Considerable variation in the pharmacokinetics of teniposide between patients has been described, which may explain some of the variation in the pharmacodynamics of the drug. Rodman et al. (1987) reported a lower plasma clearance rate (12 versus 21 mL/min per m^2) and a longer elimination half-time (12 versus 6.6 h) in responding than in non-responding cancer patients receiving a 72-h teniposide infusion. This resulted in a > 50% increase in systemic exposure, as measured by the steady-state plasma concentration (15.2 versus 6.2 mg/L).

Few studies have investigated the metabolism of teniposide in cancer patients. In children given teniposide, the main metabolite in serum and urine was reported to be the hydroxy acid, formed by opening of the lactone ring; the cis-isomer, which may be a degradation product formed during storage, was also detected. The aglycone, formed by loss of the glucopyranoside moiety, was not detected (Evans et al., 1982). The hydroxy acid has not been found in plasma or urine in other studies with high doses of teniposide, and no changes in the measured concentration of teniposide in these samples was found after incubation with glucuronidase, indicating formation of little or none of the proposed glucuronide metabolites (Holthuis et al., 1987). In another study, however, 6% of the administered dose of teniposide was excreted in the urine as parent drug over 24 h, and a further 8% as a proposed aglycone glucuronide, which was not formally identified (Rossi et al., 1984).

In patients given [^{3}H]teniposide, urinary excretion accounted for about 45% of the administered radiolabel and biliary excretion for < 10% (Creaven & Allen, 1975). With high-performance liquid chromatography assays specific for teniposide, urinary excretion accounted for only 4–14% of the dose up to 24 h (Rossi et al., 1984; D'Incalci et al., 1985; Holthuis et al., 1987). The fate of most of an administered dose of teniposide therefore remains unknown.

Teniposide was detected in one patient who died three days after a cumulative intravenous dose of 576 mg, the highest concentrations occurring in the spleen, prostate, heart, large bowel, liver and pancreas. Teniposide was not detected in any tissue from four patients who died 5–52 days (median, eight days) after their last treatment with teniposide, for a cumulative dose of 234–1577 mg, indicating a relatively short tissue half-time (Stewart et al., 1993). Teniposide was detected in intracerebral tumours at concentrations of 0.05–1.12 µg/g tissue in 11 patients given 100–150 mg/m^2 teniposide 1.5–3 h before tumour resection. The concentrations in adjacent normal brain tissue were low (< 0.9 μg/g tissue) in three patients and undetectable (< 0.05 μg/g tissue) in the others (Zucchetti et al., 1991).

After intravenous administration of teniposide, the integrated area under the curve of concentration–time (AUC) in malignant ascites fluid was 12–90% of that measured in plasma (Canal et al., 1985). In one patient in whom serial cerebrospinal fluid and plasma samples were collected after administration of teniposide at doses up to 1000 mg/m^2, the concentrations of the drug in eight samples of cerebrospinal fluid were only 0.03–0.55% of the simultaneous plasma concentrations (mean, 0.17%) (Holthuis et al., 1987). Teniposide was not detected in samples of cerebrospinal fluid collected 97–740 min after dosing of patients with 100–150 mg/m^2 intravenously (Zucchetti et al., 1991). The concentrations in serial saliva samples from two patients were only 0.37% (n = 22) and 0.42% (n = 29) of the corresponding plasma concentrations (Holthuis et al., 1987). These results are in line with the reported protein binding of teniposide of 99% or higher (Allen & Creaven, 1975; Evans et al., 1992). The binding of the drug to protein decreased with decreasing serum albumin concentration and increasing bilirubin concentration, with a resultant increase in free drug, from 0.44 to 1.25% in newly diagnosed and relapsed patients. The percentage decrease in leukocyte count correlated with the AUC for free teniposide rather than with that for total teniposide (Evans et al., 1992).

Concurrent administration of ciclosporin at 5 mg/kg bw over 2 h, followed by 30 mg/kg bw over 48 h intravenously, increased the AUC for teniposide by 50%, due to a reduction in clearance (Toffoli et al., 1997). Conversely, concurrent administration of phenytoin increased the clearance rate of teniposide to 32 mL/min per m^2 from 13 mL/min per m^2 for control patients (Baker et al., 1992).

The oral bioavailability of teniposide was around 40% at doses of 60 and 120 mg/m^2, and 29% at a dose of 250 mg/m^2, with marked differences among patients (Splinter et al., 1992).

4.1.2 Experimental systems

The pharmacokinetics of teniposide and etoposide differed in tumour-bearing mice, teniposide having a lower clearance rate (12 versus 17 mL/kg per min), a longer terminal elimination half-time (77 versus 33 min) and a larger volume of distribution (1400 versus 820 mL/kg) (Broggini et al., 1983; Colombo et al., 1986). A similar, rapid distribution half-time of about 2 min was observed for both drugs.

Studies of cellular uptake suggested that the passage of teniposide into leukaemic cells in culture was linear up to 5 min and reached a steady state by 20 min, the intracellular concentrations being about 20 times higher than the extracellular concentrations. When the drug was removed, an exponential efflux was observed (Allen, 1978). Other authors have reported greater cellular accumulation of teniposide than etoposide at the same extracellular concentration of the two drugs in Lewis lung carcinoma cells in vitro, with intracellular concentrations of 1.6 nmol/8 × 10^6 cells and

0.1 nmol/8 × 10⁶ cells, respectively, for teniposide and etoposide after a 30-min incubation at 17 μmol/L (Colombo *et al.*, 1986).

The ratios of the AUC for tissue to that for plasma in mice suggest that teniposide concentrates in a number of tissues, and particularly in the liver (AUC ratio, 4.8), intestine (AUC ratio, 5.7) and kidney (AUC ratio, 3.8) (Colombo *et al.*, 1986).

Although few published data are available on the metabolism of teniposide in experimental systems, it appears to be similar to that of etoposide (see section 4.1 of the monograph on etoposide). In isolated human liver preparations, cytochrome P450 mixed-function isozymes catalysed metabolism of the (pendant) E-ring to *O*-demethylated and catechol metabolites (Relling *et al.*, 1992). This metabolism was subsequently attributed primarily to CYP3A4 activity and to a lesser degree to CYP3A5 (Relling *et al.*, 1994). Peroxidase-mediated *O*-demethylation of teniposide has also been reported (Haim *et al.*, 1986).

4.2 Toxic effects

4.2.1 *Humans*

The toxic effects in 1069 patients entered into 25 early phase I and II studies with teniposide as a single agent have been summarized (Macbeth, 1982). With the more commonly used five-day regime (30–60 mg/m² per day), bone-marrow suppression was the dose-limiting toxic effect, with leukopenia reported in 28–38% of patients and thrombocytopenia in 7–30%. The lowest blood counts typically occurred around day 10, with recovery by day 21. Nausea and vomiting were reported as mild, occurring in up to 20% of patients, with occasional reports of diarrhoea. Less common toxic effects in this group included increased liver enzyme activity (11 patients), acute hypotension (10 patients), fever (six patients) and anaphylaxis (five patients).

More recent studies of patients given 50–80 mg/m² per day for five days confirmed these findings, haematological effects occurring most commonly. Severe neutropenia or leukopenia occurred in 30–50% of patients (Cox *et al.*, 1988; Boas *et al.*, 1990; Oishi *et al.*, 1990; Sørensen *et al.*, 1991; Berenberg *et al.*, 1993; Grozea *et al.*, 1997). Episodes of nausea, vomiting and diarrhoea occurred occasionally but were generally mild, and some degree of alopecia was observed in most patients. Less common effects in these studies included transient increases in liver enzyme activity, anaphylaxis, hypotension and hypertension, which in one study was attributed to the vegetable oil base used in the formulation (Oishi *et al.*, 1990). Single doses of 100 mg/m² given once weekly are generally less toxic (Tirelli *et al.*, 1984; Sorio *et al.*, 1990).

Because of the reports of hypotension and anaphylaxis in the early studies, reports of 82 hypersensitivity reactions in 2250 patients (3.6% incidence) were reviewed (O'Dwyer *et al.*, 1986). Of these reactions, 45% occurred in patients with neuroblastoma or brain tumour, a much higher incidence than in patients with other tumour types. These reactions are manifest as respiratory difficulty, changes in blood pressure, urticaria and flushing.

When teniposide was given at a high total dose of 300–1000 mg/m² over three days, haematological toxic effects were dose-limiting, with leukocyte counts of < 0.5–10^9/L in all three patients at 1000 mg/m². These patients also developed an intensely pruritic erythematous rash with purpura four to seven days after the start of chemotherapy, which involved the upper part of the chest and the upper part of the legs. In two of these patients, ulceration was also seen. The rash cleared spontaneously within one week and, in two patients who were treated again at 500 mg/m², no rash occurred. In the one patient who received a second dose of 1000 mg/m², paraesthesia and an abnormal electromyography were seen (de Vries et al., 1986).

In one study, the intravenous formulation was tested orally after dilution in 100 mL of syrup or orange juice (Smit et al., 1992). Several patients retched during administration, 12 received antiemetics, and vomiting persisted in five patients. The dose-limiting toxic effect was myelosuppression, and gastrointestinal toxicity was also common.

4.2.2 Experimental systems

In cell lines, teniposide was 6–10 times more toxic than etoposide, but in a murine model in vivo, it was only three times more toxic, with LD_{10} values of 9.4 mg/kg bw for etoposide and 3.4 mg/kg bw for teniposide. At equitoxic doses, the two drugs had equivalent anti-tumour activity in a murine tumour model in vivo (Jensen et al., 1990).

4.3 Reproductive and prenatal effects

4.3.1 Humans

A woman in whom Burkitt lymphoma was diagnosed in the 22nd week of pregnancy was treated with a number of anticancer agents, including teniposide given intravenously at 75–100 mg every 2.5–3 weeks until delivery in the 37th week (a total of six courses of treatment). The infant was fully developed and normal in all respects, the examinations including electrocardiography and blood counts. The mother died seven weeks after delivery (Lowenthal et al., 1982).

4.3.2 Experimental systems

Groups of 3–14 pregnant Swiss albino mice were given a single dose of teniposide at 0.5, 0.75 or 1.0 mg/kg bw intraperitoneally on day 6, 7 or 8 of gestation (vaginal plug, day 0), and the fetuses were removed and examined on day 17. No effect on maternal body-weight gain was seen in any group. In animals injected on day 6, no embryotoxicity was seen with 0.5 mg/kg bw, but 0.75 mg/kg bw reduced fetal weights, and 1.0 mg/kg bw increased the frequencies of intrauterine death and fetal malformations and reduced fetal body weight. Injection on day 7 caused embryolethality only at the high dose, and increased the frequency of fetal malformations and reduced fetal weights at the intermediate and high doses. Injection on day 8 caused no embryotoxicity or effect on fetal body weight at the low and intermediate doses, but the frequencies of embryolethality and fetal malformations were increased at 1.0 mg/kg bw. Teniposide was considerably more embryotoxic and teratogenic than etoposide, which was also included in this investigation (see the monograph on etoposide). The commonest malformations observed at the highest dose were dextrocardia, seen in 9.4% and 10% of fetuses of dams injected on days 6 and 7, respectively, and exencephaly in 5.7% and 14% of fetuses after injection on days 7 and 8, respectively (Sieber *et al.* 1978).

4.4 Genetic and related effects

4.4.1 *Humans*

Teniposide has been associated with leukaemias that show translocations similar to those seen with etoposide. In a case report, Secker-Walker *et al.* (1985) suggested that acute lymphoblastic leukaemia with translocation t(4;11) was a complication of treatment of neuroblastoma with a regimen that included teniposide. A second case of treatment-related acute lymphoblastic leukaemia with t(4;11) was reported after primary treatment for acute lymphoblastic leukaemia with a teniposide-containing regimen (Brizard *et al.*, 1991). Weh *et al.* (1986) described a case of acute monoblastic leukaemia with translocation t(9;11)(p21;q23) that arose subsequent to treatment of neuroblastoma with a teniposide-containing regimen. Teniposide has been used most often in the treatment of childhood acute lymphoblastic leukaemia, sometimes in combination with etoposide; the observations of specific leukaemia-associated chromosomal translocations in this situation, most of which involve chromosome band 11q23, are described in the monograph on etoposide (see also Pui *et al.*, 1991). In patients receiving another primary treatment regimen for acute lymphoblastic leukaemia that included teniposide as the only DNA topoisomerase II inhibitor, Verdeguer *et al.* (1992) observed three cases of treatment-related acute monoblastic leukaemia; the karyotype was normal in one case, revealed +8, t(3;17)(p11;q25), t(4;11)(q21;q23) in the second case and +8, -15, del(11)(q23)+der(15)t(15;7)(p11;7) in the third, again showing consistent involvement of chromosome band 11q23.

Hawkins *et al.* (1992) reported 10 cases of leukaemia after treatment with epipodophyllotoxin (see section 2); teniposide was used in nine cases and etoposide in one. Cytogenetic studies were performed in six cases, and translocations of chromosome band 11q23 were observed in two of these. In one case, the treatment-related leukaemia was acute lymphoblastic leukaemia with t(4;11)(q21;q23). In the other case, the translocation partner was at band 16p13. The karyotype was normal in the other four cases.

Hunger *et al.* (1992) used Southern blot analysis to examine 10 cases of leukaemia that arose after combination chemotherapy that included teniposide in eight cases and doxorubicin in two. Rearrangements of the *MLL* gene at chromosome band 11q23 were identified in seven cases with known karyotypic abnormalities and in two cases in which the karyotyping was unsuccessful. The break-points were localized in the cluster region between exons 5 and 11 of the *MLL* gene. Partner genes involved in translocations with *MLL* at the karyotypic level were located at bands 9p22, 16p13 and 19p13. In one case, the karyotype of the leukaemic cells was shown to be t(3;13)(q26;q12), and *MLL* was not rearranged.

To investigate the translocation mechanism, Atlas *et al.* (1998) examined the genomic break-point sequences in four cases of DNA topoisomerase II inhibitor-related leukaemia with translocation t(9;11)(p22;q23), which fuses *MLL* to *AF-9*. Two patients had received teniposide as the only DNA topoisomerase II inhibitor, and the karyotype showed t(9;11)(p22;q23). In one patient who received teniposide and etoposide, the karyotype showed t(9;11)(p22;q23), +der(9)t(9;11)(p22q23). The *MLL* break-points were at positions 3173, 6230 and 6784, indicating heterogeneity in the break-point distribution in the 3′ and 5′ cluster region. These break-points were proximal to regions of homology to a putative DNA topoisomerase II binding site identified *in vitro*, suggesting that DNA topoisomerase II may have played a mechanistic role in the translocation process. Evidence that such regions of homology may not accurately predict functional sites of cleavage by DNA topoisomerase II *in vivo* (Felix *et al.*, 1995) has also been presented. In one case of leukaemia, there was homology to seven of eight bases of a χ-like sequence element. Another case showed homology to VDJ recombinase signal sequences and to TRANSLIN binding sequences near the break-points in both *MLL* and *AF-9*. In addition, one of the break-points fell within an *Alu* sequence. The presence of these sequences near the translocation break-points may facilitate recombination.

In an assay for DNA topoisomerase II cleavage *in vitro*, Felix *et al.* (1995) showed that multiple cleavage sites within the *MLL* break-point cluster region are enhanced by teniposide.

4.4.2 *Experimental systems*

General reviews on the mutagenicity of inhibitors of DNA topoisomerase II enzymes, including teniposide, have been published (Anderson & Berger, 1994; Ferguson & Baguley, 1994, 1996; Baguley & Ferguson, 1998: Ferguson, 1998). The results are summarized in Table 3.

Teniposide gave mainly negative responses in a range of assays in prokaryotes and lower eukaryotes. Thus, in most studies, it did not induce significant increases in reverse mutation frequency as measured in *Salmonella typhimurium* strains TA1535, TA1537, TA1538, TA98 and TA100, *Escherichia coli* WP2 *uvr*A, and in other *E. coli* assays, in the presence or absence of exogenous metabolic activation. It also gave negative results in the SOS chromotest with *E. coli* TK104. Teniposide caused about a twofold increase in the frequency of revertant colonies in *S. typhimurium* strain

Table 3. Genetic and related effects of teniposide

Test system	Result[a] Without exogenous metabolic system	Result[a] With exogenous metabolic system	Dose[b] (LED/HID)	Reference
Prophage induction, *Escherichia coli*	–	NT	50	DeMarini & Lawrence (1992)
Escherichia coli, TK104, SOS chromotest	–	NT	8	Albertini et al. (1995)
Bacillus subtilis rec strains, differential toxicity	+	+	10 µg/disc	Nakanomyo et al. (1986)
T4 bacteriophage, reverse mutation	–	NT	660	DeMarini & Lawrence (1988)
Salmonella typhimurium TA102, reverse mutation	(+)	NT	100 µg/plate	Gupta et al. (1987)
Salmonella typhimurium TA102, reverse mutation	+	NT	250 µg/plate	Albertini et al. (1995)
Salmonella typhimurium TA1535, reverse mutation	–	–	400 µg/plate	Nakanomyo et al. (1986)
Salmonella typhimurium TA1537, reverse mutation	(+)	–	50 µg/plate	Nakanomyo et al. (1986)
Salmonella typhimurium TA1538 and TA98, reverse mutation	(+)	(+)	100 µg/plate	Nakanomyo et al. (1986)
Salmonella typhimurium TA100, reverse mutation	–	(+)	200 µg/plate	Nakanomyo et al. (1986)
Escherichia coli WP2 *uvr*A, reverse mutation	–	–	400 µg/plate	Nakanomyo et al. (1986)
Neurospora crassa, forward mutation, *ad-3A* frameshift strain	–	NT	100	Gupta (1990)
Neurospora crassa, reverse mutation, *ad-3A* frameshift strain	–	NT	525 µg/plate	Gupta (1990)
Drosophila melanogaster, somatic mutation and recombination	+		50 in feed	Frei & Würgler (1996)
DNA double-strand breaks in mouse L1210 cells *in vitro*	+	NT	0.66	Ross et al. (1984)
DNA single-strand breaks in mouse L1210 cells *in vitro*	+	NT	0.66	Kerrigan et al. (1987)
DNA–protein cross-links in mouse L1210 cells *in vitro*	+	NT	0.66	Kerrigan et al. (1987)
Mutation, Chinese hamster ovary cells, *Hprt* locus *in vitro*	+	NT	0.04	Singh & Gupta (1983)
Mutation, Chinese hamster ovary cells, *Ak* locus *in vitro*	(+)	NT	0.04	Singh & Gupta (1983)
Mutation, Chinese hamster ovary CHO-D422 cells, *Aprt* locus *in vitro*	+	NT	0.02	Han et al. (1993)
Mutation, mouse lymphoma L5178Y cells, *Tk* locus *in vitro*	+	NT	0.0005	DeMarini et al. (1987)
Mutation, mouse lymphoma L5178Y cells, *Tk* locus *in vitro*	+	NT	0.005	Albertini et al. (1995)

Table 3 (contd)

Test system	Result[a]		Dose[b] (LED/HID)	Reference
	Without exogenous metabolic system	With exogenous metabolic system		
Mutation, mouse lymphoma L5178Y cells, *Hprt* locus *in vitro*	–	NT	0.02	Albertini *et al.* (1995)
Mutation, mouse L cells, *Hprt* locus *in vitro*	+	NT	0.05	Gupta *et al.* (1987)
Sister chromatid exchange, Chinese hamster lung V79 cells *in vitro*	+	NT	0.66	Lim *et al.* (1986)
Micronucleus formation, Chinese hamster ovary CHO-K5 cells *in vitro*	+	NT	0.015	Albertini *et al.* (1995)
Chromosomal aberrations, Chinese hamster ovary cells *in vitro*	+	NT	0.005	Charron & Hancock (1991)
Chromosomal aberrations, Chinese hamster Don cells *in vitro*	+	NT	0.05	Fernández *et al.* (1995)
Chromosomal aberrations, mouse lymphoma L5178Y cells *in vitro*	+	NT	0.0005	DeMarini *et al.* (1987)
Aneuploidy[c], Chinese hamster ovary cells *in vitro*	+	NT	0.05	Charron & Hancock (1991)
Polyploidy, murine erythroleukaemic (T3CL2) cells *in vitro*	+	NT	1	Zucker *et al.* (1991)
DNA single-strand breaks, human lung carcinoma A459 cells *in vitro*	+	NT	0.066	Long *et al.* (1984)
DNA single- and double-strand breaks, human lung carcinoma A459 cells *in vitro*	+	NT	0.066	Long *et al.* (1985)
DNA double-strand breaks, Raji (Burkitt's lymphoma) cells *in vitro*	+	NT	1.32	Johnson & Beerman (1994)
DNA single-strand breaks in human colon carcinoma HT-29 and human embryonic VA-13 cells *in vitro*	+	NT	0.66	Kerrigan *et al.* (1987)
DNA–protein cross-links in human colon carcinoma HT-29 and human embryonic VA-13 cells *in vitro*	+	NT	0.66	Kerrigan *et al.* (1987)
DNA single- and double-strand breaks, human breast cancer MCF-7 cells *in vitro*	+	NT	0.66	Gewirtz *et al.* (1993)
DNA double-strand breaks, human leukaemia HL60 cells *in vitro*	+	NT	0.05	Binaschi *et al.* (1997)

Table 3 (contd)

Test system	Result[a]		Dose[b] (LED/HID)	Reference
	Without exogenous metabolic system	With exogenous metabolic system		
Micronucleus formation, bone-marrow cells of mice in vivo	+		0.5 ip × 2	Nakanomyo et al. (1986)
Chromosomal aberrations, bone marrow of pregnant Swiss mice and cells of their embryos in vivo	+		1 ip × 3	Sieber et al. (1978)
Chromosomal aberration, spermatogonial cells from Xenopus laevis, spermatocytes and spermatid stages to nuclear elongation stages observed	+	NT	3.3	Morse-Gaudio & Risley (1994)

[a] +, positive; (+), weak positive; −, negative; NT, not tested
[b] LED, lowest effective dose; HID, highest ineffective dose; in-vitro tests, μg/mL; in-vivo tests, mg/kg bw per day; ip, intraperitoneally
[c] Formation of quadriradial chromosomes due to defective segregation

TA102 and caused differential toxicity in *Bacillus subtilis* H17 rec^+ and M45 rec^-. In several of these bacterial tests, toxicity but not mutagenicity occurred at a dose of 250 µg/plate, which is higher than those studied in mammalian cells.

Teniposide did not induce prophage in *E. coli* or revert a frameshift mutant of T4 bacteriophage. The drug induced neither forward nor reverse mutations in *Neurospora crassa*.

Teniposide induced DNA breakage in mammalian cells both *in vitro* and *in vivo*. It caused protein-masked DNA double-strand breaks, DNA–protein cross-links and a small proportion of DNA single-strand breaks in various animal cells and in human cell lines. The damage induced by teniposide was found in genomic DNA in preference to episomal (Epstein-Barr virus) DNA in the Raji Burkitt lymphoma cell line. Teniposide has been suggested to inactivate DNA synthesis by inhibiting replicon cluster initiation (Suciu, 1990). Gewirtz *et al*. (1993) showed that teniposide reduced the expression of the c-*myc* oncogene in a MCF-7 human breast cancer cell line.

Teniposide caused chromosomal aberrations in cultured Chinese hamster cells and in mouse lymphoma cell lines, and micronuclei in Chinese hamster ovary (CHO-K5) cells. Teniposide induced the formation of quadriradial chromosomes and affected accurate chromosomal segregation in Chinese hamster ovary cells. Fluorescence in-situ hybridization techniques revealed that about 40% of the rearrangement sites in teniposide-induced quadriradial and triradial chromosomal configurations in Chinese hamster Don cells involved a telomere-like block of base sequences (Fernández *et al*., 1995). Teniposide induced micronuclei and chromosomal aberrations in the bone marrow of mice.

The drug induced sister chromatid exchange in V79 Chinese hamster cells and mutation and somatic recombination in *Drosophila melanogaster* in the wing spot test. It did not induce mutations at the *Hprt* locus in mouse lymphoma L5178Y cells, although it had weak effects at the same locus in Chinese hamster ovary cells. It induced primarily small colony mutants at the *Tk* locus in L5178Y cells; these mutants are usually caused by chromosomal mutations, and teniposide induced a series of deletions and duplications in the *Aprt* gene of Chinese hamster ovary cells.

Cytogenetic changes were measured in bone marrow and embryonic tissue from pregnant mice given a single intraperitoneal injection of 1.0 mg/kg bw teniposide on day 6, 7 or 8 of gestation and killed 48 h later. Treatment on day 7 or 8 increased the frequency of embryonic cells with structural aberrations, one-fourth or more of which were stable, consisting of chromosomes with metacentric or submetacentric markers. Teniposide increased the percentage of embryonic cells with numerical aberrations, but this was statistically significant only on day 8. Most of the aberrations were hypoploidy (usually monosomy) and hyperploidy (usually trisomy) (Sieber *et al*., 1978).

Whether cellular damage results in mutation or apoptosis depends on a number of factors (Ferguson & Baguley, 1994). Teniposide-induced apoptosis has been demonstrated in various cell types including unstimulated mouse splenic lymphocytes (Roy *et al*., 1992), human Hl-60 and MOLT-4 cells (Gorczyca *et al*., 1993) and human

HT-29 and HL-60 cells (Bertrand *et al.*, 1991). Teniposide can cause a widespread DNA degradative process in nuclear DNA, but mitochondrial DNA appears to be resistant (Tepper & Studzinski, 1992). Aratani *et al.* (1996) used gene transfer assays to assess whether teniposide affects non-homologous (illegitimate) recombination and found that it stimulated integration of closed circular or linearized plasmids carrying the wild-type *Aprt* gene into *Aprt*-deficient Chinese hamster cells by non-homologous (illegitimate) recombination. Treatment of simian virus 40 (SV40)-infected monkey BSC-1 cells with teniposide resulted in DNA of high relative molecular mass, which Bodley *et al.* (1993) showed to consist of recombinant SV40 DNA sequences covalently joined with cellular DNA. Their results suggest a direct role for DNA topoisomerase II in viral integration. Polyploidy induced by teniposide was demonstrated by flow cytometry techniques in Chinese hamster ovary cells (Zucker *et al.*, 1991). Teniposide induced differentiation of human HL-60 leukaemia cells (Gieseler *et al.*, 1993). It caused hypomethylation of DNA at CpG dinucleotides, resulting in altered patterns of distribution of 5-methylcytosine residues at these sites, thereby potentially modifying gene expression (Nyce, 1989; Wachsman, 1997).

In general, the effects of teniposide in mammalian cells *in vitro* occurred in the absence of exogenous metabolic activation. Various metabolic species of teniposide have been identified, but their mutagenic properties have not been studied.

Teniposide affects not only somatic cells but also germ cells. Incubation of isolated spermatogonial cells from *Xenopus laevis* with this drug led to dose-dependent induction of DNA breaks in all spermatocytes and spermatid stages to nuclear elongation stages. Spermatogonia B, meiotic divisions and pachytene spermatocytes appeared to be particularly sensitive to teniposide-induced DNA damage and production of morphological abnormalities (Morse-Gaudio & Risley, 1994).

4.5 Mechanistic considerations

Teniposide has two properties that are likely to lead to mutation.

1. It is an inhibitor of DNA topoisomerase II enzymes: Teniposide is a DNA topoisomerase II poison that has been shown to promote DNA cleavage, with a strong preference for a C or T at position -1 (Pommier *et al.*, 1991). Most of the mutational events reported in mammalian cells, including point mutations, chromosomal deletions and exchanges and aneuploidy, can be explained by this activity. Teniposide does not inhibit bacterial topoisomerases and may not mutate bacterial cells by the same mechanism as mammalian cells. Unlike many other DNA topoisomerase II poisons, teniposide does not bind to DNA, either covalently or by intercalation. Instead, it appears to interact directly with the DNA topoisomerase II enzyme (Burden & Osheroff, 1998).

2. It possesses readily oxidizable functions: Teniposide formed phenoxy radical intermediates in the presence of horseradish peroxidase or prostaglandin synthase (Haim *et al.*, 1986), but none of the mutations induced by teniposide is of the type usually associated with reactive oxygen species.

Regimens containing teniposide and other DNA topoisomerase II inhibitors are associated with leukaemias with chromosomal translocations. The role of DNA topoisomerase II inhibitors in translocations associated with leukaemia is unknown. Two possibilities are plausible. The first is that teniposide itself causes the translocations, perhaps through a cytotoxic action. The planar ring structures of epipodophyllotoxins confer an ability to form stable, stacked complexes with DNA and DNA topoisomerase II. It has been proposed that DNA cleavage induced directly by DNA topoisomerase II or by the drug-induced apoptotic cellular response is responsible for the nonrandom chromosomal translocations that lead to leukaemogenesis (Dassonneville & Bailly, 1998). In one model in which the drug causes the translocations, the process involves drug-induced DNA topoisomerase II-mediated chromosomal breakage and formation of the translocations by further processing and resolution of the breakage through cellular mechanisms of DNA repair (Felix *et al.*, 1998).

The second possibility for the role of teniposide in causing translocations is that it selects for cells that already have translocations. Indeed, *MLL* tandem duplications, a form of translocation, have been identified in peripheral blood and bone marrow of healthy adults (Schnittger *et al.*, 1998). Chemotherapy has profound effects on the kinetics of the marrow: it causes cell death, forcing many marrow stem cells to divide, which might select for the rare stem cells with a translocation (Knudson, 1992).

In favour of the first possibility is the specificity of the association between DNA topoisomerase II inhibitors, but not other forms of chemotherapy that cause cell death in the marrow (such as alkylating agents), and leukaemias characterized by translocations.

5. Summary of Data Reported and Evaluation

5.1 Exposure data

Teniposide is a semi-synthetic podophyllotoxin derivative that has been used in cancer treatment since the late 1970s. This DNA topoisomerase II inhibitor has been used in combination with other chemotherapeutic agents in the treatment of adult and childhood leukaemia, brain tumours in adults and neuroblastoma in children and, to a lesser extent, a number of other cancers.

5.2 Human carcinogenicity data

One large, well-conducted cohort study of acute lymphoblastic leukaemia in the USA and one case–control study of childhood cancer in United Kingdom found strong positive associations between the incidence of acute myeloid leukaemia and treatment with teniposide. A dose–response relationship was found in the case–control study. In both studies, teniposide was administered with other cytotoxic drugs. Although some of the other agents may have contributed to the positive association seen in the cohort study, use of these agents has not been associated with acute myeloid leukaemia in other large studies of childhood cancer. In the case–control study, the use of other potentially leukaemogenic agents was adjusted for in the analysis; however, the possibility cannot be excluded that interaction occurred between teniposide and those agents. It is unlikely that the large excess risk for acute myeloid leukaemia can be explained fully by misclassification or phenotypic change of the initial haematological malignancy.

Other cohort studies have also reported strongly increased risks for acute myeloid leukaemia after treatment of various primary malignancies with teniposide-containing regimens that also included alkylating agents or teniposide-containing regimens in combination with etoposide. In these studies, the possibility cannot be excluded that the excess risk for leukaemia was partly or wholly due to the other agents.

5.3   Animal carcinogenicity data

No data were available to the Working Group.

5.4   Other relevant data

In humans, teniposide is eliminated biphasically, with a terminal half-time of 6–10 h in adults and children. The pharmacokinetics of teniposide is linear at doses up to 1000 mg/m^2. The oral bioavailability is about 40%. About 45% of a radiolabelled dose of teniposide was excreted in the urine, 4–14% occurring as the parent drug. There are few data on the metabolism of teniposide in humans. Teniposide is highly protein-bound in plasma (99%).

In mice, the pharmacokinetics of teniposide differs from that of etoposide, a closely related drug, with lower clearance, a larger volume of distribution and a longer terminal elimination half-time. The accumulation of teniposide in leukaemic cells *in vitro* was some 15 times higher than that of etoposide applied at the same concentration. Metabolism to the catechol and quinone metabolites *in vitro* has been described.

The major dose-limiting toxic effect of teniposide in clinical trials is myelosuppression, manifest mainly as leukopenia. Less severe effects, including nausea and vomiting, diarrhoea and alopecia, are common; less common effects include transient increases in liver enzyme activity, hypertension and hypersensitivity reactions. Embryotoxicity and teratogenicity, especially in the heart and central nervous system, have been observed in mice.

Teniposide is orders of magnitude more toxic in mammalian than in microbial cells and is mutagenic in mammalian cells. The effects in mammals arise primarily because teniposide is a poison of DNA topoisomerase II enzymes. Teniposide causes accumulation of protein-masked double-stranded DNA breaks in cells and, with time, a variety of chromosomal aberrations. It is also an effective recombinogen. The predominant mutagenic effects in mammalian cells appear to involve deletion and/or interchange of large DNA segments. Teniposide also induces aneuploidy and polyploidy. It may affect gene expression through hypomethylation of DNA.

Teniposide-containing regimens are strongly related to leukaemia in which the cells contain chromosomal translocations similar to those induced by etoposide and other DNA topoisomerase II inhibitors. The translocations are key events in leukaemogenesis.

5.5 Evaluation

There is *limited evidence* in humans for the carcinogenicity of teniposide.

There is *inadequate evidence* in experimental animals for the carcinogenicity of teniposide.

Overall evaluation

Teniposide is *probably carcinogenic to humans (Group 2A)*.

In reaching this conclusion, the Working Group noted that teniposide causes distinctive cytogenetic lesions in leukaemic cells that can be readily distinguished from those induced by alkylating agents. The short latency of these leukaemias contrasts with that of leukaemia induced by alkylating agents. Potent protein-masked DNA breakage and clastogenic effects occur in human cells *in vitro* and animal cells *in vivo*.

6. References

Albertini, S., Chételat, A.-A., Miller, B., Muster, W., Pujadas, E., Strobel, R. & Gocke, E. (1995) Genotoxicity of 17 gyrase- and four mammalian topoisomerase II-poisons in prokaryotic and eukaryotic test systems. *Mutagenesis*, **10**, 343–351

Allen, L.M. (1978) Comparison of uptake and binding of two epipodophyllotoxin glucopyranosides, 4′-demethyl epipodophyllotoxin thenylidene-β-D-glucoside and 4′-demethyl epipodophyllotoxin ethylidene-β-D-glucoside, in the L1210 leukemia cell. *Cancer Res.*, **38**, 2549–2554

Allen, L.M. & Creaven, P.J. (1975) Comparison of the human pharmacokinetics of VM-26 and VP-16, two antineoplastic epipodophyllotoxin glucopyranoside derivatives. *Eur. J. Cancer*, **11**, 697–707

American Hospital Formulary Service (1997) *AHFS Drug Information® 97*, Bethesda, MD, American Society of Health-System Pharmacists, pp. 866–868

Anderson, R.D. & Berger, N.A. (1994) Mutagenicity and carcinogenicity of topoisomerase-interactive agents. *Mutat. Res.*, **309**, 109–142

Aratani, Y., Andoh, T. & Koyama, H. (1996) Effects of DNA topoisomerase inhibitors on non-homologous and homologous recombination in mammalian cells. *Mutat. Res.*, **362**, 181–191

Atlas, M., Head, D., Behm, F., Schmidt, E., Zeleznik-Le, N.J., Roe, B.A., Burian, D. & Domer, P.H. (1998) Cloning and sequence analysis of four t(9;11) therapy-related leukemia breakpoints. *Leukemia*, **12**, 1895–1902

Baguley, B.C. & Ferguson, L.R. (1998) Mutagenic properties of topoisomerase-targeted drugs. *Biochim. biophys. Acta*, **1400**, 213–222

Baker, D.K., Relling, M.V., Pui, C.-H., Christensen, M.L., Evans, W.E. & Rodman, J.H. (1992) Increased teniposide clearance with concomitant anticonvulsant therapy. *J. clin. Oncol.*, **10**, 311–315

Berenberg, J.L., Tangen, C., Macdonald, J.S., Barlogie, B. & Laufman, L.R. (1993) VM-26 in gastric cancer. A Southwest Oncology Group study. *Invest. new Drugs*, **11**, 333–334

Bertrand, R., Sarang, M., Jenkin, J., Kerrigan, D. & Pommier, Y. (1991) Differential induction of secondary DNA fragmentation by topoisomerase II inhibitors in human tumor cell lines with amplified c-*myc* expression. *Cancer Res.*, **51**, 6280–6285

Binaschi, M., Capranico, G., Dal Bo, L. & Zunino, F. (1997) Relationship between lethal effects and topoisomerase II mediated double strand breaks produced by anthracyclines with different sequence specificity. *Am. Soc. Pharmacol. exp. Ther.*, 51, 1053–1059

Boas, J., Rasmussen, D., Hansen, O.P., Engelholm, S.A. & Dombernowsky, P. (1990) Phase II study of teniposide in advanced breast cancer. *Cancer Chemother. Pharmacol.*, **25**, 463–464

Bodley, A.L., Huang, H.-C., Yu, C. & Liu, L.F. (1993) Integration of simian virus 40 into cellular DNA occurs at or near topoisomerase II cleavage hot spots induced by VM-26 (teniposide). *Mol. cell. Biol.*, **13**, 6190–6200

Brizard, A., Huret, J.L., Benz-Lemoine, E., Guilhot, F., Giraud, C. & Tanzer, J. (1991) Two cases of t(4;11) acute lymphoblastic leukemia (ALL) following ALL without the t(4;11): second or secondary leukemias? *Br. J. Haematol.*, **79**, 130–131

Broggini, M., Colombo, T. & D'Incalci, M. (1983) Activity and pharmacokinetics of teniposide in Lewis lung carcinoma-bearing mice. *Cancer Treat. Rep.*, **67**, 555–559

Budavari, S., ed. (1996) *The Merck Index*, 12th Ed., Whitehouse Station, NJ, Merck & Co., pp. 1562–1563

Burden, D.A. & Osheroff, N. (1998) Mechanism of action of eukaryotic topoisomerase II and drugs targeted to the enzyme. *Biochim. biophys. Acta*, **1400**, 139–154

Canadian Pharmaceutical Association (1997) *CPS Compendium of Pharmaceuticals and Specialties*, 32nd Ed., Ottawa, pp. 1740–1741

Canal, P., Bugat, R., Michel, C., Roche, H., Soula, G. & Combes, P.F. (1985) Pharmacokinetics of teniposide (VM 26) after iv administration in serum and malignant ascites of patients with ovarian carcinoma. *Cancer Chemother. Pharmacol.*, **15**, 149–152

Charron, M. & Hancock, R. (1991) Chromosome recombination and defective genome segregation induced in Chinese hamster cells by the topoisomerase II inhibitor VM-26. *Chromosoma*, **100**, 97–102

CIS Information Services (1998) *Worldwide Bulk Drug Users Directory, 1997/98 Edition*, Dallas, TX [CD-ROM]

Clark, P.I. & Slevin, M.L. (1987) The clinical pharmacology of etoposide and teniposide. *Clin. Pharmacokinet.*, **12**, 223–252

Colombo, T., Broggini, M., Vaghi, M., Amato, G., Erba, E. & D'Incalci, M. (1986) Comparison between VP 16 and VM 26 in Lewis lung carcinoma of the mouse. *Eur. J. Cancer clin. Oncol.*, **22**, 173–179

Cox, E.B., Vogel, C.L., Carpenter, J.T., Jr & Raney, M. (1988) Phase II evaluation of teniposide (VM-26) in metastatic breast carcinoma. A Southeastern Cancer Study Group trial. *Invest. new Drugs*, **6**, 37–39

Creaven, P.J. & Allen, L.M. (1975) PTG, a new antineoplastic epipodophyllotoxin. *Clin. Pharmacol. Ther.*, **18**, 227–233

Dassonneville, L. & Bailly, C. (1998) [Chromosomal translocations and leukaemias induced by anticarcinogenic drugs that inhibit topoisomerase II.] *Bull. Cancer*, **85**, 254–261 (in French)

DeMarini, D.M. & Lawrence, B.K. (1988) Mutagenicity of topoisomerase-active agents in bacteriophage T4. *Teratog. Carcinog. Mutag.*, **8**, 293–301

DeMarini, D.M. & Lawrence, B.K. (1992) Prophage induction by DNA topoisomerase II poisons and reactive-oxygen species: Role of DNA breaks. *Mutat. Res.*, **267**, 1–17

DeMarini, D.M., Brock, K.H., Doerr, C.L. & Moore, M.M. (1987) Mutagenicity and clastogenicity of teniposide (VM-26) in L5178Y/TK$^{+/-}$-3.7.2C mouse lymphoma cells. *Mutat. Res.*, **187**, 141–149

D'Incalci, M., Rossi, C., Sessa, C., Urso, R., Zucchetti, M., Farina, P. & Mangioni, C. (1985) Pharmacokinetics of teniposide in patients with ovarian cancer. *Cancer Treat. Rep.*, **69**, 73–77

Evans, W.E., Sinkule, J.A., Crom, W.R., Dow, L., Look, A.T. & Rivera, G. (1982) Pharmacokinetics of teniposide (VM26) and etoposide (VP16-213) in children with cancer. *Cancer Chemother. Pharmacol.*, **7**, 147–150

Evans, W.E., Crom, W.R., Sinkule, J.A., Yee, G.C., Stewart, C.F. & Hutson, P.R. (1983) Pharmacokinetics of anticancer drugs in children. *Drug Metab. Rev.*, **14**, 847–886

Evans, W.E., Rodman, J.H., Relling, M.V., Petros, W.P., Stewart, C.F., Pui, C.-H. & Rivera, G.K. (1992) Differences in teniposide disposition and pharmacodynamics in patients with newly diagnosed and relapsed acute lymphocytic leukemia. *J. Pharmacol. exp. Ther.*, **260**, 71–77

Felix, C.A., Lange, B.J., Hosler, M.R., Fertala, J. & Bjornsti, M.-A. (1995) Chromosome band 11q23 translocation breakpoints are DNA topoisomerase II cleavage sites. *Cancer Res.*, **55**, 4287–4292

Felix, C.A., Walker, A.H., Lange, B.J., Williams, T.M., Winick, N.J., Cheung, N.-K.V., Lovett, B.D., Nowell, P.C., Blair, I.A. & Rebbeck, T.R. (1998) Association of *CYP3A4* genotype with treatment-related leukemia. *Proc. natl Acad. Sci. USA*, **95**, 13176–13181

Ferguson, L.R. (1998) Inhibitors of topoisomerase II enzymes: A unique group of environmental mutagens and carcinogens. *Mutat. Res.*, **400**, 271–278

Ferguson, L.R. & Baguley, B.C. (1994) Topoisomerase II enzymes and mutagenicity. *Environ. mol. Mutag.*, **24**, 245–261

Ferguson, L.R. & Baguley, B.C. (1996) Mutagenicity of anticancer drugs that inhibit topoisomerase enzymes. *Mutat. Res.*, **355**, 91–101

Fernández, J.L., Gosálvez, J. & Goyanes, V. (1995) High frequency of mutagen-induced chromatid exchanges at interstitial telomere-like DNA sequence blocks of Chinese hamster cells. *Chromosome Res.*, **3**, 281–284

Frei, H. & Würgler, F.E. (1996) Induction of somatic mutation and recombination by four inhibitors of eukaryotic topoisomerases assayed in the wing spot test of *Drosophila melanogaster*. *Mutagenesis*, **11**, 315–325

Gennaro, A.R. (1995) *Remington: The Science and Practice of Pharmacy*, 19th Ed., Easton, PA, Mack Publishing, Vol. II, p. 1260

Gewirtz, D.A., Orr, M.S., Fornari, F.A., Randolph, J.K., Yalowich, J.C., Ritke, M.K., Povirk, L.F. & Bunch, R.T. (1993) Dissociation between bulk damage to DNA and the antiproliferative activity of teniposide (VM-26) in the MCF-7 breast tumor cell line: Evidence for induction of gene-specific damage and alterations in gene expression. *Cancer Res.*, **53**, 3547–3554

Giaccone, G. (1992) Teniposide alone and in combination chemotherapy in small cell lung cancer. *Semin. Oncol.*, **19**, 75–80

Giaccone, G., Splinter, T.A.W., Kirkpatrick, A., Dalesio, O., van Zandwijk, N. & McVie, J. G. (1992) The European organization for research and treatment of cancer experience with teniposide: Preliminary results of a randomized study in non-small lung cancer. *Semin. Oncol.*, **19**, 98–102

Gieseler, F., Boege, F., Clark, M. & Meyer, P. (1993) Correlation between the DNA-binding affinity of topoisomerase inhibiting drugs and their capacity to induce hematopoetic cell differentiation. *Toxicol. Lett.*, **67**, 331–340

Gigante, M., Sorio, R., Colussi, A.M., Sandrin, A., De Appollonia, L., Galligioni, E., Freschi, A., Talamini, R., Toffoli, G. & Boiocchi, M. (1995) Effect of cyclosporine on teniposide pharmacokinetics and pharmacodynamics in patients with renal cell cancer. *Anticancer Drugs*, **6**, 479–482

Gorczyca, W., Gong, J. & Darzynkiewicz, Z. (1993) Detection of DNA strand breaks in individual apoptotic cells by the *in situ* terminal deoxynucleotidyl transferase and nick translation assays. *Cancer Res.*, **53**, 1945–1951

Grozea, P.N., Crowley, J.J., Canfield, V.A., Kingsbury, L., Ross, S.W., Beltran, G.S., Laufman, L.R., Weiss, G.R. & Livingston, R.B. (1997) Teniposide (VM-26) as a single drug treatment for patients with extensive small cell lung carcinoma: A phase II study of the Southwest Oncology Group. *Cancer*, **80**, 1029–1033

Gupta, R. (1990) Tests for the genotoxicity of m-AMSA, etoposide, teniposide and ellipticine in *Neurospora crassa*. *Mutat. Res.*, **240**, 47–58

Gupta, R.S., Bromke, A., Bryant, D.W., Gupta, R., Singh, B. & McCalla, D.R. (1987) Etoposide (VP16) and teniposide (VM26): Novel anticancer drugs, strongly mutagenic in mammalian but not prokaryotic test systems. *Mutagenesis*, **2**, 179–186

Haim, N., Roman, J., Nemec, J. & Sinha, B.K. (1986) Peroxidative free radical formation and O-demethylation of etoposide(VP-16) and teniposide(VM-26). *Biochem. biophys. Res. Commun.*, **135**, 215–220

Han, Y.-H., Austin, M.J.F., Pommier, Y. & Povirk, L.F. (1993) Small deletion and insertion mutations induced by the topoisomerase II inhibitor teniposide in CHO cells and comparison with sites of drug-stimulated DNA cleavage *in vitro*. *J. mol. Biol.*, **229**, 52–66

Hawkins, M.M., Kinnier Wilson, L.M., Stovall, M.A., Marsden, H.B., Potok, M.H.N., Kingston, J.E. & Chessells, J.M. (1992) Epipodophyllotoxins, alkylating agents, and radiation and risk of secondary leukaemia after childhood cancer. *Br. med. J.*, **304**, 951–958

Hirsch, F.R., Dombernowsky, P. & Hansen, H.H. (1994) Treatment of small cell lung cancer: The Copenhagen experience. *Anticancer Res.*, **14**, 317–320

Holthuis, J.J.M., de Vries, L.G.E., Postmus, P.E., van Oort, W.W.J., Verleun, H., Hulshoff, A., Sleijfer, D.T. & Mulder, N.H. (1987) Pharmacokinetics of high-dose teniposide. *Cancer Treat. Rep.*, **71**, 599–603

Hunger, S.P., Sklar, J. & Link, M.P. (1992) Acute lymphoblastic leukemia occurring as a second malignant neoplasm in childhood: Report of three cases and review of the literature. *J. clin. Oncol.*, **10**, 156–163

IARC (1987) *IARC Monographs on the Evaluation of Carcinogenic Risks to Humans*, Suppl. 7, *Overall Evaluations of Carcinogenicity: An Updating of* IARC Monographs *Volumes 1–42*, Lyon, IARC*Press*, pp. 254–259

Imbert, T.F. (1998) Discovery of podophyllotoxins. *Biochimie*, **80**, 207–222

Jensen, P.B., Roed, H., Skovsgaard, T., Friche, E., Vindelov, L., Hansen, H.H. & Spang-Thomsen, M. (1990) Antitumor activity of the two epipodophyllotoxin derivatives VP-16 and VM-26 in preclinical systems: A comparison of in vitro and in vivo drug evaluation. *Cancer Chemother. Pharmacol.*, **27**, 194–198

Johnson, P.G. & Beerman, T.A. (1994) Damage induced in episomal EBV DNA in Raji cells by antitumor drugs as measured by pulsed field gel electrophoresis. *Anal. Biochem.*, **220**, 103–114

Keller-Juslén, C., Kuhn, M., Stahelin, H. & von Wartburg, A. (1971) Synthesis and antimitotic activity of glycosidic lignan derivatives related to podophyllotoxin. *J. med. Chem.*, **14**, 936–940

Kerrigan, D., Pommier, Y. & Kohn, K.W. (1987) Protein-linked DNA strand breaks produced by etoposide and teniposide in mouse L1210 and human VA-13 and HT-29 cell lines: Relationship to cytotoxicity. *Natl Cancer Inst. Monogr.*, **4**, 117–121

Kettenes-van den Bosch, J.J., Holthuis, J.J.M. & Bult, A. (1990) Teniposide. In: Florey, K., ed., *Analytical Profiles of Drug Substances*, New York, Academic Press, Vol. 19, pp. 575–600

Knudson, A.G. (1992) Stem cell regulation, tissue ontogeny, and oncogenic events. *Semin. Cancer Biol.*, **3**, 99–106

Kreissman, S.G., Gelber, R.D., Cohen, H.J., Clavell, L.A., Leavitt, P. & Sallan, S.E. (1992) Incidence of secondary acute myelogenous leukemia after treatment of childhood acute lymphoblastic leukemia. *Cancer*, **70**, 2208–2213

van Leeuwen, F.E., Chorus, A.M.J., van den Belt-Dusebout, A.W., Hagenbeek, A., Noyon, R., van Kerkhoff, E.H.M., Pinedo, H.M. & Somers, R. (1994) Leukemia risk following Hodgkin's disease: Relation to cumulative dose of alkylating agents, treatment with teniposide combinations, number of episodes of chemotherapy, and bone marrow damage. *J. clin. Oncol.*, **12**, 1063–1073

Lim, M., Liu, L.F., Jacobson-Kram, D. & Williams, J.R. (1986) Induction of sister chromatid exchanges by inhibitors of topoisomerases. *Cell Biol. Toxicol.*, **2**, 485–494

LINFO Läkemedelsinformation AB (1998) *FASS 1998 Läkemedel i Sverige*, Stockholm, pp. 1258–1260

Long, B.H., Musial, S.T. & Brattain, M.G. (1984) Comparison of cytotoxicity and DNA breakage activity of congeners of podophyllotoxin including VP16-213 and VM26: A quantitative structure–activity relationship. *Biochemistry*, **23**, 1183–1188

Long, B.H., Musial, S.T. & Brattain, M.G. (1985) Single- and double-strand DNA breakage and repair in human lung adenocarcinoma cells exposed to etoposide and teniposide. *Cancer Res.*, **45**, 3106–3112

Lowenthal, R.M., Funnell, C.F., Hope, D.M., Stewart, I.G. & Humphrey, D.C. (1982) Normal infant after combination chemotherapy including teniposide for Burkitt's lymphoma in pregnancy. *Med. pediatr. Oncol.*, **10**, 165–169

Macbeth, F.R. (1982) VM26: Phase I and II studies. *Cancer Chemother. Pharmacol.*, **7**, 87–91

Medical Economics Data Production (1999) *PDR®: Physicians' Desk Reference*, 53rd Ed., Montvale, NJ, pp. 810–812

Morse-Gaudio, M. & Risley, M.S. (1994) Topoisomerase II expression and VM-26 induction of DNA breaks during spermatogenesis in *Xenopus laevis*. *J. Cell Sci.*, **107**, 2887–2898

Muggia, F.M. (1994) Teniposide: Overview of its therapeutic potential in adult cancers. *Cancer Chemother. Pharmacol.*, **34** (Suppl.), 127–133

Nakanomyo, H., Hiraoka, M. & Shiraya, M. (1986) [Mutagenicity tests of etoposide and teniposide.] *J. toxicol. Sci.*, **11**, 301–310 (in Japanese)

Neglia, J.P., Meadows, A.T., Robison, L.L., Kim, T.H., Newton, W.A., Ruymann, F.B., Sather, H.N. & Hammond, G.D. (1991) Second neoplasms after acute lymphoblastic leukemia in childhood. *New Engl. J. Med.*, **325**, 1330–1336

Nyce, J. (1989) Drug-induced DNA hypermethylation and drug resistance in human tumors. *Cancer Res.*, **49**, 5829–5836

O'Dwyer, P.J., King, S.A., Fortner, C.L. & Leyland-Jones, B. (1986) Hypersensitivity reactions to teniposide (VM-26): An analysis. *J. clin. Oncol.*, **4**, 1262–1269

Oishi, N., Fleming, T.R., Laufman, L., Ungerleider, J.S., Natale, R.B., Einstein, A.B., Jr, Von Hoff, D.D. & Macdonald, J.S. (1990) VM-26 in colorectal carcinoma: A Southwest Oncology Group study. *Invest. new Drugs*, **8**, 93–95

Petros, W.P., Rodman, J.H., Mirro, J., Jr & Evans, W.E. (1991) Pharmacokinetics of continuous-infusion amsacrine and teniposide for the treatment of relapsed childhood acute non-lymphocytic leukemia. *Cancer Chemother. Pharmacol.*, **27**, 397–400

Pommier, Y., Capranico, G., Orr, A. & Kohn, K.W. (1991) Local base sequence preferences for DNA cleavage by mammalian topoisomerase II in the presence of amsacrine or teniposide. *Nucleic Acids Res.*, **19**, 5973–5980

Pui, C.H., Behm, F.G., Raimondi, S.C., Dodge, R.K., George, S.L., Rivera, G.K., Mirro, J., Jr, Kalwinsky, D.K., Dahl, G.V. & Murphy, S.B. (1989) Secondary acute myeloid leukemia in children treated for acute lymphoid leukemia. *New Engl. J. Med.*, **321**, 136–142

Pui, C.-H., Ribeiro, R.C., Hancock, M.L., Rivera, G.K., Evans, W.E., Raimondi, S.C., Head, D.R., Behm, F.G., Mahmoud, M.H., Sandlund, J.T. & Crist, W.M. (1991) Acute myeloid leukemia in children treated with epipodophyllotoxins for acute lymphoblastic leukemia. *New Engl. J. Med.*, **325**, 1682–1687

Relling, M.V., Evans, R., Dass, C., Desiderio, D.M. & Nemec, J. (1992) Human cytochrome P450 metabolism of teniposide and etoposide. *J. Pharmacol. exp. Ther.*, **261**, 491–496

Relling, M.V., Nemec, J., Schuetz, E.G., Schuetz, J.D., Gonzalez, F.J. & Korzekwa, K.R. (1994) *O*-Demethylation of epipodophyllotoxins is catalyzed by human cytochrome P450 3A4. *Mol. Pharmacol.*, **45**, 352–358

Rivera, G.K., Pui, C.-H., Santana, V.M., Pratt, C.B. & Crist, W.M. (1994) Epipodophyllotoxins in the treatment of childhood cancer. *Cancer Chemother. Pharmacol.*, **34** (Suppl.), 89–95

Rodman, J.H., Abromowitch, M., Sinkule, J.A., Hayes, F.A., Rivera, G.K. & Evans, W.E. (1987) Clinical pharmacodynamics of continuous infusion teniposide: Systemic exposure as a determinant of response in a phase I trial. *J. clin. Oncol.*, **5**, 1007–1014

Ross, W., Rowe, T., Glisson, B., Yalowich, J. & Liu, L. (1984) Role of topoisomerase II in mediating epipodophyllotoxin-induced DNA cleavage. *Cancer Res.*, **44**, 5857–5860

Rossi, C., Zucchetti, M., Sessa, C., Urso, R., Mangioni, C. & D'Incalci, M. (1984) Pharmacokinetic study of VM26 given as a prolonged IV infusion to ovarian cancer patients. *Cancer Chemother. Pharmacol.*, **13**, 211–214

Rote Liste Sekretariat (1998) *Rote Liste 1998*, Frankfurt, Rote Liste Service GmbH, p. 86–120

Roy, C., Brown, D.L., Little, J.E., Valentine, B.K., Walker, P.R., Sikorska, M., Leblanc, J. & Chaly, N. (1992) The topoisomerase II inhibitor teniposide (VM-26) induces apoptosis in unstimulated mature murine lymphocytes. *Exp. Cell Res.*, **200**, 416–424

Royal Pharmaceutical Society of Great Britain (1999) *Martindale, The Extra Pharmacopoeia*, 13th Ed., London, The Pharmaceutical Press [MicroMedex Online: Health Care Series]

Schnittger, S., Wormann, B., Hiddemann, W. & Griesinger, F. (1998) Partial tandem duplications of the *MLL* gene are detectable in peripheral blood and bone marrow of nearly all healthy donors. *Blood*, **92**, 1728–1734

Secker-Walker, L.M., Stewart, E.L. & Todd, A. (1985) Acute lymphoblastic leukaemia with t(4;11) follows neuroblastoma: A late effect of treatment? *Med. pediatr. Oncol.*, **13**, 48–50

Sieber, S.M., Whang-Peng, C., Botkin, C. & Knutsen, T. (1978) Teratogenic and cytogenic effects of some plant derived antitumor agents (vincristine, colchicine, maytansine, VP-16-213 and VM-26) in mice. *Teratology*, **18**, 31–47

Singh, B. & Gupta, R.S. (1983) Comparison of the mutagenic responses of 12 anticancer drugs at the hypoxanthine-guanine phosphoribosyl transferase and adenosine kinase loci in Chinese hamster ovary cells. *Environ Mutag.*, **5**, 871–880

Sinkule, J.A., Stewart, C.F., Crom, W.R., Melton, E.T., Dahl, G.V. & Evans, W.E. (1984) Teniposide (VM26) disposition in children with leukemia. *Cancer Res.*, **44**, 1235–1237

Smit, E.F., Ousterhuis, B.E., Berendsen, H.H., Sleijfer, D.T. & Postmus, P.E. (1992) Phase I study of oral teniposide (VM-26). *Semin. Oncol.*, **19**, 35–39

Smith, M.A., Rubinstein, L., Anderson, J.R., Arthur, D., Catalano, P.J., Freidlin, B., Heyn, R., Khayat, A., Krailo, M., Land, V.J., Miser, J., Shuster, J. & Vena, D. (1999) Secondary leukemia or myelodysplastic syndrome after treatment with epipodophyllotoxins. *J. clin. Oncol.*, **17**, 569–577

Sørensen, J.B., Bach, F., Dombernowsky, P. & Hansen, H.H. (1991) Phase II study of teniposide in adenocarcinoma of the lung. *Cancer Chemother. Pharmacol.*, **27**, 487–489

Sorio, R., Tirelli, U., Zagonel, V., Carbone, A. & Monfardini, S. (1990) Phase II study of teniposide (VM26) in cutaneous T-cell lymphomas. *Am. J. clin. Oncol.*, **13**, 14–16

Splinter, T.A.W., Holthuis, J.J.M., Kok, T.C. & Post, M.H. (1992) Absolute bioavailability and pharmacokinetics of oral teniposide. *Semin. Oncol.*, **19**, 28–34

Stewart, D.J., Grewaal, D., Redmond, M.D., Mikhael, N.Z., Montpetit, V.A.J., Goel, R. & Green, R.M. (1993) Human autopsy tissue distribution of the epipodophyllotoxins etoposide and teniposide. *Cancer Chemother. Pharmacol.*, **32**, 368–372

Suciu, D. (1990) Inhibition of DNA synthesis and cytotoxic effects of some DNA topoisomerase II and gyrase inhibitors in Chinese hamster V79 cells. *Mutat. Res.*, **243**, 213–218

Swiss Pharmaceutical Society, ed. (1999) *Index Nominum, International Drug Directory*, 16th Ed., Stuttgart, Medpharm Scientific Publishers [MicroMedex Online: Health Care Series]

Tepper, C.G. & Studzinski, G.P. (1992) Teniposide induces nuclear but not mitochondrial DNA degradation. *Cancer Res.*, **52**, 3384–3390

Thomas, J., ed. (1998) *Australian Prescription Products Guide*, 27th Ed., Victoria, Australian Pharmaceutical Publishing, Vol. 1, pp. 2954–2956

Tirelli, U., Carbone, A., Crivellari, D., Volpe, R., Franchin, G., Veronesi, A., Galligioni, E., Trovò, M., Tumolo, S. & Grigoletto, E. (1984) A phase II trial of teniposide (VM 26) in advanced non-Hodgkin's lymphoma, with emphasis on the treatment of elderly patients. *Cancer*, **54**, 393–396

Toffoli, G., Sorio, R., Gigante, M., Corona, G., Galligioni, E. & Boiocchi, M. (1997) Cyclosporin A as a multidrug-resistant modulator in patients with renal cell carcinoma treated with teniposide. *Br. J. Cancer*, **75**, 715–721

Verdeguer, A., Ruiz, J.G., Ferris, J., Esquembre, C., Tasso, M.J., Fernandez, J.M., Prieto, F. & Castel, V. (1992) Acute nonlymphoblastic leukemia in children treated for acute lymphoblastic leukemia with an intensive regimen including teniposide. *Med. pediat. Oncol.*, **20**, 48–52

de Vries, E.G., Mulder, N.H., Postmus, P.E., Vriesendorp, R., Willemse, P.H. & Sleijfer, D.T. (1986) High-dose teniposide for refractory malignancies: A phase I study. *Cancer Treat. Rep.*, **70**, 595–598

Wachsman, J.T. (1997) DNA methylation and the association between genetic and epigenetic changes: Relation to carcinogenesis. *Mutat. Res.*, **375**, 1–8

Weh, H.J., Kabisch, H., Landbeck, G. & Hossfeld, D.K. (1986) Translocation (9;11)(p21;q23) in a child with acute monoblastic leukemia following 2½ years after successful chemotherapy for neuroblastoma. *J. clin. Oncol.*, **4**, 1518–1520

Zucchetti, M., Rossi, C., Knerich, R., Donelli, M.G., Butti, G., Silvani, V., Gaetani, P. & D'Incalci, M. (1991) Concentrations of VP16 and VM26 in human brain tumors. *Ann. Oncol.*, **2**, 63–66

Zucker, R.M., Adams, D.J., Bair, K.W. & Elstein, K.H. (1991) Polyploidy induction as a consequence of topoisomerase inhibition. A flow cytometric assessment. *Biochem. Pharmacol.*, **42**, 2199–2208

MITOXANTRONE

1. Exposure Data

1.1 Chemical and physical data

1.1.1 Nomenclature

Mitoxantrone

Chem. Abstr. Serv. Reg. No.: 65271-80-9
Chem. Abstr. Name: 1,4-Dihydroxy-5,8-bis[{2-[(2-hydroxyethyl)amino]ethyl}-amino]- 9,10-anthracenedione
IUPAC Systematic Name: 1,4-Dihydroxy-5,8-bis-[{2-[(2-hydroxyethyl)amino]-ethyl}-amino]anthraquinone
Synonyms: DHAQ; dihydroxyanthraquinone; mitoxanthrone; mitozantrone

Mitoxantrone dihydrochloride

Chem. Abstr. Serv. Reg. No.: 70476-82-3
Chem. Abstr. Name: 1,4-Dihydroxy-5,8-bis[{2-[(2-hydroxyethyl)amino]ethyl}-amino]- 9,10-anthracenedione, dihydrochloride
IUPAC Systematic Name: 1,4-Dihydroxy-5,8-bis-[{2-[(2-hydroxyethyl)amino]-ethyl}-amino]anthraquinone dihydrochloride
Synonyms: CL 232315; DHAD; mitoxanthrone dihydrochloride; mitozantrone hydrochloride

1.1.2 Structural and molecular formulae and relative molecular mass

Mitoxantrone

$C_{22}H_{28}N_4O_6$ Relative molecular mass: 444.49

Mitoxantrone dihydrochloride

$C_{22}H_{28}N_4O_6 \cdot 2HCl$ Relative molecular mass: 517.41

1.1.3 *Chemical and physical properties of the pure substances*

Mitoxantrone

(a) *Description*: Crystalline solid (Budavari, 1996)
(b) *Melting-point*: 160–162 °C (Budavari, 1996)
(c) *Solubility*: Sparingly soluble in water; slightly soluble in methanol; practically insoluble in acetone, acetonitrile and chloroform (Budavari, 1996)

Mitoxantrone dihydrochloride

(a) *Description*: Hygroscopic blue–black solid (Budavari, 1996)
(b) *Melting-point*: 203–205 °C (Budavari, 1996)
(c) *Spectroscopy data*: Ultraviolet, infrared, nuclear magnetic resonance (proton and ^{13}C) and mass spectral data have been reported (Beijnen *et al.*, 1988)
(d) *Solubility*: Sparingly soluble in water; slightly soluble in methanol; practically insoluble in acetone, acetonitrile and chloroform (Budavari, 1996)
(e) *Dissociation constants*: pK_a, 5.99, 8.13 (Gennaro, 1995)

1.1.4 *Technical products and impurities*

Mitoxantrone hydrochloride is the common name for the dihydrochloride salt. It is available mainly as 5-, 10-, 12.5- and 15-mL solutions for intravenous infusion containing 2.33 mg/mL mitoxantrone hydrochloride, equivalent to 2 mg/mL of mitoxantrone. The injection solution may also contain acetic acid, sodium acetate, sodium chloride, sodium metabisulfite and sodium sulfate as excipients (Gennaro, 1995; Canadian Pharmaceutical Association, 1997; British Medical Association/Royal Pharmaceutical Society of Great Britain, 1998; Editions du Vidal, 1998; LINFO Läkemedelsinformation AB, 1998; Rote Liste Sekretariat, 1998; Thomas, 1998; US Pharmacopeial Convention, 1998a).

The following impurities in mitoxantrone hydrochloride are limited by the requirements of *The European Pharmacopoeia*: 1-amino-5,8-dihydroxy-4-[{2-[(2-hydroxyethyl)amino]ethyl}amino]anthracene-9,10-dione; 5-hydroxy-1,4-bis[{2-[(2-hydroxyethyl)amino]ethyl}amino]anthracene-9,10-dione; 2-chloro-1,4-dihydroxy-5,8-bis[{2-[(2-hydroxyethyl)amino]ethyl}amino]anthracene-9,10-dione; and 8,11-dihydroxy-4-(2-hydroxyethyl)-6-[{2-[(2-hydroxyethyl)amino]ethyl}amino]-1,2,3,4-tetrahydronaphtho-[2,3-*f*]quinoxaline-7,12-dione (Council of Europe, 1998).

Trade names for mitoxantrone hydrochloride include Mitoxantrona Filaxis, Mitoxantrona Raffo, Mitoxantron AWD, Mitoxantrone, Novanthrone, Novantron, Novantrone and Pralifan (Swiss Pharmaceutical Society, 1999).

1.1.5 *Analysis*

Several international pharmacopoeias specify infrared absorption spectrophotometry with comparison to standards as the method for identifying mitoxantrone hydrochloride; liquid chromatography is used to assay its purity. In pharmaceutical preparations, mitoxantrone hydrochloride is identified by ultraviolet absorption spectrophotometry, and liquid chromatography is used to assay for its content (US Pharmacopeial Convention, 1994; Council of Europe, 1998; US Pharmacopeial Convention, 1998b).

High-performance liquid chromatography is the most useful analytical tool for analysing mitoxantrone and its metabolites in biological matrices. Ion-pair chromatography and radioimmunoassay have also been used (Beijnen *et al.*, 1988).

1.2 Production

The synthesis of mitoxantrone hydrochloride involves reacting leuco-1,4,5,8-tetrahydroxyanthraquinone with 2-[(2-aminoethyl)amino]ethanol to form 1,4-dihydroxy-6,7-dihydro-5,8-bis[{2-[(2-hydroxyethyl)amino]ethyl}amino]-9,10-anthracenedione. This product is aromatized with chloranil as the oxidant, and it is converted into mitoxantrone hydrochloride by treatment with hydrogen chloride in ethanol (Beijnen *et al.*, 1988).

Information available in 1999 indicated that mitoxantrone and mitoxantrone hydrochloride were manufactured and/or formulated in seven and 31 countries, respectively (CIS Information Services, 1998; Royal Pharmaceutical Society of Great Britain; 1999; Swiss Pharmaceutical Society, 1999).

1.3 Use

Mitoxantrone is a cytotoxic drug used in the treatment of malignant disease in humans and animals. It is an inhibitor of DNA topoisomerase II. In the 1970s, analogues of the anthracenedione dyes (originally developed for use in the textile industry) were investigated as possible cytotoxic agents on the basis of the ability of the parent compounds to intercalate DNA. Mitoxantrone, a dihydroxyanthracenedione derivative, was the most active of a series of compounds synthesized (Zee-Cheng & Cheng, 1978; Dunn & Goa, 1996).

Mitoxantrone entered clinical trials in 1980 and has been used in cancer treatment since the mid-1980s. It was found to have anti-tumour activity in advanced breast cancer (often in patients in whom other treatments have failed), non-Hodgkin lymphoma and certain leukaemias. It is still most commonly used in these tumours, typically in combination with other cytotoxic drugs, and has also been used in the treatment of other cancers such as ovarian, prostate and lung cancer (Faulds *et al.*, 1991). The typical dose is the equivalent of 12–14 mg/m^2 mitoxantrone once every three weeks in patients with lymphomas and tumours of solid tissues, and 12 mg/m^2 per day for five days in patients with leukaemia. When mitoxantrone is used in combination with other cytotoxic drugs, these doses are often lower (Dunn & Goa, 1996; Royal Pharmaceutical Society of Great Britain, 1999). In recent years, mitoxantrone has been used to a limited extent in the treatment of multiple sclerosis, typically at doses lower than those used in malignant disease and on a monthly schedule (Gonsettte, 1996; Millefiorini *et al.*, 1997).

1.4 Occurrence

Mitoxantrone is not known to occur as a natural product. No data on occupational exposure were available to the Working Group.

1.5 Regulations and guidelines

Mitoxantrone hydrochloride is included in the European and US pharmacopoeias (Council of Europe, 1998; Swiss Pharmaceutical Society, 1999).

2. Studies of Cancer in Humans

The Working Group considered only studies in which mitoxantrone was given to patients who did not receive treatments with alkylating agents, with the exception of low doses of cyclophosphamide.

2.1 Case reports

Detourmignies *et al.* (1992) described two cases of acute promyelocytic leukaemia in France in patients who had previously received mitoxantrone. A woman, 51 years old, with a primary breast tumour had received a combination of mitoxantrone, vincristine, 5-fluorouracil, cyclophosphamide and radiotherapy (chest and axillary); she developed acute promyelocytic leukaemia nine months later. Another woman, 42 years old, with a primary breast tumour had received a combination of mitoxantrone, vincristine, 5-fluorouracil and radiotherapy (chest) and developed acute promyelocytic leukaemia after

17 months. [The Working Group noted that there was no information on dose, treatment schedule or duration of mitoxantrone treatment.]

Philpott et al. (1993) reported two cases of acute myeloid leukaemia following treatment of advanced breast cancer in the United Kingdom. The first case was that of a woman (aged 56 years) who received eight cycles of mitoxantrone (7 mg/m^2), methotrexate and mitomycin, local radiotherapy to the breast and axilla and tamoxifen. She was disease-free for 18 months but then developed acute myeloid leukaemia. The second patient (aged 39 years) was also treated with eight cycles of mitoxantrone (7 mg/m^2), methotrexate and mitomycin and in addition received radiotherapy to the breast. Thirteen months later she developed acute myeloid leukaemia.

Melillo et al. (1997) described three cases of acute myeloid leukaemia in 1996 in Italy in women who were treated with five to seven intravenous courses of methotrexate (30 mg/m^2 every three weeks), mitoxantrone (8 mg/m^2 every three weeks) and mitomycin (8 mg/m^2 every six weeks) for recurrent breast cancer at the age of 44, 52 and 60. They had previously received radical mastectomy and either cyclophosphamide, methotrexate and 5-fluorouracil or radiotherapy or both. Treatment with methotrexate, mitoxantrone and mitomycin was followed by tamoxifen, medroxyprogesterone acetate or medroxyprogesterone acetate and radiation therapy. Acute myeloid leukaemia (one case of acute monoblastic leukaemia, one of acute promyelocytic leukaemia and one of acute undifferentiated leukaemia) occurred 12–30 months after the start of treatment with the mitoxantrone-containing regimen. [The Working Group noted that the standard treatment for breast cancer with cyclophosphamide (< 20 g/m^2), methotrexate and 5-fluorouracil has not been associated with leukaemia (Curtis et al., 1992) and that the bone marrow is unlikely to have been affected by radiotherapy of the breast area.]

Vicari et al. (1998) reported on a 36-year-old man in Italy with acute promyelocytic leukaemia after treatment with mitoxantrone for multiple sclerosis. The patient had been treated with high doses of corticosteroids during exacerbation of the multiple sclerosis. Five years before the diagnosis of acute promyelocytic leukaemia, the patient had received an intravenous dose of mitoxantrone (10 mg/m^2) once a month for five months (total dose, 87.5 mg). The patient was reported to have no history of exposure to known leukaemogenic risk factors or a personal or family history of malignancy.

Partridge and Lowdell (1999) reported the development of myelodysplastic syndrome in a 62-year-old woman treated for advanced breast cancer with five courses of mitoxantrone (7 mg/m^2), methotrexate and mitomycin. In addition, she had received radiotherapy to the breast and axilla and tamoxifen. After 22 months, myelodysplastic syndrome was diagnosed.

2.2 Cohort study

In a pilot study to determine the toxicity of adjuvant treatment for early-stage breast cancer in a single hospital in Ireland, Cremin et al. (1996) reported on cases of acute myeloid leukaemia in 59 premenopausal women (32–54 years of age at diagnosis) with early-stage breast cancer who were treated between 1986 and 1992 with adjuvant regimens containing mitoxantrone and methothrexate with or without mitomycin. The planned doses for the intravenous regimen that included mitomycin ($n = 30$) were: mitoxantrone, 8 mg/m^2 every three weeks (total dose, 64 mg); mitomycin, 8 mg/m^2 every six weeks (total dose, 32 mg) and methothrexate, 30 mg/m^2 every three weeks (total dose, 240 mg). The planned doses for the intravenous regimen that did not include mitomycin ($n = 29$) were: mitoxantrone, 12 mg/m^2 every three weeks (total dose, 96 mg) and methothrexate, 35 mg/m^2 every three weeks (total dose, 280 mg). During follow-up for a median of 72 months, two cases of acute myeloid leukaemia (one of acute myelomonocytic leukaemia and one of acute myeloblastic leukaemia) and one case of myelodysplastic syndrome occurred. All three patients had received treatment without mitomycin in combination with tamoxifen (three cases), radiotherapy (one case) or other cytostatic drugs (one case). The interval between treatment and diagnosis was 17 and 18 months for the cases of acute myeloid leukaemia and 36 months for the case of myelodysplastic syndrome. The frequency of acute myeloid leukaemia and myelodysplastic syndrome was 3/59 (5%) in the two treatment groups combined and 3/29 in the group given treatment without mitomycin, who had received a higher dose of mitoxantrone and a slightly higher dose of methotrexate than the group treated with mitomycin. [The Working Group noted that the risk for leukaemia was not compared with the risk of the general population; however, it is clear that 2/59 is substantially more than the expected number. On the basis of an incidence of 3–4 per 100 000 persons per year (Parkin *et al.*, 1997), the Working Group calculated a relative risk of about 200. The cumulative risk for leukaemia at five years was not reported. The dose of mitoxantrone associated with leukaemia was higher than that usually given in the treatment of advanced breast cancer.]

[The Working Group was aware of a number of cohort studies (Powles *et al.*, 1991; Stein *et al.*, 1992; Smith & Powles, 1993; Gregory *et al.*, 1997) in which the combination of methotrexate, mitoxantrone and mitomycin was used in the second- or third-line treatment of advanced breast cancer. These were not considered further because the follow-up was rarely longer than one year and the patients would previously have been treated with leukaemogenic agents and/or radiation.]

3. Studies of Cancer in Experimental Animals

No data were available to the Working Group.

4. Other Data Relevant to and Evaluation of Carcinogenicity and its Mechanisms

4.1 Absorption, distribution, metabolism and excretion

4.1.1 *Humans*

The pharmacokinetics of mitoxantrone in humans has been reviewed (Batra *et al.*, 1986; Ehninger *et al.*, 1990; Dunn & Goa, 1996). There are no published data on the bioavailability of orally administered mitoxantrone in humans, but a number of studies have reported the pharmacokinetics of mitoxantrone given as an intravenous infusion over 3–60 min at doses of 1–80 mg/m^2. All showed an initial rapid phase representing distribution of the drug into blood cells, with a half-time of about 5 min (range, 2–16 min) and a long terminal half-time of about 30 h (range, 19–72 h) (Savaraj *et al.*, 1982; Alberts *et al.*, 1983; Smyth *et al.*, 1986; Van Belle *et al.*, 1986; Larson *et al.*, 1987; Hu *et al.*, 1992; Richard *et al.*, 1992; Feldman *et al.*, 1993). Many early studies reported much shorter terminal half-times, but suitably sensitive assays may not have been used or adequate numbers of late samples collected. Tri-exponential elimination has been reported, the second distribution phase having a half-time of about 1 h (Alberts *et al.*, 1983; Smyth *et al.*, 1986; Van Belle *et al.*, 1986; Hu *et al.*, 1992), representing re-distribution from blood cells into tissues. The extent of the distribution into blood cells is illustrated by the observation that at the end of a 1-h infusion, the concentrations of mitoxantrone in leukocytes were 10 times higher than those in plasma (Sundman-Engberg *et al.*, 1993), while 2–5 h after the dose the leukocyte or leukaemic cell concentrations were 350 times higher than those in plasma. The typical peak plasma concentration after a 30–60-min infusion of 12 mg/m^2 was about 500 ng/mL (Smyth *et al.*, 1986; Van Belle *et al.*, 1986; Larson *et al.*, 1987). The rapid disappearance from plasma results in a total plasma clearance rate of about 500 mL/min, while the large volume of distribution of 500–4000 L/m^2 indicates tissue sequestration of the drug (Savaraj *et al.*, 1982; Alberts *et al.*, 1983; Smyth *et al.*, 1986; Hu *et al.*, 1992; Richard *et al.*, 1992; Feldman *et al.*, 1993).

Studies of patients given mitoxantrone at doses up to 80 mg/m^2 (standard dose, 12 mg/m^2) suggest that the kinetics is linear up to this dose (Alberts *et al.*, 1983; Feldman *et al.*, 1993).

Studies of the urinary excretion of mitoxantrone concur that little of the administered dose is cleared renally. Urinary recovery has been reported variously as < 7% within 24 h (Savaraj *et al.*, 1982; Alberts *et al.*, 1983; Van Belle *et al.*, 1986), 3.3% within 48 h and < 8% within 72 h (Alberts *et al.*, 1983; Smyth *et al.*, 1986). In one study, urinary recovery of radiolabel after intravenous administration of [^{14}C]mitoxantrone accounted for 6.7% of the dose after 24 h and 10% after 72 h, with 3.9% and 5.1% as unchanged drug, respectively (Savaraj *et al.*, 1982). Urinary recovery of intravenously administered mitoxantrone over five days accounted for 6.5% of the dose, most of which (90%) was recovered during the first 24 h (Alberts et al., 1983).

The elimination half-time of mitoxantrone in two patients with impaired liver function was 63 h, whereas that in patients with normal liver function was 23 h (Smyth et al., 1986); in five patients with hepatic dysfunction, ascites or oedema, the terminal half-time was 71 h, while that in control patients was 37 h; and in two patients with oedema, the integrated area under the curve (AUC) of plasma concentration–time was double that of control patients (Rentsch et al., 1998). Faecal recovery of radiolabel after a single 12 mg/m^2 dose was 18% (range, 14–25%) over five days (Alberts et al., 1983). These results suggest that the liver is important in the elimination of mitoxantrone and that patients with impaired liver function or an abnormal fluid compartment may be at increased risk for toxic effects.

With infusion of mitoxantrone at a dose of 1.2 mg/m^2 per day for 21 days instead of the standard regimen of 12 mg/m^2 every three weeks, although the plasma concentrations reached a plateau after 35 h, the concentrations of mitoxantrone in leukocytes continued to increase throughout the 21 days suggesting that prolonged infusion may increase intracellular exposure to the drug (Greidanus et al., 1989).

After intraperitoneal administration of mitoxantrone, high peritoneal concentrations but low systemic availability were reported, with a ratio of the AUC for peritoneal fluid to that for plasma of about 1000:1 (Alberts et al., 1988; Nagel et al., 1992).

The sequestration of mitoxantrone by body tissues results in retention of the drug for long periods. The characteristic blue–green colour of mitoxantrone has been observed on the surface of the peritoneum more than one month after intraperitoneal administration, and the concentrations in peritoneal tissue 6–22 weeks after intraperitoneal dosing ranged from < 0.1 to 14 µg/g tissue (Markman et al., 1993). Mitoxantrone was readily detectable in post-mortem tissue samples from all 11 patients who had received mitoxantrone intravenously between 10 and 272 days before death. The highest concentrations were found in the thyroid, liver and heart and the lowest in brain tissue (Stewart et al., 1986). In one patient given [^{14}C]mitoxantrone intravenously, who died 35 days after the dose, as much as 15% of the administered dose could be accounted for in the liver, bone marrow, lungs, spleen, kidney and thyroid glands (Alberts et al., 1983).

Limited data are available on the protein binding of mitoxantrone in humans. In one study, the fraction of unbound drug in plasma at the end of a 30-min infusion was only 3.0% (Hu et al., 1992).

Because of its limited urinary excretion, little information is available on the metabolism of mitoxantrone. Two inactive metabolites were identified in urine as the mono- and dicarboxylic acid derivatives resulting from oxidation of the terminal hydroxy groups of the side-chains (Figure 1) (Chiccarelli et al., 1986; Rentsch et al., 1998). The concentrations of mitoxantrone in urine were not altered by pre-incubation with a β-glucuronidase or sulfatase, suggesting that the drug is not excreted renally as either the glucuronide or sulfate conjugate (Smyth et al., 1986).

Figure 1. Metabolism of mitoxantrone

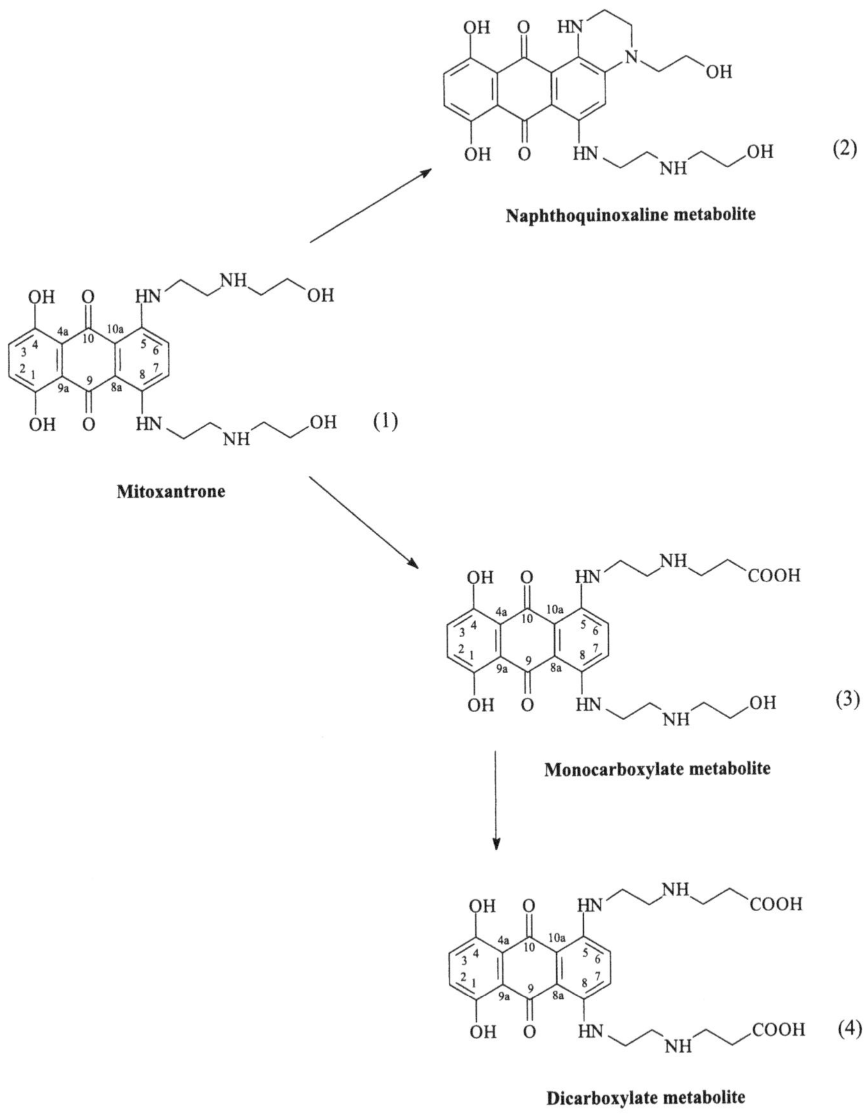

Mitoxantrone (1)

Naphthoquinoxaline metabolite (2)

Monocarboxylate metabolite (3)

Dicarboxylate metabolite (4)

Adapted from Ehninger *et al.* (1986) and Mewes *et al.* (1993)

Studies with HepG2 hepatoma cells and rat hepatocytes suggest that mitoxantrone can be oxidized to an active naphthoquinoxaline metabolite which can bind covalently to RNA and DNA (Blanz *et al.*, 1991; Mewes *et al.*, 1993; Panousis *et al.*, 1995). This metabolite has been identified in the urine of patients given mitoxantrone (Blanz *et al.*, 1991), and two studies of cell systems suggest that it may contribute to the cytotoxic activity of mitoxantrone (Duthie & Grant, 1989; Mewes *et al.*, 1993).

A 28-year-old woman in whom acute promyelocytic leukaemia was diagnosed during the 24th week of pregnancy was treated successfully with a variety of drugs and was given mitoxantrone prior to caesarean section at 34 weeks of gestation. After two further courses of 6 mg/m² mitoxantrone, her breast milk contained 120 ng/mL mitoxantrone 3–4 h after dosing and 18 ng/mL by five days, and the concentration remained at this level for 28 days. This finding indicates that the drug is slowly released from a deep tissue compartment (Azuno et al., 1995).

4.1.2 *Experimental systems*

There are no published studies of the pharmacokinetics of mitoxantrone given orally to laboratory animals. The drug was not developed for oral use, and in a review mitoxantrone was described as being poorly absorbed when administered orally [species not mentioned] (Batra et al., 1986).

In rats, dogs and monkeys, the disappearance of intravenously administered [^{14}C]-mitoxantrone from plasma was rapid, followed by a slow terminal elimination phase (James et al., 1983). In monkeys, the terminal half-time was eight days. Extensive tissue binding was indicated, with 50, 25 and 30% of the dose still retained 10 days after intravenous administration in rats, dogs and monkeys, respectively. In beagle dogs, tri-exponential elimination from plasma was reported, with a very rapid initial distribution phase with a half-time of 6.5 min, a longer distribution phase of 1.3 h and a slow terminal elimination of 28 h. Less than 4% of the dose was excreted in the urine during the first 48 h. Extensive tissue retention was again reported, the higher concentrations 24 h after dosing being found in the liver, kidney and spleen. Plasma protein binding was reported to be 70–80%. Two metabolites were detected, accounting for 30% of the radiolabel in plasma and 50% in urine, but were not identified (Lu et al., 1984).

A rapid distribution and a slow elimination phase were also observed in mice, with retention in body tissues, particularly liver and kidney (Rentsch et al., 1997), and in rabbits (Hulhoven et al., 1983).

A naphthoquinoxaline metabolite of mitoxantrone has been reported in rats and pigs, resulting from the oxidation of the phenylenediamine substructure (Blanz et al., 1991; Figure 1). In general, mitoxantrone is believed to be active in mammalian cells *in vitro* in the absence of exogenous metabolic activation; however, inhibition of cytochrome P450 mixed-function oxidase by metyrapone in HepG2 hepatoxic cells and rat hepatocytes blocked the cytotoxic activity of mitoxantrone, suggesting that conversion to reactive species might be important (Duthie & Grant, 1989; Mewes et al., 1993).

Panousis et al. (1995) reported that mitoxantrone is readily oxidized by myeloperoxidase or hydrogen peroxide and that the metabolites bind covalently to DNA. Various metabolic species and various DNA adducts have been chemically characterized, but their mutagenic properties have not been studied (Mewes et al., 1993; Dackiewicz et al., 1995).

4.2 Toxic effects

4.2.1 *Humans*

The acute toxicity of mitoxantrone has been reviewed (Smith, 1983; Faulds *et al.*, 1991; Dunn & Goa, 1996). Leukopenia is the main dose-limiting effect, the lowest leukocyte counts typically being found 10–14 days after a single dose, with recovery by day 21. Thrombocytopenia occurs but is less common. Of 505 patients treated in phase II studies at the standard dose of 12–14 mg/m^2, 5% experienced very severe leukopenia (leukocyte count, $< 1 \times 10^9$/L), and 0.8% experienced very severe thrombocytopenia (platelet count, $< 25 \times 10^9$/L) (Smith, 1983). Patients with AIDS and Kaposi sarcoma treated at a dose of 12 mg/m^2 all experienced severe neutropenia, possibly related to impaired bone-marrow function (Kaplan & Volberding, 1985).

Like other anthracyclines, mitoxantrone is associated with cardiotoxicity. In large phase II studies, summarized by Smith (1983), 15 of 543 patients experienced cardiotoxicity (3%), reported as congestive cardiac failure, pulmonary oedema or unspecified. In a large European trial, seven of 264 patients experienced cardiac abnormalities (3%). Risk factors that may be predictive of the cardiotoxicity of this drug are previous anthracycline therapy, mediastinal radiotherapy and a history of cardiovascular disease (Crossley, 1983). The number of cardiotoxic events increases with cumulative doses of mitoxantrone > 120 mg/m^2 in patients who have previously been treated with anthracyclines, and > 160 mg/m^2 in patients who were not previously treated. Henderson *et al.* (1989) reported moderate to severe decreases in left-ventricular ejection fraction in eight of 132 patients treated with mitoxantrone, all of whom had received cumulative doses > 100 mg/m^2. The cumulative dose at which a patient has a 50% probability of having to discontinue treatment because of cardiotoxicity was estimated to be 182 mg/m^2, representing approximately 13 courses of treatment.

Other toxic effects seen with standard doses of mitoxantrone (12–14 mg/m^2) include nausea and vomiting (in approximately 50% of patients), diarrhoea (15%), stomatitis and mucositis (20%) and alopecia (50%), although these effects are usually mild and transient (Crossley, 1983). As the drug is an intense blue colour, discolouration of urine and skin is not uncommon. Cases of onycholysis have been reported (Creamer *et al.*, 1995).

With higher doses (40–90 mg/m^2 or 12 mg/m^2 on days 1–3), the toxic effects are typically more severe, and hepatotoxicity has been reported (Feldman *et al.*, 1993; Ballestrero *et al.*, 1997; Feldman *et al.*, 1997), manifest as transient increases in serum bilirubin concentration and in the activity of liver enzymes, and becoming more common with increasing dose (Feldman *et al.*, 1993).

After intraperitoneal dosing, peritonitis is the dose-limiting toxic effect (Alberts *et al.*, 1988).

4.2.2 *Experimental systems*

Much of the information on the toxicity of mitoxantrone in experimental animals has not been published in detail. The LD_{50} was reported to be about 5 mg/kg bw in rats and 10 mg/kg bw in mice, and the single minimum lethal dose in beagle dogs was 10 mg/m^2 (Henderson *et al.*, 1982).

Many of the studies of the toxicity of mitoxantrone have focused on its cardiac effects, particularly in comparison with doxorubicin, another anthracycline known to be toxic to the heart. Beagle dogs given half the lethal dose (5.15 mg/m^2) had decreased leukocyte counts, haematocrit and haemoglobin concentration, diarrhoea, cutaneous sores and inactivity, one animal dying of pneumonia, but there was no evidence of cardiotoxicity at this dose (Henderson *et al.*, 1982). At doses > 2 mg/kg bw, mitoxantrone induced cardiovascular and renal toxicity in rabbits (Hulhoven *et al.*, 1983). In cats given mitoxantrone at doses of 2.5–6.5 mg/m^2 for the treatment of malignant tumours, the most common toxic effects were vomiting, anorexia, diarrhoea, lethargy, sepsis secondary to myelosuppression and seizures. Two cats died of complications that may have been attributable to mitoxantrone: one of cardiomyopathy and the other of pulmonary oedema (Ogilvie *et al.*, 1993).

Hepatotoxicity was observed in mice given 15 mg/kg bw (Llesuy & Arnaiz, 1990).

Mitoxantrone at clinically relevant concentrations was toxic to cultured heart cells from Sprague-Dawley rats, an effect that could be prevented by the chelating agent ICRF-187 (Shipp & Dorr, 1991; Shipp *et al.*, 1993).

4.3 Reproductive and prenatal effects

4.3.1 *Humans*

A woman aged 39 who was treated for 14 weeks with mitoxantrone at 20 mg intravenously every three weeks for cystic adenoma of the adenoids became amenorrhoeic and had hot flushes after a cumulative dose of 100 mg. She had received no other treatment and had not taken hormones or oral contraceptives. Measurement of luteinizing hormone, follicle-stimulating hormone and oestradiol in her blood showed that their concentrations were in the menopausal range (Shenkenberg & Von Hoff, 1986). [The Working Group noted that ovarian biopsy was not performed and that the lack of ovarian function might have been related to the woman's age.]

A 26-year-old woman in the 20th week of pregnancy was treated with cytarabine and daunorubicin for acute myeloblastic leukaemia. Three weeks later, she received mitoxantrone at 12 mg/m^2 for three days in combination with cytarabine. The pregnancy continued, with normal fetal growth, for 60 days when she had complete remission. She was then given idarubicin and cytarabine for two days. Two days later, the fetus was found to be dead *in utero* (Reynoso & Huerta, 1994).

4.3.2 *Experimental systems*

In a brief review of the toxicology of mitoxantrone, an increased frequency of fetal resorptions and decreased fetal body weights were observed in pregnant rats dosed intravenously with 0.25 mg/kg bw, but no effects were observed in rabbits at intravenous doses up to 0.5 mg/kg bw [no details of treatment times or numbers of animals used were given] (James *et al.*, 1983).

4.4 Genetic and related effects

4.4.1 *Humans*

There are few studies of the genotoxicity of mitoxantrone in humans. Liang *et al.* (1993) evaluated the induction of chromosomal breaks and sister chromatid exchange in cultured lymphocytes from 42 patients with Hodgkin disease, collected before and during treatment with mitoxantrone in combination with vincristine, vinblastine and prednisone. The authors found no evidence of increased frequencies of chromosome or single-stranded DNA breaks or sister chromatid exchange.

Vicari *et al.* (1998) detected the PML-RAR-α fusion transcript, consistent with translocation t(15;17), in a case of acute promyelocytic leukemia that occurred five years after a cumulative dose of 50 mg/m^2 mitoxantrone administered as a single agent for the treatment of multiple sclerosis. It should be noted, however, that this translocation occurs in nearly all cases of de-novo acute promyelocytic leukaemia. In a review, Quesnel *et al.* (1993) mentioned a case of acute myeloid leukaemia with a complex karyotype including t(8;21) after treatment with mitoxantrone as a single agent for breast cancer.

Leblanc *et al.* (1994) identified a *MLL* gene rearrangement by Southern blot analysis in a case of acute monoblastic leukaemia with translocation t(1;11)(q13;q23) that followed chemotherapy with a mitoxantrone-containing protocol for primary acute myeloid leukaemia with inv(16). The therapy for the primary leukaemia included induction with cytarabine and mitoxantrone, two consolidations with cytarabine, daunorubicin and etoposide and then cytarabine and amsacrine followed by maintanence therapy with 6-mercaptopurine and cytarabine. The regimen thus contained three DNA topoisomerase II inhibitors. Which, if any, can be linked to the translocation t(1;11)(q13;q23) is uncertain.

Similarly, Bredeson *et al.* (1993) observed a case of acute monoblastic leukaemia with t(9;11)(p22;q23) 47 months after the initiation of treatment for primary non-Hodgkin lymphoma with a mitoxantrone-containing regimen that also included alkylating agents and other DNA topoisomerase II inhibitors.

Pedersen-Bjergaard and Philip (1991) reported a balanced translocation involving chromosome band 21q22 in a case of acute myeloid leukaemia that followed mitoxantrone-containing therapy.

Izumi et al. (1996) described a case of acute myeloblastic leukaemia with t(2;21)(q21;q22), t(8;21)(q22;q22) and add (13)(q34) after treatment for non-Hodgkin lymphoma with mitoxantrone, other DNA topoisomerase II inhibitors and alkylating agents.

Detourmignies et al. (1992) reported a case of acute promyelocytic leukaemia that occurred nine months after initiation of treatment of breast cancer with mitoxantrone, vincristine, cyclophosphamide and 5-fluorouracil, but karyotype analysis was not performed. Melillo et al. (1997) observed three cases of acute myeloid leukaemia after therapy with mitoxantrone, mitomycin and methotrexate for advanced breast cancer. In one case, the karyotype was normal. In the second case, which was an acute promyelocytic leukaemia, the karyotype revealed t(15;17)(q22;q12), typical of this leukaemia, and the PML-RAR-α fusion transcript was detected by reverse transcriptase polymerase chain reaction. The karyotype of the third case showed del(3)(q12;q25), –7, –19, +mar.

4.4.2 Experimental systems

General reviews on the mutagenicity of inhibitors of DNA topoisomerase II enzymes, including mitoxantrone, have been published (Anderson & Berger, 1994; Ferguson & Baguley, 1994, 1996; Baguley & Ferguson, 1998; Ferguson, 1998). Jackson et al. (1996) collated a genetic activity profile for this drug. The results are summarized in Table 1.

Limited data are available on the mutagenic effects of mitoxantrone in microbial assays, but, by analogy with other DNA topoisomerase II inhibitors, it probably gives weak or negative responses in assays in prokaryotes and lower eukaryotes. Mitoxantrone weakly induced reverse mutation in *Salmonella typhimurium* TA98 and TA1537, and these effects did not depend on metabolic activation. It did not induce reverse mutation in *S. typhimurium* TA1535 or TA100 in the presence or absence of metabolic activation. In another study, mitoxantrone induced reverse mutation in strains TA98, TA1538 and TA1978 in the absence of metabolic activation.

Mitoxantrone is a potent inducer of DNA breakage in mammalian cells *in vitro* and *in vivo*. It caused protein-masked DNA double-strand breaks and DNA–protein cross-links in various animal and human cell lines at a concentration of about 1 μmol/L. These strand breakage effects could be enhanced in T-47D human breast cancer cells by prior stimulation with oestrogen. In a single study, mitoxantrone did not induce DNA breakage in peripheral blood cells obtained from leukaemia patients treated with the drug.

Mitoxantrone was highly effective in causing chromosomal aberrations in cultured Chinese hamster cells and in human peripheral blood lymphocytes in tissue culture. These effects were reduced when an exogenous metabolic activation system was added to the cells. Mitoxantrone induced chromosomal aberrations in the bone marrow of rats.

Table 1. Genetic and related effects of mitoxantrone

Test system	Result[a] Without exogenous metabolic system	Result[a] With exogenous metabolic system	Dose[b] (LED or HID)	Reference
Salmonella typhimurium TA1537, TA98, reverse mutation	+	+	32.5 mmol/L[c]	Au *et al.* (1981)
Salmonella typhimurium TA100, TA1535, reverse mutation	–	–	130 mmol/L[c]	Au *et al.* (1981)
Salmonella typhimurium TA1538, reverse mutation	+	NT	50 µg/plate	Matney *et al.* (1985)
Salmonella typhimurium TA98, reverse mutation	(+)	NT	200 µg/plate	Matney *et al.* (1985)
Salmonella typhimurium TA1978, reverse mutation	+	NT	20 µg/plate	Matney *et al.* (1985)
Drosophila melanogaster, somatic mutation and recombination	+		2000 in feed	Clements *et al.* (1990)
Drosophila melanogaster, somatic mutation and recombination	+		445 in feed	Frei *et al.* (1992)
Drosophila melanogaster, sex-linked recessive lethal mutation	(+)		1335 in feed	Frei *et al.* (1992)
DNA single-strand breaks, Chinese hamster ovary cells *in vitro*	+	NT	0.05	Štětina & Veselá (1991)
DNA–protein cross-linkage, Chinese hamster ovary and UV-5 (excision repair-deficient) cells *in vitro*	+	NT	0.5	Štětina & Veselá (1991)
Unscheduled DNA synthesis, Sprague-Dawley rat primary hepatocytes *in vitro*	+	NT	0.1	Manandhar *et al.* (1986)
Gene mutation, L5178Y mouse lymphoma cells, *Tk* locus *in vitro*	+	+	0.0003	Manandhar *et al.* (1986)
Sister chromatid exchange, Chinese hamster ovary cells *in vitro*	+	+	0.022	Au *et al.* (1981)
Sister chromatid exchange, Chinese hamster ovary cells *in vitro*	+	NT	0.0004	Nishio *et al.* (1982)
Sister chromatid exchange, Chinese hamster ovary cells *in vitro*	+	+	0.0003	Manandhar *et al.* (1986)
Chromosomal aberrations, Chinese hamster ovary cells *in vitro*	+	(+)	0.004	Au *et al.* (1981)
Chromosomal aberrations, Chinese hamster ovary cells *in vitro*	+	NT	0.0004	Nishio *et al.* (1982)
Chromosomal aberrations, Chinese hamster ovary cells *in vitro*	+	NT	0.1	Rosenberg & Hittelman (1983)
Chromosomal aberrations, Chinese hamster lung cells *in vitro*	+	NT	0.01	Suzuki & Nakane (1994)
Polyploidy, Chinese hamster ovary cells *in vitro*	+	NT	9	Sumner (1995)
Cell transformation, C3H 10T1/2 mouse cells	–	NT	0.0005	Manandhar *et al.* (1986)

Table 1 (contd)

Test system	Result[a]		Dose[b] (LED or HID)	Reference
	Without exogenous metabolic system	With exogenous metabolic system		
DNA double-strand breaks, human leukaemia and lymphoma cell lines *in vitro*	+	NT	0.1	Ho *et al.* (1987)
DNA double-strand breaks, T-47D human breast cancer cells *in vitro*	+	NT	0.05	Epstein & Smith (1988)
DNA single and double-strand breaks, human LoVo cell line *in vitro*	+	NT	0.11	Capolongo *et al.* (1990)
DNA single-strand breaks, human lung carcinoma cells *in vitro*	+	NT	0.04	De Isabella *et al.* (1993)
DNA double-strand breaks, NCI-H69 human cells *in vitro*	+	NT	0.125	Smith *et al.* (1990)
DNA double-strand breaks, human astrocytoma and glioblastoma cell lines *in vitro*	+	NT	0.01	Senkal *et al.* (1997)
Chromosomal aberrations, human lymphocytes *in vitro*	+	NT	12×10^{-6}	Medeiros & Takahashi (1994)
Chromosomal aberrations, Sprague-Dawley rat bone-marrow cells *in vivo*	+		1 ip × 5	Manandhar *et al.* (1986)
Dominant lethal mutation, male and female Sprague-Dawley rats	−		1 ip × 5	Manandhar *et al.* (1986)
DNA single-strand breaks, human leukaemia cells *in vivo*	−		5 mg/m² iv × 3	Heinemann *et al.* (1988)

[a] +, positive; (+), weak positive; −, negative; NT, not tested
[b] LED, lowest effective dose; HID, highest ineffective dose; in-vitro tests, μg/mL; in-vivo tests, mg/kg bw per day; d, day
[c] Unclear what this concentration refers to

Mitoxantrone induced sister chromatid exchange in Chinese hamster cells. It also induced mutation and somatic recombination in the *Drosophila white–ivory* test for somatic mutation and in the wing spot test.

Mitoxantrone induced primarily small colony mutants at the *Tk* locus in mouse lymphoma L5178Y cells, in the presence or absence of exogenous metabolic activation. Small colony mutants in L5178Y cells are generally considered to be caused by chromosomal mutations (DeMarini *et al.*, 1987).

Some discrepancies with regard to the activity of mitoxantrone have been found in various assays. Although apoptosis may eliminate cells that appear to be mutated (Ferguson & Baguley, 1994), short-term (2–6 h) exposure of the human myeloid leukaemia line HL-60 and of MOLT-4 cells to 0.02–0.4 μg/mL mitoxantrone induced cell cycle arrest rather than apoptosis in experiments reported by Del Bino and Darzynkiewicz (1991). In other studies, incubation of the human myeloid leukaemia lines HL-60 and KG-1 with mitoxantrone for only 1 h at concentrations between 0.1 and 10 μmol/L gave clear indications of apoptosis (Bhalla *et al.*, 1993). The culture media and conditions differed between the two laboratories, and serum levels and types of media affect apoptosis (Ferguson & Baguley, 1996). Mitoxantrone-induced apoptosis was demonstrated in cultured B lymphocytes from a patient with chronic lymphoblastic leukaemia (Bellosillo *et al.*, 1998).

Mitoxantrone-induced polyploidy was demonstrated by cytogenetic techniques in Chinese hamster ovary cells by Sumner (1995). Although not directly studied for induction of aneuploidy, mitoxantrone inhibited the polymerization of microtubule assembly (Ho *et al.*, 1991) and almost certainly would act as an aneuploidogen. It did not induce transformation in C3H 10T1/2 cells (Manandhar *et al.*, 1986).

Equivocal results were found in studies of germ cells in *Drosophila*. A clinical preparation of mitoxantrone weakly induced sex-linked recessive mutation, but the response failed to reach statistical significance (Frei *et al.*, 1992). Similarly, assays for dominant lethal mutation in male and female Sprague-Dawley rats showed signs of reduced pregnancy rates but no clear statistical trend in dominant lethal events in either sex. [The Working Group noted that, given the unusual timing of the effects of etoposide on germ cells (Russell *et al.*, 1998), these experiments would bear repetition with different schedules, as the available data must be considered equivocal.]

4.5   Mechanistic considerations

Mitoxantrone has three properties that are likely to induce mutation.

1. It inhibits DNA topoisomerase II enzymes: Mitoxantrone is a DNA topoisomerase II poison that has been shown to resemble etoposide and teniposide in promoting DNA cleavage, with a strong preference for C or T at position –1 (Capranico *et al.*, 1993; De Isabella *et al.*, 1993). Most of the mutational events reported in mammalian cells, including point mutations, chromosomal deletions and exchanges and aneuploidy, can be explained by this activity. Mitoxantrone does not inhibit bacterial topoisomerases and may not mutate bacterial cells by the same mechanism as mammalian cells. Instead, it has two other activities that may be responsible for other types of mutation.

2. *It possesses readily oxidizable functions*: Oxidation of the substituted anthraquinone skeleton leads to biotransformation of mitoxantrone (Mewes *et al.*, 1993). Panousis *et al.* (1995) reported that myeloperoxidase oxidizes mitoxantrone to metabolites that bind covalently to DNA. Dackiewicz *et al.* (1995) reported formation of several different DNA adducts when mitoxantrone was incubated with a peroxidase/hydrogen peroxide system. Nevertheless, none of the mutations seen with mitoxantrone is of the type usually associated with oxygen radicals.

3. *It intercalates into, but does not covalently interact with, DNA*: By analogy with other frameshift mutagens, mitoxantrone causes the frameshift mutagenicity seen in bacteria by DNA intercalation (Ferguson & Denny, 1990). A frameshift event was observed in both strains of *S. typhimurium* in which it caused reverse mutation (Au *et al.*, 1981).

Mitoxantrone-containing regimens are associated with chromosomal translocations in leukaemic cells similar to those observed with other DNA topoisomerase II inhibitors. The role of DNA topoisomerase II inhibitors in translocations associated with leukaemia is unknown. Two possibilities are plausible. The first is that mitoxantrone itself causes the translocations. It has been proposed that DNA cleavage induced directly by DNA topoisomerase II or by the drug-induced apoptotic cellular response is responsible for the nonrandom chromosomal translocations that lead to leukaemogenesis (Dassonneville & Bailly, 1998). The second possibility for the role of mitoxantrone in causing translocations is that it selects for cells that already have translocations. Indeed, *MLL* tandem duplications, a form of translocation, have been identified in peripheral blood and bone marrow of healthy adults (Schnittger *et al.*, 1998). Chemotherapy has profound effects on the kinetics of the bone marrow; it causes cell death, forcing many bone-marrow stem cells to divide, which might select for the rare stem cells with a translocation (Knudson, 1992). In favour of the first possibility is the specificity of the association between DNA topoisomerase II inhibitors, but not other forms of chemotherapy that cause cell death in the bone marrow (such as alkylating agents), and leukaemias characterized by translocations.

5. Summary of Data Reported and Evaluation

5.1 Exposure data

Mitoxantrone is a synthetic DNA topoisomerase II inhibitor of the anthracenedione class that has been used in cancer treatment since the mid-1980s. It is used mainly in the treatment of advanced breast cancer, non-Hodgkin lymphoma and certain leukaemias. Recently, it has been used in the treatment of multiple sclerosis.

5.2 Human carcinogenicity data

In the one available, small cohort study of women with early-stage premenopausal breast cancer who had been treated with mitoxantrone in the absence of known or suspected leukaemogenic agents, a substantially increased risk for acute myeloid leukaemia was observed.

Case reports of acute myeloid leukaemia developing in patients treated with mitoxantrone are compatible with the association found in the cohort study.

5.3 Animal carcinogenicity data

No data were available to the Working Group.

5.4 Other relevant data

In humans, mitoxantrone is eliminated biphasically or triphasically, with a terminal half-time of 19–72 h. The drug is rapidly taken up by blood cells and is extensively distributed in body tissues. The pharmacokinetics of mitoxantrone is linear up to 80 mg/m^2 (standard dose, 12 mg/m^2). The elimination half-life was prolonged in patients with impaired hepatic function and in patients with ascites or oedema. Urinary recovery of mitoxantrone as the parent drug or radiolabel is low (< 10%), and significant amounts are still present in body tissues weeks or months after dosing. Few data are available on the metabolism of mitoxantrone in humans, but two inactive metabolites have been reported.

A long elimination phase and tissue retention are also seen in animal species. Active naphthoquinoxaline mitoxantrone metabolites have been reported in some experimental systems.

The main dose-limiting toxic effect of mitoxantrone is myelosuppression, manifest mostly as leukopenia. Other toxic effects include nausea and vomiting, diarrhoea, stomatitis, mucositis and alopecia. Cardiotoxicity is reported in about 3% of patients and is more common with cumulative doses of 160 mg/m^2 in previously untreated patients and 120 mg/m^2 in previously treated patients, particularly in those who have received anthracyclines.

Mitoxantrone can mutate cells through one of three mechanisms. It intercalates into DNA and causes frameshift mutations in bacteria through that mechanism. Although the drug *per se* does not interact covalently with the DNA, it is readily oxidized to a species which does form DNA adducts; however, there is currently little evidence that DNA adduct formation is critical for mutagenic events in mammalian cells. The drug is orders of magnitude more toxic in mammalian than in microbial cells. Most of the effects in mammals arise because mitoxantrone is an effective poison of DNA topoisomerase II enzymes. The predominant effects seen to date involve the deletion and/or interchange of large DNA segments. Additionally, mitoxantrone induces polyploidy.

Chromosomal translocations characteristic of those that occur after administration of DNA topoisomerase II inhibitors have been observed in leukaemic cells of patients treated with mitoxantrone-containing regimens. The mode of action of this compound is similar to that of others for which evidence of a leukaemogenic effect is more compelling.

5.5 Evaluation

There is *limited evidence* in humans for the carcinogenicity of mitoxantrone.

There is *inadequate evidence* in experimental animals for the carcinogenicity of mitoxantrone.

Overall evaluation

Mitoxantrone is *possibly carcinogenic to humans (Group 2B)*.

6. References

Alberts, D.S., Peng, Y.-M., Leigh, S., Davis, T.P. & Woodward, D.L. (1983) Disposition of mitoxantrone in patients. *Cancer Treat. Rev.*, **10** (Suppl. B), 23–27

Alberts, D.S., Surwit, E.A., Peng, Y.-M., McCloskey, T., Rivest, R., Graham, V., McDonald, L. & Roe, D. (1988) Phase I clinical and pharmacokinetic study of mitoxantrone given to patients by intraperitoneal administration. *Cancer Res.*, **48**, 5874–5877

Anderson, R.D. & Berger, N.A. (1994) Mutagenicity and carcinogenicity of topoisomerase-interactive agents. *Mutat. Res.*, **309**, 109–142

Au, W.W., Butler, M.A., Matney, T.S. & Loo, T.L. (1981) Comparative structure–genotoxicity study of three aminoanthraquinone drugs and doxorubicin. *Cancer Res.*, **41**, 376–379

Azuno, Y., Kaku, K., Fujita, N., Okubo, M., Kaneko, T. & Matsumono, N. (1995) Mitoxantrone and etoposide in breast milk (Letter to the Editor). *Am. J. Hematol.*, **48**, 131–132

Baguley, B.C. & Ferguson, L.R. (1998) Mutagenic properties of topoisomerase-targeted drugs. *Biochim. biophys. Acta*, **1400**, 213–222

Ballestrero, A., Ferrando, F., Garuti, A., Basta, P., Gonella, R., Esposito, M., Vannozzi, M.O., Sorice, G., Friedman, D., Puglisi, M., Brema, F., Mela, G.S., Sessarego, M. & Patrone, F. (1997) High-dose mitoxantrone with peripheral blood progenitor cell rescue: Toxicity, pharmacokinetics and implications for dosage and schedule. *Br. J. Cancer*, **76**, 797–804

Batra, V.K., Morrison, J.A., Woodward, D.L., Siverd, N.S. & Yacobi, A. (1986) Pharmacokinetics of mitoxantrone in man and laboratory animals. *Drug Metab. Rev.*, **17**, 311–329

Beijnen, J.H., Bult, A. & Underberg, W.J.M. (1988) Mitoxantrone hydrochloride. In: Florey, K., ed., *Analytical Profiles of Drug Substances*, New York, Academic Press, Vol. 17, pp. 221–258

Bellosillo, B., Colomer, D., Pons, G. & Gil, J. (1998) Mitoxantrone, a topoisomerase II inhibitor, induces apoptosis of B-chronic lymphocytic leukaemia cells. *Br. J. Haematol.*, **100**, 142–146

Bhalla, K., Ibrado, A.M., Tourkina, E., Tang, C., Grant, S., Bullock, G., Huang, Y., Ponnathpur, V. & Mahoney, M.E. (1993) High-dose mitoxantrone induces programmed cell death or apoptosis in human myeloid leukemia cells. *Blood*, **82**, 3133–3140

Blanz, J., Mewes, K., Ehninger, G., Proksch, B., Waidelich, D., Greger, B. & Zeller, K.-P. (1991) Evidence for oxidative activation of mitoxantrone in human, pig, and rat. *Drug Metab. Dispos.*, **19**, 871–880

Bredeson, C.N., Barnett, M.J., Horsman, D.E., Dalal, B.I., Ragaz, J. & Phillips, G.L. (1993) Therapy-related acute myelogenous leukemia associated with 11q23 chromosomal abnormalities and topoisomerase II inhibitors: Report of four additional cases and brief commentary. *Leuk. Lymphoma*, **11**, 141–145

British Medical Association/Royal Pharmaceutical Society of Great Britain (1998) *British National Formulary*, No. 36, London, p. 373

Budavari, S., ed. (1996) *The Merck Index*, 12th Ed., Whitehouse Station, NJ, Merck & Co., p. 1064

Canadian Pharmaceutical Association (1997) *CPS Compendium of Pharmaceuticals and Specialties*, 32nd Ed., Ottawa, pp. 1071–1072

Capolongo, L., Belvedere, G. & D'Incalci, M. (1990) DNA damage and cytotoxicity of mitoxantrone and doxorubicin in doxorubicin-sensitive and -resistant human colon carcinoma cells. *Cancer Chemother. Pharmacol.*, **25**, 430–434

Capranico, G., De Isabella, P., Tinelli, S., Bigioni, M. & Zunino, F. (1993) Similar sequence specificity of mitoxantrone and VM-26 stimulation of in vitro DNA cleavage by mammalian DNA topoisomerase II. *Biochemistry*, **32**, 3038–3046

Chiccarelli, F.S., Morrison, J.A., Cosulich, D.B., Perkinson, N.A., Ridge, D.N., Sum, F.W., Murdock, K.C., Woodward, D.L. & Arnold, E.T. (1986) Identification of human urinary mitoxantrone metabolites. *Cancer Res.*, **46**, 4858–4861

CIS Information Services (1998) *Worldwide Bulk Drug Users Directory 1997/98 Edition*, Dallas, TX [CD-ROM]

Clements, J., Howe, D., Lowry, A. & Phillips, M. (1990) The effects of a range of anti-cancer drugs in the *white–ivory* somatic mutation test in *Drosophila*. *Mutat. Res.*, **228**, 171–176

Council of Europe (1998) *European Pharmacopoeia*, 3rd Ed., Supplement 1998, Strasbourg, pp. 387–388

Creamer, J.D., Mortimer, P.S. & Powles, T.J. (1995) Mitozantrone-induced onycholysis. A series of five cases. *Clin. exp. Dermatol.*, **20**, 459–461

Cremin, P., Flattery, M., McCann, S.R. & Daly, P.A. (1996) Myelodysplasia and acute myeloid leukaemia following adjuvant chemotherapy for breast cancer using mitoxantrone and methothrexate with or without mitomycin (Short report). *Ann. Oncol.*, **7**, 745–746

Crossley, R.J. (1983) Clinical safety and tolerance of mitoxantrone (Novantrone). *Cancer Treat. Rev.*, **10**, 29–36

Curtis, R.E., Boice, J.D., Jr, Stovall, M., Bernstein, L., Greenberg, R.S., Flannery, J.T., Schwartz, A.G., Weyer, P., Moloney, W.C. & Hoover, R.N. (1992) Risk of leukemia after chemotherapy and radiation treatment for breast cancer. *New Engl. J. Med.*, **326**, 1745–1751

Dackiewicz, P., Skladanowski, A. & Konopa, J. (1995) ^{32}P-postlabelling analysis of adducts formed by mitoxantrone and ametantrone with DNA and homopolydeoxyribonucleotides after enzymatic activation. *Chem.-biol. Interactions*, **98**, 153–166

Dassonneville, L. & Bailly, C. (1998) [Chromosomal translocations and secondary leukaemias induced by topoisomerase II inhibitors.] *Bull. Cancer*, **85**, 254–261 (in French)

De Isabella, P., Capranico, G., Palumbo, M., Sissi, C., Krapcho, A.P. & Zunino, F. (1993) Sequence selectivity of topoisomerase II DNA cleavage stimulated by mitoxantrone derivatives: Relationships to drug DNA binding and cellular effects. *Mol. Pharmacol.*, **43**, 715–721

Del Bino, G. & Darzynkiewicz, Z. (1991) Camptothecin, teniposide, or 4'-(9-acridinylamino)-3-methanesulfon-*m*-anisidide, but not mitoxantrone or doxorubicin, induces degradation of nuclear DNA in the S phase of HL-60 cells. *Cancer Res.*, **51**, 1165–1169

DeMarini, D.M., Brock, K.H., Doerr, C.L. & Moore, M.M. (1987) Mutagenicity and clastogenicity of teniposide (VM-26) in L5178Y/TK$^{+/-}$-3.7.2C mouse lymphoma cells. *Mutat. Res.*, **187**, 141–149

Detourmignies, L., Castaigne, S., Stoppa, A.M., Harousseau, J.L., Sadoun, A., Janvier, M., Demory, J.L., Sanz, M., Berger, R., Bauters, F., Chomienne, C. & Fenaux, P. (1992) Therapy-related acute promyelocytic leukemia: A report on 16 cases. *J. clin Oncol.*, **10**, 1430–1435

Dunn, C.J. & Goa, K.L. (1996) Mitoxantrone. A review of its pharmacological properties and use in acute nonlymphoblastic leukaemia. *Drugs Aging*, **9**, 122–147

Duthie, S.J. & Grant, M.H. (1989) The role of reductive and oxidative metabolism in the toxicity of mitoxantrone, adriamycin and menadione in human liver derived Hep G2 hepatoma cells. *Br. J. Cancer*, **60**, 566–571

Editions du Vidal (1998) *Dictionnaire Vidal 1998*, 74th Ed., Paris, OVP, p. 1321

Ehninger, G., Proksch, B., Heinzel, G. & Woodward, D.L. (1986) Clinical pharmacology of Mitoxantrone. *Cancer Treat. Rep.*, **70**, 1373–1378

Ehninger, G., Schuler, U., Proksch, B., Zeller, K.-P. & Blanz, J. (1990) Pharmacokinetics and metabolism of mitoxantrone. A review. *Clin. Pharmacokinet.*, **18**, 365–380

Epstein, R.J. & Smith, P.J. (1988) Estrogen-induced potentiation of DNA damage and cytotoxicity in human breast cancer cells treated with topoisomerase II-interactive antitumor drugs. *Cancer Res.*, **48**, 297–303

Faulds, D., Balfour, J.A., Chrisp, P. & Langtry, H.D. (1991) Mitoxantrone. A review of its pharmacodynamic and pharmacokinetic properties, and therapeutic potential in the chemotherapy of cancer. *Drugs*, **41**, 400–449

Feldman, E.J., Alberts, D.S., Arlin, Z., Ahmed, T., Mittelman, A., Baskind, P., Peng, Y.-M., Baier, M. & Plezia, P. (1993) Phase I clinical and pharmacokinetic evaluation of high-dose mitoxantrone in combination with cytarabine in patients with acute leukemia. *J. clin. Oncol.*, **11**, 2002–2009

Feldman, E.J., Seiter, K., Damon, L., Linker, C., Rugo, H., Ries, C., Case, D.C., Jr, Beer, M. & Ahmed, T. (1997) A randomized trial of high- vs standard-dose mitoxantrone with cytarabine in elderly patients with acute myeloid leukemia. *Leukemia*, **11**, 485–489

Ferguson, L.R. (1998) Inhibitors of topoisomerase II enzymes: A unique group of environmental mutagens and carcinogens. *Mutat. Res.*, **400**, 271–278

Ferguson, L.R. & Baguley, B.C. (1994) Topoisomerase II enzymes and mutagenicity. *Environ. mol. Mutag.*, **24**, 245–267

Ferguson, L.R. & Baguley, B.C. (1996) Mutagenicity of anticancer drugs that inhibit topoisomerase enzymes. *Mutat. Res.*, **355**, 91–101

Ferguson, L.R. & Denny, W.A. (1990) Frameshift mutagenesis by acridines and other reversibly-binding DNA ligands. *Mutagenesis*, **5**, 529–540

Frei, H., Clements, J., Howe, D. & Würgler, F.E. (1992) The genotoxicity of the anti-cancer drug mitoxantrone in somatic and germ cells of *Drosophila melanogaster*. *Mutat. Res.*, **279**, 21–33

Gennaro, A.R. (1995) *Remington: The Science and Practice of Pharmacy*, 19th Ed., Easton, PA, Mack Publishing, Vol. II, p. 1257

Gonsette, R.E. (1996) Mitoxantrone immunotherapy in multiple sclerosis. *Multiple Sclerosis*, **1**, 329–332

Gregory, R.K., Powles, T.J., Chang, J.C., & Ashley, S. (1997) A randomized trial of six versus twelve courses of chemotherapy in metastatic carcinoma of the breast. *Eur. J. Cancer*, **33**, 2194–2197

Greidanus, J., de Vries, E.G.E., Mulder, N.H., Sleijfer, D.T., Uges, D.R.A., Oosterhuis, B. & Willemse, P.H.B. (1989) A phase I pharmacokinetic study of 21-day continuous infusion mitoxantrone. *J. clin. Oncol.*, **7**, 790–797

Heinemann, V., Murray, D., Walters, R., Meyn, R.E. & Plunkett, W. (1988) Mitoxantrone-induced DNA damage in leukemia cells is enhanced by treatment with high-dose arabinosylcytosine. *Cancer Chemother. Pharmacol.*, **22**, 205–210

Henderson, B.M., Dougherty, W.J., James, V.C., Tilley, L.P. & Noble, J.F. (1982) Safety assessment of a new anticancer compound, mitoxantrone, in beagle dogs: Comparison with doxorubicin. I. Clinical observations. *Cancer Treat. Rep.*, **66**, 1139–1143

Henderson, I.C., Allegra, J.C., Woodcock, T., Wolff, S., Bryan, S., Cartwright, K., Dukart, G. & Henry, D. (1989) Randomized clinical trial comparing mitoxantrone with doxorubicin in previously treated patients with metastatic breast cancer. *J. clin. Oncol.*, **7**, 560–571

Ho, A.D., Seither, E., Ma, D.D.F. & Prentice, H.G. (1987) Mitoxantrone-induced toxicity and DNA strand breaks in leukaemic cells. *Br. J. Haematol.*, **65**, 51–55

Ho, C.-K., Law, S.-L., Chiang, H., Hsu, M.-L., Wang, C.-C. & Wang, S.-Y. (1991) Inhibition of microtubule assembly is a possible mechanism of action of mitoxantrone. *Biochem. biophys. Res. Commun.*, **180**, 118–123

Hu, O.Y.-P., Chang, S.-P., Law, C.-K., Jian, J.-M. & Chen, K.-Y. (1992) Pharmacokinetic and pharmacodynamic studies with mitoxantrone in the treatment of patients with nasopharyngeal carcinoma. *Cancer*, **69**, 847–853

Hulhoven, R., Dumont, E. & Harvengt, C. (1983) Acute cardiovascular and renal changes induced by mitoxantrone in rabbits. A pharmacokinetic approach. *Toxicol. Lett.*, **18**, 19–26

Izumi, T., Ohtsuki, T., Ohya, K.-I., Ogawa, Y., Yoshida, M., Muroi, K., Imagawa, S., Hatake, K., Kuriki, K., Saito, K. & Miura, Y. (1996) Therapy-related leukemia with a novel 21q22 rearrangement. *Cancer Genet. Cytogenet.*, **90**, 45–48

Jackson, M.A., Stack, H.F. & Waters, M.D. (1996) Genetic activity profiles of anticancer drugs. *Mutat. Res.*, **355**, 171–208

James, V., Chiccarelli, F., Dougherty, W., Hall, C., Henderson, B., Iatropoulos, M., Morrison, J., Nicolau, G., Noble, J., Sparano, B., Gordon, G. & Wu, H. (1983) Preclinical toxicity studies on mitoxantrone and bisantrene. In: Rozencweig, M., Von Hoff, D.D. & Staquet, M.J., eds, *New Anticancer Drugs: Mitoxantrone and Bisantrene*, New York, Raven Press, pp. 47–69

Kaplan, L. & Volberding, P.A. (1985) Failure (and danger) of mitozantrone in AIDS-related Kaposi's sarcoma (Letter to the Editor). *Lancet*, **ii**, 396

Knudson, A.G. (1992) Stem cell regulation, tissue ontogeny, and oncogenic events. *Semin. Cancer Biol.*, **3**, 99–106

Larson, R.A., Daly, K.M., Choi, K.E., Han, D.S. & Sinkule, J.A. (1987) A clinical and pharmacokinetic study of mitoxantrone in acute nonlymphocytic leukemia. *J. clin. Oncol.*, **5**, 391–397

Leblanc, T., Hillion, J., Derré, J., Le Coniat, M., Baruchel, A., Daniel, M.-T. & Berger, R. (1994) Translocation t(11;11)(q13;q23) and HRX gene rearrangement associated with therapy-related leukemia in a child previously treated with VP16. *Leukemia*, **8**, 1646–1648

Liang, J.C., Bailey, N.M., Gabriel, G.J., Kattan, M.W., Wang, R.Y., Hagemeister, F.B., Cabanillas, F.F. & Fuller, L.M. (1993) A new chemotherapy regimen for treatment of Hodgkin's disease associated with minimal genotoxicity. *Leuk. Lymphoma*, **9**, 503–508

LINFO Läkemedelsinformation AB (1998) *FASS 1998 Läkemedel i Sverige*, Stockholm, p. 894

Llesuy, S.F. & Arnaiz, S.L. (1990) Hepatotoxicity of mitoxantrone and doxorubicin. *Toxicology*, **63**, 187–198

Lu, K., Savaraj, N. & Loo, T.L. (1984) Pharmacological disposition of 1,4-dihydroxy-5-8-bis[{2 [(2-hydroxyethyl)amino]ethyl}amino]-9,10-anthracenedione dihydrochloride in the dog. *Cancer Chemother. Pharmacol.*, **13**, 63–66

Manandhar, M., Cheng, M., Iatropoulos, M.J. & Noble, J.F. (1986) Genetic toxicology profile of the new antineoplastic drug mitoxantrone in the mammalian test systems. *Arzneimittelforschung*, **36**, 1375–1379

Markman, M., Alberts, D., Rubin, S., Hakes, T., Lewis, J.L., Jr, Reichman, B., Jones, W., Curtin, J., Barakat, R., Brodar, F., Peng, Y.-M., Pennie, K., Almadrones, L. & Hoskins, W. (1993) Evidence for persistence of mitoxantrone within the peritoneal cavity following intraperitoneal delivery. *Gynecol. Oncol.*, **48**, 185–188

Matney, T.S., Nguyen, T.V., Connor, T.H., Dana, W.J. & Theiss, J.C. (1985) Genotoxic classification of anticancer drugs. *Teratog. Carcinog. Mutag.*, **5**, 319–328

Medeiros, M. das G. & Takahashi, C.S. (1994) Effects of treatment with mitoxantrone in combination with novobiocin, caffeine and ara-C on human lymphocytes in culture. *Mutat. Res.*, **307**, 285–292

Melillo, L.M.A., Sajeva, M.R., Musto, P., Perla, G., Cascavilla, N., Minervi, M.M., D'Arena, G. & Carotenuto, M. (1997) Acute myeloid leukemia following 3M (mitoxantrone, mitomycin and methotrexate) chemotherapy for advanced breast cancer (Letter to the Editor). *Leukemia*, **11**, 2211–2213

Mewes, K., Blanz, J., Ehninger, G., Gebhardt, R. & Zeller, K.-P. (1993) Cytochrome P-450-induced cytotoxicity of mitoxantrone by formation of electrophilic intermediates. *Cancer Res.*, **53**, 5135–5142

Millefiorini, E., Gasperini, C., Pozzilli, C., D'Andrea, F., Bastianello, S., Trojano, M., Morino, S., Morra, V.B., Bozzao, A., Cao, A., Bernini, M.L., Gambi, D. & Prencipe, M. (1997) Randomized placebo-controlled trial of mitoxantrone in relapsing–remitting multiple sclerosis: 24-month clinical and MRI outcome. *J. Neurol.*, **244**, 153–159

Nagel, J.D., Varossieau, F.J., Dubbelman, R., ten Bokkel Huinink, W.W. & McVie, J.G. (1992) Clinical pharmacokinetics of mitoxantrone after intraperitoneal administration. *Cancer Chemother. Pharmacol.*, **29**, 480–484

Nishio, A., DeFeo, F., Cheng, C.C. & Uyeki, E.M. (1982) Sister-chromatid exchange and chromosomal aberrations by DHAQ and related anthraquinone derivatives in Chinese hamster ovary cells. *Mutat. Res.*, **101**, 77–86

Ogilvie, G.K., Moore, A.S., Obradovich, J.E., Elmslie, R.E., Vail, D.M., Straw, R.C., Salmon, M.D., Klein, M.K., Atwater, S.W. & Ciekot, P.E. (1993) Toxicoses and efficacy associated with administration of mitoxantrone to cats with malignant tumors. *J. Am. vet. Med. Assoc.*, **202**, 1839–1844

Panousis, C., Kettle, A.J. & Phillips, D.R. (1995) Myeloperoxidase oxidizes mitoxantrone to metabolites which bind covalently to DNA and RNA. *Anticancer Drug Des.*, **10**, 593–605

Parkin, D.M., Whelan, S.L., Ferlay, J., Raymond, L. & Young, J., eds (1997) *Cancer Incidence in Five Continents, Vol. VII* (IARC Scientific Publications No. 143), Lyon, IARC*Press*

Partridge, S.E. & Lowdell, C.P. (1999) Myelodysplastic syndrome as a complication of neo-adjuvant triple M chemotherapy and radiotherapy. *Clin. Oncol.*, **11**, 187–189

Pedersen-Bjergaard, J. & Philip, P. (1991) Balanced translocations involving chromosome bands 11q23 and 21q22 are highly characteristic of myelodysplasia and leukemia following therapy with cytostatic agents targeting at DNA-topoisomerase II (Letter to the Editor). *Blood*, **78**, 1147–1148

Philpott, N.J., Bevan, D.H. & Gordon-Smith, E.C. (1993) Secondary leukaemia after MMM combined modality therapy for breast carcinoma (Letter to the Editor). *Lancet*, **341**, 1289

Powles, T.J., Jones, A.L., Judson, I.R., Hardy, J.R. & Ashley, S.E. (1991) A randomized trial comparing combination chemotherapy using mitomycin C, mitozantrone and methotrexate (3M) with vincristine, anthracycline and cyclophosphamide (VAC) in advanced breast cancer. *Br. J. Cancer*, **64**, 406–410

Quesnel, B., Kantarjian, H., Pedersen Bjergaard, J., Brault, P., Estey, E., Lai, J.L., Tilly, H., Stoppa, A.M., Archimbaud, E., Harousseau, J.L., Bauters, F. & Fenaux, P. (1993) Therapy-related acute myeloid leukemia with t(8;21), inv(16), and t(8;16): A report on 25 cases and review of the literature. *J. clin. Oncol.*, **11**, 2370–2379

Rentsch, K.M., Horber, D.H., Schwendener, R.A., Wunderli-Allenspach, H. & Hänseler, E. (1997) Comparative pharmacokinetic and cytotoxic analysis of three different formulations of mitoxantrone in mice. *Br. J. Cancer*, **75**, 986–992

Rentsch, K.M., Schwendener, R.A., Pestalozzi, B.C., Sauter, C., Wunderli-Allenspach, H. & Hänseler, E. (1998) Pharmacokinetic studies of mitoxantrone and one of its metabolites in serum and urine in patients with advanced breast cancer. *Eur. J. clin. Pharmacol.*, **54**, 83–89

Reynoso, E.E. & Huerta, F. (1994) Acute leukemia and pregnancy—Fatal fetal outcome after exposure to idarubicin during the second trimester. *Acta oncol.*, **33**, 709–710

Richard, B., Launay-Iliadis, M.-C., Iliadis, A., Just-Landi, S., Blaise, D., Stoppa, A.-M., Viens, P., Gaspard, M.-H., Maraninchi, D., Cano, J.P. & Carcassone, Y. (1992) Pharmacokinetics of mitoxantrone in cancer patients treated by high-dose chemotherapy and autologous bone marrow transplantation. *Br. J. Cancer*, **65**, 399–404

Rosenberg, L.J. & Hittelman, W.N. (1983) Direct and indirect clastogenic activity of anthracenedione in Chinese hamster ovary cells. *Cancer Res.*, **43**, 3270–3275

Rote Liste Sekretariat (1998) *Rote Liste 1998*, Frankfurt, Rote Liste Service GmbH, pp. 86-111–86-112

Royal Pharmaceutical Society of Great Britain (1999) *Martindale, The Extra Pharmacopoeia*, 13th Ed., London, The Pharmaceutical Press [MicroMedex Online: Health Care Series]

Russell, L.B., Hunsicker, P.R., Johnson, D.K. & Shelby, M.D. (1998) Unlike other chemicals, etoposide (a topoisomerase-II inhibitor) produces peak mutagenicity in primary spermatocytes of the mouse. *Mutat. Res.*, **400**, 279–286

Savaraj, N., Lu, K., Manuel, V. & Loo, T.L. (1982) Pharmacology of mitoxantrone in cancer patients. *Cancer Chemother. Pharmacol.*, **8**, 113–117

Schnittger, S., Wormann, B., Hiddemann, W. & Griesinger, F. (1998) Partial tandem duplications of the *MLL* gene are detectable in peripheral blood and bone marrow of nearly all healthy donors. *Blood*, **92**, 1728–1734

Senkal, M., Tonn, J.C., Schönmayr, R., Schachenmayr, W., Eickhoff, U., Kemen, M. & Kollig, E. (1997) Mitoxantrone-induced DNA strand breaks in cell-cultures of malignant human astrocytoma and glioblastoma tumors. *J. Neuro-oncol.*, **32**, 203–208

Shenkenberg, T.D. & Von Hoff, D.D. (1986) Possible mitoxantrone-induced amenorrhea. *Cancer Treat. Rep.*, **70**, 659–661

Shipp, N.G. & Dorr, R.T. (1991) Biochemical effects and toxicity of mitoxantrone in cultured heart cells. *Adv. exp. Med. Biol.*, **283**, 821–825

Shipp, N.G., Dorr, R.T., Alberts, D.S., Dawson, B.V. & Hendrix, M. (1993) Characterization of experimental mitoxantrone cardiotoxicity and its partial inhibition by ICRF-187 in cultured neonatal rat heart cells. *Cancer Res.*, **53**, 550–556

Smith, I.E. (1983) Mitoxantrone (novantrone): A review of experimental and early clinical studies. *Cancer Treat. Rev.*, **10**, 103–115

Smith, I.E. & Powles, T.J. (1993) MMM (mitomycin/mitoxantrone/methotrexate): An effective new regimen in the treatment of metastatic breast cancer. *Oncology*, **50** (Suppl. 1), 9–15

Smith, P.J., Morgan, S.A., Fox, M.E. & Watson, J.V. (1990) Mitoxantrone–DNA binding and the induction of topoisomerase II associated DNA damage in multi-drug resistant small cell lung cancer cells. *Biochem. Pharmacol.*, **40**, 2069–2078

Smyth, J.F., Macpherson, J.S., Warrington, P.S., Leonard, R.C.F. & Wolf, C.R. (1986) The clinical pharmacology of mitozantrone. *Cancer Chemother. Pharmacol.*, **17**, 149–152

Stein, R.C., Bower, M., Law, M., Bliss, J.M., Barton, C., Gaset, J.-C., Ford, H.T. & Coombes, R.C. (1992) Mitozantrone and methotrexate chemotherapy with and without mytomycin C in the treatment of advanced breast cancer: A randomized clinical trial. *Eur. J. Cancer*, **28A**, 1963–1965

Štetina, R. & Veselá, D. (1991) The influence of DNA-topoisomerase II inhibitors novobiocin and fostriecin on the induction and repair of DNA damage in Chinese hamster ovary (CHO) cells treated with mitoxantrone. *Neoplasma*, **38**, 109–117

Stewart, D.J., Green, R.M., Mikhael, N.Z., Montpetit, V., Thibault, M. & Maroun, J.A. (1986) Human autopsy tissue concentrations of mitoxantrone. *Cancer Treat. Rep.*, **70**, 1255–1261

Sumner, A.T. (1995) Inhibitors of topoisomerase II delay progress through mitosis and induce a doubling of the DNA content in CHO cells. *Exp. Cell Res.*, **217**, 440–447

Sundman-Engberg, B., Tidefelt, U., Gruber, A. & Paul, C. (1993) Intracellular concentrations of mitoxantrone in leukemic cells *in vitro* vs *in vivo*. *Leuk. Res.*, **17**, 347–352

Suzuki, H. & Nakane, S. (1994) Differential induction of chromosomal aberrations by topoisomerase inhibitors in cultured Chinese hamster cells. *Biol. pharm. Bull.*, **17**, 222–226

Swiss Pharmaceutical Society, ed. (1999) *Index Nominum, International Drug Directory*, 16th Ed., Stuttgart, Medpharm Scientific Publishers [MicroMedex Online: Health Care Series]

Thomas, J., ed. (1998) *Australian Prescription Products Guide*, 27th Ed., Victoria, Australian Pharmaceutical Publishing, Vol. 1, pp. 2060–2063

US Pharmacopeial Convention (1994) *The 1995 US Pharmacopeia*, 23rd Rev./*The National Formulary*, 18th Rev., Rockville, MD, pp. 1034–1036

US Pharmacopeial Convention (1998a) *Drug Information for the Health Care Professional, USP Dispensing Information*, 18th Ed., Rockville, MD, Vol. I, pp. 2050–2053

US Pharmacopeial Convention (1998b) *The 1995 US Pharmacopeia*, 23rd Rev./*The National Formulary*, 18th Rev., Supplement 8, Rockville, MD, pp. 4230–4232

Van Belle, S.J.P., de Planque, M.M., Smith, I.E., van Oosterom, A.T., Schoemaker, T.J., Deneve, W. & McVie, J.G. (1986) Pharmacokinetics of mitoxantrone in humans following single-agent infusion or intra-arterial injection therapy or combined-agent infusion therapy. *Cancer Chemother. Pharmacol.*, **18**, 27–32

Vicari, A.M., Ciceri, F., Folli, F., Lanzi, R., Colombo, B., Comi, G. & Camba, L. (1998) Acute promyelocytic leukemia following mitoxantrone as single agent for the treatment of multiple sclerosis (Letter to the Editor). *Leukemia*, **12**, 441–442

Zee-Cheng, R.K.-Y. & Cheng, C.C. (1978) Antineoplastic agents. Structure–activity relationship study of bis(substituted aminoalkylamino)anthraquinones. *J. med. Chem.*, **21**, 291–294

AMSACRINE

1. Exposure Data

1.1 Chemical and physical data

1.1.1 Nomenclature

Chem. Abstr. Serv. Reg. No.: 51264-14-3
Chem. Abstr. Name: *N*-[4-(9-Acridinylamino)-3-methoxyphenyl]methane-sulfonamide
IUPAC Systematic Name: 4'-(9-Acridinylamino)methanesulfon-*meta*-anisidide
Synonyms: Acridinylanisidide; *meta*-AMSA; *meta*-Amsacrine
[Note: Amsacrine was incorrectly referred to as AMSA in some early reports (Cain & Atwell, 1974). AMSA has an -OH instead of an -OCH$_3$ at the 3-position of the anilino ring.]

1.1.2 *Structural and molecular formulae and relative molecular mass*

$C_{21}H_{19}N_3O_3S$ Relative molecular mass: 393.47

1.1.3 *Chemical and physical properties of the pure substance*

(a) *Description*: Yellow crystalline powder (Parke-Davis Canada, 1984)
(b) *Melting-point*: 230–240 °C (Parke-Davis Canada, 1984)
(c) *Spectroscopy data*: Infrared, ultraviolet and nuclear magnetic resonance spectral data have been reported (Dubicki *et al.*, 1981).

(d) *Solubility*: Insoluble in water (< 1.0 mg/mL); slightly soluble in chloroform, ethanol and methanol (National Cancer Institute, 1992)

(e) *Reactivity*: Incompatible with saline solutions; 5% dextrose is the only recommended infusion fluid; may react with certain plastic syringes (Thomas, 1998)

1.1.4 Technical products and impurities

Three intravenous formulations have been used in clinical studies: amsacrine lactate, amsacrine lactate plus anhydrous *N,N*-dimethylacetamide and amsacrine gluconate (Hornedo & Van Echo, 1985; Louie & Issell, 1985). Amsacrine is formulated as two sterile liquids in separate ampoules, one containing 75 mg of the drug in 1.5 mL *N,N*-dimethylacetamide, the other containing 13.5 mL of 0.0353 mol/L lactic acid. On mixing, the resulting solution contains 5 mg/mL of amsacrine. Amsacrine is typically used in combination with other antileukaemic agents, including cytarabine, thioguanine, 5-azacytidine, vincristine and prednisone (Gennaro, 1995; Editions du Vidal, 1998; Rote Liste Sekretariat, 1998; Thomas, 1998).

Trade names for amsacrine include Amekrin, AMSA P-D, Amsacrina, Amsacrine, Amsidil, Amsidine, Amsidyl and Lamasine (Swiss Pharmaceutical Society, 1999).

1.1.5 Analysis

Amsacrine has been determined in plasma by gas chromatography combined with flame ionization or nitrogen–phosphorus detection. With the latter method of detection, the limit of sensitivity was approximately 50 ng/mL; with the former, it was 125 ng/mL (Emonds *et al.*, 1981).

Amsacrine has been measured in human nucleated haematopoietic cells by high-performance liquid chromatography (HPLC) after the leukocytes have been separated from the erythrocytes by dextran sedimentation (Brons *et al.*, 1987). Amsacrine has also been determined in blood and urine by HPLC. The plasma samples were extracted with hexane at pH 3–4 and re-extracted with diethyl ether at pH 9 in the presence of borate present at a high concentration. Hexane extraction is not required for urine samples. After drying, the residue was dissolved in methanol before injection into the chromatograph. Absorbance was detected at 254 nm for plasma and simultaneously at 254 nm and 405 nm for urine samples (Paxton, 1984). Amsacrine has also been determined in serum by HPLC with a methanol:dichloromethane:acetate/diethylamine buffer (10:90:0.15) as eluent and ultraviolet detection at 254 nm. The limit of quantification with this method was 20 μg/L (Uges, 1990).

1.2 Production

Amsacrine is synthesized from 2′-methoxy-4′-nitrobutyranilide. The nitro group is reduced to the amine and converted to the methanesulfonamide, and the resulting free amino group is reacted with 9-acridinyl chloride to yield amsacrine (Dubicki et al., 1981; Gennaro, 1995).

Information available in 1999 indicated that amsacrine was manufactured and/or formulated in 18 countries (CIS Information Services, 1998; Swiss Pharmaceutical Society, 1999).

1.3 Use

Amsacrine is a cytotoxic drug used in the treatment of malignant disease. Its antitumour activity was first described in 1974 (Cain & Atwell, 1974), and the drug entered clinical trials in 1976 (Hornedo & Van Echo, 1985; Louie & Issell, 1985). It is an inhibitor of DNA topoisomerase II (Malonne & Atassi, 1997).

The use of amsacrine is limited almost exclusively to the treatment of leukaemia in adults and children, in which it has been included in a number of combination chemotherapy regimens at cumulative doses of 450–600 mg/m^2 (Arlin et al., 1991; Berman, 1992). In phase II trials in patients with a variety of solid tumours, amsacrine showed little or no activity at typical doses of 90–150 mg/m^2, except in Hodgkin disease (Louie & Issell, 1985).

Amsacrine is formulated as two sterile liquids that are combined before intravenous administration, diluted in 500 mL dextrose and typically infused over 30–90 min (Editions du Vidal, 1998; Thomas, 1998).

1.4 Occurrence

Amsacrine is not known to occur as a natural product. No data were available to the Working Group on occupational exposure.

1.5 Regulations and guidelines

Amsacrine is not listed in any international pharmacopoeias. Information from an industry representative indicated that amsacrine is approved for use in at least 18 countries (Parke-Davis Canada, 1999).

2. Studies of Cancer in Humans

No data were available to the Working Group.

3. Studies of Cancer in Experimental Animals

3.1 Intraperitoneal administration

Mouse: In a bioassay for lung tumours, groups of 26 male and 26 female A/J mice, six to eight weeks of age, received seven weekly intraperitoneal injections of amsacrine [purity unspecified] in dimethyl sulfoxide and tricaprylin at a dose of 0 (vehicle control), 2, 5 or 10 mg/kg bw. Positive controls received a single intraperitoneal injection of 500 or 1000 mg/kg bw urethane. The mice were held for 17 weeks after the last injection. In the groups treated with amsacrine, no significant increase in the number of mice with lung adenomas was observed [tumour incidence and multiplicity not reported] (de la Iglesia *et al.*, 1984).

3.2 Intravenous administration

Rat: Groups of 50 male and 50 female Wistar [Crl:(WI)BR] rats, six to eight weeks old, were given amsacrine (purity, 98.9%) intravenously into the lateral tail vein at a dose of 0 (vehicle control), 0.25, 1 or 3 mg/kg bw per day for five days, followed by a 23-day recovery period. This cycle of dosing and recovery was repeated six times. The animals were then maintained without dosing for the remainder of the 104-week study. The mortality rates were 44% of male controls, 48% at the low dose, 66% at the intermediate dose and 100% at the high dose; and 36% of female controls, 54% at the low dose, 46% at the intermediate dose and 96% at the high dose. None of the males at the high dose survived beyond week 90 of study. The incidences of small intestinal adenomas were 0/50, 0/50, 1/50 and 7/50 ($p < 0.01$, trend test) in male controls and those at the low, intermediate and high doses, and 0/50, 0/50, 0/50 and 7/50 ($p < 0.01$, trend test) in these groups of females, respectively. The incidences of small intestinal adenocarcinomas were 0/50, 1/50, 7/50 and 10/50 ($p < 0.01$, trend test) in the male groups and 0/50, 1/50, 1/50 and 9/50 ($p < 0.01$, trend test) in the female groups, respectively. Two adenocarcinomas and one adenoma of the large intestine were observed in males at the high dose and none in the other groups of males; two adenocarcinomas of the large intestine were observed in females at the high dose and none in the other groups. Squamous-cell carcinomas of the skin were observed in 1/50, 0/50, 4/50 and 10/50 ($p < 0.01$, trend test) rats in the four groups of males and in 0/50, 0/50, 0/50 and 4/50 ($p < 0.01$, trend test) rats in the four groups of females, respectively. Squamous-cell papillomas were observed at increased incidence in male rats (3/50 controls, 20/50 at the high dose; $p < 0.01$, Fisher's exact test) and in female rats (0/50 controls, 12/50 at the high dose; $p < 0.01$, Fisher's exact test). The incidences of keratocanthoma of the skin were significantly higher in male rats (3/50, 2/50, 7/50 and 12/50 in controls and at the low, intermediate and high doses, respectively; $p < 0.01$, trend test), but not in females. Fibromas of the skin occurred at significantly higher incidences in male rats (0/50, 8/50, 15/10 and 11/50; $p < 0.01$, trend test), but not in females. In females, the incidences of mammary adenocarcinomas were 4/50, 2/50, 5/50 and 14/50 ($p < 0.01$, trend test) and the incidences of mammary fibroadenomas were 9/50, 9/50, 17/50 and 17/50 ($p < 0.01$, trend test) in the four groups, respectively (Gough *et al.*, 1994; Graziano *et al.*, 1996).

4. Other Data Relevant to an Evaluation of Carcinogenicity and its Mechanisms

4.1 Absorption, distribution, metabolism and excretion

4.1.1 *Humans*

In cancer patients, amsacrine undergoes biphasic elimination, with a distribution half-time of 0.25–1.6 h (Van Echo *et al.*, 1979; Jurlina *et al.*, 1985; Linssen *et al.*, 1993) and an elimination half-time of 4.7–9 h (Van Echo *et al.*, 1979; Hall *et al.*, 1983; Jurlina *et al.*, 1985; Linssen *et al.*, 1993). The total plasma clearance rate is 200–300 mL/min per m², and the apparent distribution volume is 70–110 L/m², suggesting concentration in tissues (Jurlina *et al.*, 1985; Linssen *et al.*, 1993). During a 1-h infusion of amsacrine at 90–200 mg/m², the peak plasma concentration was 10–15 μmol/L (Van Echo *et al.*, 1979; Jurlina *et al.*, 1985).

Although not fully reported, early trials in which amsacrine was given orally failed to reach the maximum tolerated dose, as shown by lack of toxicity even at doses as high as 500 mg/m² per day, suggesting incomplete or erratic absorption. In subsequent studies, the intravenous route was used, with which the maximum tolerated dose in patients with solid tumours is 100–150 mg/m² when administered over 1–3 h (described by Louie & Issell, 1985).

The elimination half-time was increased to 17 h in patients with impaired liver function, but it was not altered significantly in patients with renal impairment. Urinary excretion of amsacrine over 72 h, typically around 12% of the dose, decreased to only 2% in patients with renal impairment and increased to 20% in patients with hepatic impairment (Hall *et al.*, 1983). After administration of [^{14}C]amsacrine, the total amount of radiolabel excreted in urine was 35% in patients with normal organ function, 49% in patients with liver impairment and 2–16% in patients with renal impairment. Patients with decreased amsacrine clearance rates experienced more toxicity. In two patients from whom biliary outflow was collected, 8% and 36% of the administered radiolabel was recovered within 72 h, < 2% being unchanged amsacrine (Hall *et al.*, 1983).

Amsacrine is taken up rapidly by nucleated blood cells *in vivo*, peak concentrations occurring shortly after the end of a 3-h infusion; the concentration was about five times greater than the peak plasma concentration. Over 24 h, the mean integrated area under the time–concentration curve (AUC) for cellular amsacrine was eight times that of the AUC for plasma. The kinetics of elimination from peripheral blast cells was similar to that from plasma (Linssen *et al.*, 1993).

In tumour samples from patients receiving amsacrine, the tumour:plasma concentration ratio ranged from 2:1 to 4.9:1 (Guo et al., 1983). High tissue concentrations of amsacrine were still present two weeks after treatment (Stewart et al., 1984), the highest concentrations occurring in the gall-bladder, liver and kidney. The concentrations in cerebrospinal fluid were < 2% of the corresponding plasma concentration in one study (Hall et al., 1983) and were undetectable in another (Guo et al., 1983).

About 97% of a dose of amsacrine is bound to protein bound in plasma in both cancer patients and healthy volunteers. Studies of human plasma *in vitro* showed no change in protein binding across a concentration range of 1–100 μmol/L. The unbound fraction increased to 21.7%, however, when the pH was changed to 6.4 (Paxton et al., 1986).

No studies of the metabolism of amsacrine in humans have been published.

4.1.2 *Experimental systems*

The pharmacokinetics of amsacrine has been described for mice (Cysyk et al., 1977; Kestell et al., 1990), rats (Cysyk et al., 1977), rabbits (Paxton & Jurlina, 1985) and dogs (Paxton et al., 1990). This typically includes biphasic elimination, with a rapid distribution phase and a more prolonged terminal elimination phase with a half-time of about 0.2 h in mice, 0.5 h in rats, 2.6 h in rabbits and 6.5 h in dogs. The pharmacokinetics was typically predictable in all species, including humans (Paxton et al., 1990).

The bioavailability of orally administered amsacrine in mice (10 mg/kg bw) and rats (100 mg/kg bw) was incomplete and variable (Cysyk et al., 1978), with high concentrations occurring in the liver and rapid excretion into the bile. In rabbits, the bioavailability of amsacrine given orally at a dose of 12.7 μmol/kg bw was 50% in fed animals but 90% in fasting rabbits (Paxton, 1986).

After intravenous administration of [^{14}C]amsacrine to mice and rats, > 50% of the radiolabel was excreted in bile within the first 2 h, and the bile:plasma ratio was > 400:1 (Cysyk et al., 1977); 74% of an intravenous dose was excreted in the faeces of mice within 72 h (Robertson et al., 1988). These studies demonstrate the importance of the liver in clearance of amsacrine.

A number of reports have described the metabolism of amsacrine in rats and mice. In mouse bile, 5′- and 6′-glutathione conjugates were present in roughly equal amounts and accounted for 70% of the excreted biliary radiolabel after administration of radiolabelled amsacrine (Robertson et al., 1988). In rats, the principal biliary metabolite was the 5′-glutathione conjugate, which accounted for 80% of the excreted radiolabel within the first 90 min and > 50% of the administered dose over 3 h (Shoemaker et al., 1982). The 6′-conjugate was also subsequently identified in rat bile (Robertson et al., 1993). In rat liver microsomes and human neutrophils, intermediate oxidation products have been identified as N1′-methanesulfonyl-N4′-(9-acridinyl)-3′-methoxy-2′,5′-cyclohexadiene-1′,4′-diimine and 3′-methoxy-4′-(9-acridinylamino-2′,5′-cyclohexadien-1′-one (Shoemaker et al., 1984; Kettle et al., 1992). These oxidation products were about

100 times more cytotoxic to cells than amsacrine *in vitro*, while the principal conjugation product in rats, the 5′-glutathione conjugate, was inactive (Shoemaker *et al.*, 1984). The same conjugation products were reported after exposure of Chinese hamster fibroblasts to amsacrine or its methanesulfonyl oxidation product in culture. The rate of glutathione conjugate formation during exposure to the oxidation product in cultured cells was rapid, whereas formation after exposure to amsacrine was slow, suggesting a low rate of oxidation of amsacrine to its oxidation products, with subsequent conjugation formation in this system (Robbie *et al.*, 1990) (see Figure 1).

Figure 1. Metabolism of amsacrine

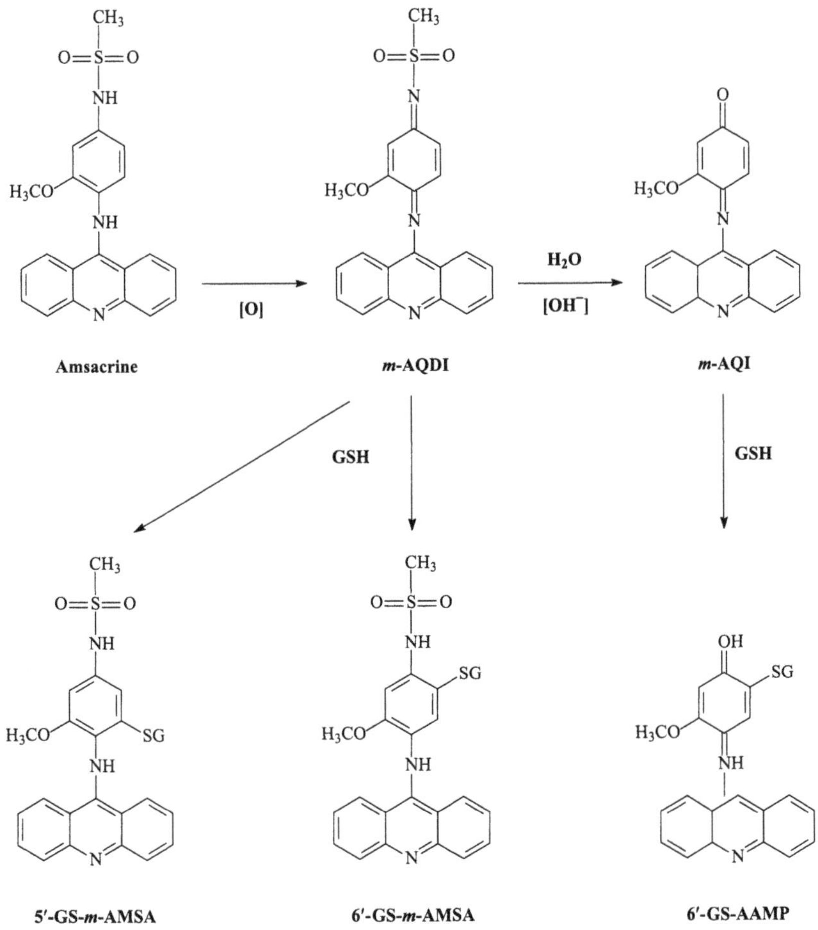

m-AQDI, N1′-methanesulfonyl-N4′-(9-acridinyl)-3′-methoxy-2′,5′-cyclohexadiene-1′,4′-diimine; *m*-AQI, 3′-methoxy-4′-(9-acridinylamino)-2′,5′-cyclohexadien-1′-one; 5′-GS-*m*-AMSA, 5′-glutathione conjugate of amsacrine; 6′-GS-*m*-AMSA, 6′-glutathione conjugate of amsacrine; 6′-GS-AAMP, 4′-(9-acridinylamino)-6′-(S-glutathionyl)-3′-methoxyphenol

4.2 Toxic effects

4.2.1 Humans

The toxicity of amsacrine in humans has been comprehensively reviewed and summarized (Hornedo & Van Echo, 1985; Louie & Issell, 1985). In all of the phase I studies, the dose-limiting toxic effect was myelosuppression, resulting mainly in leukopenia. Other effects included nausea, vomiting, fever, injection-site reaction, skin rash and discolouration (due to the yellow colour of the drug), mucositis and alopecia. Paraesthesia and hepatoxicity were seen in a few patients, but cardiac toxicity was not observed in one study (Louie & Issell, 1985).

In phase II studies with amsacrine as a single agent in patients with solid tumours, myelosuppression was again the dose-limiting effect (90–120 mg/m^2 once every three to four weeks), with leukopenia and thrombocytopenia occurring in almost all patients. Anaemia is also common. At these doses, the leukopenia is mild to moderate in most patients but more severe in around 30% of patients (Hornedo & Van Echo, 1985). The lowest counts usually occur at about day 10, with recovery by day 21. Myelosuppression is usually more severe in previously treated patients, and is much more severe with high doses of amsacrine (600–1000 mg/m^2).

Nausea, vomiting and mucositis are common after administration of amsacrine. Diarrhoea occurs in about 10–20% of patients (Louie & Issell, 1985). Stomatitis and mucositis become more frequent with higher doses (> 120 mg/m^2) (Slevin et al., 1981).

Hepatotoxicity has been reported, typically manifest as transient increases in serum bilirubin concentration and/or hepatic enzyme activity, but lethal hepatotoxicity has also been reported (Appelbaum & Shulman, 1982).

Phlebitis occurred in up to 17% of patients in early studies with amsacrine (Legha et al., 1978; Louie & Issell, 1985), but the incidence has been reduced by administering the drug in a more dilute solution.

Eighty-two cases of amsacrine-associated cardiotoxicity were observed among over 6000 patients in phase II studies who had received amsacrine up until 1986, giving a total incidence of just over 1%. The more common effects were alterations in the electrocardiogram and arrhythmia, but cardiomyopathy and congestive heart failure also occurred (Weiss et al., 1986). Amsacrine has been used safely in patients with pre-existing arrhythmia when a serum potassium concentration of > 4 mmol/L was maintained (Arlin et al., 1991).

4.2.2 Experimental systems

In dogs given single doses, the toxic effects at the highest non-lethal dose (3.1 mg/kg bw) were leukopenia, anaemia and increased serum activity of liver enzymes. Controls receiving 100 mg/mL N,N-dimethylacetamide and 2.8 mg/mL L-lactic acid (pH 3.2) also showed signs of liver toxicity. Similar toxic effects were seen at the highest non-lethal regimes of five daily doses of 0.39 mg/kg bw in dogs and five daily doses of 5.2 mg/kg bw in rhesus monkeys (Henry et al., 1980).

Toxic effects on the gastrointestinal and central nervous system were observed at lethal doses in dogs (6.25 mg/kg bw as a single dose, 0.78 mg/kg with five daily doses), but no cardiac toxic effects were reported in any species (Henry et al., 1980). In subsequent studies, evidence of cardiotoxicity was not seen in rats (Kim et al., 1985), but cardiac rhythm abnormalities and ectopic pulses were seen in rabbits at doses of 2.5–7.5 mg/kg bw and in an isolated rabbit heart preparation, in which dose-related negative ionotropic effects were seen at therapeutically relevant concentrations (D'Alessandro et al., 1983).

Intravenous dosing of rats at 1 or 3 mg/kg bw per day for five days resulted in hair loss, diarrhoea and leukopenia; these effects were reversible (Pegg et al., 1996).

Local tissue reactions were seen when the drug was administered subcutaneously or intramuscularly to guinea-pigs or rabbits, but similar effects were seen after administration of the vehicle alone, suggesting that the acidity of the vehicle (see above) may have been responsible (Henry et al., 1980). Skin rashes in personnel involved in bulk formulation of amsacrine prompted further studies in experimental animals. In the Magnussen and Kligman maximization test, amsacrine was extremely sensitizing to the skin of guinea-pigs when given as a challenge dose by direct application, while the vehicle alone produced almost no response. The animals were not sensitized for systemic anaphylaxis, however, and there was no detectable induction of antibodies in rabbits (Watson et al., 1981).

4.3 Reproductive and prenatal effects

4.3.1 *Humans*

Amsacrine at a dose of 40 mg/m^2 per day for three days every three weeks led to a marked reduction in sperm count in a patient with melanoma (da Cunha et al., 1982). As in mice (da Cunha et al., 1985), however, the sperm count returned to normal during a 10-week gap in treatment, indicating that amsacrine has only a temporary, reversible effect on differentiating germinal cells and is not toxic to stem cells.

4.3.2 *Experimental systems*

In mice given total doses of 7.5–30 mg/kg bw amsacrine intraperitoneally as three daily doses or as a single dose of 15 mg/kg bw, substantial killing of differentiating spermatogonia (types A_2 to B) was seen. There was no effect on post-spermatogonial stages and little effect on stem cells, and the sperm counts had recovered by day 56 (da Cunha et al., 1985).

Amsacrine was reported in an abstract to be embryotoxic, fetotoxic and teratogenic in groups of 20 CD rats dosed intraperitoneally with 0.1, 0.5 or 1.0 mg/kg bw per day amsacrine lactate on days 6–15 of gestation. Maternal weight gain was reduced at the high dose only. Eye, jaw and other skeletal malformations were observed in the fetuses at all doses. An increased frequency of resorptions and decreased fetal weight were observed at the intermediate and high doses (Ng et al. 1987).

Day-10 rat embryos [strain not specified] cultured for 24 h *in vitro* were exposed for the first 3 h to amsacrine at concentrations of 10 nmol/L to 1 μmol/L. A dose-related increase in the frequency of malformations was observed at doses of 50–500 nmol/L, and 100% of the embryos were malformed at 500 nmol/L. At 1 μmol/L, all embryos were killed. Embryonic growth was reduced at concentrations from 200 nmol/L. The malformations consisted mainly of hypoplasia of the prosencephalon, microphthalmia and oedema of the rhombencephalon. Similar malformations were observed in the same system with etoposide (see the monograph on etoposide). Comparison of the concentrations necessary to produce lethality and malformations in 50% of fetuses showed that amsacrine was 10 times and 20 times more potent, respectively, than etoposide (Mirkes & Zwelling, 1990).

In a study reported only as an abstract, male mice were treated with a maximum tolerated dose of 15 mg/kg bw [no further details given] amsacrine and showed no signs of dominant lethal mutation. Female mice treated with a maximum tolerated dose of 12.5 mg/kg bw amsacrine in a test for total reproductive capacity showed reduced litter size at the first mating interval, suggesting a dominant lethal effect (Bishop et al., 1997).

4.4 Genetic and related effects

4.4.1 *Humans*

No data were available to the Working Group.

4.4.2 *Experimental systems*

General reviews on the mutagenicity of inhibitors of DNA topoisomerase II enzymes, including amsacrine, have been published (Anderson & Berger, 1994; Ferguson & Baguley, 1994, 1996; Baguley & Ferguson, 1998). Jackson et al. (1996) collated a genetic activity profile for this drug. The results are summarized in Table 1.

Amsacrine was mutagenic in some strains of *Salmonella typhimurium*, causing an increased number of revertants in TA1537, a small increase (about twofold) in revertants in TA102 but no increase in revertants in TA1535, TA98 or TA100. Addition of an exogenous metabolic system reduced but did not eliminate the mutagenic effects in TA1537. The positive effects required a dose of about 800 μg/plate, which is higher than those tested in mammalian cells.

Amsacrine reverted a frameshift mutant of T4 and induced prophage λ in *Escherichia coli* WP2, suggesting an 'SOS' repair response. In *Saccharomyces cerevisiae* strain D5, amsacrine failed to induce the mitochondrial 'petite' mutation, but it was an effective mitotic recombinogen when testing was done under conditions permitting cell growth. It did not induce either forward or reverse mutations in *Neurospora crassa*.

Table 1. Genetic and related effects of amsacrine

Test system	Result[a] Without exogenous metabolic system	Result[a] With exogenous metabolic system	Dose[b] (LED or HID)	Reference
Escherichia coli WP2s (λ) prophage induction, SOS response	−	+	312	DeMarini & Lawrence (1992)
Bacteriophage T4, reverse mutation (frameshift)	+	NT	1	DeMarini & Lawrence (1988)
Salmonella typhimurium TA100, TA98, reverse mutation	−	−	1000 µg/plate	Ferguson et al. (1988)
Salmonella typhimurium TA102, reverse mutation	(+)	(+)	800 µg/plate	Ferguson et al. (1988)
Salmonella typhimurium TA102, reverse mutation	−	NT	3.33 µg/plate	Albertini et al. (1995)
Salmonella typhimurium TA1535, reverse mutation	−	NT	50 µg/plate	Iwamoto et al. (1992a)
Salmonella typhimurium TA1537, reverse mutation	+	+	100 µg/plate	Ferguson et al. (1988)
Salmonella typhimurium TA1537, reverse mutation	+	NT	225 µg/plate	Iwamoto et al. (1992a,b)
Saccharomyces cerevisiae D5, mitotic recombination	+	NT	500	Ferguson & Turner (1988a)
Saccharomyces cerevisiae D5, mitochondrial petite mutation	−	NT	> 2000	Ferguson & Turner (1988b)
Neurospora crassa, forward mutation, *ad-3A* frameshift strain	−	NT	100	Gupta (1990)
Neurospora crassa reverse mutation, *ad-3A* frameshift strain	−	NT	315 µg/plate	Gupta (1990)
Drosophila melanogaster, genetic crossing-over or recombination (white–ivory assay)	−		790 in feed	Ferreiro et al. (1997)
Drosophila melanogaster, somatic mutation and recombination	−		1970	Torres et al. (1998)
DNA single-strand breaks and DNA–protein cross-links, mouse L1210 cells *in vitro*	+	NT	0.04	Minford et al. (1984)
DNA single- and double-strand breaks, Chinese hamster lung V79 cells *in vitro*	+	NT	0.04	Pommier et al. (1985)

Table 1 (contd)

Test system	Result[a]		Dose[b] (LED or HID)	Reference
	Without exogenous metabolic system	With exogenous metabolic system		
DNA single-strand breaks (protein-linked), mouse embryo 3T3 fibroblasts in vitro	+	NT	0.2	Markovits et al. (1987)
DNA single-strand breaks, mouse leukaemia L1210 cells in vitro	+	NT	4.0	Covey et al. (1988)
DNA–protein cross-links, mouse leukaemia L1210 cells in vitro	+	NT	0.4	Covey et al. (1988)
DNA double-strand breaks, mouse fibrosarcoma 935.1 cells in vitro	+	NT	NR	Woynarowski et al. (1994)
DNA–protein cross-links and double-strand breaks, Chinese hamster ovary CHO-K1 and xrs-1 cells in vitro	+	NT	0.2	Caldecott et al. (1990)
Gene mutation, Chinese hamster lung V79 cells, ouabain resistance in vitro	–	NT	0.2	Wilson et al. (1984)
Gene mutation, Chinese hamster lung V79 cells, Hprt locus in vitro	+	NT	0.004–0.04	Wilson et al. (1984)
Mutation, Chinese hamster lung V79 cells, Hprt locus in vitro	+	NT	0.08	Pommier et al. (1985)
Gene mutation, Chinese hamster ovary AA8 cells, Hprt locus in vitro	+	NT	NR	Ferguson et al. (1992)
Mutation, Chinese hamster ovary AA8 cells, cytosine arabinoside resistance in vitro	(+)	NT	NR	Ferguson et al. (1992)
Mutation, A$_L$ (human × hamster) hybrid cell line, Hprt locus in vitro	(+)	NT	0.016	Shibuya et al. (1994)
Mutation, A$_L$ (human × hamster) hybrid cell line, S1 phenotype in vitro	+	NT	0.004	Shibuya et al. (1994)
Mutation, Chinese hamster ovary D422 cells, Aprt locus in vitro	+	NT	0.4	Zhou et al. (1997)

Table 1 (contd)

Test system	Result[a]		Dose[b] (LED or HID)	Reference
	Without exogenous metabolic system	With exogenous metabolic system		
Mutation, mouse lymphoma L5178Y cells, *Tk* locus *in vitro*	+	NT	0.001	DeMarini *et al.* (1987)
Mutation, mouse lymphoma L5178Y cells, *Tk* locus *in vitro*	+	NT	0.001	Doerr *et al.* (1989)
Mutation, mouse lymphoma L5178Y cells, *Tk* locus *in vitro*	+	NT	0.001	Backer *et al.* (1990)
Gene mutation, mouse lymphoma L5178Y cells, *Tk* locus *in vitro*	–	NT	0.05	Albertini *et al.* (1995)
Gene mutation, mouse lymphoma L5178Y cells, *Hprt* locus *in vitro*	+	NT	0.001	Albertini *et al.* (1995)
Mutation, AS52 Chinese hamster cells, bacterial *Gpt* locus *in vitro*	+	NT	0.04	Ferguson *et al.* (1998)
Sister chromatid exchange, Chinese hamster lung V79 cells *in vitro*	+	NT	0.4	Lim *et al.* (1986)
Sister chromatid exchange, Chinese hamster cells *in vitro*	+	NT	0.08	Pommier *et al.* (1985)
Sister chromatid exchange, Chinese hamster lung DC3F cells	+[c]	NT	0.4	Pommier *et al.* (1988)
Sister chromatid exchange, Chinese hamster AA8 and EM9 cells *in vitro*	+	NT	0.4	Cortés *et al.* (1993)
Sister chromatid exchange, Chinese hamster CHO6 cells	+	NT	0.1	Cortés & Piñero (1994)
Sister chromatid exchange, Chinese hamster CHO6 cells	+	NT	0.04	Piñero *et al.* (1996)
Micronucleus formation, mouse C3H10T1/2 cells *in vitro*	+	NT	0.005	Ferguson *et al.* (1986)
Micronucleus formation, mouse lymphoma L5178Y cells	+	NT	0.001	Doerr *et al.* (1989)
Micronucleus formation, mouse lymphoma L5178Y cells *in vitro*	+	NT	0.001	Backer *et al.* (1990)

Table 1 (contd)

Test system	Result[a]		Dose[b] (LED or HID)	Reference
	Without exogenous metabolic system	With exogenous metabolic system		
Chromosomal aberrations (anaphase/telophase test), Chinese hamster ovary cells *in vitro*	+	NT	0.1	Larripa *et al.* (1984)
Chromosomal aberrations, Chinese hamster lung V79 cells *in vitro*	+	NT	0.005	Ferguson *et al.* (1988)
Chromosomal aberrations, Chinese hamster lung V79 cells *in vitro*	+	NT	0.08	Pommier *et al.* (1985)
Chromosomal aberrations, Chinese hamster lung DC3F cells *in vitro*	+[c]	NT	0.4	Pommier *et al.* (1988)
Chromosomal aberrations, Chinese hamster AA8 and EM9 cells *in vitro*	+	NT	0.4	Cortés *et al.* (1993)
Chromosomal aberrations, Chinese hamster CHO6 cells *in vitro*	+	NT	0.1	Cortés & Piñero (1994)
Chromosomal aberrations, mouse L1210 cells *in vitro*	+	NT	0.04	Ferguson & Baguley (1984)
Chromosomal aberrations, C3H10T1/2 mouse cells *in vitro*	+	NT	0.0025	Ferguson *et al.* (1986)
Chromosomal aberrations, mouse lymphoma L5178Y cells *in vitro*	+	NT	0.001	Doerr *et al.* (1989)
Chromosomal aberrations, mouse lymphoma L5178Y cells *in vitro*	+	NT	0.0005	DeMarini *et al.* (1987)
Chromosomal aberrations, mouse lymphoma L5178Y cells *in vitro*	+	NT	0.0001	Backer *et al.* (1990)
Aneuploidy/polyploidy, Chinese hamster–human hybrid GM10115A cell line *in vitro*	+	NT	0.004	Ferguson *et al.* (1996a)
Polyploidy, Chinese hamster ovary cells *in vitro*	+	NT	16	Sumner (1995)
Polyploidy, murine erythroleukaemic cells *in vitro*	+	NT	1	Zucker *et al.* (1991)

Table 1 (contd)

Test system	Result[a]		Dose[b] (LED or HID)	Reference
	Without exogenous metabolic system	With exogenous metabolic system		
Cell transformation, C3H10T1/2 mouse cells	+	NT	0.01	Ferguson et al. (1986)
Protein-associated DNA strand breaks, human leukaemic myeloblasts and normal lymphocytes in vitro	+	NT	0.1	Brox et al. (1986)
DNA double-strand breaks, human breast cancer T-47D cells in vitro	+	NT	0.15	Epstein & Smith (1988)
DNA double-strand breaks, human breast cancer MCF-7 cells in vitro	+	NT	0.2	Bunch et al. (1994)
DNA single- and double-strand breaks, Raji (Burkitt lymphoma) cells in vitro	+	NT	1.2	Johnson & Beerman (1994)
DNA double-strand breaks within the AML1 locus, various human leukaemia cell lines in vitro	+	NT	12	Stanulla et al. (1997)
Sister chromatid exchange, human lymphocytes in vitro	+	NT	0.005	Kao-Shan et al. (1984)
Sister chromatid exchange, human lymphocytes in vitro	+	NT	0.2	Andersson & Kihlman (1989)
Sister chromatid exchange, human lymphocytes in vitro	+	NT	3.2	Ribas et al. (1996)
Micronucleus formation, human lymphocytes from neonatal cord blood in vitro	+	NT	0.01	Slavotinek et al. (1993)
Chromosomal aberrations, human lymphocytes in vitro	+	NT	0.005	Kao-Shan et al. (1984)
Chromosomal aberrations, human lymphocytes in vitro	+	NT	0.6	Andersson & Kihlman (1989)
Chromosomal aberrations, human lymphocytes in vitro	+	NT	0.4	Mosesso et al. (1998)
Chromosomal aberrations, Hela cells in vitro	+	NT	0.25	Ferguson & Baguley (1984)
DNA breaks preferentially in episomal regulatory regions in tumour-bearing mRIII S/J mice in vivo	+		15 iv × 1	Cullinan et al. (1990)

Table 1 (contd)

Test system	Result[a]		Dose[b] (LED or HID)	Reference
	Without exogenous metabolic system	With exogenous metabolic system		
Chromosomal aberrations, host-mediated assay, L1210 leukaemia cells grown intraperitoneally in male DBA/2J mice	+		5 ip × 1	Ferguson & Baguley (1984)
Sister chromatid exchange, bone-marrow cells of male C57BL/6J mice in vivo	+		1.5 ip × 1	Backer et al. (1990)
Micronucleus formation, bone-marrow cells of male and female CFW mice in vivo	+		1.5 ip × 1	Larripa et al. (1984)
Micronucleus formation, bone marrow of male and female CD-1 mice in vivo	+		1.5 ip × 1	Holmström & Winters (1992)
Micronucleus formation, hepatocytes and peripheral blood reticulocytes of male ddY mice in vivo	+		10 ip × 1	Igarashi & Shimada (1997)
Chromosomal aberrations, bone marrow of male C57BL/6J mice in vivo	+		3 ip × 1	Backer et al. (1990)
Dominant lethal mutations, female C3H × C57BL mice	+		12.5[d]	Bishop et al. (1996)
Dominant lethal mutations, male C3H × C57BL mice	–		15[d]	Bishop et al. (1996)
Sister chromatid exchange, human lymphocytes in vivo	–		30 mg/m^2 per day; continuous iv, 3–4 d	Kao-Shan et al. (1984)

Table 1 (contd)

Test system	Result[a]		Dose[b] (LED or HID)	Reference
	Without exogenous metabolic system	With exogenous metabolic system		
Chromosomal aberrations, human lymphocytes *in vivo*	+		30 mg/m² per day; continuous iv, 3–4 d	Kao-Shan *et al.* (1984)

[a] +, positive; (+), weak positive; −, negative; NT, not tested
[b] LED, lowest effective dose; HID, highest ineffective dose; in-vitro tests, μg/mL; in-vivo tests, mg/kg bw per day; NR, not reported; ip, intraperitoneally; iv, intravenously; d, day
[c] Negative in topoisomerase II-resistant DC3F/9-OHE cells
[d] Route not specified

Amsacrine is a clastogen in mammalian cells. It caused DNA double-strand breaks and DNA–protein cross-links in various animal cells and in human cell lines at a concentration of about 1 μmol/L. Amsacrine caused DNA breaks preferentially in episomal regulatory regions in tumour-bearing mRIII S/J mice and at a very specific site within the *AML*1 locus in several human cell lines. The Chinese hamster cell line xrs-1 was hypersensitive to amsacrine treatment (Caldecott *et al.*, 1990). The drug appears to inactivate DNA synthesis by inhibiting replicon cluster initiation (Suciu, 1991).

Amsacrine caused chromosomal aberrations in cultured Chinese hamster cells, in various rodent cell lines, in HeLa cells and in cultured human peripheral blood lymphocytes. It also induced micronuclei in neonatal human lymphocytes. Fluorescence in-situ hybridization techniques revealed a high frequency of dicentrics and stable translocations in amsacrine-treated human peripheral blood lymphocytes. Various chromosomal aberrations were also observed in mouse leukaemia L1210 cells that were grown intraperitoneally in male DBA/2J mice and treated with amsacrine at doses and schedules that effectively reduced the tumour burden. Additionally, amsacrine induced micronuclei and chromosomal aberrations in the bone marrow of non-tumour-bearing male and female mice. In male ddY mice, amsacrine increased the incidence of micronuclei in both hepatocytes and peripheral blood reticulocytes. In one study, amsacrine caused chromosomal aberrations, but no sister chromatid exchange in blood lymphocytes of patients treated with this drug by intravenous infusion.

Amsacrine induced sister chromatid exchange in Chinese hamster cells and in human lymphocytes *in vitro*. This effect was also seen *in vivo*. It had no effect in *Drosophila melanogaster* in the wing spot test or in the *white–ivory* assay, which provide a measure of somatic crossing-over or recombination.

Although there is evidence that amsacrine causes point mutations in bacteria, it does not appear to do so in mammalian cells, possibly because the concentrations necessary to evoke these events would be lethal to mammalian cells. Amsacrine did not induce resistance to ouabain (a known measure of base-pair substitution mutagenesis) in Chinese hamster lung V79 cells, although it induced mutations at the *Hprt* locus in these cells, in Chinese hamster ovary cells and in A_L (human × hamster) hybrid cell lines. It was a potent mutagen at the *MIC*1 locus in the last cell line and a moderate inducer of cytarabine resistance (by an unknown mechanism) in Chinese hamster AA8 cells. Amsacrine caused mutations at the *Aprt* locus in Chinese hamster ovary D422 cells. In two of three studies, it induced primarily small colony mutants at the *Tk* locus in mouse lymphoma L5178Y cells; although these events were classified as gene mutations (Jackson *et al.*, 1996), they are probably chromosomal events. Mutations at the *Hprt* locus in V79 cells paralleled chromosomal events as measured by micronucleus formation (Wilson *et al.*, 1984), strand breakage (single or double strands) and sister chromatid exchange. The differential sensitivity of the *MIC*1 locus (studied with the S1 antigen) and the *Hprt* locus in A_L cells suggests that amsacrine produces megabase-pair deletions at the *Hprt* locus that would prove lethal. Amsacrine primarily increased small colony mutants in mouse lymphoma L5178Y cells, and these are known to be caused by chromosomal mutations (DeMarini et al., 1987).

The molecular nature of amsacrine-induced mutations to 6-thioguanine resistance was studied in late log-phase Chinese hamster AS52 cells (Ferguson et al., 1998). Neither frameshift nor base pair-substitution mutational events could be unequivocally associated with this treatment. In the study of Ferguson et al. (1998), amsacrine caused major chromosomal deletions and illegitimate recombination in Chinese hamster ovary cells, detectable by Southern blotting. On the basis of the size of the deletions observed, Shibuya et al. (1994) speculated that amsacrine-induced deletions are mediated by a series of subunit exchanges between overlapping DNA topoisomerase II dimers at the bases of replicons or larger chromosomal structures such as replicon clusters or chromosomal minibands. Zhou et al. (1997) also showed reciprocal exchanges involving the *Aprt* locus after amsacrine treatment and suggested a model similar to that of Shibuya et al. (1994).

The extent of amsacrine-induced mutation varies among cell lines, depending on their susceptibility to apoptosis, or programmed cell death, which is a means of ensuring that genetically damaged cells do not survive to form progeny and acts as an alternative pathway to mutagenesis. For example, treatment of human lymphoblastoid AHH-1 $TK^{+/-}$ cells with amsacrine led to cell cycle arrest at the G_2/M phase, and conditions that enhance apoptosis led to a low recovery of viable mutants (Morris et al., 1995, 1996). Cells may be particularly susceptible to apoptosis by DNA topoisomerase II inhibitors such as amsacrine, which cause apoptosis through both *p53*-dependent and -independent routes (Ferguson, 1998).

Fluorescence in-situ hybridization techniques revealed that amsacrine caused both aneuploidy and polyploidy in a Chinese hamster–human cell hybrid. Polyploidy was also demonstrated by cytogenetic techniques in Chinese hamster ovary cells and, by flow cytometry, in murine erythroleukaemic cells. Amsacrine caused cell transformation in mouse C3H10T1/2 cells *in vitro* and prevented the dimethyl sulfoxide-induced differentiation of human leukaemia HL-60 cells.

Amsacrine also mutates germ cells: dominant lethal events were seen in female but not in male mice. Treatment of meiotic cells with amsacrine can disrupt the structure of the synaptonemal complex, a meiosis-specific structure that is essential for accurate recombination and chromosomal segregation. For example, exposure of preleptotene mouse germ cells to amsacrine led to an aberrant multi-axial configuration of the synaptonemal complex (Ferguson et al., 1996b). This provides indirect evidence that amsacrine interferes with meiotic recombination and is a probable aneuploidogen in meiotic cells.

4.5 Mechanistic considerations

In general, the events caused by amsacrine in mammalian cells *in vitro* occurred in the absence of exogenous metabolic activation, although a possible mechanism for oxidative metabolism has been identified (Kettle *et al.*, 1992). Three mechanisms have been identified to explain the mutagenicity and carcinogenicity of amsacrine.

It has three activities that may be responsible for mutation.

1. It inhibits DNA topoisomerase II enzymes: Amsacrine is a DNA topoisomerase II poison that has been shown to promote DNA cleavage, with a strong preference for a site one base away from adenine (Marsh *et al.*, 1996). Most of the mutational events reported in mammalian cells, including point mutations, chromosomal deletions and exchanges and aneuploidy, can be explained by this activity. Amsacrine does not inhibit bacterial topoisomerases and may not mutate bacterial cells by the same mechanism as mammalian cells.

2. It possesses readily oxidizable functions: The anilino ring of amsacrine can be reversibly oxidized, either chemically or microsomally, to produce a quinone diimine (Jurlina *et al.*, 1987). DeMarini and Lawrence (1992) suggested that the induction of prophage reflects this activity of the drug. Nevertheless, none of the mutations seen with amsacrine is of the type usually associated with reactive oxygen species.

3. It intercalates into, but does not interact covalently with, DNA: DNA intercalation, but not DNA topoisomerase II inhibition, is probably responsible for the frameshift mutagenicity seen in bacteria (Ferguson & Baguley, 1981; Ferguson & Denny, 1990).

5. Summary of Data Reported and Evaluation

5.1 Exposure data

Amsacrine is a synthetic DNA topoisomerase II inhibitor used primarily in the treatment of leukaemia in adults and children.

5.2 Human carcinogenicity data

No data were available to the Working Group.

5.3 Animal carcinogenicity data

Amsacrine was tested by intraperitoneal administration in one assay for lung adenomas in mice; no increase in incidence was reported. In a single study in rats given amsacrine by intravenous administration, small-intestinal adenomas and adenocarcinomas were induced in a dose-dependent fashion in males and females, and a few adenocarcinomas of the large intestine were seen in males and females at the high dose. The incidences of squamous-cell papillomas and carcinomas of the skin were increased in males and females, those of keratoacanthomas and of fibromas of the skin were increased in males, and those of mammary fibroadenomas and adenocarcinomas were increased in females. All of these increases were dose-dependent.

The occurrence of intestinal carcinomas in rats of each sex and the occurrence of skin tumours after intravenous administration of a chemical are unusual.

5.4 Other relevant data

In humans, amsacrine is eliminated biphasically, with an elimination half-time of 5–9 h. The drug is rapidly taken up by nucleated blood cells, with an overall cell:plasma ratio over 24 h of 8:1, and is distributed to other tissues. Preliminary studies suggest that the oral bioavailability of amsacrine is poor, and there is currently no oral formulation of the drug. About 35% of an intravenous dose was excreted renally over 72 h, with 12% as unchanged amsacrine; biliary recovery in two patients was up to 36%. Biphasic elimination was also observed in a number of animal species. In mice and rats, > 50% of a radiolabelled dose was excreted in the bile within 2 h, and 74% of the dose was recovered in the faeces of mice by 72 h. The results of studies in humans and animals demonstrate the importance of renal and hepatic function in amsacrine clearance. In animals, much of a radiolabelled dose of amsacrine was excreted as metabolites, some of which were cytotoxic. There are currently no data on the metabolism of amsacrine in humans.

In human and animal species, the main toxic effect of amsacrine is myelosuppression, especially leukopenia. Other common toxic effects are nausea and vomiting, mucositis, alopecia and diarrhoea. Less common effects include hepatotoxicity and cardiotoxicity.

Amsacrine does not bind covalently to DNA. It appears to mutate cells through two mechanisms. In mammals, amsacrine is an effective poison of DNA topoisomerase II enzymes, leading to cellular accumulation of protein-masked double-stranded DNA breaks and, with time, a variety of chromosomal aberrations. It is also an effective recombinogen, its predominant effects appearing to involve the deletion and/or interchange of large DNA segments. Amsacrine also induces both polyploidy and aneuploidy. It is a frameshift mutagen in bacteria and bacteriophages, and this property may be related to its intercalating action.

Potent protein-masked DNA breakage and clastogenic effects occur in human cells *in vitro* and in animal cells *in vivo*.

5.5 Evaluation

There is *inadequate evidence* in humans for the carcinogenicity of amsacrine.

There is *sufficient evidence* in experimental animals for the carcinogenicity of amsacrine.

Overall evaluation

Amsacrine is *possibly carcinogenic to humans (Group 2B)*.

6. References

Anderson, R.D. & Berger, N.A. (1994) Mutagenicity and carcinogenicity of topoisomerase-interactive agents. *Mutat. Res.*, **309**, 109–142

Andersson, H.C. & Kihlman, B.A. (1989) The production of chromosomal alterations in human lymphocytes by drugs known to interfere with the activity of DNA topoisomerase II. I. *m*-AMSA. *Carcinogenesis*, **10**, 123–130

Appelbaum, F.R. & Shulman, H.M. (1982) Fatal hepatotoxicity associated with AMSA therapy. *Cancer Treat. Rep.*, **66**, 1863–1865

Arlin, Z.A., Feldman, E.J., Mittelman, A., Ahmed, T., Puccio, C., Chun, H.G., Cook, P., Baskind, P., Marboe, C. & Mehta, R. (1991) Amsacrine is safe and effective therapy for patients with myocardial dysfunction and acute leukemia. *Cancer*, **68**, 1198–1200

Backer, L.C., Allen, J.W., Harrington-Brock, K., Campbell, J.A., DeMarini, D.M., Doerr, C.L., Howard, D.R., Kligerman, A.D. & Moore, M.M. (1990) Genotoxicity of inhibitors of DNA topoisomerases I (camptothecin) and II (*m*-AMSA) *in vivo* and *in vitro*. *Mutagenesis*, **5**, 541–547

Baguley, B.C. & Ferguson, L.R. (1998) Mutagenic properties of topoisomerase-targeted drugs. *Biochim. biophys. Acta*, **1400**, 213–222

Berman, E. (1992) New drugs in acute myelogenous leukemia: A review. *J. clin. Pharmacol.*, **32**, 296–309

Bishop, J.B., Hughes, L.A., Ferguson, L.R. & Generoso, W.M. (1996) Amsacrine: A topoisomerase inhibitor which is a female specific germ cell mutagen (Abstract). *Environ. mol. Mutag.*, **27**, 8

Bishop, J.B., Hughes, L.A., Ferguson, L.R., Wei, X. & Generoso, W.M. (1997) Reproductive and developmental effects induced in mice by amsacrine, a topoisomerase inhibitor (Abstract No. 21). *Teratology*, **55**, 39

Brons, P.P.T., Wessels, J.M.C., Linssen, P.C.M., Haanen, C. & Speth, P.A.J. (1987) Determination of amsacrine in human nucleated hematopoietic cells. *J. Chromatogr.*, **422**, 175–185

Brox, L.W., Belch, A., Ng, A. & Pollock, E. (1986) Loss of viability and induction of DNA damage in human leukemic myeloblasts and lymphocytes by *m*-AMSA. *Cancer Chemother. Pharmacol.*, **17**, 127–132

Bunch, R.T., Povirk, L.F., Orr, M.S., Randolph, J.K., Fornari, F.A. & Gewirtz, D.A. (1994) Influence of amsacrine (m-AMSA) on bulk and gene-specific DNA damage and c-*myc* expression in MCF-7 breast tumor cells. *Biochem. Pharmacol.*, **47**, 317–329

Cain, B.F. & Atwell, G.J. (1974) The experimental antitumour properties of three congeners of the acridylmethanesulphonanilide (AMSA) series. *Eur. J. Cancer.*, **10**, 539–549

Caldecott, K., Banks, G. & Jeggo, P. (1990) DNA double-strand break repair pathways and cellular tolerance to inhibitors of topoisomerase II. *Cancer Res.*, **50**, 5778–5783

CIS Information Services (1998) *Worldwide Bulk Drug Users Directory 1997/98 Edition*, Dallas, TX [CD-ROM]

Cortés, F. & Piñero, J. (1994) Synergistic effect of inhibitors of topoisomerase I and II on chromosome damage and cell killing in cultured Chinese hamster ovary cells. *Cancer Chemother. Pharmacol.*, **34**, 411–415

Cortés, F., Piñero, J. & Palitti, F. (1993) Cytogenetic effects of inhibition of topoisomerase I or II activities in the CHO mutant EM9 and its parental line AA8. *Mutat. Res.*, **288**, 281–289

Covey, J.M., Kohn, K.W., Kerrigan, D., Tilchen, E.J. & Pommier, Y. (1988) Topoisomerase II-mediated DNA damage produced by 4'-(9-acridinylamino)methanesulfon-*m*-anisidide and related acridines in L1210 cells and isolated nuclei: Relation to cytotoxicity. *Cancer Res.*, **48**, 860–865

Cullinan, E.B., Gawron, L.S., Rustum, Y.M. & Beerman, T.A. (1990) Topoisomerase II-mediated DNA damage of episomes in tumor-bearing mice. *Cancer Res.*, **50**, 6154–6157

da Cunha, M.F., Meistrich, M.L., Haq, M.M., Gordon, L.A. & Wyrobek, A.J. (1982) Temporary effects of AMSA [4'-(9-acridinylamino) methanesulfon-*m*-anisidide] chemotherapy on spermatogenesis. *Cancer*, **49**, 2459–2462

da Cunha, M.F., Meistrich, M.L. & Finch-Neimeyer, M.V. (1985) Effects of AMSA, an antineoplastic agent, on spermatogenesis in the mouse. *J. Androl.*, **6**, 225–229

Cysyk, R.L., Shoemaker, D. & Adamson, R.H. (1977) The pharmacologic disposition of 4'-(9-acridinylamino)methanesulfon-*m*-anisidide in mice and rats. *Drug Metab. Dispos.*, **5**, 579–590

Cysyk, R.L., Shoemaker, D.D., Ayers, O.C. & Adamson, R.H. (1978) Oral absorption and selective tissue localization of 4'-(9-acridinylamino)-methanesulfon-*m*-anisidide. *Pharmacology*, **16**, 206–213

D'Alessandro, N., Gebbia, N., Crescimanno, M., Flandina, C., Leto, G., Tumminello, F.M. & Messina, L. (1983) Effects of amsacrine (*m*-AMSA), a new aminoacridine antitumor drug, on the rabbit heart. *Cancer Treat. Rep.*, **67**, 467–474

DeMarini, D.M. & Lawrence, B.K. (1988) Mutagenicity of topoisomerase-active agents in bacteriophage T4. *Teratog. Carcinog. Mutag.*, **8**, 293–301

DeMarini, D.M. & Lawrence, B.K. (1992) Prophage induction by DNA topoisomerase II poisons and reactive-oxygen species: Role of DNA breaks. *Mutat. Res.*, **267**, 1–17

DeMarini, D.M., Doerr, C.L., Meyer, M.K., Brock, K.H., Hozier, J. & Moore, M.M. (1987) Mutagenicity of *m*-AMSA and *o*-AMSA in mammalian cells due to clastogenic mechanism: Possible role of topoisomerase. *Mutagenesis*, **2**, 349–355

Doerr, C.L., Harrington-Brock, K. & Moore, M.M. (1989) Micronucleus, chromosome aberration, and small-colony TK mutant analysis to quantitate chromosomal damage in L5178Y mouse lymphoma cells. *Mutat. Res.*, **222**, 191–203

Dubicki, H., Parsons, J.L. & Starks, F.W. (1981) *Multi-step Process for the Production of Methanesulfon-m-anisidide, 4'-(9-acridinylamino)-*, US Patent No. 4,258,191

Editions du Vidal (1998) *Dictionnaire Vidal 1998*, 74th Ed., Paris, OVP, p. 87

Emonds, A., Driessen, O., De Bruijn, E.A. & Van Oosterom, A.T. (1981) Gas-chromatographic determination of amsacrine (AMSA) in plasma. *Fresenius Z. anal. Chem.*, **307**, 286–287

Ferguson, L.R. (1998) Inhibitors of topoisomerase II enzymes: A unique group of environmental mutagens and carcinogens. *Mutat. Res.*, **400**, 271–278

Ferguson, L.R. & Baguley, B.C. (1981) The relationship between frameshift mutagenicity and DNA-binding affinity in a series of acridine-substituted derivatives of the experimental antitumour drug 4'-(9-acridinylamino)methanesulphonanilide (AMSA). *Mutat. Res.*, **82**, 31–39

Ferguson, L.R. & Baguley, B.C. (1984) Relationship between the induction of chromosome damage and cytotoxicity for amsacrine and congeners. *Cancer Treat. Rep.*, **68**, 625–630

Ferguson, L.R. & Baguley, B.C. (1994) Topoisomerase II enzymes and mutagenicity. *Environ. mol. Mutag.*, **24**, 245–261

Ferguson, L.R. & Baguley, B.C. (1996) Mutagenicity of anticancer drugs that inhibit topoisomerase enzymes. *Mutat. Res.*, **355**, 91–101

Ferguson, L.R. & Denny, W.A. (1990) Frameshift mutagenesis by acridines and other reversibly-binding DNA ligands. *Mutagenesis*, **5**, 529–540

Ferguson, L.R. & Turner, P.M. (1988a) Mitotic crossing-over by anticancer drugs in *Saccharomyces cerevisiae* strain D5. *Mutat. Res.*, **204**, 239–249

Ferguson, L.R. & Turner, P.M. (1988b) 'Petite' mutagenesis by anticancer drugs in *Saccharomyces cerevisiae*. *Eur. J. Cancer clin. Oncol.*, **24**, 591–596

Ferguson, L.R., van Zijl, P. & Nesnow, S. (1986) Morphological transformation and chromosome damage by amsacrine in C3H/10T1/2 clone 8 cells. *Mutat. Res.*, **170**, 133–143

Ferguson, L.R., van Zijl, P. & Baguley, B.C. (1988) Comparison of the mutagenicity of amsacrine with that of a new clinical analogue, CI-921. *Mutat. Res.*, **204**, 207–217

Ferguson, L.R., Hill, C.L. & Morecombe, P. (1992) Induction of resistance to 6-thioguanine and cytarabine by a range of anticancer drugs in Chinese hamster AA8 cells. *Eur. J. Cancer*, **28A**, 736–742

Ferguson, L.R., Whiteside, G., Holdaway, K.M. & Baguley, B.C. (1996a) Application of fluorescence in situ hybridisation to study the relationship between cytotoxicity, chromosome aberrations, and changes in chromosome number after treatment with the topoisomerase II inhibitor amsacrine. *Environ. mol. Mutag.*, **27**, 255–262

Ferguson, L.R., Allen, J.W. & Mason, J.M. (1996b) Meiotic recombination and germ cell aneuploidy. *Environ. mol. Mutag.*, **28**, 192–210

Ferguson, L.R., Turner, P.M., Hart, D.W. & Tindall, K.R. (1998) Amsacrine-induced mutations in AS52 cells. *Environ. mol. Mutag.*, **32**, 47–55

Gennaro, A.R. (1995) *Remington: The Science and Practice of Pharmacy*, 19th Ed., Easton, PA, Mack Publishing, Vol. II, p. 1242

Gough, A., Courtney, C. & Graziano, M. (1994) Induction of small intestinal adenocarcinoma in Wistar rats administered amsacrine. *Exp. Toxicol. Pathol.*, **46**, 275–281

Graziano, M.J., Courtney, C.L., Meierhenry, E.F., Kheoh, T., Pegg, D.G. & Gough, A.W. (1996) Carcinogenicity of the anticancer topoisomerase inhibitor, amsacrine, in Wistar rats. *Fundam. appl. Toxicol.*, **32**, 53–65

Guo, Z., Savaraj, N., Feun, L.G., Lu, K., Stewart, D.J., Luna, M., Benjamin, R.S. & Loo, T.L. (1983) Tumor penetration of AMSA in man. *Cancer Invest.*, **1**, 475–478

Gupta, R. (1990) Tests for the genotoxicity of m-AMSA, etoposide, teniposide and ellipticine in *Neurospora crassa*. *Mutat. Res.*, **240**, 47–58

Hall, S.W., Friedman, J., Legha, S.S., Benjamin, R.S., Gutterman, J.U. & Loo, T.L. (1983) Human pharmacokinetics of a new acridine derivative, 4'-(9-acridinylamino)methanesulfon-*m*-anisidide (NSC 249992). *Cancer Res.*, **43**, 3422–3426

Henry, M.C., Port, C.D. & Levine, B.S. (1980) Preclinical toxicologic evaluation of 4'-(9-acridinylamino)methanesulfon-*m*-anisidide (AMSA) in mice, dogs, and monkeys. *Cancer Treat. Rep.*, **64**, 855–860

Holmström, M. & Winters, V. (1992) Micronucleus induction by camptothecin and amsacrine in bone marrow of male and female CD-1 mice. *Mutagenesis*, **7**, 189–193

Hornedo, J. & Van Echo, D.A. (1985) Amsacrine (m-AMSA): A new antineoplastic agent. Pharmacology, clinical activity and toxicity. *Pharmacotherapy*, **5**, 78–90

Igarashi, M. & Shimada, H. (1997) An improved method for the mouse liver micronucleus test. *Mutat. Res.*, **391**, 49–55

de la Iglesia, F.A., Fitzgerald, J.E., McGuire, E.J., Kim, S.N., Heifetz, C.L. & Stoner, G.D. (1984) Bacterial and mammalian cell mutagenesis, sister-chromatid exchange, and mouse lung adenoma bioassay with the antineoplastic acridine derivative amsacrine. *J. Toxicol. environ. Health*, **14**, 667–681

Iwamoto, Y., Ferguson, L.R., Pogai, H.B., Uzuhashi, T., Kurita, A., Yangihara, Y. & Denny, W.A. (1992a) Mutagenic activities of azido analogues of amsacrine and other 9-anilino-acridines in *Salmonella typhimurium* and their enhancement by photoirradiation. *Mutat. Res.*, **280**, 233–244

Iwamoto, Y., Ferguson, L.R., Pearson, A. & Baguley, B.C. (1992b) Photo-enhancement of the mutagenicity of 9-anilinoacridine derivatives related to the antitumour agent amsacrine. *Mutat. Res.*, **268**, 35–41

Jackson, M.A., Stack, H.F. & Waters, M.D. (1996) Genetic activity profiles of anticancer drugs. *Mutat. Res.*, **355**, 171–208

Johnson, P.G. & Beerman, T.A. (1994) Damage induced in episomal EBV DNA in Raji cells by antitumor drugs as measured by pulsed field gel electrophoresis. *Anal. Biochem.*, **220**, 103–114

Jurlina, J.L., Varcoe, A.R. & Paxton, J.W. (1985) Pharmacokinetics of amsacrine in patients receiving combined chemotherapy for treatment of acute myelogenous leukemia. *Cancer Chemother. Pharmacol.*, **14**, 21–25

Jurlina, J.L., Lindsay, A., Packer, J.E., Baguley, B.C. & Denny, W.A. (1987) Redox chemistry of the 9-anilinoacridine class of antitumor agents. *J. med. Chem.*, **30**, 473–480

Kao-Shan, C.S., Micetich, K., Zwelling, L.A. & Whang-Peng, J. (1984) Cytogenetic effects of amsacrine on human lymphocytes *in vivo* and *in vitro*. *Cancer Treat. Rep.*, **68**, 989–997

Kestell, P., Paxton, J.W., Evans, P.C., Young, D., Jurlina, J.L., Robertson, I.G.C. & Baguley, B.C. (1990) Disposition of amsacrine and its analogue 9-([2-methoxy-4-[(methylsulfonyl)-amino]phenyl]amino)-N,5-dimethyl-4- acridinecarboxamide (CI-921) in plasma, liver, and Lewis lung tumors in mice. *Cancer Res.*, **50**, 503–508

Kettle, A.J., Robertson, I.G.C., Palmer, B.D., Anderson, R.F., Patel, K.B. & Winterbourn, C.C. (1992) Oxidative metabolism of amsacrine by the neutrophil enzyme myeloperoxidase. *Biochem. Pharmacol.*, **44**, 1731–1738

Kim, S.N., Watkins, J.R., Jayasekara, U., Anderson, J.A., Fitzgerald, J.E. & de la Iglesia, F.A. (1985) Cardiotoxicity study of amsacrine in rats. *Toxicol. appl. Pharmacol.*, **77**, 369–373

Larripa, I., Mudry de Pargament, M., Labal de Vinuesa, M., Demattei, A. & Brieux de Salum, S. (1984) In vivo and in vitro cytogenetic effects of the anti-tumor agent amsacrina (AMSA). *Mutat. Res.*, **138**, 87–91

Legha, S.S., Gutterman, J.U., Hall, S.W., Benjamin, R.S., Burgess, M.A., Valdivieso, M. & Bodey, G.P. (1978) Phase 1 clinical investigation of 4′-(9-acridinylamino)methanesulfon-*m*-anisidide (NSC 249992), a new acridine derivative. *Cancer Res.*, **38**, 3712–3716

Lim, M., Liu, L.F., Jacobson-Kram, D. & Williams, J.R. (1986) Induction of sister chromatid exchanges by inhibitors of topoisomerases. *Cell Biol. Toxicol.*, **2**, 485–494

Linssen, P., Brons, P., Knops, G., Wessels, H. & de Witte, T. (1993) Plasma and cellular pharmacokinetics of m-AMSA related to in vitro toxicity towards normal and leukemic clonogenic bone marrow cells (CFU-GM, CFU-L). *Eur. J. Haematol.*, **50**, 149–154

Louie, A.C. & Issell, B.F. (1985) Amsacrine (AMSA)—A clinical review. *J. clin. Oncol.*, **3**, 562–592

Malonne, H. & Atassi, G. (1997) DNA topoisomerase targeting drugs: Mechanisms of action and perspectives. *Anticancer Drugs*, **8**, 811–822

Markovits, J., Pommier, Y., Kerrigan, D., Covey, J.M., Tilchen, E.J. & Kohn, K.W. (1987) Topoisomerase II-mediated DNA breaks and cytotoxicity in relation to cell proliferation and the cell cycle in NIH 3T3 fibroblasts and L1210 leukemia cells. *Cancer Res.*, **47**, 2050–2055

Marsh, K.L., Willmore, E., Tinelli, S., Cornarotti, M., Meczes, E.L., Capranico, G., Fisher, L.M. & Austin, C.A. (1996) Amsacrine-promoted DNA cleavage site determinants for the two human DNA topoisomerase II isoforms α and β. *Biochem. Pharmacol.*, **52**, 1675–1685

Minford, J., Kerrigan, D., Nichols, M., Shackney, S. & Zwelling, L.A. (1984) Enhancement of the DNA breakage and cytotoxic effects of intercalating agents by treatment with sublethal doses of 1-β-D-arabinofuranosylcytosine or hydroxyurea in L1210 cells. *Cancer Res.*, **44**, 5583–5593

Mirkes, P.E. & Zwelling, L.A. (1990) Embryotoxicity of the intercalating agents m-AMSA and *o*-AMSA and the epipodophyllotoxin VP-16 in postimplantation rat embryos in vitro. *Teratology*, **41**, 679–688

Morris, S.M., Domon, O.E., McGarrity, L.J., Chen, J.J. & Casciano, D.A. (1995) Programmed cell death and mutation induction in AHH-1 human lymphoblastoid cells exposed to *m*-amsa. *Mutat. Res.*, **329**, 79–96

Morris, S.M., McGarrity, L.J., Domon, O.E., Chen, J.J. & Casciano, D.A. (1996) Cell cycle traverse in AHH-1 *tk* +/− human lymphoblastoid cells exposed to the chromosomal mutagen, *m*-amsa. *Environ. mol. Mutag.*, **27**, 10–18

Mosesso, P., Darroudi, F., van den Berg, M., Vermeulen, S., Palitti, F. & Natarajan, A.T. (1998) Induction of chromosomal aberrations (unstable and stable) by inhibitors of topoisomerase II, m-AMSA and VP16, using conventional Giemsa staining and chromosome painting techniques. *Mutagenesis*, **13**, 39–43

National Cancer Institute (1992) *NCI Investigational Drugs—Chemical information—1992* (NIH Publication No. 92-2654), Bethesda, MD, National Institutes of Health, pp. 16–18

Ng, W.W., Anderson, J.A. & Sakowski, R. (1987) Teratogenicity of amsacrine lactate given ip to rats during the entire organogenesis period (Abstract No. 87). *Teratology*, **35**, 76A

Parke-Davis Canada (1984) *Product Monograph: AMSA P-D, Amsacrine for Infusion, 75 mg Ampoule, Antineoplastic Agent* (Report No. WP2-710), Scarborough, Ontario

Parke-Davis Canada (1999) *Amsacrine*, Scarborough, Ontario

Paxton, J.W. (1984) Determination of the anti-cancer drug amsacrine in biological fluids by HPLC. *Meth. Surv. biochem. Anal.*, **14**, 201–209

Paxton, J.W. (1986) The effect of food on the bioavailability and kinetics of the anticancer drug amsacrine and a new analogue, N-5-dimethyl-9-[(2-methoxy-4-methylsulphonylamino)-phenylamino]-4 acridinecarboxamide in rabbits. *J. pharm. Pharmacol.*, **38**, 837–840

Paxton, J.W. & Jurlina, J.L. (1985) Elimination kinetics of amsacrine in the rabbit: Evidence of nonlinearity. *Pharmacology*, **31**, 50–56

Paxton, J.W., Jurlina, J.L. & Foote, S.E. (1986) The binding of amsacrine to human plasma proteins. *J. pharm. Pharmacol.*, **38**, 432–438

Paxton, J.W., Kim, S.N. & Whitfield, L.R. (1990) Pharmacokinetic and toxicity scaling of the antitumor agents amsacrine and CI-921, a new analogue, in mice, rats, rabbits, dogs, and humans. *Cancer Res.*, **50**, 2692–2697

Pegg, D.G., Watkins, J.R., Graziano, M.J. & McKenna, M.J. (1996) Subchronic intravenous toxicity of the antineoplastic drug, amsacrine, in male Wistar rats. *Fundam. appl. Toxicol.*, **32**, 45–52

Piñero, J., López, B.M., Ortiz, T. & Cortés, F. (1996) Sister chromatid exchange induced by DNA topoisomerases poisons in late replicating heterochromatin: Influence of inhibition of replication and transcription. *Mutat. Res.*, **354**, 195–201

Pommier, Y., Zwelling, L.A., Kao-Shan, C.-S., Whang-Peng, J. & Bradley, M.O. (1985) Correlations between intercalator-induced DNA strand breaks and sister chromatid exchanges, mutations, and cytotoxicity in Chinese hamster cells. *Cancer Res.*, **45**, 3143–3149

Ribas, G., Xamena, N., Creus, A. & Marcos, R. (1996) Sister-chromatid exchanges (SCE) induction by inhibitors of DNA topoisomerases in cultured human lymphocytes. *Mutat. Res.*, **368**, 205–211

Robbie, M.A., Palmer, B.D., Denny, W.A. & Wilson, W.R. (1990) The fate of $N1'$-methane-sulphonyl-$N4'$-(9-acridinyl)-3'-methoxy-2',5'-cyclohexadiene-1',4'-diimine (m-AQDI), the primary oxidative metabolite of amsacrine, in transformed Chinese hamster fibroblasts. *Biochem. Pharmacol.*, **39**, 1411–1421

Robertson, I.G.C., Kestell, P., Dormer, R.A. & Paxton, J.W. (1988) Involvement of glutathione in the metabolism of the anilinoacridine antitumour agents CI-921 and amsacrine. *Drug Metab. Drug Interactions*, **6**, 371–381

Robertson, I.G., Palmer, B.D. & Shaw, G.J. (1993) The characterization of two biliary glutathione conjugates of amsacrine using liquid secondary ion mass spectrometry. *Biol. mass Spectrom.*, **22**, 661–665

Rote Liste Sekretariat (1998) *Rote Liste 1998*, Frankfurt, Rote Liste Service GmbH, p. 86-098

Shibuya, M.L., Ueno, A.M., Vannais, D.B., Craven, P.A. & Waldren, C.A. (1994) Megabase pair deletions in mutant mammalian cells following exposure to amsacrine, an inhibitor of DNA topoisomerase II. *Cancer Res.*, **54**, 1092–1097

Shoemaker, D.D., Cysyk, R.L., Padmanabhan, S., Bhat, H.B. & Malspeis, L. (1982) Identification of the principal biliary metabolite of 4'-(9-acridinylamino)methanesulfon-m-anisidide in rats. *Drug Metab. Dispos.*, **10**, 35–39

Shoemaker, D.D., Cysyk, R.L., Gormley, P.E., DeSouza, J.J.V. & Malspeis, L. (1984) Metabolism of 4'-(9-acridinylamino)methanesulfon-m-anisidide by rat liver microsomes. *Cancer Res.*, **44**, 1939–1945

Slavotinek, A., Perry, P.E. & Sumner, A.T. (1993) Micronuclei in neonatal lymphocytes treated with the topoisomerase II inhibitors amsacrine and etoposide. *Mutat. Res.*, **319**, 215–222

Slevin, M.L., Shannon, M.S., Prentice, H.G., Goldman, A.J. & Lister, T.A. (1981) A phase I and II study of m-AMSA in acute leukaemia. *Cancer Chemother. Pharmacol.*, **6**, 137–140

Stanulla, M., Wang, J., Chervinsky, D.S. & Aplan, P.D. (1997) Topoisomerase II inhibitors induce DNA double-strand breaks at a specific site within the *AML1* locus. *Leukemia*, **11**, 490–496

Stewart, D.J., Zhengang, G., Lu, K., Savaraj, N., Feun, L.G., Luna, M., Benjamin, R.S., Keating, M.J. & Loo, T.L. (1984) Human tissue distribution of 4'-(9-acridinylamino)-methanesulfon-m-anisidide (NSC 141549, AMSA). *Cancer Chemother. Pharmacol.*, **12**, 116–119

Suciu, D. (1991) Reproductive death of Chinese hamster V79 cells after exposure to chemical inhibitors of DNA synthesis. *Int. J. Biochem.*, **23**, 1245–1249

Sumner, A.T. (1995) Inhibitors of topoisomerase II delay progress through mitosis and induce a doubling of the DNA content in CHO cells. *Exp. Cell Res.*, **217**, 440–447

Swiss Pharmaceutical Society, ed. (1999) *Index Nominum, International Drug Directory*, 16th Ed., Stuttgart, Medpharm Scientific Publishers [MicroMedex Online: Health Care Series]

Thomas, J., ed. (1998) *Australian Prescription Products Guide*, 27th Ed., Victoria, Australian Pharmaceutical Publishing, Vol. 1, pp. 368–369

Torres, C., Creus, A. & Marcos, R. (1998) Genotoxic activity of four inhibitors of DNA topoisomerases in larval cells of *Drosophila melanogaster* as measured in the wing spot assay. *Mutat. Res.*, **413**, 191–203

Uges, D.R.A. (1990) [Methods for the analysis of some xenobiotics in body fluids. XII. Amsacrine, pentazocine and platinum.] *Ziekenhuisfarmacie*, **6**, 30–32 (in Dutch)

Van Echo, D.A., Chiuten, D.F., Gormley, P.E., Lichtenfeld, J.L., Scoltock, M. & Wiernik, P.H. (1979) Phase I clinical and pharmacological study of 4'-(9-acridinylamino)-methanesulfon-*m*-anisidide using an intermittent biweekly schedule. *Cancer Res.*, **39**, 3881–3884

Watson, E.S., Murphy, J.C., King, B.S. & Harland, E.C. (1981) Antigenicity and cutaneous toxicity of *N*-(4'-(9-acridinylamino)-3-methoxyphenyl)-methanesulfonamide (AMSA; NSC-249992) in guinea pigs and rabbits. *Toxicol. appl. Pharmacol.*, **59**, 476–482

Weiss, R.B., Grillo-López, A.J., Marsoni, S., Posada, J.G., Jr, Hess, F. & Ross, B.J. (1986) Amsacrine-associated cardiotoxicity: An analysis of 82 cases. *J. clin. Oncol.*, **4**, 918–928

Wilson, W.R., Harris, N.M. & Ferguson, L.R. (1984) Comparison of the mutagenic and clastogenic activity of amsacrine and other DNA-intercalating drugs in cultured V79 Chinese hamster cells. *Cancer Res.*, **44**, 4420–4431

Woynarowski, J.M., McCarthy, K., Reynolds, B., Beerman, T.A. & Denny, W.A. (1994) Topoisomerase II mediated DNA lesions induced by acridine-4-carboxamide and 2-(4-pyridyl)-quinoline-8-carboxamide. *Anticancer Drug Des.*, **9**, 9–24

Zhou, R.-H., Wang, P., Zou, Y., Jackson-Cook, C. & Povirk, L.F. (1997) A precise interchromosomal reciprocal exchange between hot spots for cleavable complex formation by topoisomerase II in amsacrine-treated Chinese hamster ovary cells. *Cancer Res.*, **57**, 4699–4702

Zucker, R.M., Adams, D.J., Bair, K.W. & Elstein, K.H. (1991) Polyploidy induction as a consequence of topoisomerase inhibition. A flow cytometric assessment. *Biochem. Pharmacol.*, **42**, 2199–2208

OTHER PHARMACEUTICAL AGENTS

HYDROXYUREA

1. Exposure Data

1.1 Chemical and physical data

1.1.1 *Nomenclature*

Chem. Abstr. Serv. Reg. No.: 127-07-1
Chem. Abstr. Name: Hydroxyurea
IUPAC Systematic Name: Hydroxyurea
Synonyms: *N*-(Aminocarbonyl)hydroxylamine; carbamohydroxamic acid; carbamohydroximic acid; carbamoyl oxime; HU; hydroxycarbamide; hydroxycarbamine; hydroxylurea

1.1.2 *Structural and molecular formulae and relative molecular mass*

$$H_2N-\underset{\underset{H}{|}}{\overset{\overset{O}{\|}}{C}}-N-OH$$

$CH_4N_2O_2$ Relative molecular mass: 76.06

1.1.3 *Chemical and physical properties of the pure substance*

(a) *Description*: White, odourless, crystalline (needles) powder (Gennaro, 1995; Budavari, 1996)
(b) *Melting-point*: 133–136 °C (Budavari, 1996)
(c) *Spectroscopy data*: Infrared (prism, [45287; 475C]; grating [30287]; FT-IR, [801C]) and nuclear magnetic resonance (proton, [33625; 671D]; C-13, [24474]) spectral data have been reported (Pouchert, 1981, 1983, 1985; British Pharmacopoeial Commission, 1993; Sadtler Research Laboratories, 1995).
(d) *Solubility*: Very soluble in water; slightly soluble in ethanol (Budavari, 1996; American Hospital Formulary Service, 1997)
(e) *Stability*: Hygroscopic and decomposes in the presence of moisture (Royal Pharmaceutical Society of Great Britain, 1999)

1.1.4 *Technical products and impurities*

Hydroxyurea is available as a 200-, 300-, 400- or 500-mg capsule; the capsule may also contain calcium citrate, citric acid, colourants (D&C Red No. 28; D&C Red No. 33; D&C Yellow No. 10; FD&C Blue No.1; FD&C Green No. 3; FD&C Red No. 40), disodium citrate, erythrosine, gelatin, indigocarmine, iron oxide, lactose, magnesium stearate, sodium lauryl sulfate, sodium monohydrogen phosphate, tartrazine and titanium dioxide (American Hospital Formulary Service, 1997; British Medical Association/Royal Pharmaceutical Society of Great Britain, 1998; Editions du Vidal, 1998; Rote Liste Sekretariat, 1998; Thomas, 1998; US Pharmacopeial Convention, 1998; Medical Economics Data Production, 1999).

Trade names for hydroxyurea include Biosupressin, Droxia, Droxiurea, Hidroks, Hidroxiurea Asofarma, Hidroxiurea Filaxis, Hidroxiurea Martian, Hydrea, Hydrea capsules, Hydreia, Hydroxycarbamid, Hydroxycarbamide capsules BP 1998, Hydroxycarbamide capsules USP 23, Hydroxyurea, Litalir, Onco-Carbide, Oxyurea and Syrea (CIS Information Services, 1998; Royal Pharmaceutical Society of Great Britain, 1999; Swiss Pharmaceutical Society, 1999).

1.1.5 *Analysis*

Several international pharmacopoeias specify infrared absorption spectrophotometry with comparison to standards as the method for identifying hydroxyurea; titration with sodium thiosulfate is used to assay its purity. Similar methods are used for identifying and assaying hydroxyurea in pharmaceutical preparations (British Pharmacopoeial Commission, 1993; US Pharmacopeial Convention, 1994).

1.2 Production

Hydroxyurea has been prepared by the reaction of calcium cyanate with hydroxylamine nitrate in absolute ethanol and by the reaction of potassium cyanate and hydroxylamine hydrochloride in aqueous solution. Hydroxyurea has also been prepared by converting a quaternary ammonium anion exchange resin from the chloride form to the cyanate form with sodium cyanate and reacting the resin in the cyanate form with hydroxylamine hydrochloride (Graham, 1955).

Information available in 1999 indicated that hydroxyurea was manufactured and/or formulated in 25 countries (CIS Information Services, 1998; Royal Pharmaceutical Society of Great Britain; 1999; Swiss Pharmaceutical Society, 1999).

1.3 Use

Hydroxyurea is a chemically simple antimetabolite, which is cytostatic by inhibiting ribonucleotide reductase, an enzyme important in creating deoxynucleosides for DNA replication in growing cells (Gao *et al.*, 1998). Hydroxyurea was initially synthesized over 120 years ago, but its potential biological significance was not recognized until 1928. In the late 1950s, the drug was evaluated in a large number of experimental murine tumour systems and shown to be active against a broad spectrum of tumours. Phase I trials with hydroxyurea began in 1960 and by the late 1960s it was in clinical use (Donehower, 1992).

Hydroxyurea has been used, or investigated for use, in the treatment of a number of diseases.

(*a*)   *Sickle-cell haemoglobinopathy*

Hydroxyurea is widely used to treat severe sickle-cell disease (Charache *et al.*, 1996; Ferster *et al.*, 1996; de Montalembert *et al.*, 1997) and beta-thalassaemia–sickle-cell disease (Voskaridou *et al.*, 1995). It was shown to induce fetal haemoglobin synthesis (Fibach *et al.*, 1993; Maier-Redelsperger *et al.*, 1998), and preliminary reports demonstrated its benefit in beta-thalassaemia–sickle-cell haemoglobinopathy (Loukopoulos *et al.*, 1998). The efficacy of hydroxyurea in sickle-cell disease is well validated, but its use appears to be limited to patients with frequent crises and hospitalizations. The doses used in patients with sickle-cell anaemia are 25 mg/kg bw per day in children (Ferster *et al.*, 1996) and up to 35 mg/kg bw per day in adults (Charache *et al.*, 1996).

(*b*)   *Myeloproliferative syndromes*

Hydroxyurea is also used as a cytostatic agent in myelodyplastic or myeloproliferative diseases, including chronic myeloid leukaemia (Donehower, 1992; Fitzgerald & McCann, 1993; Guilhot *et al.*, 1993), polycythemia vera (Najean & Rain, 1997a,b), myelodysplastic syndrome (Nair *et al.*, 1993) and essential thrombocythaemia and corticosteroid-resistant hypereosinophilia (Donehower, 1992). The risks and benefits of hydroxyurea in haematological disease are debated and have been reviewed (Donehower, 1992). It is used most commonly in chronic myeloid leukaemia to prevent or delay the onset of blast crises, and complete responses have been seen occasionally (Tanaka *et al.*, 1997).

(*c*)   *With didanosine in the treatment of HIV/AIDS*

Hydroxyurea is given as an adjunct with didanosine (see monograph, this volume) in treatment of human immunodeficiency virus (HIV) infection. Several case series and randomized trials have shown dramatic results with the combination (Biron *et al.*, 1996; Montaner *et al.*, 1997; Foli *et al.*, 1998), although not without exception (Simonelli *et al.*, 1997). Trials in which didanosine and hydroxyurea were given in combination with other agents (Lisziewicz *et al.*, 1998; Rutschmann *et al.*, 1998) led to large-scale controlled trials which are currently under way. Intriguing reports of prolonged periods without rebound viraemia after didanosine and hydroxyurea therapy, especially in patients who began treatment shortly after HIV infection, have led to intensive investigation (Vila et al., 1997; Lisziewicz et al., 1998). The doses of hydroxyurea used in combination with didanosine are 500–1000 mg/day (Montaner et al., 1997; Rutschmann et al., 1998).

Hydroxyurea itself has no antiviral effect (Lori et al., 1997a). Its mechanism of action with didanosine appears to be selective inhibition of ribonucleotide reductase, thus decreasing endogenous dATP concentrations, leading to increased generation of dATP from the pro-drug didanosine. Hydroxyurea thus improves the antiviral potency of didanosine (Lori et al., 1997b; De Boer et al., 1998; Johns & Gao, 1998). The effect is likely to be greater with dATP analogues such as didanosine than with other antiviral nucleoside analogues (Gandhi et al., 1998).

Increased cytokine levels (Navarra et al., 1995, 1996) and adrenal activity have been seen in hydroxyurea-treated patients (Navarra et al., 1990, 1998) but not in HIV-infected patients treated with hydroxyurea and didanosine.

(d) *Psoriasis*

Hydroxyurea can be administered over long periods to treat psoriasis (Moschella & Greenwald, 1973; Boyd & Neldner, 1991), although it is currently used relatively infrequently.

(e) *Solid tumours*

Hydroxyurea is used as a radiosensitizing agent in carcinoma of the cervix (Stehman, 1992; Stehman et al., 1997) and glioma (Levin & Prados, 1992). Other malignancies in which use of hydroxyurea as an adjunct has been studied (Wadler et al., 1996) include meningioma (Schrell et al., 1997), uterine leiomyosarcoma (Currie et al., 1996a) and uterine mixed mesodermal tumours (Currie et al., 1996b).

1.4 Occurrence

Hydroxyurea is not known to occur as a natural product. No data on occupational exposure were available to the Working Group.

1.5 Regulations and guidelines

Hydroxyurea is listed in the British, French and US pharmacopoeias (Royal Pharmaceutical Society of Great Britain, 1999; Swiss Pharmaceutical Society, 1999).

2. Studies of Cancer in Humans

The carcinogenic potential of hydroxyurea has been studied in patients with chronic myeloproliferative disorders, which include chronic myeloid leukaemia, ideopathic myelofibrosis, polycythaemia vera and essential thrombocythaemia. An assessment of the carcinogenicity of this agent is hampered by an inherent tendency of chronic myeloproliferative disorders to undergo spontaneous transformation to myelodysplastic syndrome or acute leukaemia. Thus, among 431 patients with polycythaemia vera who were randomized to one of three treatment arms, phlebotomy ($n = 134$), chlorambucil ($n = 141$) or radioactive phosphorus ($n = 156$), patients in the phlebotomy arm were found to have a cumulative risk for acute leukaemia after 11–18 years of follow-up of 1.5% on the basis of two observed cases. The rates for acute myeloid leukaemia in the US population indicate that about 0.13 cases would have been expected (Landaw, 1986).

Although hydroxyurea is used in the treatment of sickle-cell anaemia and of psoriasis, these conditions are not suspected to predispose to cancer.

2.1 Case reports

Several case reports have been published on the occurrence of multiple squamous-cell and basal-cell carcinomas of the skin in patients who received prolonged treatment with hydroxyurea for chronic myeloid leukaemia (Disdier *et al.*, 1991; Stasi *et al.*, 1992; Best & Petitt, 1998; De Simone *et al.*, 1998), essential thrombocythaemia or polycythaemia vera (Callot-Mellot *et al.*, 1996; Best & Petitt, 1998). The skin carcinomas were typically seen in sun-exposed areas and had been preceded by other degenerative cutaneous manifestations.

Reiffers *et al.* (1985), van den Anker-Lugtenburg and Sizoo (1990) and Furgerson *et al.* (1996) described the occurrence of acute leukaemia in patients who had been treated with hydroxyurea for long periods for essential thrombocythaemia and had not received other treatments.

2.2 Cohort studies

These studies are summarized in Table 1.

2.2.1 *Polycythaemia vera* (see also section 2.2.3)

Sharon *et al.* (1986) reported the results of a prospective study conducted in Israel of 36 patients with polycythaemia vera who were treated with hydroxyurea at a daily dose of 500–1500 mg for 1–5.6 years. Nineteen of the patients had previously been treated with other myelosuppressive drugs. During treatment, no cases of leukaemia or other malignant neoplasms were seen.

Table 1. Cohort studies of acute leukaemia (AL) and myelodysplastic syndrome (MDS) in patients treated with hydroxyurea

Country (reference)	Study design (no. of cases); period	Daily dose (mg/kg bw)[a]	Follow-up (years) average (range)	Cases of AL and MDS	Proportion with blast transformation	Comments
Polycythaemia vera						
Israel (Sharon et al., 1986)	Prospective (36); not reported	[7–21]	Duration of treatment (1–5.6)	AL: 0	0%	19 patients with other prior myelosuppressive treatment
USA (West, 1987)	Prospective (100); 1963–83	[10]	Duration of treatment 5.4 (0.3–18)	AL: 1	1%	Possibly one additional case of chronic leukaemia
USA (Kaplan et al., 1986)	Prospective (51); 1979–86 (Nand et al., 1990)	~15	Duration of treatment 4.7 (0.1–7.5)	AL: 3	5.9%	Another case of AL diagnosed 19 years after first diagnosis (Holcombe et al., 1991)
USA (Nand et al., 1990)	Retrospective (18); 1975–87	1.7 ± 1.7 g/day, 1 year	Duration of treatment: 12	AL: 5	27.8%	10 patients also received other myelosuppressive treatment. Patients considered in a study of MDS
Sweden (Weinfeld et al., 1994)	Prospective (21); since 1976	[7–21]	(5–>10)	AL: 3	14%	Patients considered in a study of MDS
USA (Nand et al., 1996)	Cross-sectional (16); 1993–95; prevalent cases	1.5 (0.5–6) g/day, 1 year	5.5 (1.5–20)	AL or MDS: 1	6.2%	Patients considered in a study of MDS
France (Najean & Rain, 1997a)	Prospective (150), since 1980	10–15	Follow-up (1–17)	AL: not given MDS: not given	Actuarial risk: 10% at 13th year	Cases of AL and MDS not distinguished according to treatment received

Table 1 (contd)

Country (reference)	Study design (no. of cases); period	Daily dose (mg/kg bw)[a]	Follow-up (years) average (range)	Cases of AL and MDS	Proportion with blast transformation	Comments
Essential thrombocythaemia						
France (Belluci et al., 1986)	Retrospective (42); 1961–82	Not reported	Follow-up (> 0–19)	AL: 2	4.8%	
France (Liozon et al., 1997)	Retrospective (53); 1981–95	4–43	Follow-up (6)	AL: 1 MDS: 2	5.7%	
France (Sterkers et al., 1998)	Retrospective (251); 1970–91	[21] (starting dose)	Follow-up; 8.2 (1.8–22)	AL: 5 MDS: 9	5.6%	50 patients also received other myelosuppressive treatment
Sweden (Löfvenberg et al., 1990)	Prospective (32); 1981–89	15–20	Treatment duration; 3.8 (1.3–6.6)	AL: 2 MDS: 1	9.4%	Patients considered in a study of MDS
Sweden (Weinfeld et al., 1994)	Prospective (9); since 1976	[7–21]	(5–> 10)	AL: 1	11%	Patients considered in a study of MDS
Chronic myeloproliferative disease						
Sweden (Löfvenberg et al., 1990)	Prospective (81); 1981–89	15–20	Treatment duration; 3.9 (0.1–8.7) (means)	AL: 3 MDS: 1	4.9%	3 patients with other prior myelosuppressive treatment, but none of AL or MDS patients
Sweden (Weinfeld et al., 1994)	Prospective (50); since 1976	7–21	(5–> 10)	AL: 9 MDS: 1	20%	13 patients with other prior myelosuppressive treatment

Table 1 (contd)

Country (reference)	Study design (no. of cases); period	Daily dose (mg/kg bw)[a]	Follow-up (years) average (range)	Cases of AL and MDS	Proportion with blast transformation	Comments
Chronic myeloproliferative disease (contd)						
USA (Nand et al., 1996)	Cross-sectional (25); prevalent cases; 1993–95	0.25–6 g/day, 1 year	5.2 (0.3–20)	AL or MDS: 2	8.0%	
Sickle-cell anaemia						
USA (Charache et al., 1995)	Prospective (152); 1992–94	0–35	1.8 (1.2–2.0)	AL: 0	0%	Treatment arm in a clinical trial
USA (Scott et al., 1996)	Prospective (13); 1992–95	10–35	Treatment: 2.0 (0.5–3.3)	AL: 0	0%	
Cyanotic congenital heart disease						
France (Triadou et al., 1994)	Prospective (64); not reported	10	5 (2–15)	AL: 0	0%	

[a] When not given in the paper, calculated assuming a body weight of 70 kg

West (1987) studied the incidence of acute leukaemia in 100 patients in Kentucky, USA, who were treated for polycythaemia vera which had been diagnosed during 1963–83. They were also treated by phlebotomy. The mean daily dose of hydroxyurea was 720 mg, and the duration of therapy ranged from three months to 18 years (mean, 5.4 years). During this time, two (2%) cases of leukaemia were observed: one chronic neutrophilic leukaemia after nine months of treatment and one acute myeloid leukaemia after five years. The authors noted that the chronic neutrophilic leukaemia might have been present before the date of recruitment.

Of 118 patients in New York, USA, with polycythaemia vera, all had received supplementary phlebotomy and hydroxyurea at a daily dose of 30 mg/kg bw for one week, then 15 mg/kg bw and then modified downwards and upwards; 59 of the patients had had no prior myelosuppressive therapy (Donovan *et al.*, 1984). Hydroxyurea was given for a mean of 4.7 years (range, one month to 7.5 years). Three out of 51 patients with no prior myelosuppressive therapy developed acute leukaemia after 1.7, 2.8 and 4.8 years of treatment (Kaplan *et al.*, 1986). Two cases of leukaemia (1.5%) were observed in the most appropriate historical control group of 134 patients who had been treated exclusively with phlebotomy (Landaw, 1986), and the difference between the two groups was not statistically significant. [The Working Group noted the reduction in numbers of hydroxyurea-treated patients from 59 to 51, which was unexplained.] In a subsequent case report, Holcombe *et al.* (1991) described an additional case of chronic myelomonocytic leukaemia (which transforms to acute myeloid leukaemia) in the group of 51 hydroxyurea-treated patients with polycythaemia vera. This case was seen 19 years from the date of initial diagnosis. No data were given on the historical control group.

Nand *et al.* (1990) conducted a retrospective study of 48 patients in Chicago, Illinois, USA, with polycythaemia vera diagnosed during 1975–87 (seven cases were diagnosed previously) and treated over a period of 12 years. Of these, 18 had been treated with hydroxyurea at doses ranging from 500 mg every other day for nine months to 1000 mg daily for seven years. Four cases of acute leukaemia were seen among 10 of the patients who had received hydroxyurea in combination with other myelosuppressive treatment including radioactive phosphorus and one case among eight patients who had received hydroxyurea alone (relative risk = 3.8; $p = 0.38$). The cases developed at a mean of 3.9 years after the start of treatment. [The Working Group noted the small size of the study.]

Two published reports are available on the results of a clinical trial of the French Polycythaemia Vera Study Group (Najean *et al.*, 1996; Najean & Rain, 1997a). The most recent report includes 292 patients with polycythaemia vera diagnosed after 1980 when the patients were aged 0–64 years. The patients were treated with either hydroxyurea ($n = 150$) at a daily dose of 25 mg/kg bw followed by a maintenance dose of 10–15 mg/kg bw, or pipobroman [1,4-bis(3-bromopropionyl)piperazine] ($n = 142$). The patients were followed for 1–17 years, during which time nine cases of acute myeloid leukaemia and four cases of myelodysplastic syndrome were observed. The precise treatment received in these 13 cases was not specified, but the authors stated that the actuarial risk for acute myeloid leukaemia or myelodysplastic syndrome was about 10% at the 13th year of follow-up, with no difference according to treatment. Four cases of non-melanoma skin cancer were seen in patients given hydroxyurea only and one in a patient given pipobroman only, while six cancers at sites other than the bone marrow and non-melanoma skin were seen in six patients given hydroxyurea and five given pipobroman. These frequencies of extracutaneous solid tumours were only slightly greater than those expected for this age group.

In a complementary trial covering the period 1979–96, Najean and Rain (1997b) recruited 461 patients with polycythaemia vera who were over 65 years of age and had not previously been treated with chemotherapeutic agents. Initially, the patients were treated with radioactive phosphorus (0.1 mCi/kg bw with a maximum of 7 mCi) administered intravenously until complete remission of the polycythaemia was obtained. They were then randomized to receive either maintenance treatment with low-dose hydroxyurea (5–10 mg/kg bw per day) ($n = 219$) or simple surveillance ($n = 242$). When the haematocrit of a patient in either treatment arm had increased to 50% and the erythrocyte volume was > 125% of the normal value during follow-up, intravenous administration of radioactive phosphorus was resumed. The median survival was 9.1 years in the group receiving maintenance therapy and 11.2 years in the surveyed group ($p = 0.10$). In a subset of 408 patients followed for more than two years (maximum follow-up time, 16 years), the mean annual dose of radioactive phosphorus was 0.009 mCi/kg bw in the group receiving hydroxyurea and 0.033 mCi/kg bw in the surveyed group [average for all study subjects, approximately 0.021 mCi/kg bw per year]. In the same subset of 408 patients, 41 haematological malignancies were observed, consisting of 15 cases of acute myeloid leukaemia, two of non-Hodgkin lymphoma, two of chronic lymphocytic leukaemia, two of multiple myeloma, three of chronic myelomonocytic leukaemia and 17 of myelodysplastic syndrome. The precise treatment schedule received in these 41 cases was not specified, but the authors stated that statistical analysis (log-rank test) showed a significantly increased risk for these tumour types combined in patients receiving maintenance treatment with hydroxyurea when compared with those under simple surveillance ($p = 0.01$ or $p = 0.03$, depending on whether outcomes were analysed according to intention to treat or the main therapy received). The dose of radioactive phosphorus received by the patients who developed leukaemia was moderately higher (0.044 mCi/kg bw per year) than that received by other patients (0.032 mCi/kg bw per year), but the difference was not statistically significant. Seven cases of non-melanoma skin cancer were observed among patients receiving hydroxyurea maintenance and two cases in the surveyed group. [The Working Group noted that the average dose of 0.032 mCi/kg bw per year received by persons without leukaemia does not concord with the average level of 0.021 mCi/kg bw per year for all study subjects followed for more than two years. The Group also noted that the distributions of haematological malignancies by type of treatment were not presented and that the cases of non-Hodgkin lymphoma, chronic lymphocytic leukaemia and multiple myeloma in these elderly people were apparently grouped with the cases of acute myeloid leukaemia and myelodysplastic syndrome before risk analyses were performed, which limits interpretation of the results.]

2.2.2   *Essential thrombocythaemia* (see also section 2.2.3)

Bellucci *et al.* (1986) reviewed the medical records of 94 patients (average age, 49.5 years; range, 6–90) in one treatment centre in Paris, France, in whom essential thrombocythaemia had been diagnosed during 1961–82. The patients were followed up for periods ranging from a few months to 19 years, during which time five cases of acute leukaemia were observed. Two of the five cases occurred in the subgroup of 42 patients who had received hydroxyurea as the only chemotherapeutic agent.

In a treatment centre in Limoges, France, Liozon *et al.* (1997) conducted a retrospective follow-up study of 58 patients (mean age, 66.5 years; range, 18–85) in whom essential thrombocythaemia had been diagnosed during 1981–95. The mean duration of follow-up was approximately five years. Among the 53 patients who had received hydroxyurea as first-line therapy (mean weekly dose, 6 g; range, 2–21 g), one developed acute myeloid leukaemia, one developed chronic myelomonocytic leukaemia and one had myelodysplastic syndrome.

Sterkers *et al.* (1998) reviewed the medical records of 357 patients (median age, 62 years; range, 30–75) with essential thrombocythaemia diagnosed between 1970 and 1991 and followed-up until 1996 at two haematological centres, in Lille and Lomme, France. Overall, 326 of the 357 patients had been treated with at least one chemotherapeutic agent, and 251 had received hydroxyurea at a starting dose of 1.5 g/day (some had received pipobroman). Within a median duration of follow-up of 8.2 years (range, 1.8–22 years), six patients had developed acute myeloid leukaemia and 11 myelodysplastic syndrome (including chronic myelomonocytic leukaemia). Fourteen of these 17 patients had received hydroxyurea at some time, while seven of the cases were seen in the subgroup of 201 patients who had been treated with hydroxyurea alone.

2.2.3   *Chronic myeloproliferative disease*

In one treatment centre in Sweden, 81 consecutive patients (age range, 31–82 years) with Philadelphia chromosome-negative chronic myeloproliferative disease, consisting of 35 cases of polycythaemia vera, 32 of essential thrombocythaemia, 12 of myelofibrosis and two of myeloproliferative syndrome [not further specified], were followed prospectively from 1981 to 1989 (Löfvenberg & Wahlin, 1988; Löfvenberg *et al.*, 1990). All had received maintenance treatment with hydroxyurea at a dose of 15–20 mg/kg bw per day. During an average follow-up of 3.9 years (range, one month to 8.7 years), three cases of acute myeloid leukaemia (two cases in patients with essential thrombocythaemia, one in a patient with myelodysplastic syndrome) and one case of myelodysplastic syndrome (in a patient with essential thrombocythaemia) were seen. None of these four cases had been treated with alkylating agents or radioactive phosphorus before treatment with hydroxyurea. No data were available on the number of cancers to be expected among these patients on the basis of incidence rates in the general population.

In another treatment centre in Sweden, Weinfeld et al. (1994) conducted a prospective follow-up of 50 consecutive patients (age range, 33–82 years) with Philadelphia chromosome-negative chronic myeloproliferative disease, consisting of 30 patients with polycythaemia vera, 10 with essential thrombocythaemia and 10 with myelofibrosis, of whom 21, 9 and 7, respectively, had been treated only with hydroxyurea at 60 mg/kg per day for the first week and then 0.5–1.5 g/day. The median observation period was > 10 years, and the minimum was five years, during which time nine cases of acute leukaemia and one case of myelodysplastic syndrome were seen. Seven of the acute leukaemias occurred among 37 patients treated with hydroxyurea only (three in patients with polycythaemia vera, one in a patient with essential thrombocythaemia and three in patients with myelofibrosis), and two of the cases of acute leukaemia and one case of myelodysplastic syndrome occurred among 13 patients treated with alkylating agents prior to entrance into the study, yielding transformation frequencies of [19%] with hydroxyurea and [23%] with previous treatment.

Forty-two patients with polycythaemia vera (16 of whom were treated with hydroxyurea only), 15 with essential thrombocythaemia, six with myelofibrosis with myeloid metaplasia and one with an unclassified myeloproliferative disorder seen at a medical centre in Illinois, USA, during 1993–95 were evaluated for subsequent development of acute leukaemia or myelodysplastic syndrome (Nand et al., 1996). At the date of entry into the study, the patients had survived for a median of 5.2 years (range, four months to 20 years) since diagnosis of their chronic myeloproliferative disease. Five (7.8%) of the 64 cases transformed into acute leukaemia or myelodysplastic syndrome; none of these were in the 11 patients who had received no treatment or aspirin, two (11%) occurred in 18 patients treated with phlebotomy alone, two (8%) in 25 patients who had received hydroxyurea and one (10%) in 10 patients who had received only other immunosuppressive therapy. [The Working Group noted that the study group was composed of prevalent cases of chronic myeloproliferative disease only and that the follow-up period for most patients must have been very short.]

2.2.4 *Sickle-cell anaemia*

In order to test the efficacy of hydroxyurea in reducing the frequency of painful crises in adults with sickle-cell anaemia, Charache et al. (1995) conducted a randomized, placebo-controlled clinical trial. Of 299 such patients, 152 were assigned to hydroxyurea, while 147 were given placebo. Because of the beneficial effects observed, the trial was stopped after a median of 21 months (range, 14–24 months). At that time, no cases of leukaemia or other neoplastic disorders were seen.

To assess the safety and efficacy of hydroxyurea for the treatment of severe sickle-cell anaemia in children, Scott *et al.* (1996) conducted a small prospective study of 15 patients in one treatment centre in Illinois, USA. Thirteen patients in whom sickle-cell anaemia had been diagnosed in 1992–95 received hydroxyurea for a median of two years (range, 0.5–3.3 years), during which time no cases of acute leukaemia or other malignancies were seen.

2.2.5 *Congenital heart disease*

Sixty-four patients ranging in age from 8 to 47 years with inoperable cyanotic congenital heart disease were included in a prospective study in a treatment centre in France (Triadou *et al.*, 1994). The patients received hydroxyurea at an initial dose of 10 mg/kg bw per day, which was adapted according to haematological tolerance and continued over a period ranging from [two to 15 years] (mean, approximately five years). No cases of acute leukaemia or other malignancies were seen.

3. Studies of Cancer in Experimental Animals

The Working Group was aware of early studies in mice (Bhide & Sirsat, 1973) and in rats (Philips & Sternberg, 1975), which were considered inadequate for evaluation.

3.1 Intraperitoneal administration

Groups of 50 mice of each sex of the XVII/G strain were treated intraperitoneally with hydroxyurea [purity not specified] starting at two days of age and then at weekly intervals for one year. The doses per mouse were: 1 mg at two days of age, 3 mg at eight days, 5 mg at 15 days and 10 mg from 30 days to one year of age. One group of 50 mice was kept untreated as controls. The incidences of pulmonary tumours were 30/50 (60%) in control and 16/35 (46%) in treated mice. In a positive control group treated with urethane, 28/30 (93%) of mice had lung tumours (Muranyi-Kovacs & Rudali, 1972).

3.2 Administration with known carcinogens

Groups of 40 female Swiss mice, six to seven weeks of age, received dermal applications of 5 μg of 7,12-dimethylbenz[*a*]anthracene followed four weeks later by treatment with 1% croton oil for 14 weeks. Hydroxyurea at a dose of 500 mg/kg bw was injected intraperitoneally once at 24 h or twice at 24 and 48 h after the first painting with croton oil. Treatment with two doses of hydroxyurea significantly reduced the incidence of skin papillomas when compared with 7,12-dimethylbenz[*a*]anthracene and croton oil treatment alone (Chan *et al.*, 1970).

Groups of 16 male and 16 female hairless (hr/hr) Oslo mice were given an intraperitoneal injection of 0 or 5 mg hydroxyurea in 0.5 mL distilled water 30 min before dermal application of 2 mg of N-methyl-N-nitrosourea (MNU). Hydroxyurea enhanced the production of skin tumours by MNU from about 50% to 80%, this effect being attributed to inhibition of DNA synthesis (Iversen, 1982a). No such effect was observed when hydroxyurea was administered simultaneously with or after dermal application of 1 mg of MNU (Iversen, 1982b).

Groups of 36–43 female Wistar rats, weighing about 200 g, were given intraperitoneal injections of hydroxyurea in 23 fractionated consecutive doses of 0.1 mg/kg bw each shortly before and during maximal urothelial cell proliferation (33–55 h after partial cystectomy) produced by MNU administered as a single intravesicular pulse dose of 5 mg/kg bw during the various cell cycle phases. Hydroxyurea inhibited MNU-induced urothelial tumour development, and the degree of this inhibition depended on the cell cycle phase during which MNU was instilled. The numbers of rats with urothelial bladder tumours were: 14/43 in the control group (G_0 phase) and 7/37, 4/43 ($p < 0.02$), 10/46, 10/38, 9/36 and 12/40 in groups receiving MNU during the late G_1, early and late S, G_2+M, and early and late postmitotic phases, respectively (Kunze et al., 1989).

4. Other Data Relevant to an Evaluation of Carcinogenicity and its Mechanisms

4.1 Absorption, distribution, metabolism and excretion

4.1.1 *Humans*

Although hydroxyurea has been in clinical use for 30 years, the pharmacokinetics of the compound has been extensively studied only recently. Two useful reviews have been published (Donehower, 1992; Gwilt & Tracewell, 1998), but the best of the limited data available come from the study of Rodriguez et al. (1998). These investigators gave 2 g of hydroxyurea either orally or by intravenous infusion over 30 min in a cross-over design to 29 patients with advanced cancers. They demonstrated clearly that oral and intravenous administration have essentially identical kinetics except for a 19.5% greater maximum plasma concentration (C_{max}) after intravenous dosing; the lag time of the peak after oral dosing was 0.22 h. Hydroxyurea is essentially completely absorbed from the human gastrointestinal tract, with a narrow range between subjects. The half-time of hydroxyurea is short, with an initial half-time of 0.63 h after intravenous administration and 1.78 h after oral administration and a terminal half-time of 3.32 h after oral administration and 3.39 h after intravenous administration. The clearance of hydroxyurea given orally or intravenously is identical and rapid, at 76 mL/min per m², with a mean distribution volume of 19.7 L/m². In this study, slightly more than one-third of the administered dose was recovered in the urine. The 2-g dose resulted in a mean C_{max} of 794 μmol/L after oral administration and 1000 μmol/L after intravenous administration and a mean integrated area under the curve of concentration–time (AUC) of 3600 μmol/L per h after intravenous and 3900 μmol/L per h after oral administration.

Belt et al. (1980) compared oral and intravenous administration of escalating doses of hydroxyurea to patients with advanced malignancies. The maximal tolerated dose was 800 mg/m² every 4 h by oral administration and 3.0 mg/m² per min when given intravenously as a continuous 72-h infusion. After oral administration of doses of 500 or 800 mg/m² every 4 h, the peak concentration in plasma ranged from 5.4 to 24.8×10^{-4} mol/L. The time to attain the peak concentrations was 30–120 min. Two- to threefold variations among patients in the C_{max} after oral dosing were found. The C_{max} values for continuous intravenous infusion of doses of 2.0–3.5 mg/min per m² were $5.0–11.5 \times 10^{-4}$ mol/L. The plasma half-times of hydroxyurea in patients given single oral doses of 400–1200 mg/m² ranged from 132 to 279 min. In pleural fluid samples obtained from two patients, the concentrations paralleled those found in plasma. The mean half-time after discontinuation of intravenous infusion was about 250 min.

Hydroxyurea enters the cerebrospinal fluid, ascites fluid and serum (Beckloff et al., 1965) and breast milk (Sylvester et al., 1987).

Villani et al. (1996) studied nine HIV-infected patients receiving hydroxyurea at 500 mg twice per day orally with or without zidovudine. The C_{max} was 0.135 mmol/L, and the C_{min} was 0.0085 mmol/L serum. The rate of clearance was 0.18 L/h per kg bw [12.6 L/h], with a half-time of 2.5 ± 0.5 h. The time to maximum clearance was approximately 0.9 h, and the bioavailability was good.

The maximum tolerated dose in a study of patients with chronic myeloid leukaemia in accelerated phase or blast crisis was 27 g/m² when given as a 24-h intravenous infusion (Gandhi et al., 1998). Intravenous doses of 8–40 g/m² resulted in plasma concentrations of 0.9–6.4 mmol/L with a half-time of approximately 3.5 h. A steady state was reached in all patients by 6 h. In this study, the dATP levels in peripheral blast cells decreased by 57%, but DNA synthesis decreased by 80–90%. The concentrations of the other deoxynucleotides were not affected.

About 30–60% of an orally administered dose of hydroxyurea is excreted unchanged by the kidneys (Donehower, 1992), although about 35% is generally excreted (Rodriguez et al., 1998).

Andrae (1984) implicated a cytochrome P450-dependent process in metabolic activation of hydroxyurea which increases its potential for genetic damage. Hydrogen peroxide was reported to be a toxic metabolic product of hydroxyurea (Andrae & Greim, 1979). DeSesso et al. (1994) found that D-mannitol, a scavenger of free radicals, decreases the genotoxic effect of hydroxyurea. Sato et al. (1997) described pathways for the generation of nitric oxide from hydroxyurea via copper-catalysed peroxidation. Hepatic and renal conversion of hydroxyurea by a cytochrome c-dependent pathway to urea may account for 30–50% of administered doses. Urease may degrade hydroxyurea to produce hydroxylamine and ultimately acetohydroxamic acid (Gwilt & Tracewell, 1998).

Both high and low doses show log-linear excretion kinetics, reflecting the predominance of renal mechanisms. The excretion of doses of 10–35 mg/kg bw diverges from linearity, probably because of an increasingly important saturable non-renal metabolic pathway (Villani *et al.*, 1996; Luzzati *et al.*, 1998).

4.1.2 *Experimental systems*

In contrast to the situation for humans, little information is available on the pharmacokinetics of hydroxyurea in animals, despite its wide use as a model teratogen and to synchronize the cell cycle in cell cultures. The lack of data may be due to the lack of a suitably sensitive assay during the early development of the drug (Donehower, 1992).

Van den Berg *et al.* (1994) gave nude mice doses of 0–200 mg/kg bw hydroxyurea by intraperitoneal injection and found a plasma concentration of 159 μmol/L within a half-time of only 11 min.

Wilson *et al.* (1975) found that the half-time of hydroxyurea in rats given 137 mg/kg bw per day intraperitoneally on days 9–12 of gestation was 15 min in the dams and 85 min in the embryos. In rhesus monkeys given 100 mg/kg bw per day intravenously on days 23–32 of gestation, the half-time was 120 min after the last injection in the mothers and 265 min in their fetuses.

4.2 Toxic effects

4.2.1 *Humans*

The major dose-limiting (and dose-related) toxic effects of hydroxyurea are granulocytopenia, which resolves relatively rapidly after withdrawal of the drug (Belt *et al.*, 1980), and myelosuppression, seen in advanced chronic myeloid leukaemia (Gandhi *et al.*, 1998). Drug-induced dermopathy with characteristics of dermatomyositis have been reported (Richard *et al.*, 1989; Velez *et al.*, 1998) as well as hyperpigmentation of the nails (Gropper *et al.*, 1993; de Montalembert *et al.*, 1997) and leg ulcers (Cox *et al.*, 1997; Weinlich *et al.*, 1998), although one large study of patients with sickle-cell anaemia found an equal rate of leg ulcers in patients given the placebo (Charache *et al.*, 1996). In two- (Charache *et al.*, 1996) and three-year (de Montalembert *et al.*, 1997) follow-up studies of patients with sickle-cell anaemia treated continuously with hydroxyurea, no serious side-effects other than mild neutropenia were observed, and this did not limit treatment.

When very high doses are given intravenously, dose-related mucositis is seen (Gandhi *et al.*, 1998), but neutropenia is usually the treatment-limiting side-effect.

4.2.2 *Experimental systems*

No formal toxicological studies on hydroxyurea in animals were available to the Working Group.

4.3 Reproductive and prenatal effects

4.3.1 *Humans*

Information on the use of hydroxyurea in pregnancy is limited to a few case reports. Five case reports involved exposure to hydroxyurea for periods ranging from seven months to four years before pregnancy and throughout gestation at doses of 0.5–3.0 g daily. One woman developed eclampsia at 26 weeks and delivered a stillborn but phenotypically normal infant (Delmer *et al.*, 1992). The other four pregnancies ended in four normal, healthy infants at 36–40 weeks of gestation, with normal blood counts and normal postnatal development up to a maximum of 32 months (Patel *et al.*, 1991; Delmer *et al.*, 1992; Tertian *et al.*, 1992; Jackson *et al.*, 1993). Three other cases have been reported: one woman received a single dose of 8 g of hydroxyurea at about 12 weeks of pregnancy and had an elective termination four weeks later of an apparently normal fetus (Doney *et al.*, 1979). Another woman was treated with an unspecified dose of hydroxyurea for six months before pregnancy and from mid-second trimester to near term, and delivered a healthy infant who developed normally during one year of follow-up (Fitzgerald & McCann, 1993). The third case involved a woman who had been treated with an unspecified dose of hydroxyurea two years before conception. She delivered a normal infant, who had normal physical and mental development at seven years of age (Pajor *et al.*, 1991). [The Working Group noted that the doses of hydroxyurea used clinically are about one-fifth to one-tenth of the teratogenic dose in rodents.]

4.3.2 *Experimental systems*

Studies on the teratogenicity of hydroxyurea in chicks, mice, rats, rabbits, cats and monkeys have been published since the original reports by Murphy and Chaube (1964) and Chaube and Murphy (1966), who showed that a single intraperitoneal dose of 250 mg/kg bw or more given to Wistar rats on one of days 9–12 of gestation produced a high proportion of fetuses with multiple gross malformations of the central nervous system, palate and skeleton.

Pregnant NMRI mice injected intraperitoneally on day 10 of gestation with 500 mg/kg bw hydroxyurea showed marked necrosis of the neuroepithelium of the spinal cord 4 h after injection. The cytotoxicity could be partially prevented by simultaneous injection of 700 mg/kg bw deoxycytidine monophosphate (Herken, 1984) and completely prevented by simultaneous injection of 1 mg/kg bw colchicine (Herken, 1985). These results suggest that the action of hydroxyurea is dependent both on DNA synthesis and on the cytoskeleton.

Pregnant Wistar-derived rats were dosed intraperitoneally on day 12 of gestation with 250, 500, 750 or 1000 mg/kg bw hydroxyurea, and the fetuses were examined on day 20. A dose-related increase in the frequency of multiple malformations of the viscera and skeleton and reduced fetal weight were observed at doses ≥ 500 mg/kg bw, but embryolethality was seen only at 1000 mg/kg bw. Hydroxyurea was shown to pass into the embryo and to persist there longer than in maternal blood. DNA synthesis, as measured by thymidine incorporation into the embryo, was depressed markedly by doses ≥ 500 mg/kg bw, and marked cytotoxicity was also observed (Scott et al., 1971).

Studies from the same laboratory with the same strain of rat showed that intraperitoneal injection of 375 or 500 mg/kg bw hydroxyurea on day 12 of pregnancy produced microscopic evidence of cytotoxicity in the neural tube, but no malformations were observed when the dams were allowed to deliver their pups at term. Nevertheless, observation of the offspring at 30–50 days of age showed locomotor and behavioural deficits at both doses (Butcher et al., 1973). Further studies from the same laboratory with the same strain of rat showed that teratogenic and embryolethal effects could be induced by a dose as low as 137 mg/kg bw, but not by 100 mg/kg bw, administered intraperitoneally on days 9–12 of gestation (Wilson et al., 1975). Behavioural effects were also observed in the offspring of Sprague-Dawley dams treated with a single intraperitoneal dose of 150 mg/kg bw hydroxyurea on various days of pregnancy (Brunner et al., 1978). The wide range of malformations induced in rats by hydroxyurea has led to its use as a positive control substance in standard testing for both teratogenicity (Aliverti et al., 1980; Price et al., 1985) and developmental toxicity (postnatal behaviour) (Vorhees et al., 1979, 1983). Comparisons of the teratogenic responses in various stocks and strains of rats showed differences in the type of malformation and the time of sensitivity in two stocks of Wistar rats (Barr & Beaudoin, 1981) and in Wistar and Fischer 344 rats (DePass & Weaver, 1982).

A group of 27 pregnant golden hamsters received an intravenous injection of 50 mg/kg bw hydroxyurea on day 8 of pregnancy. The embryos were examined for external malformations only. A high rate of fetal death and malformations, especially of the central nervous system, was observed (Ferm, 1966).

The teratogenicity of hydroxyurea in pregnant New Zealand white rabbits was demonstrated by subcutaneous injection of 750 mg/kg bw once on day 12 of gestation, with embryo and fetal examination 15 min to 32 h later by histology and on day 29 for malformations. Treatment produced marked cytotoxicity and a high percentage of resorptions (61%), reduced fetal weight and malformations in all surviving fetuses affecting most organ systems and the skeleton, as observed in rats (DeSesso & Jordan, 1977; DeSesso, 1981a). The mechanism by which hydroxyurea produces its teratogenic action was investigated in detail by DeSesso and his co-workers, who showed in rabbits that hydroxyurea is not only cytotoxic and inhibits DNA synthesis but also causes a very rapid, marked reduction in uterine–placental blood flow, which may be responsible for some of the teratogenic effects (Millicovsky et al., 1981). In addition, the teratogenic effects can be inhibited by simultaneous administration of the anti-oxidant propyl gallate, which reduces the cytotoxicity (DeSesso, 1981b). This activity occurs within the embryo and is independent of the inhibition of DNA synthesis (DeSesso & Goeringer, 1990). Inhibition of the cytotoxicity and teratogenicity of hydroxyurea by D-mannitol, a potent scavenger of hydroxyl free radicals, suggests that these radicals are the proximate cytotoxins and teratogens (DeSesso *et al.*, 1994).

Groups of 17 mated cats of European and Persian breeds were dosed orally with 50 or 100 mg/kg bw hydroxyurea on days 10–22 of gestation, and the fetuses were examined on day 43. At 50 mg/kg bw, fetal weight and survival were not affected, but a high proportion of the fetuses were malformed, with a wide range of malformations similar to those seen in other species. At 100 mg/kg bw, a large proportion of the cats were not pregnant, but maternal and fetal weights were reduced, the frequency of resorptions increased and one of two live fetuses was malformed (cyclopia) (Khera, 1979).

Of 22 pregnant female rhesus monkeys (*Macaca mulatta*) dosed intravenously with 50–500 mg/kg bw hydroxyurea for various times between days 18 and 45 of gestation, eight aborted or had intrauterine deaths; 10 had fetuses with multiple malformations mostly of the axial skeleton, but also genitourinary, cardiac, brain, eye and intestinal defects; and the infants of three were growth retarded and one was normal (Theisen *et al.*, 1973; Wilson, 1974; Wilson *et al.*, 1975). [The Working Group noted that little detailed information is given in these reports.]

The teratogenicity of hydroxyurea was compared in mouse embryos *in vivo* and *in vitro*, to study the effects of varying the concentration of drug and the duration of exposure. Mated ICR mice were injected intraperitoneally with 300 mg/kg bw hydroxyurea on day 9 of pregnancy (vaginal plug = day 1), and the embryos were removed 48 h later for examination for malformations and for protein content. The embryos of untreated mice were removed on day 9 and cultured *in vitro* in various concentrations of hydroxyurea for various lengths of time, followed by culture in drug-free medium up to 48 h. *In vivo*, 45% of the embryos showed malformations, including exencephaly and phocomelia, and the peak plasma concentration of hydroxyurea was 311 ± 22 μg/mL 7 min after injection, with a half-time of 30 min. Culture *in vitro* with hydroxyurea at 300 μg/mL for 30 min resulted in malformations in 41% of the embryos that were similar to those found *in vivo*. Culture at a concentration of 500 μg/mL for 30 min or at 250 μg/mL for 1 h resulted in 100% malformed embryos, but culture at 125 μg/mL for 1 h resulted in no malformations (Warner *et al.*, 1983). Culture of 10-day CD rat embryos and eight-day CD-1 mouse embryos with 300 μg/mL hydroxyurea for 1 h followed by 43 h in drug-free medium resulted in impaired development, and the embryos had reduced DNA and protein contents. Addition of various concentrations of dAMP to the culture medium did not inhibit the action of hydroxyurea, and addition of dCMP had minimal inhibitory activity. Hydroxyurea decreased all nucleotide pools, and addition of dAMP increased the pools but not to control levels (Hansen *et al.*, 1995).

Malformations were also produced in chicks injected *in ovo* on day 4 with 800 μg of hydroxyurea (Iwama *et al.*, 1983).

Seven groups of at least six male C57BL/6J×C3H/HeJ F_1 mice were injected when 13–15 weeks of age with 0, 25, 50, 100, 200, 400 or 500 mg/kg bw hydroxyurea intraperitoneally daily for five consecutive days. The epididymides and testes were examined eight and 29 days after the last injection. Body weight was not affected in any of the animals, but the testis weight was reduced in a dose-related manner at all doses except the lowest. A dose-related reduction in DNA synthesis was seen, resulting in depletion of pachytene spermatocytes and a consequent reduction in later cell stages and spermiogenesis. Spermatogonial stem cells were not affected, and showed repopulation of cell stages with normal differentiation kinetics (Evenson & Jost, 1993). Similar results were reported in B6C3/F_1/BOM M mice aged six to eight weeks injected intraperitoneally with 200 mg/kg bw hydroxyurea for five days (Wiger et al., 1995).

4.4 Genetic and related effects

4.4.1 Humans

In studies of genetic alterations in leukaemic cells of patients treated with hydroxyurea, a statistically non-significant association was seen between treatment with hydroxyurea alone or in combination and the occurrence of leukaemia and myelodysplastic syndrome characterized by abnormalities of chromosome 17 in patients with essential thrombocythaemia [$p = 0.11$, Fisher's exact test]. As discussed in section 2, Sterkers et al. (1998) monitored the occurrence of acute leukaemia and myelodysplastic syndrome in 251 patients with essential thrombocythemia who were treated with hydroxyurea. The findings in the leukaemic cells are summarized in Table 2. In seven cases of leukaemia treated with hydroxyurea, including three given the drug alone, there were rearrangements of chromosome 17, including unbalanced translocations, partial or complete deletions and isochromosome 17q, which resulted in 17p deletion in the leukaemic cells. P53 mutation was observed in six cases, including two treated with hydroxyurea alone. The authors suggested that the molecular characteristics of these

Table 2. Karyotypic findings in the bone marrow of patients with essential thrombocythaemia treated with hydroxyurea

Treatment	Leukaemia or myelodysplastic syndrome			No leukaemia	Total no. of patients
	17p deletion	No 17p deletion	Karyotype unavailable		
Hydroxyurea	3	2	2	194	201
Hydroxyurea plus other agents	4	1	2	43	50
No hydroxyurea	0	3	0	104	107

Derived from Sterkers et al. (1998)

leukaemias are consistent with 17p⁻ syndrome and that prolonged use of hydroxyurea in patients with essential thrombocythaemia may lead to acute myeloid leukaemia and myelodysplastic syndrome with loss of chromosome 17p material and *P53* mutation. A review of the literature by these authors revealed similar 17p deletions in four of 11 patients treated for essential thrombocythaemia with hydroxyurea alone but in only one of 24 patients who did not receive this treatment. Tefferi (1998) cautioned, however, that the results of bone-marrow and cytogenetic investigations before treatment were not available for some of the patients. Monosomy 17 was also observed in complex karyotypes in two of three cases of leukaemia reported by Liozon *et al.* (1997) among 58 patients with essential thrombocythaemia treated with hydroxyurea; in the third case, which was chronic myelomonocytic leukaemia, the karyotype was normal.

Quesnel *et al.* (1993) identified the t(8;21) translocation in a case of leukaemia in which essential thrombocythaemia had been treated with hydroxyurea alone. The t(8;21) is associated with the French–American–British M2 (acute myeloblastic) subtype of de-novo and treatment-related acute myeloid leukaemia. The complex karyotype, which also contained monosomy 17, was 46, XX[3]/47, XX, +8 [2]/43–44,XX,der(7)t(7;dup5), t(8;21)(q22;q22), –16,–17,t(18;?)(q;?)[10].

Ören *et al.* (1999) described a case of acute promyelocytic leukaemia with i(17q) after treatment of Philadelphia chromosome-positive chronic myeloid leukaemia with combination therapy including hydroxyurea, but i(17q) may occur in chronic myeloid leukaemia in blast crisis.

Diverse chromosomal aberrations have been seen in human bone-marrow cells after hydroxyurea treatment. Diez-Martin *et al.* (1991) reviewed studies of the chromosomes of 104 patients at various stages of polycythaemia vera. The bone-marrow cells of five of six patients treated with hydroxyurea alone had abnormalities, including an unbalanced t(1;7)(p11;p11), which can be associated with treatment-related myelodysplastic syndrome, but this abnormality may occur without prior treatment. Cytogenetic analyses in these five patients were performed only on bone-marrow samples obtained after treatment. One each of the other four abnormal marrows had t(8;13)(p21;q12), +9, del(6)(q13q21) and t(1;?)(q12;?). Furthermore, the authors observed several de-novo abnormalities in untreated patients which they related to the disease itself rather than to the therapy, including +9, +8 and 20q–, and suggested that the 13q– abnormality is related to disease progression.

Löfvenberg *et al.* (1990) examined 81 hydroxyurea-treated patients with Philadelphia chromosome-negative chronic myeloproliferative disorders, comprising 35 with polycythaemia vera, 32 with essential thrombocythaemia, 12 with myelofibrosis and two with myeloproliferative syndromes. Only three had received prior therapy with alkylating agents or radioactive phosphorus. Four of the 81 developed acute myeloid leukaemia or myelodysplastic syndrome. Five of 53 evaluable patients (9%) had clonal cytogenetic abnormalities involving chromosomes 1, 9, 20 and 21 before treatment, and 15% had these abnormalities at follow-up, during or after hydroxyurea treatment. Treatment was thus associated with a low frequency of cytogenetic abnormalities in a heterogeneous population, and the abnormalities observed before and after treatment were similar.

The series later reported on by Weinfeld *et al.* (1994) included 30 patients with polycythaemia vera, 10 with essential thrombocythaemia and 10 with myelofibrosis who were treated with hydroxyurea. Acute leukaemia developed in nine patients and myelodysplastic syndrome in one; seven of the leukaemia patients had been treated with hydroxyurea alone. The duration of therapy for patients who developed leukaemia or myelodysplastic syndrome was 5–111 months. Seven of 19 previously untreated patients with initially normal karyotypes treated with hydroxyurea alone developed clonal chromosomal abnormalities during therapy (37%).

Davidovitz *et al.* (1998) observed evolution of polycythaemia vera to myelofibrosis with a t(1;20)(q32;q13.3) in a patient who received chronic low-dose hydroxyurea. The t(1;20) affected the same region of chromosome 20 as the 20q– abnormality; it could not be determined whether the translocation was related to the treatment. Furgerson *et al.* (1996) described a patient in whom essential thrombocythaemia evolved to acute myeloid leukaemia after hydroxyurea treatment. The karyotype was normal at the time of diagnosis of essential thrombocythaemia but revealed del(5)(q23), del(7)(q31), inv(16)(p13;q22),+8 when acute myeloid leukaemia emerged.

4.4.2 *Experimental systems*

Early studies on the mutagenicity of hydroxyurea were summarized by Timson (1975). Reviews on the mutagenicity of anticancer drugs in general, including hydroxyurea, were provided by Ferguson (1995) and Jackson *et al.* (1996). Ferguson and Denny (1995) commented on some practical issues in testing antimetabolites, which may limit the usefulness (and meaning) of some types of in-vitro assays.

The results of tests for genotoxicity with hydroxyurea are summarized in Table 3.

Hydroxyurea was inactive as either a frameshift or base-pair substitution mutagen in *Salmonella typhimurium* strains TA1537, TA1535, TA98 and TA100, and addition of an exogenous metabolic activation system did not affect these results. Hydroxyurea induced SOS repair in *Escherichia coli* K12 cells. In various *Saccharomyces cerevisiae* strains, hydroxyurea induced mitotic crossing over, mitotic gene conversion, intrachromosomal recombination and aneuploidy, but not 'petite' mutations. It also increased the frequency of ultraviolet-induced mitotic gene conversion and induced recombination in dividing but not G1 or G2 arrested cells of the RS112 strain of yeast. In meiotic yeast cells, hydroxyurea increased the frequency of meiotic recombination.

Hydroxyurea is a clastogen in mammalian cells *in vitro* and *in vivo*.

Hydroxyurea caused chromosomal aberrations in cultured Chinese hamster cells, in mouse cells and in various human cell lines. Karon and Benedict (1972) found that hydroxyurea induced chromosomal aberrations when given during S phase but not when given during G2 phase. It did not induce micronuclei in human peripheral blood lymphocytes but increased the frequency of sister chromatid exchange and of gene

Table 3. Genetic and related effects of hydroxyurea

Test system	Result[a] Without exogenous metabolic system	Result[a] With exogenous metabolic system	Dose[b] (LED or HID)	Reference
Escherichia coli K12, SOS repair response	+	NT	7600	Barbé et al. (1987)
Salmonella typhimurium TA100, TA1535, TA1537, TA98, reverse mutation	–	–	10 000 µg/plate	Haworth et al. (1983)
Saccharomyces cerevisiae D5, petite mutations	–	NT	10 000	Ferguson & Turner (1988a)
Saccharomyces cerevisiae D5, mitotic crossing-over	+	NT	2400	Ferguson & Turner (1988b)
Saccharomyces cerevisiae D61.M, mitotic gene conversion	+	NT	7600	Mayer et al. (1986)
Saccharomyces cerevisiae D61.M, aneuploidy	+	NT	7600	Mayer et al. (1986)
Saccharomyces cerevisiae RS112, intrachromosomal recombination	+	NT	380	Galli & Schiestl (1996)
Saccharomyces cerevisiae SBTD and D7, increased frequency of ultraviolet-induced mitotic gene conversion	+	NT	2280	Zaborowska et al. (1983)
Saccharomyces cerevisiae 419 and 580, meiotic recombination	+	NT	3040	Simchen et al. (1976)
Drosophila melanogaster larvae, chromosomal aberrations, mitotic brain ganglion cells *in vitro*	+	NT	7.6	Banga et al. (1986)
Drosophila melanogaster larvae, chromosomal aberrations, brain ganglia *in vivo*	+	NT	6080	Banga et al. (1986)
Unscheduled DNA synthesis, rat primary hepatocytes *in vitro*	+	NT	760	Rossberger & Andrae (1985)
Mutation, mouse lymphoma L5178Y cells, *Tk* locus *in vitro*	+	NT	3	Amacher & Turner (1987)
Mutation, mouse lymphoma L5178Y cells, *Tk* locus *in vitro*	+	NT	0.7	Wangenheim & Bolcsfoldi (1988)
Mutation, mouse lymphoma L5178Y cells, *Tk* locus *in vitro*	+[c]	+[c]	20	Sofuni et al. (1996)
Sister chromatid exchange, Chinese hamster lung V79-4 cells *in vitro*	–	NT	0.5	Popescu et al. (1977)

Table 3 (contd)

Test system	Result[a]		Dose[b] (LED or HID)	Reference
	Without exogenous metabolic system	With exogenous metabolic system		
Sister chromatid exchange, Chinese hamster lung V79 B-1 cells in vitro	+	NT	7.6	Ishii & Bender (1980)
Sister chromatid exchange, Chinese hamster lung V79 and ovary cells in vitro	+	NT	76	Mehnert et al. (1984)
Sister chromatid exchange, Chinese hamster ovary CHO-B11 cells in vitro	+	NT	23	Hahn et al. (1986)
Sister chromatid exchange, mouse lymphoma L5178Y Jsens and C3 cells in vitro	+	NT	76	Hill & Schimke (1985)
Sister chromatic exchange, Chinese hamster ovary CHO-K1 cells in vitro	+	NT	76	Tohda & Oikawa (1990)
Chromosomal aberrations, Chinese hamster lung V79-4 cells in vitro	+	NT	0.5	Popescu et al. (1977)
Chromosomal aberrations, Chinese hamster ovary CHO-B11 cells in vitro	+	NT	23	Hahn et al. (1986)
Chromosomal aberrations, Chinese hamster Don-C cells in vitro (S phase)	+	NT	100	Karon & Benedict (1972)
Chromosomal aberrations, mouse lymphoma L5178Y Jsens and C3 cells in vitro	+	NT	76	Hill & Schimke (1985)
Cell transformation, cultures of embryonic cells from BN/a mice, with confirmation in newborn mice	–	NT	0.76	Chlopkiewicz & Koriorowska (1983)
Cell transformation, cultures of embryonic cells from DBA/2 and Swiss mice		NT	Not reported	Chlopkiewicz & Koriorowska (1983)
Cell transformation, BALB/c 3T3 cells mouse cells	–	NT	7.6	Chlopkiewicz & Koriorowska (1983)
DNA single-strand breaks, Ehrlich ascites tumour cells in vitro	+	NT	38	Li & Kaminskas (1987)

Table 3 (contd)

Test system	Result[a] Without exogenous metabolic system	Result[a] With exogenous metabolic system	Dose[b] (LED or HID)	Reference
DNA single-strand breaks, human T lymphoma CCRF-CEM cells *in vitro*	+	NT	4.6	Skog *et al.* (1992)
Mutation, human T-lymphoblast cell line, *HPRT* locus *in vitro*	–	NT	19	Mattano *et al.* (1990)
Micronucleus formation, human primary lymphocytes *in vitro*	–	NT	1520	Fenech *et al.* (1994)
Chromosomal aberrations, human lymphocytes *in vitro*	+	NT	150	Kihlman & Andersson (1985)
Chromosomal aberrations, human Hep.2 cell line *in vitro*	+	NT	190	Strauss *et al.* (1972)
Chromosomal aberrations, human B lymphoblast TK6, WI-L2-NS and WTK1 cell lines *in vitro*	+	NT	76	Greenwood *et al.* (1998)
Specific locus mutation, (101/H male × C3H/HeH female)F₁ mice	–		500 ip × 2	Cattanach *et al.* (1989)
Micronucleus formation, bone-marrow cells, male NMRI mice *in vivo*	+		400 ip × 1	Hart & Hartley-Asp (1983)
Micronucleus formation, bone-marrow cells, female C57BL/6 × C3H/He hybrid mice *in vivo*	–		250 ip × 5	Bruce & Heddle (1979)
Chromosomal aberrations, spermatogonial cells, male Swiss mice	–		500 ip × 1	van Buul & Bootsma (1994)
Dominant lethal assay, male ICR/Ha Swiss mice	–		1000 ip × 1	Epstein *et al.* (1972)
Sperm morphology, C57BL/6 × C3H/He hybrid mice *in vivo*	+		250 ip × 5	Bruce & Heddle (1979)

[a] +, positive; (+), weak positive; –, negative; NT, not tested; ?, inconclusive
[b] LED, lowest effective dose; HID, highest ineffective dose; in-vitro tests, μg/mL; in-vivo tests, mg/kg bw per day; ip, intraperitoneally
[c] Same result in two laboratories

amplification in L5178Y mouse lymphoma cells. Hydroxyurea induced sister chromatid exchange in various Chinese hamster cell lines *in vitro*. It caused DNA strand breaks in Ehrlich ascites tumour cells and in human T lymphoma cells *in vitro*.

It did not induce mutations at the *HPRT* locus in a cultured human T-lymphocyte cell line at doses of 50–250 μmol/L, which had substantial effects on DNA synthesis, but induced mutants at the *Tk* locus in L5178Y cells.

Hydroxyurea caused cell transformation in mass cultures of embryonic cells from BN/a, mice, but not in cultures derived from two other strains of mice—DBA/2 and Swiss, nor in BALB/c 3T3 cells. Although hydroxyurea alone did not induce morphological transformation in Syrian hamster embryo cells, the cell cycle arrest caused by the drug led to enhancement of cell transformation by bromodeoxyuridine (Tsutsui *et al.*, 1979). Hydroxyurea did not enhance metabolic cooperation between V79 cells (Toraason *et al.*, 1992).

Hydroxyurea treatment led to hypermethylation of DNA in hamster fibrosarcoma cells (Nyce *et al.*, 1986). In rats, this resulted in nitric oxide production (Jiang *et al.*, 1997) and induced a cytokine response (Navarra *et al.*, 1995, 1997). These effects may indicate an enhanced effect on chromosomal damage in certain situations *in vivo*. Hydroxyurea also induced DNA hypermethylation in normal human embryonic lung fibroblasts (WI-38) and their simian virus 40-transformed counterparts (SVWI-38) (De Haan & Parker, 1988).

Hydroxyurea induced micronuclei in the bone marrow of non-tumour-bearing male NMRI mice but did not induce micronucleated cells in female C57BL/6 × C3H/He hybrid mice, although it produced sperm abnormalities in male mice of this strain.

Although hydroxyurea is a mutagen in somatic cells, there is no evidence that it mutates germ cells. It did not cause dominant lethal mutation or specific locus mutation in mice. It did not induce chromosomal damage in spermatogonial cells of male Swiss mice, although it enhanced damage induced by X-rays.

Minford *et al.* (1984) showed that hydroxyurea at 0.1 mmol/L enhanced both DNA breakage and cytotoxicity caused by the intercalating DNA topoisomerase II inhibitor, amsacrine. Lambert *et al.* (1983) found similar results in relation to adriamycin. Palitti *et al.* (1984a) showed that treatment with hydroxyurea after mitomycin C enhanced the frequencies of chromosomal aberrations and sister chromatid exchange induced by mitomycin C alone in both Chinese hamster cells and human lymphocytes. Hydroxyurea had a synergistic effect on ultraviolet-induced sister chromatid exchange (Ishii & Bender, 1980) and enhanced X-radiation-induced damage in spermatogonial cells of Swiss mice (van Buul & Bootsma, 1994).

4.5 Mechanistic considerations

Hydroxyurea does not bind or bond to DNA but acts by inhibiting ribonucleotide reductase, which converts ribonucleoside diphosphates to deoxyribonucleotide diphosphates, the precursors for de-novo DNA synthesis. Hydroxyurea depletes intracellular deoxyribonucleotide pools and is known and used as an inhibitor of DNA synthesis (Timson, 1975).

The differences in the results of various studies may depend on the exact cell culture conditions, especially in regard to the amounts of deoxyribonucleotides available. Hansen *et al.* (1995) found that they could partially attenuate the embryotoxic effects of hydroxyurea by providing additional deoxyribonucleotides.

In a number of experiments, hydroxyurea appeared to enhance the susceptibility of cells to mutagenesis by other agents (e.g. Palitti *et al.*, 1983, 1984a,b; Ferguson, 1990; Jelmert *et al.*, 1992). There are three possible reasons for this:
1. It halts the progression of cells in the late G1 phase of the cycle, allowing synchronization of the culture (e.g. Tsutsui *et al.*, 1979). Thus, if cells are sensitive to a certain agent in a particular phase of the cell cycle, hydroxyurea may reveal this effect.
2. Although hydroxyurea inhibits normal DNA synthesis, it does not appear to inhibit unscheduled DNA synthesis at the same doses after treatment with various genotoxic agents, including X-rays (e.g. Painter & Cleaver, 1967). This justifies its inclusion in protocols of unscheduled DNA synthesis.
3. Prempree and Merz (1969) suggested that hydroxyurea could inhibit the repair of chromosomal breaks without itself inducing breaks.

5. Summary of Data Reported and Evaluation

5.1 Exposure data

Hydroxyurea is a chemically simple antimetabolite that inhibits the enzyme ribonucleotide reductase. It has been in clinical use since the 1960s and is widely used for the treatment of severe sickle-cell disease, chronic myeloid leukaemia, myeloproliferative disorders such as polycythaemia vera and essential thrombocythaemia and, increasingly, in combination with didanosine in HIV infection. Hydroxyurea is sometimes used for the treatment of psoriasis and various solid tumours.

5.2 Human carcinogenicity data

The risk for leukaemia associated with administration of hydroxyurea in the treatment of chronic myeloproliferative disorders has been evaluated in a number of small cohort studies. Overall, 5–6% of patients developed either acute leukaemia or myelodysplastic syndrome subsequent to the start of hydroxyurea treatment. Large variation in the length of active follow-up was not taken into account in the analyses. The risk for leukaemia in patients with chronic myeloproliferative disorders who were not treated with hydroxyurea or other agents (e.g. polycythaemia vera patients treated with phlebotomy alone) was also increased in comparison with that of the general population. The available data do not allow a conclusion about whether the occurrence of acute leukaemia and myelodysplastic syndrome in the hydroxyurea-treated patients represents progression of the myeloproliferative process or an effect of the treatment.

5.3 Animal carcinogenicity data

Hydroxyurea was tested in one experiment in mice by intraperitoneal administration beginning at two days of age. No increase in the incidence of tumours was reported. Hydroxyurea has also been tested in combination with other chemical carcinogens to assess the effect of inhibition of DNA synthesis on carcinogenesis. The experiments are inadequate to assess the carcinogenicity of hydroxyurea.

5.4 Other relevant data

Hydroxyurea is readily absorbed after oral administration. In one study, 35% of an administered dose was excreted unchanged in the urine of humans. Hydroxyurea is widely distributed in tissues. Its main toxic effect is neutropenia.

Hydroxyurea is teratogenic and causes postnatal behavioural deficits after prenatal exposure in all species of animals in which it has been tested. It has commonly been used as positive control substance in studies of developmental toxicity.

In one study of patients treated with hydroxyurea for essential thrombocythaemia who developed leukaemia, a statistically non-significant association was found with a 17p chromosomal deletion in leukaemic cells.

Hydroxyurea neither bonds chemically nor otherwise binds to DNA. Instead, it inhibits ribonucleotide reductase, which converts ribonucleoside diphosphates to deoxyribonucleotide diphosphate precursers for de-novo DNA synthesis. Hydroxyurea does not induce gene mutation in bacteria and does not cause mutation at the *Hprt* locus in mammalian cells. It causes chromosomal mutations and mutagenic effects at the *Tk* locus in mouse lymphoma cells. It is an effective recombinogen in yeast and induces sister chromatid exchange in mammalian cells. It also causes gene amplification in mammalian cells and may lead to transformation of some but not all cell lines. Although it has been reported to be ineffective in causing germ-cell mutation, it has not been extensively tested for that end-point.

5.5 Evaluation

There is *inadequate evidence* in humans for the carcinogenicity of hydroxyurea.

There is *inadequate evidence* in experimental animals for the carcinogenicity of hydroxyurea.

Overall evaluation

Hydroxyurea is *not classifiable as to its carcinogenicity to humans (Group 3)*.

6. References

Aliverti, V., Bonanomi, L. & Giavini, E. (1980) Hydroxyurea as a reference standard in teratological screening. Comparison of the embryotoxic and teratogenic effects following single intraperitoneal or repeated oral administrations to pregnant rats. *Arch. Toxicol.*, **Suppl. 4**, 239–247

Amacher, D.E. & Turner, G.N. (1987) The mutagenicity of 5-azacytidine and other inhibitors of replicative DNA synthesis in the L5178Y mouse lymphoma cell. *Mutat. Res.*, **176**, 123–131

American Hospital Formulary Service (1997) *AHFS Drug Information® 97*, Bethesda, MD, American Society of Health-System Pharmacists, pp. 766–770

Andrae, U. (1984) Evidence for the involvement of cytochrome P-450-dependent monooxygenase(s) in the formation of genotoxic metabolites from N-hydroxyurea. *Biochem. biophys. Res. Commun.*, **118**, 409–415

Andrae, U. & Greim, H. (1979) Induction of DNA repair replication by hydroxyurea in human lymphoblastoid cells mediated by liver microsomes and NADPH. *Biochem. biophys. Res. Commun.*, **87**, 50–58

van den Anker-Lugtenburg, P.J. & Sizoo, W. (1990) Myelodysplastic syndrome and secondary acute leukemia after treatment of essential thrombocythemia with hydroxyurea. *Am. J. Hematol.*, **33**, 152

Banga, S.S., Shenkar, R. & Boyd, J.B. (1986) Hypersensitivity of Drosophila *mei-41* mutants to hydroxyurea is associated with reduced mitotic chromosome stability. *Mutat. Res.*, **163**, 157–165

Barbé, J., Villaverde, A. & Guerrero, R. (1987) Induction of the SOS response by hydroxyurea in *Escherichia coli* K12. *Mutat. Res.*, **192**, 105–108

Barr, M., Jr & Beaudoin, A.B. (1981) An exploration of the role of hydroxyurea injection time in fetal growth and terartogenesis in rats. *Teratology*, **24**, 163–167

Beckloff, G.L., Lerner, H.J., Frost, D., Russo-Alesi, F.M. & Gitomer, S. (1965) Hydroxyurea in biologic fluids: Dose–concentration relationship. *Cancer Chemother. Rep.*, **48**, 57–58

Bellucci, S., Janvier, M., Tobelem, G., Flandrin, G., Charpak, Y., Berger, R. & Boiron, M. (1986) Essential thrombocythemias. Clinical evolutionary and biological data. *Cancer*, **58**, 2440–2447

Belt, R.J., Haas, C.D., Kennedy, J. & Taylor, S. (1980) Studies of hydroxyurea administered by continuous infusion: Toxicity, pharmacokinetics, and cell synchronization. *Cancer*, **46**, 455–462

Best, P.J.M. & Petitt, R.M. (1998) Multiple skin cancers associated with hydroxyurea therapy. *Mayo Clin. Proc.*, **73**, 961–963

Bhide, S.V. & Sirsat, M.V. (1973) Delayed effects of a single treatment of hydroxyurea to newborn mice. *Indian J. Cancer*, **10**, 26–30

Biron, F., Lucht, F., Peyramond, D., Fresard, A., Vallet, T., Nugier, F., Grange, J., Malley, S., Hamedi-Sangsari, F. & Vila, J. (1996) Pilot clinical trial of the combination of hydroxyurea and didanosine in HIV-1 infected individuals. *Antiviral Res.*, **29**, 111–113

Boyd, A.S. & Neldner, K.H. (1991) Hydroxyurea therapy. *J. am. Acad. Dermatol.*, **25**, 518–524

British Medical Association/Royal Pharmaceutical Society of Great Britain (1998) *British National Formulary*, No. 36, London, p. 377

British Pharmacopoeial Commission (1993) *British Pharmacopoeia 1993*, London, Her Majesty's Stationery Office, Vols I & II, pp. 343, 954, S68

Bruce, W.R. & Heddle, J.A. (1979) The mutagenic activity of 61 agents as determined by the micronucleus, *Salmonella*, and sperm abnormality assays. *Can. J. Genet. Cytol.*, **21**, 319–334

Brunner, R.L., McLean, M., Vorhees, C.V. & Butcher, R.E. (1978) A comparison of behavioral and anatomical measures of hydroxyurea induced abnormalities. *Teratology*, **18**, 379–384

Budavari, S., ed. (1996) *The Merck Index*, 12th Ed., Whitehouse Station, NJ, Merck & Co., p. 833

Butcher, R.E., Scott, W.J., Kazmaier, K. & Ritter, E.J. (1973) Postnatal effects in rats of prenatal treatment with hydroxyurea. *Teratology*, **7**, 161–165

van Buul, P.P. & Bootsma, A.L. (1994) The induction of chromosomal damage and cell killing in mouse spermatogonial stem cells following combined treatments with hydroxyurea, 3-aminobenzamide and X-rays. *Mutat. Res.*, **311**, 217–224

Callot-Mellot, C., Bodemer, C., Chosidow, O., Frances, C., Azgui, Z., Varet, B. & de Prost, Y. (1996) Cutaneous carcinoma during long-term hydroxyurea therapy: A report of 5 cases. *Arch. Dermatol.*, **132**, 1395–1397

Cattanach, B.M., Peters, J. & Rasberry, C. (1989) Induction of specific locus mutations in mouse spermatogonial stem cells by combined chemical X-ray treatments. *Mutat. Res.*, **212**, 91–101

Chan, P.C., Goldman, A. & Wynder, E.L. (1970) Hydroxyurea: Suppression of two-stage carcinogenesis in mouse skin. *Science*, **168**, 130–132

Charache, S., Terrin, M.L., Moore, R.D., Dover, G.J., Barton, F.B., Eckert, S.V., McMahon, R.P., Bonds, D.R. & the Investigators of the Multicenter Study of Hydroxyurea in Sickle Cell Anemia (1995) Effect of hydroxyurea on the frequency of painful crises in sickle cell anemia. *New Engl. J. Med.*, **332**, 1317–1322

Charache, S., Barton, F.B., Moore, R.D., Terrin, M.L., Steinberg, M.H., Dover, G.J., Ballas, S.K., McMahon, R.P., Castro, O., Orringer, E.P. & the Investigators of the Multicenter Study of Hydroxyurea in Sickle Cell Anemia (1996) Hydroxyurea and sickle cell anemia. Clinical utility of a myelosuppressive 'switching' agent. *Medicine*, **75**, 300–326

Chaube, S. & Murphy, M.L. (1966) The effects of hydroxyurea and related compounds on the rat fetus. *Cancer Res.*, **26**, 1448–1457

Chlopkiewicz, B. & Koziorowska, J.H. (1983) Transforming activities of methotrexate, hydroxyurea and 5-fluorouracil in different cell systems. *Neoplasma*, **30**, 295–302

CIS Information Services (1998) *Worldwide Bulk Drug Users Directory 1997/98 Edition*, Dallas, TX [CD-ROM]

Cox, C., Nowicky, D. & Young, R. (1997) Hydroxyurea-related ankle ulcers in patients with myeloproliferative disorders: A case report and review of the literature. *Ann. plast. Surg.*, **39**, 546–549

Currie, J.L., Blessing, J.A., Muss, H.B., Fowler, J., Berman, M. & Burke, T.W. (1996a) Combination chemotherapy with hydroxyurea, dacarbazine (DTIC), and etoposide in the treatment of uterine leiomyosarcoma: A Gynecologic Oncology Group study. *Gynecol. Oncol.*, **61**, 27–30

Currie, J.L., Blessing, J.A., McGehee, R., Soper, J.T. & Berman, M. (1996b) Phase II trial of hydroxyurea, dacarbazine (DTIC), and etoposide (VP-16) in mixed mesodermal tumors of the uterus: A Gynecologic Oncology Group study. *Gynecol. Oncol.*, **61**, 94–96

Davidovitz, Y., Lev, D., Ballin, A., Tsudik, A. & Meytes, D. (1998) Short communication. Translocation (1;20)(q32;q13.3) in myelofibrosis following polycythemia vera. *Cancer Genet. Cytogenet.*, **101**, 156–158

De Boer, R.J., Boucher, C.A. & Perelson, A.S. (1998) Target cell availability and the successful suppression of HIV by hydroxyurea and didanosine. *AIDS*, **12**, 1567–1570

De Haan, J.B. & Parker, M.I. (1988) Differential effects of DNA synthesis inhibitors on DNA methylation in normal and transformed cells. *Anticancer Res.*, **8**, 617–620

Delmer, A., Rio, B., Bauduer, F., Ajchenbaum, F., Marie, J.-P. & Zittoun, R. (1992) Pregnancy during myelosuppressive treatment for chronic myelogenous leukaemia (Letter to the Editor). *Br. J. Haematol.*, **82**, 783–784

DePass, L.R. & Weaver, E.V. (1982) Comparison of teratogenic effects of aspirin and hydroxyurea in the Fischer 344 and Wistar strains. *J. Toxicol. environ. Health*, **10**, 297–305

DeSesso, J.M. (1981a) Comparative ultrastructural alterations in rabbit limb-buds after a teratogenic dose of either hydroxyurea or methotrexate. *Teratology*, **23**, 197–215

DeSesso, J.M. (1981b) Amelioration of teratogenesis. I. Modification of hydroxyurea-induced teratogenesis by the antioxidant propyl gallate. *Teratology*, **24**, 19–35

DeSesso, J.M. & Goeringer, G.C. (1990) The nature of the embryo-protective interaction of propyl gallate with hydroxyurea. *Reprod. Toxicol.*, **4**, 145–152

DeSesso, J.M. & Jordan, R.L. (1977) Drug-induced limb dysplasias in fetal rabbits. *Teratology*, **15**, 199–211

DeSesso, J.M., Scialli, A.R. & Goeringer, G.C. (1994) D-Mannitol, a specific hydroxyl free radical scavenger, reduces the developmental toxicity of hydroxyurea in rabbits. *Teratology*, **49**, 248–259

De Simone, C., Guerriero, C., Guidi, B., Rotoli, M., Venier, A. & Tartaglione, R. (1998) Multiple squamous cell carcinomas of the skin during long-term treatment with hydroxyurea. *Eur. J. Dermatol.*, **8**, 114–115

Diez-Martin, J.L., Graham, D.L., Petitt, R.M. & Dewald, G.W. (1991) Chromosome studies in 104 patients with polycythemia vera. *Mayo Clin. Proc.*, **66**, 287–299

Disdier, P., Harle, J.R., Grob, J.J., Weiller-Merli, C., Magalon, G. & Weiller, P.J. (1991) Rapid development of multiple squamous-cell carcinomas during chronic granulocytic leukemia. *Dermatologica*, **183**, 47–48

Donehower, R.C. (1992) An overview of the clinical experience with hydroxyurea. *Semin. Oncol.*, **19** (Suppl. 9), 11–19

Doney, K.C., Kraemer, K.G. & Shepard, T.H. (1979) Combination chemotherapy for acute myelocytic leukemia during pregnancy: Three case reports. *Cancer Treat. Rep.*, **63**, 369–371

Donovan, P.B., Kaplan, M.E., Goldberg, J.D., Tatarsky, I., Najean, Y., Silberstein, E.B., Knospe, W.H., Laszlo, J., Mack, K., Berk, P.D. & Wasserman, L.R. (1984) Treatment of polycythemia vera with hydroxyurea. *Am. J. Hematol.*, **17**, 329–334

Editions du Vidal (1998) *Dictionnaire Vidal 1998*, 74th Ed., Paris, OVP, pp. 889–890

Epstein, S.S., Arnold, E., Andrea, J., Bass, W. & Bishop, Y. (1972) Detection of chemical mutagens by the dominant lethal assay in the mouse. *Toxicol. appl. Pharmacol.*, **23**, 288–325

Evenson, D.P. & Jost, L.K. (1993) Hydroxyurea exposure alters mouse testicular kinetics and sperm chromatin structure. *Cell Prolif.*, **26**, 147–159

Fenech, M., Rinaldi, J. & Surralles, J. (1994) The origin of micronuclei induced by cytosine arabinoside and its synergistic interaction with hydroxyurea in human lymphocytes. *Mutagenesis*, **9**, 273–277

Ferguson, L.R. (1990) Mutagenic and recombinogenic consequences of DNA-repair inhibition during treatment with 1,3-bis(2-chloroethyl)-1-nitrosourea in *Saccharomyces cerevisiae*. *Mutat. Res.*, **241**, 369–377

Ferguson, L.R. (1995) Mutagenic properties of anticancer drugs. In: Ponder, B.A.J. & Waring, M.J., eds, *The Genetics of Cancer*, Lancaster, Kluwer Academic Publisher, pp. 177–216

Ferguson, L.R. & Denny, W.A. (1995) Anticancer drugs: An underestimated risk or an underutilised resource in mutagenesis. *Mutat. Res.*, **331**, 1–26

Ferguson, L.R. & Turner, P.M. (1988a) 'Petite' mutagenesis by anticancer drugs in *Saccharomyces cerevisiae*. *Eur. J. Cancer clin. Oncol.*, **24**, 591–596

Ferguson, L.R. & Turner, P.M. (1988b) Mitotic crossing-over by anticancer drugs in *Saccharomyces cerevisiae* strain D5. *Mutat. Res.*, **204**, 239–249

Ferm, V.H. (1966) Severe developmental malformations. *Arch. Pathol.*, **81**, 174–177

Ferster, A., Vermylen, C., Cornu, G., Buyse, M., Corazza, F., Devalck, C., Fondu, P., Toppet, M. & Sariban, E. (1996) Hydroxyurea for treatment of severe sickle cell anemia: A pediatric clinical trial. *Blood*, **88**, 1960–1964

Fibach, E., Burke, K.P., Schechter, A.N., Noguchi, C.T. & Rodgers, G.P. (1993) Hydroxyurea increases fetal hemoglobin in cultured erythroid cells derived from normal individuals and patients with sickle cell anemia or beta-thalassemia. *Blood*, **81**, 1630–1635

Fitzgerald, J.M. & McCann, S.R. (1993) The combination of hydroxyurea and leucapheresis in the treatment of chronic myeloid leukaemia in pregnancy. *Clin. Lab. Haematol.*, **15**, 63–65

Foli, A., Maserati, R., Minoli, L., Wainberg, M.A., Gallo, R.C., Lisziewicz, J. & Lori, F. (1998) Therapeutic advantage of hydroxyurea and didanosine combination therapy in patients previously treated with zidovudine. *AIDS*, **12**, 1113–1114

Furgerson, J.L., Vukelja, S.J., Baker, W.J. & O'Rourke, T.J. (1996) Acute myeloid leukemia evolving from essential thrombocythemia in two patients treated with hydroxyurea. *Am. J. Hematol.*, **51**, 137–140

Galli, A. & Schiestl, R.H. (1996) Hydroxyurea induces recombination in dividing but not in G1 or G2 cell cycle arrested yeast cells. *Mutat. Res.*, **354**, 69–75

Gandhi, V., Plunkett, W., Kantarjian, H., Talpaz, M., Robertson, L.E. & O'Brien, S. (1998) Cellular pharmacodynamics and plasma pharmacokinetics of parenterally infused hydroxyurea during a phase I clinical trial in chronic myelogenous leukemia. *J. clin. Oncol.*, **16**, 2321–2331

Gao, W.Y., Zhou, B.S., Johns, D.G., Mitsuya, H. & Yen, Y. (1998) Role of the M2 subunit of ribonucleotide reductase in regulation by hydroxyurea of the activity of the anti-HIV-1 agent 2',3'-dideoxyinosine. *Biochem. Pharmacol.*, **56**, 105–112

Gennaro, A.R. (1995) *Remington: The Science and Practice of Pharmacy*, 19th Ed., Easton, PA, Mack Publishing Co., Vol. II, p. 1252

Graham, P.J. (1955) *Synthesis of Ureas*. US Patent No. 2,705,727. Assigned to E.I. du Pont de Nemours & Co., Wilmington, DE

Greenwood, S.K., Armstrong, M.J., Hill, R.B., Bradt, C.I., Johnson, T.E., Hilliard, C.A. & Galloway, S.M. (1998) Fewer chromosome aberrations and earlier apoptosis induced by DNA synthesis inhibitors, a topoisomerase II inhibitor or alkylating agents in human cells with normal compared with mutant p53. *Mutat. Res.*, **401**, 39–53

Gropper, C.A., Don, P.C. & Sadjadi, M.M. (1993) Nail and skin hyperpigmentation associated with hydroxyurea therapy for polycythemia vera. *Int. J. Dermatol.*, **32**, 731–733

Guilhot, F., Abgrall, J.-F., Harousseau, J.-L., Bauters, F., Brice, P., Dine, G., Tilly, H., Ifrah, N., Cassasus, P., Rochant, H., Christian, B., Guerci, A., Lamagnere, J.-P., Le Prise, P.-Y., Duclos, B. & Tanzer, J. (1993) A multicentric randomised study of alpha 2b interferon (IFN) and hydroxyurea (HU) with or without cytosine-arabinoside (Ara-c) in previously untreated patients with Ph+ chronic myelocytic leukemia (CML): Preliminary cytogenetic results. *Leuk. Lymphoma*, **11** (Suppl. 1), 181–183

Gwilt, P.R. & Tracewell, W.G. (1998) Pharmacokinetics and pharmacodynamics of hydroxyurea. *Clin. Pharmacokinet.*, **34**, 347–358

Hahn, P., Kapp, L.N., Morgan, W.F. & Painter, R.B. (1986) Chromosomal changes without DNA overproduction in hydroxyurea-treated mammalian cells: Implications for gene amplification. *Cancer Res.*, **46**, 4607–4612

Hansen, D.K., Grafton, T.F., Cross, D.R. & James, S.J. (1995) Partial attenuation of hydroxyurea-induced embryotoxicity by deoxyribonucleotides in mouse and rat embryos treated *in vitro*. *Toxicol. in Vitro*, **9**, 11–19

Hart, J.W. & Hartley-Asp, B. (1983) Induction of micronuclei in the mouse. Revised timing of the final stage of erythropoiesis. *Mutat. Res.*, **120**, 127–132

Haworth, S., Lawlor, T., Mortelmans, K., Speck, W. & Zeiger, E. (1983) *Salmonella* mutagenicity test results for 250 chemicals. *Environ. Mutag.*, **5** (Suppl. 1), 3–142

Herken, R. (1984) The influence of deoxycytidine monophosphate (dCMP) on the cytotoxicity of hydroxyurea in the embryonic spinal cord of the mouse. *Teratology*, **30**, 83–90

Herken, R. (1985) Ultrastructural changes in the neural tube of 10-day-old mouse embryos exposed to colchicine and hydroxyurea. *Teratology*, **31**, 345–352

Hill, A.B. & Schimke, R.T. (1985) Increased gene amplification in L5178Y mouse lymphoma cells with hydroxyurea-induced chromosomal aberrations. *Cancer Res.*, **45**, 5050–5057

Holcombe, R.F., Treseler, P.A. & Rosenthal, D.S. (1991) Chronic myelomonocytic leukemia transformation in polycythemia vera. *Leukemia*, **5**, 606–610

Ishii, Y. & Bender, M.A. (1980) Effects of inhibitors of DNA synthesis on spontaneous and ultraviolet light-induced sister-chromatid exchanges in Chinese hamster cells. *Mutat. Res.*, **79**, 19–32

Iversen, O.H. (1982a) Enhancement of methylnitrosourea skin carcinogenesis by inhibiting cell proliferation with hydroxyurea or skin extracts. *Carcinogenesis*, **3**, 881–889

Iversen, O.H. (1982b) Hydroxyurea enhances methylnitrosourea skin carcinogenesis when given shortly before, but not after, the carcinogen. *Carcinogenesis*, **3**, 891–894

Iwama, M., Sakamoto, Y., Honda, A. & Mori, Y. (1983) Limb deformity induced in chick embryo by hydroxyurea. *J. Pharmacobiodyn.*, **6**, 836–843

Jackson, H., Shukri, A. & Ali, K. (1993) Hydroxyurea treatment for chronic myeloid leukaemia during pregnancy. *Br. J. Haematol.*, **85**, 203–204

Jackson, M.A., Stack, H.F. & Waters, M.D. (1996) Genetic activity profiles of anticancer drugs. *Mutat. Res.*, **355**, 171–208

Jelmert, Ø., Hansteen, I.-L. & Langård, S. (1992) Enhanced cytogenetic detection of previous in vivo exposure to mutagens in human lymphocytes after treatment with inhibitors of DNA synthesis and DNA repair *in vitro*. *Mutat. Res.*, **271**, 289–298

Jiang, J., Jordan, S.J., Barr, D.P., Gunther, M.R., Maeda, H. & Mason, R.P. (1997) In vivo production of nitric oxide in rats after administration of hydroxyurea. *Mol. Pharmacol.*, **52**, 1081–1086

Johns, D.G. & Gao, W.Y. (1998) Selective depletion of DNA precursors: An evolving strategy for potentiation of dideoxynucleoside activity against immunodeficiency virus. *Biochem. Pharmacol.*, **55**, 1551–1556

Kaplan, M.E., Mack, K., Goldberg, J.D., Donovan, P.B., Berk, P.D. & Wasserman, L.R. (1986) Long-term management of polycythemia vera with hydroxyurea: A progress report. *Semin. Hematol.*, **23**, 167–171

Karon, M. & Benedict, W.F. (1972) Chromatid breakage: Differential effect of inhibitors of DNA synthesis during G2 phase. *Science*, **178**, 62

Khera, K.S. (1979) A teratogenicity study on hydroxyurea and diphenylhydantoin in cats. *Teratology*, **20**, 447–452

Kihlman, B.A. & Andersson, H.C. (1985) Synergistic enhancement of the frequency of chromatid aberrations in cultured human lymphocytes by combinations of inhibitors of DNA repair. *Mutat. Res.*, **150**, 313–325

Kunze, E., Graewe, T., Scherber, S., Weber, J. & Gellhar, P. (1989) Cell cycle dependence of *N*-methyl-*N*-nitrosourea-induced tumour development in the proliferating, partially resected urinary bladder. *Br. J. exp. Pathol.*, **70**, 125–142

Lambert, B., Sten, M., Söderhäll, S., Ringborg, U. & Lewensohn, R. (1983) DNA repair replication, DNA breaks and sister-chromatid exchange in human cells treated with adriamycin *in vitro*. *Mutat. Res.*, **111**, 171–184

Landaw, S.A. (1986) Acute leukemia in polycythemia vera. *Semin. Hematol.*, **23**, 156–165

Levin, V.A. & Prados, M.D. (1992) Treatment of recurrent gliomas and metastatic brain tumors with a polydrug protocol designed to combat nitrosourea resistance. *J. clin. Oncol.*, **10**, 766–771

Li, J.C. & Kaminskas, E. (1987) Progressive formation of DNA lesions in cultured Ehrlich ascites tumor cells treated with hydroxyurea. *Cancer Res.*, **47**, 2755–2758

Liozon, E., Brigaudeau, C., Trimoreau, F., Desangles, F., Fermeaux, V., Praloran, V. & Bordessoule, D. (1997) Is treatment with hydroxyurea leukemogenic in patients with essential thrombocythemia? An analysis of three new cases of leukaemic transformation and review of the literature. *Hematol. Cell Ther.*, **39**, 11–18

Lisziewicz, J., Jessen, H., Finzi, D., Siliciano, R.F. & Lori, F. (1998) HIV-1 suppression by early treatment with hydroxyurea, didanosine, and a protease inhibitor. *Lancet*, **352**, 199–200

Löfvenberg, E. & Wahlin, A. (1988) Management of polycythaemia vera, essential thrombocythaemia and myelofibrosis with hydroxyurea. *Eur. J. Haematol.*, **41**, 375–381

Löfvenberg, E., Nordenson, I. & Wahlin, A. (1990) Cytogenetic abnormalities and leukemic transformation in hydroxyurea-treated patients with Philadelphia chromosome negative chronic myeloproliferative disease. *Cancer Genet. Cytogenet.*, **49**, 57–67

Lori, F., Gallo, R.C., Malykh, A., Cara, A., Romano, J., Markham, P. & Franchini, G. (1997a) Didanosine but not high doses of hydroxyurea rescue pigtail macaque from a lethal dose of SIV (smmpbj14). *AIDS Res. hum. Retroviruses*, **13**, 1083–1088

Lori, F., Malykh, A.G., Foli, A., Maserati, R., De Antoni, A., Minoli, L., Padrini, D., Degli Antoni, A., Barchi, E., Jessen, H., Wainberg, M.A., Gallo, R.C. & Lisziewicz, J. (1997b) Combination of a drug targeting the cell with a drug targeting the virus controls human immunodeficiency virus type 1 resistance. *AIDS Res. hum. Retroviruses*, **13**, 1403–1409

Loukopoulos, D., Voskaridou, E., Stamoulakatou, A., Papassotiriou, Y., Kalotychou, V., Loutradi, A., Cozma, G., Tsiarta, H. & Pavlides, N. (1998) Hydroxyurea therapy in thalassemia. *Ann. N.Y. Acad. Sci.*, **850**, 120–128

Luzzati, R., Di-Perri, G., Fendt, D., Ramarli, D., Broccali, G. & Concia, E. (1998) Pharmacokinetics, safety and anti-human immunodeficiency virus (HIV) activity of hydroxyurea in combination with didanosine (Letter). *J. antimicrob. Chemother.*, **42**, 565–566

Maier-Redelsperger, M., de Montalembert, M., Flahault, A., Neonato, M.G., Ducrocq, R., Masson, M.P., Girot, R. & Elion, J. for the French Study Group on Sickle Cell Disease (1998) Fetal hemoglobin and F-cell responses to long-term hydroxyurea treatment in young sickle cell patients. *Blood*, **91**, 4472–4479

Mattano, S.S., Palella, T.D. & Mitchell, B.S. (1990) Mutations induced at the hypoxanthine–guanine phosphoribosyltransferase locus of human T-lymphoblasts by perturbations of purine deoxyribonucleoside triphosphate pools. *Cancer Res.*, **50**, 4566–4571

Mayer, V.W., Goin, C.J. & Zimmermann, F.K. (1986) Aneuploidy and other genetic effects induced by hydroxyurea in *Saccharomyces cerevisiae*. *Mutat. Res.*, **160**, 19–26

Medical Economics Data Production (1999) *PDR®: Physicians' Desk Reference*, 53rd Ed., Montvale, NJ, Medical Economics

Mehnert, K., Vogel, W., Benz, R. & Speit, G. (1984) Different effects of mutagens on sister chromatid exchange induction in three Chinese hamster cell lines. *Environ. Mutag.*, **6**, 573–583

Millicovsky, G., DeSesso, J.M., Kleinman, L.I. & Clark, K.E. (1981) Effects of hydroxyurea on hemodynamics of pregnant rabbits: A maternally mediated mechanism of embryotoxicity. *Am. J. Obstet. Gynecol.*, **140**, 747–752

Minford, J., Kerrigan, D., Nichols, M., Shackney, S. & Zwelling, L.A. (1984) Enhancement of the DNA breakage and cytotoxic effects of intercalating agents by treatment with sublethal doses of 1-beta-D-arabinofuranosylcytosine or hydroxyurea in L1210 cells. *Cancer Res.*, **44**, 5583–5593

de Montalembert, M., Belloy, M., Bernaudin, F., Gouraud, F., Capdeville, R., Mardini, R., Philippe, N., Jais, J.P., Bardakdjian, J., Ducrocq, R., Maier-Redelsperger, M., Elion, J., Labie, D. & Girot, R. for the French Study Group on Sickle Cell Disease (1997) Three-year follow-up of hydroxyurea treatment in severely ill children with sickle cell disease. *J. pediatr. Hematol./Oncol.*, **19**, 313–318

Montaner, J.S., Zala, C., Conway, B., Raboud, J., Patenaude, P., Rae, S., O'Shaughnessy, M.V. & Schechter, M.T. (1997) A pilot study of hydroxyurea among patients with advanced human immunodeficiency virus (HIV) disease receiving chronic didanosine therapy: Canadian HIV trials network protocol 080. *J. infect. Dis.*, **175**, 801–806

Moschella, S.L. & Greenwald, M.A. (1973) Psoriasis with hydroxyurea. An 18-month study of 60 patients. *Arch. Dermatol.*, **107**, 363–368

Muranyi-Kovacs, I. & Rudali, G. (1972) Comparative study of carcinogenic activity of hydroxyurea and urethane in XVII-G mice. *Rev. Eur. Etud. clin. biol.*, **17**, 93–95

Murphy, M.L. & Chaube, S. (1964) Preliminary survey of hydroxyurea (NSC-32065) as a teratogen. *Cancer Chemother. Rep.*, **40**, 1–7

Nair, R., Iyer, R.S., Nair, C.N., Kurkure, P.A., Pai, S.K., Saikia, T.K., Nadkarni, K.S., Pai, V.R., Gopal, R. & Advani, S.H. (1993) Myelodysplastic syndrome. A clinical and pathological analysis of 88 patients. *Indian J. Cancer*, **30**, 169–175

Najean, Y. & Rain, J.-D. (1997a) Treatment of polycythemia vera: The use of hydroxyurea and pipobroman in 292 patients under the age of 65 years. *Blood*, **90**, 3370–3377

Najean, Y. & Rain, J.D. for the French Polycythemia Study Group (1997b) Treatment of polycythemia vera: Use of ^{32}P alone or in combination with maintenance therapy using hydroxyurea in 461 patients greater than 65 years of age. *Blood*, **89**, 2319–2327

Najean, Y., Rain, J.-D., Dresch, C., Goguel, A., Lejeune, F., Echard, M. & Grange, M.-J. (1996) Risk of leukaemia, carcinoma, and myelofibrosis in ^{32}P- or chemotherapy-treated patients with polycythemia vera: A prospective analysis of 682 cases. *Leuk. Lymphoma*, **22**, 111–119

Nand, S., Messmore, H., Fisher, S.G., Bird, M.L., Schulz, W. & Fisher, R.I. (1990) Leukemic transformation in polycythemia vera: Analysis of risk factors. *Am. J. Hematol.*, **34**, 32–36

Nand, S., Stock, W., Godwin, J. & Fisher, S.G. (1996) Leukemogenic risk of hydroxyurea therapy in polycythemia vera, essential thrombocythemia, and myeloid metaplasia with myelofibrosis. *Am. J. Hematol.*, **52**, 42–46

Navarra, P., Del Carmine, R., Ciabattoni, G., D'Amato, M., Ragazzoni, E., Vacca, M., Volpe, A.R. & Preziosi, P. (1990) Hydroxyurea: Relationship between toxicity and centrally-induced adrenal activation. *Pharmacol. Toxicol.*, **67**, 209–215

Navarra, P., Puccetti, P., Riccardi, C. & Preziosi, P. (1995) Anticancer drug toxicity via cytokine production: The hydroxyurea paradigm. *Toxicol. Lett.*, **82–83**, 167–171

Navarra, P., Tringali, G. & Preziosi, P. (1996) The effects of inhibitors of cyclo-oxygenase, lipoxygenase and nitric oxide synthase pathways on the toxicity of hydroxyurea in adrenalectomized rats. *Toxicol. Lett.*, **86**, 13–18

Navarra, P., Grohmann, U., Nocentini, G., Tringali, G., Puccetti, P., Riccardi, C. & Preziosi, P. (1997) Hydroxyurea induces the gene expression and synthesis of proinflammatory cytokines *in vivo*. *J. Pharmacol. exp. Ther.*, **280**, 477–482

Navarra, P., Tringali, G. & Preziosi, P. (1998) Hydroxyurea influences adrenocortical function in humans. *Eur. J. clin. Pharmacol.*, **54**, 491–492

Nyce, J., Liu, L. & Jones, P.A. (1986) Variable effects of DNA-synthesis inhibitors upon DNA methylation in mammalian cells. *Nucleic Acids Res.*, **14**, 4353–4367

Ören, H., Düzovali, O., Yüksel, E., Sakizli, M. & Irken, G. (1999) Development of acute promyelocytic leukemia with isochromosome 17q after BCR/ABL positive chronic myeloid leukemia. *Cancer Genet. Cytogenet.*, **109**, 141–143

Painter, R.B. & Cleaver, J.E. (1967) Radiobiology. Repair replication in HeLa cells after large doses of X-irradiation. *Nature*, **216**, 369–370

Pajor, A., Zimonyi, I., Koos, R., Lehoczky, D. & Ambrus, C. (1991) Pregnancies and offspring in survivors of acute lymphoid leukemia and lymphoma. *Eur. J. Obstet. Gynecol. reprod. Biol.*, **40**, 1–5

Palitti, F., Tanzarella, C., Degrassi, F., De Salvia, R., Fiore, M. & Natarajan, A.T. (1983) Formation of chromatid-type aberrations in G2 stage of the cell cycle. *Mutat. Res.*, **110**, 343–350

Palitti, F., Tanzarella, C., Degrassi, F., De Salvia, R. & Fiore, M. (1984a) Enhancement of induced sister chromatid exchange and chromosomal aberrations by inhibitors of DNA repair processes. *Toxicol. Pathol.*, **12**, 269–273

Palitti, F., Degrassi, F., De Salvia, R., Tanzarella, C. & Fiore, M. (1984b) Potentiation of induced sister chromatid exchanges and chromatid-type aberrations by inhibitors of DNA synthesis and repair in G2. *Basic Life Sci.*, **29A**, 313–318

Patel, M., Dukes, I.A.F. & Hull, J.D. (1991) Use of hydroxyurea in chronic myeloid leukemia during pregnancy: A case report. *Am. J. Obstet. Gynecol.*, **165**, 565–566

Philips, F.S. & Sternberg, S.S. (1975) Tests for tumour induction by antitumor agents. *Recent Results Cancer Res.*, **52**, 29–35

Popescu, N.C., Turnbull, D. & DiPaolo, J.A. (1977) Sister chromatid exchange and chromosome aberration analysis with the use of several carcinogens and noncarcinogens. *J. natl Cancer Inst.*, **59**, 289–293

Pouchert, C.J. (1981) *The Aldrich Library of Infrared Spectra*, 3rd Ed., Milwaukee, WI, Aldrich Chemical Co., p. 475

Pouchert, C.J. (1983) *The Aldrich Library of NMR Spectra*, 2nd Ed., Milwaukee, WI, Aldrich Chemical Co., Vol. 1, p. 671

Pouchert, C.J. (1985) *The Aldrich Library of FT-IR Spectra*, Milwaukee, WI, Aldrich Chemical Co., Vol. 1, p. 801

Prempree, T. & Merz, T. (1969) Does hydroxyurea inhibit chromosome repair in cultured human lymphocytes? *Nature*, **224**, 603–604

Price, C.J., Tyl, R.W., Marks, T.A., Taschke, L.L., Ledoux, T.A. & Reel, J.R. (1985) Teratologic and postnatal evaluation of aniline hydrochloride in the Fischer 344 rat. *Toxicol. appl. Pharmacol.*, **77**, 465–478

Quesnel, B., Kantarjian, H., Pedersen Bjergaard, J., Brault, P., Estey, E., Lai, J.L., Tilly, H., Stoppa, A.M., Archimbaud, E., Harousseau, J.L., Bauters, F. & Fenaux, P. (1993) Therapy-related acute myeloid leukemia with t(8;21), inv(16), and t(8;16): A report on 25 cases and review of the literature. *J. clin. Oncol.*, **11**, 2370–2379

Reiffers, J., Dachary, D., David, B., Bernard, P., Marit, G., Boisseau, M. & Brousted, A. (1985) Megakaryoblastic transformation of primary thrombocythemia. *Acta haematol.*, **73**, 228–231

Richard, M., Truchetet, F., Friedel, J., Leclech, C. & Heid, E. (1989) Skin lesions simulating chronic dermatomyositis during long-term hydroxyurea therapy. *J. Am. Acad. Dermatol.*, **21**, 797–799

Rodriguez, G.I., Kuhn, J.G., Weiss, G.R., Hilsenbeck, S.G., Eckardt, J.R., Thurman, A., Rinaldi, D.A., Hodges, S., Von Hoff, D.D. & Rowinsky, E.K. (1998) A bioavailability and pharmacokinetic study of oral and intravenous hydroxyurea. *Blood*, **91**, 1533–1541

Rossberger, S. & Andrae, U. (1985) DNA repair synthesis induced by N-hydroxyurea, acetohydroxamic acid, and N-hydroxyurethane in primary rat hepatocyte cultures: Comparative evaluation using the autoradiographic and the bromodeoxyuridine density-shift method. *Mutat. Res.*, **145**, 201–207

Rote Liste Sekretariat (1998) *Rote Liste 1998*, Frankfurt, Rote Liste Service GmbH, pp. 86–106, 86–115

Royal Pharmaceutical Society of Great Britain (1999) *Martindale, The Extra Pharmacopoeia*, 13th Ed., London, The Pharmaceutical Press [MicroMedex Online: Health Care Series]

Rutschmann, O.T., Opravil, M., Iten, A., Malinverni, R., Vernazza, P.L., Bucher, H.C., Bernasconi, E., Sudre, P., Leduc, D., Yerly, S., Perrin, L.H. & Hirschel, B. for the Swiss HIV Cohort Study (1998) A placebo-controlled trial of didanosine plus stavudine, with and without hydroxyurea, for HIV infection. *AIDS*, **12**, F71–F77

Sadtler Research Laboratories (1995) *Sadtler Standard Spectra, 1981–1995 Supplementary Index*, Philadelphia, PA, p. 1

Sato, K., Akaike, T., Sawa, T., Miyamoto, Y., Suga, M., Ando, M. & Maeda, H. (1997) Nitric oxide generation from hydroxyurea via copper-catalyzed peroxidation and implications for pharmacological actions of hydroxyurea. *Jpn. J. Cancer Res.*, **88**, 1199–1204

Schrell, U.M., Rittig, M.G., Anders, M., Koch, U.H., Marschalek, R., Kiesewetter, F. & Fahlbusch, R. (1997) Hydroxyurea for treatment of unresectable and recurrent meningiomas. II. Decrease in the size of meningiomas in patients treated with hydroxyurea. *J. Neurosurg.*, **86**, 840–844

Scott, W.J., Ritter, E.J. & Wilson, J.G. (1971) DNA synthesis inhibition and cell death associated with hydroxyurea teratogenesis in rat embryos. *Dev. Biol.*, **26**, 306–315

Scott, J.P., Hillery, C.A., Brown, E.R., Misiewicz, V. & Labotka, R.J. (1996) Hydroxyurea therapy in children severely affected with sickle cell disease. *J. Pediatr.*, **128**, 820–828

Sharon, R., Tatarsky, I. & Ben-Arieh, Y. (1986) Treatment of polycythemia vera with hydroxyurea. *Cancer*, **57**, 718–720

Simchen, G., Idar, D. & Kassir, Y. (1976) Recombination and hydroxyurea inhibition of DNA synthesis in yeast meiosis. *Mol. Gen. Genet.*, **144**, 21–27

Simonelli, C., Comar, M., Zanussi, S., De Paoli, P., Tirelli, U. & Giacca, M. (1997) No therapeutic advantage from didanosine (ddI) and hydroxyurea versus ddI alone in patients with HIV infection. *AIDS*, **11**, 1299–1300

Skog, S., Heiden, T., Eriksson, S., Wallström, B. & Tribukait, B. (1992) Hydroxyurea-induced cell death in human T lymphoma cells as related to imbalance in DNA/protein cycle and deoxyribonucleotide pools and DNA strand breaks. *Anticancer Drugs*, **3**, 379–386

Sofuni, T., Honma, M., Hayashi, M., Shimada, H., Tanaka, N., Wakuri, S., Awogi, T., Yamamoto, K.I., Nishi, Y. & Nakadate, M. (1996) Detection of in vitro clastogens and spindle poisons by the mouse lymphoma assay using the microwell method: Interim report of an international collaborative study. *Mutagenesis*, **11**, 349–355

Stasi, R., Cantonetti, M., Abruzzese, E., Papi, M., Didona, B., Cavalieri, R. & Papa, G. (1992) Multiple skin tumors in long-term treatment with hydroxyurea (Letter to the Editor). *Eur. J. Haematol.*, **48**,121–122

Stehman, F.B. (1992) Experience with hydroxyurea as a radiosensitizer in carcinoma of the cervix. *Semin. Oncol.*, **19**, 48–52

Stehman, F.B., Bundy, B.N., Kucera, P.R., Deppe, G., Reddy, S. & O'Connor, D.M. (1997) Hydroxyurea, 5-fluorouracil infusion, and cisplatin adjunct to radiation therapy in cervical carcinoma: A phase I–II trial of the Gynecologic Oncology Group. *Gynecol. Oncol.*, **66**, 262–267

Sterkers, Y., Preudhomme, C., Laï, J.-L., Demory, J.-L., Caulier, M.-T., Wattel, E., Borderssoule, D., Bauters, F. & Fenaux, P. (1998) Acute myeloid leukemia and myelodysplastic syndromes following essential thrombocythemia treated with hydroxyurea: High proportion of cases with 17p deletion. *Blood*, **91**, 616–622

Strauss, B., Coyle, M., McMahon, M., Kato, K. & Dolyniuk, M. (1972) DNA synthesis, repair and chromosome breaks in eucaryotic cells. *Johns Hopkins med. J.*, **1**, 111–124

Swiss Pharmaceutical Society, ed. (1999) *Index Nominum, International Drug Directory*, 16th Ed., Stuttgart, Medpharm Scientific Publishers [MicroMedex Online: Health Care Series]

Sylvester, R.K., Lobell, M., Teresi, M.E., Brundage, D. & Dubowy, R. (1987) Excretion of hydroxyurea into milk. *Cancer*, **60**, 2177–2178

Tanaka, M., Yamazaki, Y., Kondo, E., Hattori, M., Tsushita, K. & Utsumi, M. (1997) Achievement of a complete cytogenetic response with hydroxyurea in a patient with chronic myelogenous leukemia. *Leuk. Res.*, **21**, 465–468

Tefferi, A. (1998) Is hydroxyurea leukemagenic in essential thrombocythemia? (Letter to the Editor). *Blood*, **92**, 1459–1460; discussion 1460–1461

Tertian, G., Tchernia, G., Papiernik, E. & Elefant, E. (1992) Hydroxyurea and pregnancy (Letter to the Editor). *Am. J. Obstet. Gynecol.*, **166**, 1868

Theisen, C.T., Fradkin, R. & Wilson, J.G. (1973) Teratogenicity of hydroxyurea in rhesus monkeys. *Teratology*, **7**, A29

Thomas, J., ed. (1998) *Australian Prescription Products Guide*, 27th Ed., Victoria, Australian Pharmaceutical Publishing, Vol. 1, p. 1406

Timson, J. (1975) Hydroxyurea. *Mutat. Res.*, **32**, 115–132

Tohda, H. & Oikawa, A. (1990) Hypoxanthine enhances hydroxyurea-induced sister-chromatid exchanges in Chinese hamster ovary cells. *Mutat. Res.*, **230**, 235–240

Toraason, M., Bohrman, J.S., Krieg, E., Combes, R.D., Willington, S.E., Zajac, W. & Langenbach, R. (1992) Evaluation of the V79 cell metabolic co-operation assay as a screen in vitro for developmental toxicants. *Toxicol. in Vitro*, **6**, 165–174

Triadou, P., Maier-Redelsperger, M., Krishnamoorty, R., Deschamps, A., Casadevall, N., Dunda, O., Ducrocq, R., Elion, J., Girot, R., Labie, D., Dover, G. & Cornu, P. (1994) Fetal haemoglobin variations following hydroxyurea treatment in patients with cyanotic congenital heart disease. *Nouv. Rev. Fr. Hematol.*, **36**, 367–372

Tsutsui, T., Barrett, J.C. & Ts'o, P.O.P. (1979) Morphological transformation, DNA damage, and chromosomal aberrations induced by a direct DNA perturbation of synchronized Syrian hamster embryo cells. *Cancer Res.*, **39**, 2356–2365

US Pharmacopeial Convention (1994) *The 1995 US Pharmacopeia*, 23rd Rev./The National Formulary, 18th Rev., Rockville, MD, pp. 776–777

US Pharmacopeial Convention (1998) *USP Dispensing Information*, Vol. I, *Drug Information for the Health Care Professional*, 18th Ed., Rockville, MD, pp. 1607–1609

Van den Berg, C.L., McGill, J.R., Kuhn, J.G., Walsh, J.T., De La Cruz, P.S., Davidson, K.K., Wahl, G.M. & Von Hoff, D.D. (1994) Pharmacokinetics of hydroxyurea in nude mice. *Anticancer Drugs*, **5**, 573–578

Velez, A., Lopez-Rubio, F. & Moreno, J.C. (1998) Chronic hydroxyurea-induced dermatomyositis-like eruption with severe dermal elastosis. *Clin. exp. Dermatol.*, **23**, 94–95

Vila, J., Nugier, F., Bargues, G., Vallet, T., Peyramond, D., Hamedi-Sangsari, F. & Seigneurin, J.M. (1997) Absence of viral rebound after treatment of HIV-infected patients with didanosine and hydroxycarbamide. *Lancet*, **350**, 635–636

Villani, P., Maserati, R., Regazzi, M.B., Giacchino, R. & Lori, F. (1996) Pharmacokinetics of hydroxyurea in patients infected with human immunodeficiency virus type I. *J. clin. Pharmacol.*, **36**, 117–121

Vorhees, C.V., Butcher, R.E., Brunner, R.L. & Sobotka, T.J. (1979) A developmental test battery for neurobehavioral toxicity in rats: A preliminary analysis using monosodium glutamate calcium carrageenan, and hydroxyurea. *Toxicol. appl. Pharmacol.*, **50**, 267–282

Vorhees, C.V., Butcher, R.E., Brunner, R.L., Wootten, V. & Sobotka, T.J. (1983) Developmental toxicity of phychotoxicity of FD and C red dye No. 40 (allura red AC) in rats. *Toxicology*, **28**, 207–217

Voskaridou, E., Kalotychou, V. & Loukopoulos, D. (1995) Clinical and laboratory effects of long-term administration of hydroxyurea to patients with sickle-cell/beta-thalassaemia. *Br. J. Haematol.*, **89**, 479–484

Wadler, S., Haynes, H., Schechner, R., Rozenblit, A. & Wiernik, P.H. (1996) Phase I trial of high-dose infusional hydroxyurea, high-dose infusional 5-fluorouracil and recombinant interferon-alpha-2a in patients with advanced malignancies. *Invest. New Drugs*, **13**, 315–320

Wangenheim, J. & Bolcsfoldi, G. (1988) Mouse lymphoma L5178Y thymidine kinase locus assay of 50 compounds. *Mutagenesis*, **3**, 193–205

Warner, C.W., Sadler, T.W., Shockey, J. & Smith, M.K. (1983) A comparison of the in vivo and in vitro response of mammalian embryos to a teratogenic insult. *Toxicology*, **28**, 271–282

Weinfeld, A., Swolin, B. & Westin, J. (1994) Acute leukaemia after hydroxyurea therapy in polycythemia vera and allied disorders: Prospective study of efficacy and leukaemogenicity with therapeutic implications. *Eur. J. Haematol.*, **52**, 134–139

Weinlich, G., Schuler, G., Greil, R., Kofler, H. & Fritsch, P. (1998) Leg ulcers associated with long-term hydroxyurea therapy. *J. Am. Acad. Dermatol.*, **39**, 372–374

West, W.O. (1987) Hydroxyurea in the treatment of polycythemia vera: A prospective study of 100 patients over a 20-year period. *South. med. J.*, **80**, 323–327

Wiger, R., Hongslo, J.K., Evenson, D.P., De Angelis, P., Schwartze, P.E. & Holme, J.A. (1995) Effects of acetaminophen and hydroxyurea on spermatogenesis and sperm chromatin structure in laboratory mice. *Reprod. Toxicol.*, **9**, 21–33

Wilson, J.G. (1974) Teratogenic causation in man and its evaluation in non-human primates. In: Motulsky, A.G. & Lenz, W., eds, *Birth Defects. Proceedings of 4th International Conference*, Amsterdam, Excerpta Medica, pp. 191–203

Wilson, J.G., Scott, W.J., Ritter, E.J. & Fradkin, R. (1975) Comparative distribution and embryotoxicity of hydroxyurea in pregnant rats and rhesus monkeys. *Teratology*, **11**, 169–178

Zaborowska, D., Swietlinska, Z. & Zuk, J. (1983) Induction of mitotic recombination by UV and diepoxybutane and its enhancement by hydroxyurea in *Saccharomyces cerevisiae*. *Mutat. Res.*, **120**, 21–26

PHENOLPHTHALEIN

1. Exposure Data

1.1 Chemical and physical data

1.1.1 *Nomenclature*

Chem. Abstr. Serv. Reg. No.: 77-09-8
Chem. Abstr. Name: 3,3-Bis(4-hydroxyphenyl)-1-(3H)-isobenzofuranone
IUPAC Systematic Name: Phenolphthalein
Synonyms: 3,3-Bis(4-hydroxyphenyl)phthalide; 3,3-bis(*para*-hydroxyphenyl)-phthalide; α-(*para*-hydroxyphenyl)-α-(4-oxo-2,5-cyclohexadien-1-ylidine)-*ortho*-toluic acid

1.1.2 *Structural and molecular formulae and relative molecular mass*

$C_{20}H_{14}O_4$ Relative molecular mass: 318.33

1.1.3 *Chemical and physical properties of the pure substance*

(a) *Description*: White or yellowish-white, triclinic crystals, often twinned (Budavari, 1996)
(b) *Melting-point*: 258–262 °C (Budavari, 1996)
(c) *Spectroscopy data*: Infrared (prism, [8113; 1471C]; grating [28037]; FT-IR, [1006B]), ultraviolet [2188] and nuclear magnetic resonance (proton, [14709]; ^{13}C, [4455]) spectral data have been reported (Sadtler Research Laboratories, 1980; Pouchert, 1981, 1985)

(d) *Solubility*: Practically insoluble in water; soluble in diethyl ether, ethanol and dilute solutions of alkali hydroxides; very slightly soluble in chloroform (Budavari, 1996)

(e) *Dissociation constant*: pK_a at 25 °C, 9.7 (Budavari, 1996)

1.1.4 Technical products and impurities

Phenolphthalein (white) is available as a 6.5-, 14-, 32.4-, 60-, 65-, 75-, 100-, 120-, 130- and 200-mg tablet, a 60- and 120-mg chewable tablet, a 30-, 65- and 90-mg capsule, a 64.8-mg wafer, a 15-, 50-, 60-, 65-, 66.7- and 200-mg/5 mL and 198 mg/15 mL liquid emulsion and a 117-mg (9%) chocolate square; phenolphthalein (yellow) is available as a 65-, 90-, 95- and 135-mg tablet, an 80-, 90-, 95- and 97.2-mg chewable tablet, a 65- and 130-mg capsule and a 97.2-mg chewing gum. The tablets may also contain aloin, aspartame, bile salts, butylparaben, cascara sagrada, cascara sagrada extract, corn starch, cocoa butter, cocoa paste from cocoa seeds, colourants (D&C Yellow No. 10 aluminium lake, D&C Red No. 28, FD&C Blue No. 1, FD&C Red No. 40, FD&C No. 40 aluminium lake), docusate sodium, dextrates, dibasic calcium phosphate dihydrate, ethyl vanillin, flavours, hydroxypropyl methylcellulose, lactose, leaves of senna, lecithin from soya beans, magnesium stearate, methylene blue, microcrystalline cellulose, oleoresin capsicum, ox bile extract, polydextrose, polyethylene glycol, polysorbate 80, potassium nitrate, povidone, propylene glycol, sodium carbonate (anhydrous), sodium saccharin, sodium starch glycolate, starch, sucrose, titanium dioxide and triacetin. The capsule may also contain dehydrocholic acid, docusate calcium, ethanol, parabens, povidone and sorbitol. The liquid emulsion may also contain agar, benzoic acid, glycerin, liquid paraffin, mineral oil, sodium cyclamate and sorbic acid (Gennaro, 1995; American Hospital Formulary Service, 1997; Canadian Pharmaceutical Association, 1997; Medical Economics Data Production, 1998; Rote Liste Sekretariat, 1998; Thomas, 1998; US Pharmacopeial Convention, 1998).

In the manufacture of phenolphthalein, a stage is reached in which certain by-products formed in the synthesis have not yet been removed, resulting in a product called yellow phenolphthalein. Compounds isolated from one sample of yellow phenolphthalein were: white phenolphthalein, 93%; fluoran, 0.32%; isophenolphthalein, 0.08%; 2-(4-hydroxybenzoyl)benzoic acid, 0.10%. Yellow phenolphthalein was reported to be 2.5 times more active as a laxative in rhesus monkeys than phenolphthalein (Budavari, 1996).

Trade names for phenolphthalein include Alophen Pills, Ap-La-Day, Bonomint, Brooklax, Caolax N.F., Certolax, Cirulaxia, Confetto Falqui, Darmol, Dilsuave, Easylax, Espotabs, Evac-Q-Tabs, Evac-U-Gen, Evac-U-Lax, Ex-Lax, Feen-A-Mint, Figsen, Fletchers Childrens Laxative, Fructines, Fructosan, Lacto-Purga, Laxative Pills, Laxen Busto, Laxettes, Lax-Pills, Lilo, Medilax, Modane, Musilaks, Neo-Prunex, Novopuren, Phenolax, Phenolphthalein Tablets USP 23, Prifinol, Prulet, Purga, Purganol, Purgante, Pürjen Sahap, Reguletts, Sure Lax and Thalinol (National Toxicology Program, 1999;

Royal Pharmaceutical Society of Great Britain, 1999; Swiss Pharmaceutical Society, 1999).

Trade names for phenolphthalein that have been discontinued include Alophen, Bom-Bon, Confetto, Euchessina, Fructine-Vichy, Koprol, Laxatone, Laxogen, Neopurghes, Phthalin, Prunetta, Purgen, Purgestol, Spulmako-lax and Trilax.

Trade names for multi-ingredient preparations of phenolphthalein include Abfuhrdragees, Agarol, Agoral, Aid-Lax, Alofedina, Alophen, Alsiline, Bicholate, Calcium Docuphen, Caroid, Carter Petites Pilules, Carters, Carters Little Pills, Cholasyn, Colax, Damalax, Dialose Plus, Disolan, Docucal-P, Doulax, Doxidan, Emuliquen Laxante, Evac-Q-Kwik, Ex-Lax Extra Gentle Pills, Ex-Lax Light, Falqui, Fam-Lax, Feen-a-mint Pills, Femilax, Ford Pills, Grains de Vals, Herbalax Forte, Juno Junipah, Kest, Kondremul with Phenolphthalein, Laxa, Laxante Bescansa, Laxante Bescansa Aloico, Laxante Olan, Laxante Salud, Laxarol, Laxo Vian, Le 100 B, Lipograsil, Mackenzies Menthoids, Mahiou, Modane Plus, Mucinum, Nylax, Obstinol, Paragar, Paragol, Petrolagar No. 2, Petrolagar with Phenolphthalein, Phillips Gelcaps, Phillips' Laxative Gelcaps, Phillips' Laxcaps, Phytolax, Pildoras Zeninas, Sanicolax, Takata, Thunas Bilettes, Triolax, Unilax, Vencipon, Veracolate and Vesilax (Royal Pharmaceutical Society of Great Britain, 1999).

Trade names for preparations containing phenolphthalein which have been discontinued include Agarbil, Amaro Lassativo, Bilagar, Boldolaxine, Boldolaxine Aloes, Confetti Lassativi, Confetto Complex, Correctol, Crisolax, Dietaid, Dragées 19, Emulsione Lassativa, Flamlax, Lactolaxine, Lax-Lorenz, Laxante Geve, Laxante Richelet, Laxativum, Laxicaps, Medimonth, Ormobyl, Pillole Lassative Aicardi, Pillole Schias, Pluribase, Reolina, Rim and Verecolene Complesso.

1.1.5 *Analysis*

Several international pharmacopoeias specify colorimetric and liquid chromatographic methods for identifying phenolphthalein; visible absorption spectrophotometry and liquid chromatography are used to assay its purity. Phenolphthalein is identified in pharmaceutical preparations by colorimetry and liquid chromatography; liquid chromatography is used to assay for content (British Pharmacopoeial Commission, 1993; US Pharmacopeial Convention, 1994).

Several methods for the analysis of phenolphthalein in various matrices have been reported, which include spectrophotometric, titrimetric, polarographic and chromatographic methods. The chromatographic methods include paper, gas, thin-layer and high-performance liquid chromatography (Al-Shammary *et al.*, 1991).

1.2 Production

Phenolphthalein can be prepared from a mixture of phenol, phthalic anhydride and sulfuric acid which is heated to 120 °C for 10–12 h. The product is extracted with boiling water, and the residue is dissolved in dilute sodium hydroxide solution, filtered, and precipitated with acid (Gennaro, 1995).

It has been reported that 197 tonnes of phenolphthalein were produced by one US manufacturer in the early 1990s (National Toxicology Program, 1999). Information available in 1999 indicated that phenolphthalein was manufactured and/or formulated in 33 countries (CIS Information Services, 1998; Royal Pharmaceutical Society of Great Britain; 1999; Swiss Pharmaceutical Society, 1999).

1.3 Use

Phenolphthalein is a stimulant laxative which has been used for the treatment of constipation and for bowel evacuation before investigational procedures or surgery. The laxative effect of phenolphthalein was discovered in 1902, and it has been widely used since that time (Mvros *et al.*, 1991). It usually has an effect within 4–8 h after oral administration, generally in tablets or capsules; it is also available as an emulsion with liquid paraffin. It is available without prescription in many countries. The usual oral laxative dose of phenolphthalein (white or yellow) is 30–200 mg daily taken at bedtime for adults and children aged $\geq$ 12 years (270 mg should not be exceeded); 30–60 mg daily for children aged 6–11 years; and 15–30 mg daily for children aged 2–5 years, given as a single or divided doses. A dose of 260 mg has been used in regimens for bowel evacuation (American Hospital Formulary Service, 1997; Royal Pharmaceutical Society of Great Britain, 1999).

The use of laxatives to relieve constipation and to maintain regularity in bowel habits is common in western cultures. Studies in Australia, the United Kingdom and the USA have found that about 20% of the general population reports regular use of laxatives (Kune, 1993). Two large surveys of the adult population in the USA found that about 10% of adults used some form of laxative at least once a month, that female users outnumbered male users and that the fraction of users increases with age (Everhart *et al.*, 1989; Harari *et al.*, 1989).

Few studies report the prevalence of use of phenolphthalein laxatives. One study of 424 cases of colon cancer and 414 controls in Washington State, USA, aged 30–62, found that 34% of the control subjects reported constipation requiring treatment (use of a laxative, enema or prunes), 2.7% reported ever having used phenolphthalein laxatives and 1.4% reported having used phenolphthalein laxatives at least 350 times in their lifetimes (Jacobs & White, 1998).

In three populations of 268–813 persons who had undergone endoscopy for colon polyps, two in North Carolina and one in California, USA, comprising approximately equal numbers of cases and controls, 0.8–4.4% of the control subjects had used phenolphthalein laxatives at least once per week. The two groups in North Carolina comprised subjects aged 30–89 years, 58% and 53% of whom were female; the group in California comprised subjects aged 50–74 years of whom 34% were female. The mean ages of the three groups were comparable (59–62 years). Among controls, the frequent users of phenolphthalein laxatives represented 5.2–30% of all frequent laxative users. In the two studies in North Carolina, 18% of case subjects and 25% of controls reported ever having used phenolphthalein laxatives, and 10% of cases and 7% of controls had used them at least once a month (Longnecker *et al.*, 1997). In a study of colorectal cancer in Melbourne, Australia (Kune, 1993), 9.7% of the 723 subjects reported ever having used phenolphthalein laxatives.

Phenolphthalein in a 1% alcoholic solution is also used as a visual indicator in titrations of mineral and organic acids and most alkalis. Phenolphthalein-titrated solutions are colourless at pH < 8.5 and pink to deep-red at pH > 9 (Budavari, 1996).

1.4 Occurrence

Phenolphthalein is not known to occur as a natural product. No data on occupational exposure were available to the Working Group.

1.5 Regulations and guidelines

Phenolphthalein is listed in the Austrian, Belgian, British, Chinese, Czech Republic, Hungarian, Italian, Swiss and US pharmacopoeias (Royal Pharmaceutical Society of Great Britain, 1999; Swiss Pharmaceutical Society, 1999).

After the publication in 1996 of the results of studies in rodents indicating that phenolphthalein was carcinogenic and genotoxic in several test systems, with damage (loss) of the *p53* tumour suppressor gene (Food & Drug Administration, 1999), many countries moved to restrict over-the-counter sales of phenolphthalein-containing laxatives. Both France and Italy have suspended use of phenolphthalein in prescription and over-the-counter pharmaceutical preparations, and the United Kingdom has changed the status of phenolphthalein from an over-the-counter to prescription agent in pharmaceutical preparations (WHO, 1997; Francesco International, 1998; WHO, 1998). Canada has suspended the sale of all products containing phenolphthalein (Canadian Pharmacists Association, 1999). The German Federal Institute for Drugs and Medical Devices recommended that holders of authorizations to market phenolphthalein-containing laxative products withdraw their products from the market because of the potential toxicological risks. The Japanese Pharmaceutical and Medical Safety Bureau of the Ministry of Health and Welfare issued a statement that laxative products containing phenolphthalein had been voluntarily withdrawn by the manufacturers (WHO, 1998). The Food and Drug Administration (1999) issued a final rule establishing that phenolphthalein is not generally recognized as safe and effective.

2. Studies of Cancer in Humans

Studies of the association between colorectal neoplasia and use of phenolphthalein-containing laxatives are summarized in Table 1.

2.1 Colon cancer

Kune (1993) analysed data on laxative use reported by 685 subjects with colorectal adenocarcinoma diagnosed in 1980–81 in Melbourne, Australia, and 723 controls frequency matched with cases on age and sex. Laxative use throughout adult life was assessed by interview. The relative risk associated with use of commercially produced laxatives was 1.0 (95% confidence interval [CI], 0.86–1.4). Eighty-seven case subjects (13%) and 70 controls (9.7%) reported having used phenolphthalein-containing laxatives (relative risk, 1.4 [95% CI, 0.96–1.9]).

In a case–control study of the association between colon cancer, constipation and use of phenolphthalein–containing laxatives in Washington State, USA (Jacobs & White, 1998), of 659 potential cases identified, 102 died before being approached and 55 were found to be ineligible. Of the 502 remaining cases, data were obtained from 424. Potentially eligible controls were selected by stratified random sampling of subjects in households identified by random-digit dialling, to approximate the distribution by age, sex and county of residence of the case subjects. Of 549 controls thus identified, data were obtained from 414 subjects. Data on laxative use were obtained by telephone interview, and subjects were also asked to complete a mailed food frequency questionnaire. The reference period was up to two years before diagnosis. Regular use was defined as a total use of more than 90 days. The relative risk for colon cancer associated with up to 349 lifetime uses of phenolphthalein-containing laxatives compared with no regular use was 1.0 (95% CI, 0.3–3.7) after adjustment for fibre as percentage of calories. The relative risk for ≥ 350 lifetime uses was 3.9 (95% CI, 1.5–10). Frequent constipation during the 10 years before the reference date (two years before diagnosis) was associated with an increased risk for colon cancer (4.4; 95% CI, 2.1–8.9). When constipation and commercial laxative use were adjusted for mutually, the association with commercial laxative use was no longer apparent, whereas the association with constipation persisted (2.7; 95% CI, 1.4–5.3). The relative risk associated with use of phenolphthalein-containing laxatives adjusted for constipation was 0.42 (95% CI, 0.10–1.7) for < 350 lifetime uses and 1.4 (95% CI, 0.47–4.3) for > 350 uses. [The Working Group noted the difficulty of excluding possible confounding by indication.]

2.2 Colorectal adenomatous polyps

The association between phenolphthalein-containing laxatives and colorectal adenomatous polyps was investigated in a case–control study in Los Angeles (California,

Table 1. Association between colorectal neoplasia and reported use of phenolphthalein-containing laxatives

Area and period of study (reference)	Source population	Exclusion criteria	Cases (no.)	Controls (no.)	Phenolphthalein-containing laxatives — Proportion of cases/controls reporting use (%)	Phenolphthalein-containing laxatives — Relative risk (95% CI)	Adjustment for:
Australia, Melbourne, 1980–81 (Kune, 1993)	Resident in Metropolitan Melbourne	Ulcerative colitis, familial polyposis, metachronous colorectal cancer, no data on bowel habits	Histologically confirmed colorectal adenocarcinoma (685)	Population, frequency matched on age and sex (723)	13/9.7	1.4 [0.96–1.9]	NR
USA, Washington State, Seattle Metropolitan area 1985–89 (Jacobs & White, 1998)	White, resident in private household with telephone in King, Pierce or Snohomish counties	History of colon or rectal cancer, polyposis or inflammatory bowel disease; inadequate ability to communicate in English	Incident invasive colon adenocarcinoma (424)	Population selected by random digit dialling (414)	6.6/2.7	<350 uses versus no regular use: 1.0 (0.3–3.7); ≥350 uses versus no regular use: 3.9 (1.5–10)	Age, sex and fibre as percentage of calories
USA, Los Angeles, 1991–93 (Longnecker et al., 1997)	Subjects undergoing sigmoidoscopy (screening, 45%; minor symptoms, 15%, not stated, 41%; response rate, 83%	Previous bowel cancer or adenoma, bowel surgery, inflammatory bowel disease, polyposis, inability to speak English, non-resident of Los Angeles or Orange County, invasive cancer	Histologically confirmed adenomatous polyps (488)	Subjects undergoing sigmoidoscopy in whom no polyps of any type were found, matched with cases on age, sex, medical facility and period of examination (488)	1.8ᵃ/0.8ᵃ	1.8 (0.5–6.2)	Alcohol, smoking, vigorous activity and intake of energy, saturated fat and fruits and vegetables

Table 1 (contd)

Area and period of study (reference)	Source population	Exclusion criteria	Cases (no.)	Controls (no.)	Phenolphthalein-containing laxatives		Adjustment for:
					Proportion of cases/controls reporting use (%)	Relative risk (95% CI)	
USA, North Carolina, 1988–90 (Longnecker et al., 1997)	Subjects undergoing colonoscopy (bleeding, 57%; anaemia, 10%; other, 33%); response rate, 83%	Previous bowel cancer or adenoma, bowel surgery, inflammatory bowel disease, inability to speak English; unsatisfactory bowel preparation, incomplete colonoscopy, colitis	Histologically confirmed adenomatous polyps ($n = 209$) or colorectal cancer ($n = 27$)	Subjects undergoing colonoscopy in whom no colorectal adenomatous polyps were found. Controls not matched to cases (409)	3.8[a]/4.4[a]	1.0 (0.4–2.2)	Age, sex, alcohol, smoking, leisure activity and intake of energy, total fat and fibre from fruits and vegetables
USA, North Carolina, 1992–95 (Longnecker et al., 1997)	Subjects undergoing colonoscopy (bleeding, 35%; anaemia, 8%; follow-up of previous non-adenomatous polyps, 17%; other, 40%): response rate, 45%	Previous bowel cancer or adenoma, bowel surgery, inflammatory bowel disease, inability to speak English; unsatisfactory bowel preparation, incomplete colonoscopy, colitis, invasive cancer	Histologically confirmed adenomatous polyps (142)	Subjects undergoing colonoscopy in whom no colorectal adenomatous polyps were found (169)	2.8[a]/1.8[a]	1.1 (0.2–5.7)	Age, sex, alcohol, smoking, hard physical activity, intake of energy, total fat and fibre from fruits and vegetables

[a] Use ≥ once a week

USA) in the period 1991–93 and in two case–control studies in North Carolina (USA) in 1988–90 and 1992–95 (Longnecker *et al.*, 1997*)*. In all three studies, cases and controls were selected from among people undergoing an endoscopic procedure (sigmoidoscopy in Los Angeles, colonoscopy in North Carolina); the cases were those found to have polyps. The main indication for this procedure was screening in the Los Angeles study and bleeding in the North Carolina studies. In the Los Angeles study, data on laxative use were collected by personal interview, and subjects were asked about use of specified agents in the year prior to sigmoidoscopy. The agents specified did not include phenolphthalein-containing laxatives but included 'other laxative preparations' as a category. If the subject reported use of laxatives in this category, the specific preparation was recorded. In North Carolina, subjects were asked over the telephone about the brand of laxative they used most often. For all three studies, the responses to questions about the preparation used were reviewed without knowledge of the subject's case or control status, and laxatives were classified as containing phenolphthalein on the basis of brand. In view of these differences between the studies and differences in the eligibility criteria and matching, the three studies were analysed separately. The relative risk for colorectal polyps associated with use of phenolphthalein-containing laxatives at least once a week was 1.8 (95% CI, 0.5–6.2) in Los Angeles (488 cases, 488 controls), 1.0 (95% CI, 0.4–2.2) in North Carolina in 1988–90 (236 cases, 409 controls) and 1.1 (95% CI, 0.2–5.7) in North Carolina in 1992–95 (142 cases, 169 controls).

[The Working Group noted the low statistical power of these studies to detect associations, resulting from the low prevalence of use of phenolphthalein-containing laxatives.]

3. Studies of Cancer in Experimental Animals

Oral administration

Mouse

Groups of 50 male and 50 female B6C3F$_1$ mice, six to seven weeks of age, were given diets containing phenolphthalein (purity, 99.9%) at a concentration of 3000, 6000 or 12 000 mg/kg for two years, equivalent to 0, 300, 600 or 1200 mg/kg bw in males and 0, 400, 800 or 1500 mg/kg bw in females. Only females treated with the highest dose had a significantly decreased rate of survival when compared with controls. The plasma concentrations of total phenolphthalein were similar at all doses. As shown in Table 2, the incidence of histiocytic sarcoma (principally in the liver but also at other sites) was significantly greater in males and females at the two higher doses than in controls. The incidence of malignant lymphoma (all types) was significantly increased in all groups of treated females, but not in males. The incidence of lymphoma of thymic origin was significantly increased in all groups of exposed

Table 2. Incidences of lesions in mice fed diets containing phenolphthalein

Sex	Dose (mg/kg diet)	No. examined	Numbers of animals with lesions					
			Histiocytic sarcoma[a]	Atypical thymic aplasia	Lymphoma of thymic origin[b]	Malignant lymphoma[c]	Ovarian hyperplasia	Benign sex cord/stromal tumour
Male	0	50	1	0	0	6		
	3000	50	3	3	4	8		
	6000	50	11**	7**	7**	12		
	12 000	49	12**	7**	2	8		
Female	0	50	0	0	1	15	4	0
	3000	50	2	7**	9**	28**	11*[d]	7**
	6000	50	7**	6**	10**	33**	10	6*
	12 000	50	7**	5**	7*	25*	17**	5*

From Dunnick & Hailey (1996); National Toxicology Program (1996); $*p < 0.05$; $**p < 0.01$, logistic regression
[a] Historical range: males, 0–2%; females, 0–4%
[b] Includes lymphomas of 'primary' or 'probable' thymic origin
[c] Includes all lymphomas
[d] 49 animals examined

females and in males at 6000 ppm. As shown in Table 2, the incidence of benign ovarian sex-cord stromal tumours was significantly increased in treated females; the mean historical incidence of all ovarian luteomas was 0.4% (Dunnick & Hailey, 1996; National Toxicology Program, 1996).

Groups of 20 female $p53^{+/-}$ heterozygous mice, 7–10 weeks of age, received diets containing phenolphthalein at a concentration of 0 (control), 200, 375, 750, 3000 or 12 000 mg/kg for 26 weeks, equivalent to average daily doses of phenolphthalein of 0, 43, 84, 174, 689 or 2375 mg/kg bw per day. The two lowest concentrations delivered doses of phenolphthalein that were approximately 0.5–1.5 times the recommended human dose based on a mg/m² body surface area comparison. The incidence of malignant lymphoma of the thymus was significantly increased in heterozygous $p53$-deficient female mice given the two higher doses. Atypical thymic hyperplasia, seen in 3/20 animals at 750 mg/kg, 3/20 at 3000 mg/kg and 5/20 at 12 000 ppm, was considered to represent proliferative change preceding lymphoma. The incidence of atypical hyperplasia or malignant lymphoma was increased in animals at 750 ppm. The incidence of malignant lymphomas was significantly increased at the two highest doses (0/19 in controls and 1/20, 0/20, 2/20, 17/20 ($p < 0.01$) and 14/20 ($p < 0.01$) at the five doses, respectively). Loss of the $p53$ wild-type allele was found in 2/2 thymic lymphomas from animals at 750 mg/kg, 13/13 at 200 mg/kg and 6/6 at 12 000 mg/kg (Dunnick et al., 1997).

In a study published as an abstract, $p53^{+/-}$ knock-out mice [age not specified] were given phenolphthalein [purity not specified] for 26 weeks by gavage at a dose of 800 or 2400 mg/kg bw per day [number of treatments per week not specified] or in the diet at 2400 mg/kg bw per day [dietary concentration not specified]. [Details of the control groups were not reported.] The experiment was terminated at 26 weeks. The incidences of thymic lymphomas were 3/15, 4/15 and 12/15 in males and 5/15, 8/15 and 14/15 in females receiving 800 (by gavage), 2400 (by gavage) and 2400 (in the diet) mg/kg bw, respectively (Furst et al., 1999).

Rat

Groups of 50 male and 50 female Fischer 344 rats, seven weeks of age, were given diets containing phenolphthalein (purity, 99.9%) at a concentration of 0, 12 000, 25 000 or 50 000 mg/kg for two years, equivalent to 0, 500, 1000 or 2000 mg/kg bw for males and 0, 500, 1000 or 2500 mg/kg bw for females. As in the mice, the total plasma concentrations of phenolphthalein did not increase with increasing dose. The survival rate in all groups of treated animals was similar to that of controls. As shown in Table 3, the incidence of benign phaeochromocytoma of the adrenal medulla was significantly increased in all treated male groups, and most were bilateral. The incidence of malignant phaeochromocytoma was not increased by treatment at any dose. The incidence of benign phaeochromocytoma was also increased in female rats given the highest dose, but the incidences of bilateral tumours and malignant phaeochromocytoma were not increased in

Table 3. Incidences of lesions in the adrenal medulla in Fischer 344 rats fed diets containing phenolphthalein

Sex	Dose (mg/kg diet)	No. examined	Numbers of animals with lesions		
			Hyperplasia	Phaeochromocytoma	
				Benign[a]	Benign and malignant[b]
Male	0	50	13	17	18
	12 500	50	22*	34**	35**
	25 000	50	18	34**	35**
	50 000	50	23*	34**	35**
Female	0	50	10	3	3
	12 500	50	18	11*	12*
	25 000	50	15	9	10*
	50 000	50	11	2	2

From Dunnick & Hailey (1996); National Toxicology Program (1996); *$p < 0.05$; ** $p < 0.01$, logistic regression
[a] Historical range: males, 10–63% (mean, 31%); females, 0–8% (mean, 4%)
[b] Historical range: females, 2–12%; mean, 5%

females. As seen in Table 4, the incidence of renal tubular adenoma (single and step sections combined) was also significantly increased in all treated male groups, and a few renal tubular carcinomas were also observed. In females, one renal tubular adenoma was observed at the highest dose (Dunnick & Hailey, 1996; National Toxicology Program, 1996). [The Working Group noted the high doses administered.]

4. Other Data Relevant to an Evaluation of Carcinogenicity and its Mechanisms

4.1 Absorption, distribution, metabolism and excretion

4.1.1 Humans

The absorption of phenolphthalein in humans has been estimated to be 15% of an oral dose (American Hospital Formulary Service, 1995). The absorbed compound is excreted primarily in the urine as phenolic-hydroxyglucuronide or sulfate conjugates. Some conjugated compound is also excreted in the faeces via the bile, and the resulting enterohepatic recirculation probably contributes to prolongation of the laxative effect (Hardman et al., 1996), a hypothesis supported by the observation that phenolphthalein is ineffective as a laxative in patients suffering from obstructive jaundice or

Table 4. Incidences of renal tubular lesions in male Fischer 344 rats fed diets containing phenolphthalein

Numbers of animals	Dose (mg/kg diet)			
	0	12 500	25 000	50 000
Examined	50	50	50	50
Original sections				
With hyperplasia	0	6**	7**	2
With adenoma	0	4	2	6*
With carcinoma	0	1	1	2
With adenoma and carcinoma[a]	0	5*	3	7**
Step sections				
With hyperplasia	3	23**	29**	27**
With adenoma	1	7*	15**	11**
With carcinoma	0	0	1	0
With adenoma and carcinoma[a]	1	7*	15**	11**
Combined (original and step sections)				
With hyperplasia	3	25**	29**	27**
With adenoma	1	10**	15**	15**
With carcinoma	0	1	2	2
With adenoma and carcinoma[a]	1	10**	16**	16**

From Dunnick & Hailey (1996); National Toxicology Program (1996); * $p < 0.05$;
** $p < 0.01$, logistic regression test
[a] Historical range, 0–6% (mean, 0.9%)

in experimental animals with ligated common bile ducts (Steigmann *et al.*, 1938). Small doses of phenolphthalein (30–60 mg) are excreted by humans entirely as conjugated metabolites in urine or faeces, while larger doses (300 mg) result in excretion of both the free and conjugated drug (Williams, 1959). Use of phenolphthalein by women during breast-feeding may cause diarrhoea in their infants (Tyson *et al.*, 1937).

4.1.2 *Experimental systems*

Phenolphthalein is absorbed in the intestine (Visek *et al.*, 1956) and is almost completely converted to its glucuronide during extensive first-pass metabolism in the intestinal epithelium and liver (Parker *et al.*, 1980) via uridine diphosphate glucuronosyltransferase (UDPGT) in rodents and dogs (Sund & Hillestad, 1982; National Toxicology Program, 1996). In guinea-pigs, small amounts of sulfate-conjugated metabolites have been detected in isolated mucosal sheets originating in the jejunum and colon (Sund & Lauterbach, 1986). Faecal excretion is the major route of elimination of phenolphthalein in rats, while in mice both urinary and faecal elimination are important. The metabolites

Figure 1. Metabolism of [^{14}C]phenolphthalein in Fischer 344 rats and B6C3F$_1$ mice

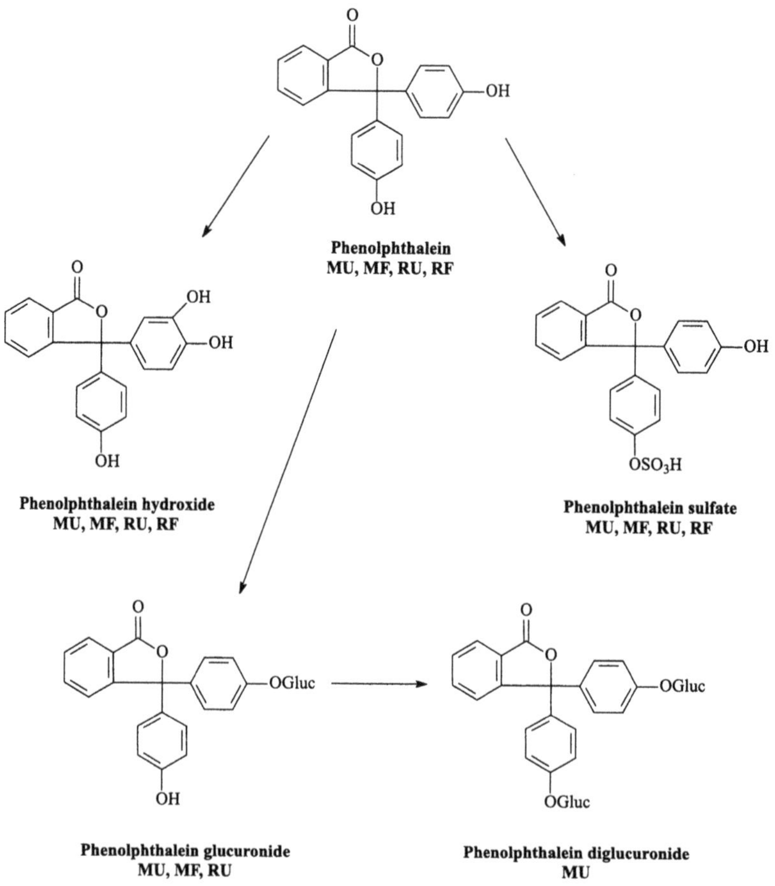

From Griffin *et al.* (1998)
Gluc, glucuronide; MU, mouse urine; MF, mouse faeces; RU, rat urine; RF, rat faeces

identified in urine and faeces are phenolphthalein glucuronide, phenolphthalein sulfate and phenolphthalein hydroxide (Griffin *et al.*, 1998; see Figure 1).

Six hours after an intravenous injection of [^{3}H]phenolphthalein to female Wistar rats, analysis of the systemic circulation showed that all of the radiolabel was associated with the glucuronide conjugate (Colburn *et al.*, 1979). Enterohepatic recirculation is limited by the rate of hydrolysis of phenolphthalein glucuronide to aglycone by intestinal bacterial β-glucuronidase (Bergan *et al.*, 1982; National Toxicology Program, 1996).

The extent of enterohepatic recirculation of phenolphthalein was examined in rats with cannulated bile ducts. Within 24 h, 95% of a dose of 25 mg/kg bw [^{3}H]phenolphthalein administered intraperitoneally to female Wistar rats was recovered as glucuronide in the bile, with 0.2% in the urine. In rats without cannulated bile ducts, 86% of the same dose was recovered in the faeces, with little glucuronide, and 10% was recovered in the urine, primarily as the glucuronide (Millburn et al., 1967; Parker et al., 1980).

In male Sprague-Dawley CR-1 strain rats with cannulated femoral veins, femoral arteries and bile ducts given an intravenous dose of 3, 30 or 60 mg phenolphthalein, 99.5% of the dose was eliminated in the bile as the glucuronide. When the same rats were given 3, 30 or 100 mg phenolphthalein glucuronide by intravenous administration, no phenolphthalein was detected in the bile (Mehendale, 1990).

Studies in dogs and mice given [^{14}C]phenolphthalein showed that the radiolabel is evenly distributed throughout the body. In newborn pups of bitches given 4.8 mg/kg bw orally 50 h before whelping, < 0.03% of the dose was found in the liver and gallbladder and none in the blood, indicating extremely limited passage across the placenta (Visek et al., 1956).

Phenolphthalein is excreted in bile, urine, faeces and milk. In mice, 56% of an oral dose was recovered from the urine within 48 h and an additional 38% from the faeces. When an intravenous dose was given, 30% was recovered from the urine and 68% from the faeces (Visek et al., 1956). Some phenolphthalein is excreted into the bile, and the prolonged cathartic effect may be due to the ensuing enterohepatic recirculation (Hardman et al., 1996). Pre-treatment with hepatic microsomal enzyme inducers increased biliary excretion of metabolites in rats, but post-treatment with enzyme inhibitors decreased it (National Toxicology Program, 1996).

Within 72 h of oral administration of 4.8 mg/kg bw [^{14}C]phenolphthalein to mongrel bitches, 51% of the radiolabel was excreted in the faeces and 36% in the urine. After an intravenous dose, 54% was found in the faeces and 37% in the urine. When the same animals received a cannula in the bile-duct and were given an oral dose, 31% of the radiolabel was found in faeces, 38% in urine and 22% in bile. After an intravenous dose, 11% was eliminated in faeces, 35% in urine and 43% in bile (Visek et al., 1956).

The profile of systemic blood concentration–time for phenolphthalein during 24 h after a single intravenous bolus injection was described by a classical compartmental pharmacokinetics model, with evidence of enterohepatic recirculation (Colburn et al., 1979).

In the two-year bioassays of the National Toxicology Program (1996), the concentrations of total phenolphthalein in plasma were 100–200 µg/mL.

Whole-body autoradiography of male BOM:NMRI mice showed high concentrations of radiolabel in the stomach, gall-bladder and small intestine 1 h after administration of an intragastric dose of 1 mL/100 g bw [^{14}C]phenolphthalein (10 µCi/100g) [10 mL/kg bw or 3.2 mg/kg bw]. As evidenced by the presence of radiolabel in peripheral organs (including the kidney, liver and skin), the compound was absorbed. After 2 h, it had arrived in the large intestine, and 4 h after administration, maximum radiolabel was observed in the rectum. Two days after administration, no radiolabel was detected (Sund et al., 1986).

4.2 Toxic effects

4.2.1 *Humans*

Until the mid-1990s, phenolphthalein was regarded as non-toxic and safe for consumption, although therapeutic oral doses occasionally produced abdominal discomfort, diarrhoea, nausea, decreased blood pressure and faintness (American Hospital Formulary Service, 1995). Serious side-effects were reported in cases of habitual phenolphthalein consumption under conditions of abuse (Cooke, 1977; Pietrusko, 1977).

The main target organ for the toxic effects of phenolphthalein is reported to be the intestine. Indiscriminate use of phenolphthalein results in chronic constipation and laxative dependence, loss of normal bowel function and bowel irritation. Habitual use for several years may cause a 'cathartic colon', i.e. a poorly functioning colon with atonic dilatation, especially on the right side, resulting in extensive retention of the bowel contents. The clinical condition, which resembles chronic ulcerative colitis both radiologically and pathologically, involves thinning of the intestinal wall and loss of the normal mucosal pattern of the terminal ileum (Cummings, 1974; Cummings *et al.*, 1974; Cooke, 1977; Pietrusko, 1977; American Hospital Formulary Service, 1995).

Anecdotal cases of long-term use or overdose of phenolphthalein have been associated with abdominal pain, diarrhoea, vomiting, electrolyte imbalance (hypokalaemia, hypocalcaemia and/or metabolic acidosis or alkalosis), dehydration, malabsorption, protein-losing gastroenteropathy, steatorrhoea, anorexia, weight loss, polydipsia, polyuria, cardiac arrhythmia, muscle weakness, prostration and histopathological lesions (Heizer *et al.*, 1968; Velentzas & Ikkos, 1971; Cummings, 1974; LaRusso & McGill, 1975; Pohl & Lowe, 1978; American Hospital Formulary Service, 1995). Kidney, muscle and central nervous system disturbances are thought to be due to electrolyte imbalance. Loss of intestinal sodium and water stimulates compensatory renin production and secondary aldosteronism, leading to sodium conservation and potassium loss by the kidney. The hypokalaemia contributes to renal insufficiency and is sometimes associated with rhabdomyolysis (Copeland, 1994).

Abuse of phenolphthalein-containing laxatives has been associated with gastrointestinal bleeding, iron-deficient anaemia (Weiss & Wood, 1982), acute pancreatitis (Lambrianides & Rosin, 1984) and multiple organ damage in cases of massive overdose, including fulminant hepatic failure and disseminated intravascular coagulation (Sidhu *et al.*, 1989).

Allergy to phenolphthalein is often manifested as cutaneous inflammatory reactions or fixed drug eruptions, i.e. solitary or multiple, well-defined, erythematous macules that may progress to vesicles and/or bullae. These lesions characteristically recur in the same location with each subsequent dose of phenolphthalein and generally leave residual hyperpigmentation that increases in intensity with each exposure; numerous melanin-containing dermal macrophages have been found in pigmented areas (Wyatt *et al.*, 1972; Davies, 1985; Stroud & Rosio, 1987; Zanolli *et al.*, 1993). In extreme cases, recurrences have involved progressively more severe lesions characterized as bullous erythema multiforme, with focal haemorrhage and necrosis and perivascular lymphocytic infiltration (Shelley *et al.*, 1972) and, in one case report, toxic epidermal necrolysis (Kar *et al.*, 1986).

A review of 204 cases of phenolphthalein ingestion in children aged five years and younger reported to the Pittsburgh Poison Center (USA) over a 30-month period indicated that ingestion of ≤ 1 g was associated with a minimal risk of developing dehydration due to excessive diarrhoea and resulting fluid loss (Mrvos *et al.*, 1991). Despite the profile of low acute toxicity documented in this study, cases of fatal poisoning of children have been reported; symptoms of pulmonary and cerebral oedema, multiple organ effects and encephalitis were attributed to hypersensitivity reactions (Cleves, 1932; Kendall, 1954; Sarcinelli *et al.*, 1970). Repeated administration of phenolphthalein-containing laxatives to children has led to serious illness and multiple hospitalizations (Sugar *et al.*, 1991; Ayass *et al.*, 1993).

4.2.2 *Experimental systems*

Fischer 344/N rats and B6C3F$_1$ mice were given an NIH 07 diet containing phenolphthalein at a concentration of 0, 3000, 6000, 12 000, 25 000 or 50 000 mg/kg *ad libitum* for 13 weeks, equivalent to intakes of 0, 200, 400, 800, 1600 or 3500 mg/kg bw for rats, 500, 1000, 2000, 4100 or 9000 mg/kg bw for male mice and 600, 1200, 2400, 5000 or 10 500 mg/kg bw for female mice. Phenolphthalein did not appear to be toxic in rats, and no laxative effect was observed. Rats at the two higher doses showed slightly lower weight gain. Treated rats showed increased relative (to body weight) kidney weights (males only) and elevated absolute and relative liver weights at concentrations of 12 000–50 000 ppm. Female rats showed no effect on body-weight gain, but those receiving concentrations of 6000–50 000 mg/kg had elevated liver weights. The primary treatment-related findings in mice involved the reproductive and haematopoietic systems. The haematopoietic changes included bone-marrow hypoplasia (at 12 000–50 000 mg/kg) and increased splenic haematopoiesis (males only; 25 000 and 50 000 mg/kg) (National Toxicology Program, 1996).

In female mice [strain not specified] fed 5, 25 or 50 mg/kg bw phenolphthalein per day orally for 135 days, no toxic manifestations or evidence of histopathological changes were found in the liver, kidney or gastrointestinal tract (Visek *et al.*, 1956).

Phenolphthalein at doses of 25 and 50 µg/mL was cytotoxic in cultured Chang liver cells, causing decreased cell growth and increased anaerobic glycolysis, i.e. increased glucose consumption and lactate production (Nishikawa, 1981).

4.3 Reproductive and prenatal effects

4.3.1 *Humans*

No data were available to the Working Group.

4.3.2 Experimental systems

Phenolphthalein is a partial oestrogen in immature rat uteri. Doses of 1–10 mg given subcutaneously twice daily for two days to female Wistar rats weighing 35–40 g induced a dose-related increase in uterine weight, but the maximum increase was only about half of that induced by oestradiol. Phenolphthalein was shown to bind to the oestrogen receptor and was a competitive antagonist to oestradiol (Nieto et al., 1990).

In a study reported in an abstract, exposure of female $B6C3F_1$ mice to 1895 mg/kg bw phenolphthalein orally [method not stated] daily for 30 or 60 days caused no changes in weight gain, oestrous cycles or the numbers of oocyte-containing follicles of any class (primordial, primary, growing or antral), or any detectable pathological change in ovarian cells (Hoyer et al., 1997).

Using a continuous breeding protocol, Chapin et al. (1997a) administered phenolphthalein in the feed of Swiss CD-1 mice at a concentration of 0.1, 0.7 or 3.0% w/v, to provide estimated intakes of 0.15, 1.0 and 4.5 g/kg bw per day (National Toxicology Program, 1996; Chapin et al., 1997b). Pairs of 40 control and 20 treated mice were housed together and allowed to produce up to five litters, the last of which was reared and their reproductive performance measured. Significant reproductive toxicity was observed at the intermediate and high doses. At the intermediate dose, the proportions of pairs producing one to five litters were 100, 89, 84, 68 and 36%, the percentages producing second to fifth litters being significantly smaller than in controls. The decrease at the high dose was more severe, only 5% of pairs producing a fifth litter. Overall, the mean number of litters per pair was reduced by 24 and 50% at the intermediate and high doses, and the number of pups per litter decreased by 58–59%. The final litters were reared on the same diets as the parents. Up to 70% of the pups at the high dose died within four days of birth. Cross-over breeding of animals at the intermediate dose with controls showed that the fertility of the females was affected, the litter sizes being reduced to half. Breeding of the F_1 offspring at the intermediate dose with controls showed that treatment halved the number of litters and the litter size. The survival of the F_2 pups was not affected. Examination of F_0 males at the intermediate dose showed a reduction in testis weight by 36% and in the epididymal sperm count by 30%, and seminiferous tubular degeneration was seen in 9 of 10 treated males. The oestrous cycles and ovarian histology of females at this dose were not affected. Very similar results were found in the F_1 adults at termination. No adverse effects were observed at the low dose.

After 13 weeks of exposure to the same doses as used in the studies of toxicity, there was no evidence of reproductive toxicity in female $B6C3F_1$ mice or male or female Fischer 344/N rats. Lower epididymal weights and lower sperm density (number of sperm/g of crude epididymal tissue) were observed in male mice at 12 000, 25 000 and 50 000 mg/kg (National Toxicology Program, 1996).

4.4 Genetic and related effects

4.4.1 *Humans*

No data were available to the Working Group.

4.4.2 *Experimental systems*

The results of these studies are summarized in Table 5.

Phenolphthalein was not mutagenic in several assays in *Salmonella typhimurium* strains TA1535, TA1537, TA1538, TA98 and TA100 in the presence or absence of exogenous metabolic activation. It did not induce DNA damage in DNA repair-deficient strains of *Bacillus subtilis*.

Phenolphthalein did not induce sister chromatid exchange in Chinese hamster ovary cells in the presence or absence of exogenous metabolic activation, but it induced a dose-related response in chromosomal aberrations in these cells only in the presence of exogenous metabolic activation.

In experiments in which a number of end-points were studied in Syrian hamster embryo cells (a mixed population of cell types that retain some endogenous metabolizing enzymic activity, including oxidation and peroxidation), phenolphthalein induced chromosomal aberrations and *Hprt* mutations, but not ouabain mutations or aneuploidy. No evidence was found for adduct formation in DNA of these cells. The data for micronuclei failed to reach statistical significance ($p = 0.057$). Phenolphthalein caused cellular transformation in the same cell line, indicating that it is metabolized appropriately in this system.

Phenolphthalein increased the incidence of micronucleated erythrocytes in male and female $B6C3F_1$ mice and in male Swiss CD-1 mice. [The Working Group noted that the doses were significantly higher than those to which humans would be exposed.]

Tice *et al.* (1998) studied the effects of phenolphthalein at various concentrations in the diet of transgenic female mice heterozygous for the *p53* gene, over a six-month period. They found significant increases in the frequency of micronucleated erythrocytes, most of which appeared to arise from whole chromosomes rather than chromosomal damage; these were observed at doses comparable to those to which humans are exposed. Inconclusive evidence was found for DNA damage in blood leukocytes, and there was no evidence for DNA damage, apoptosis or necrosis in liver parenchymal cells.

In phenolphthalein-induced thymic lymphomas in $B6C3F_1$ mice, p53 protein accumulated in most tumour cell nuclei, but detectable p53 protein was not seen in control thymuses in this model (Dunnick *et al.*, 1997). Other studies have shown that accumulation of p53 protein results from *p53* gene alterations (Hegi *et al.*, 1993).

In $p53^{+/-}$ heterozygous mice, phenolphthalein induced atypical hyperplasia and malignant lymphomas of thymic origin within six months in 0% of controls, 5% of animals at 200 mg/kg, 5% at 375 mg/kg, 25% at 750 mg/kg, 100% at 3000 mg/kg and

Table 5. Genetic and related effects of phenolphthalein

Test system	Result[a] Without exogenous metabolic system	Result[a] With exogenous metabolic system	Dose[b] (LED or HID)	Reference
Bacillus subtilis rec strains, differential toxicity	–	–	1000[c]	Kada et al. (1972)
Salmonella typhimurium TA100, TA1535, TA1537, TA1538, TA98, reverse mutation	–	–	320 µg/plate	Bonin et al. (1981)
Salmonella typhimurium TA100, TA1535, TA1537, TA98, reverse mutation	–	–	333 µg/plate	Mortelmans et al. (1986)
Gene mutation, Syrian hamster embryo cells, oubain resistance *in vitro*	–	NT	12.8	Tsutsui et al. (1997)
Gene mutation, Syrian hamster embryo cells *in vitro*, *Hprt* locus	+	NT	6.4	Tsutsui et al. (1997)
Sister chromatid exchange, Chinese hamster ovary cells *in vitro*	–	–	50	National Toxicology Program (1995)
Micronucleus formation, Syrian hamster embryo cells *in vitro*	–	NT	25	Gibson et al. (1997)
Chromosomal aberrations, Chinese hamster ovary cells *in vitro*	–	+	40	Witt et al. (1995)
Chromosomal aberrations, Syrian hamster embryo cells *in vitro*	+	NT	12.8	Tsutsui et al. (1997)
Aneuploidy, Syrian hamster embryo cells *in vitro*	–	NT	12.8	Tsutsui et al. (1997)
Binding (covalent) to DNA, Syrian hamster embryo cells *in vitro*	–	NT	12.8	Tsutsui et al. (1997)
Cell transformation, Syrian hamster embryo cells *in vitro*	+	NT	20	Kerckaert et al. (1996)
Cell transformation, Syrian hamster embryo cells *in vitro*	+	NT	3.2	Tsutsui et al. (1997)
Micronucleus formation, AHH-1 *Tk*[+/–] human lymphoblastoid cells *in vitro*	–	NT	10	Bishop et al. (1998)
Micronucleus formation, MCL-5 human lymphoblastoid cells *in vitro*	+	NT	0.5	Bishop et al. (1998)
DNA damage in blood leukocytes, transgenic female TSG-*p53* mice (comet assay) *in vivo*	?		2074; in diet, 6 mo	Tice et al. (1998)

Table 5 (contd)

Test system	Result[a]		Dose[b] (LED or HID)	Reference
	Without exogenous metabolic system	With exogenous metabolic system		
Micronucleus formation, peripheral blood erythrocytes, male and female B6C3F$_1$ mice in vivo	+		~1000[d]; in diet, 13 wk	Dietz et al. (1992)
Micronucleus formation, peripheral blood erythrocytes, male Swiss CD-1 mice in vivo	+		120; in diet, 14 wk	Witt et al. (1995)
Micronucleus formation, peripheral blood erythrocytes, transgenic female TSG-p53 mice in vivo	+		37; in diet, 6 mo	Tice et al. (1998)

[a] +, positive; −, negative; NT, not tested; ?, inconclusive
[b] LED, lowest effective dose; HID, highest ineffective dose; in-vitro tests, μg/mL; in-vivo tests, mg/kg bw per day; d, day; mo, month; wk, week
[c] Absorbed onto paper disc
[d] LED represents the average dose in male and female mice for the formation of normochromatic erythrocytes.

95% of animals at 12 000 mg/kg. Two of two thymic lymphomas examined from animals at 750 mg/kg, 13/13 from those at 3000 mg/kg and 6/6 from those at 12 000 mg/kg had lost the remaining *p53* wild-type allele (Dunnick *et al.*, 1997). No spontaneous thymic lymphomas were found in control mice in these studies, but in other studies in *p53*$^{+/-}$ mice of spontaneous tumours (which may occur in mice after one year of age), only 55% showed loss of the remaining functional *p53* allele (Harvey *et al.*, 1993). The presence of functional p53 protein is essential for normal cell growth. When this protein is absent, as is the case in phenolphthalein-induced thymic lymphomas, regulation of cell cycle electrophoresis is lost and malignant progression may be enhanced.

4.5 Mechanistic considerations

Analogy with related biphenolic compounds suggests that phenolphthalein has oestrogenic activity; however, studies with MCF-7 human breast cancer cells in tissue culture (Ravdin *et al.*, 1987) and in rat uterus *in vivo* (Nieto *et al.*, 1990) suggested only a weak oestrogenic response. Tsutsui *et al.* (1997) used the nuclease P1 enhancement version of the ^{32}P-postlabelling assay to investigate whether (and what type of) DNA adducts were responsible for the morphological transformation induced by phenolphthalein. Although they found no adducts, they recognized the possible limitations of the techniques and suggested that small DNA adducts formed by free radicals could be involved in the effects. Sipe *et al.* (1997) showed free radical metabolism of phenolphthalein by peroxidases *in vitro*.

The observation of Witt *et al.* (1995) that chromosomal damage in Chinese hamster ovary cells occurred only when exogenous metabolic activation was added suggests that some as yet unidentified metabolite is responsible for these effects. Bishop *et al.* (1998) also interpreted differences in the micronucleus response between the two human lymphoblastoid cell lines, MCL-5 and AHH-1 *TK*$^{+/-}$, as being likely to reflect the importance of a metabolite in chromosome-damaging effects.

Tice *et al.* (1998) suggested that numerical chromosomal loss is responsible for the enhanced incidence of thymic tumours seen after treatment with phenolphthalein in *p53* heterozygous mice. Dunnick *et al.* (1997) noted that these tumours uniformly showed loss of heterozygosity for the *p53* allele rather than point mutations, suggesting either chromosome loss or deletions of large chromosomal segments.

The ability to detect micronuclei but not mutations at the *TK* locus in AHH cells may indicate that cells containing phenolphthalein-induced lesions are susceptible to apoptosis (Bishop *et al.*, 1998).

5. Summary of Data Reported and Evaluation

5.1 Exposure data

Phenolphthalein has been widely used as a laxative for nearly a century. Generally available without prescription, it is now being withdrawn from the market in many countries because of recent toxicological concern. Phenolphthalein has also long been used in the laboratory as an indicator in acid–base titrations.

5.2 Human carcinogenicity data

In the few available studies, there was no consistent association between the occurrence of colon cancer or adenomatous colorectal polyps and use of phenolphthalein-containing laxatives. Cancers at other sites have not been studied.

5.3 Animal carcinogenicity data

Phenolphthalein was tested for carcinogenicity by oral administration in two experiments in mice and in one experiment in rats. In one experiment in mice, it induced histiocytic sarcomas and lymphomas in both males and females and benign ovarian tumours in females. In an experiment in mice lacking one allele of the *p53* tumour suppressor gene, it increased the incidence of lymphomas. This result was confirmed in a separate study reported as an abstract. It induced benign renal tumours in male rats and benign phaeochromocytomas in males and females.

5.4 Other relevant data

Phenolphthalein is absorbed in the small bowel and is conjugated in the liver to form phenolphthalein glucuronide, which is eliminated in the bile. As it passes through the small intestine, it is partially deconjugated and reabsorbed.

Phenolphthalein and its glucuronide enhance oxygen radical production and cause oxidative damage *in vitro*. Phenolphthalein has also been shown to have low oestrogenic activity in some model systems. Phenolphthalein induced micronucleated erythrocytes in mice given multiple but not single treatments by gavage or in feed. Abnormal spermatozoa were induced in male mice but not male rats treated with phenolphthalein in the feed for 13 weeks. The malignant thymic lymphomas induced by phenolphthalein in female heterozygous *p53*-deficient mice showed loss of the normal *p53* allele.

Phenolphthalein induced chromosomal aberrations, *Hprt* gene mutations and morphological transformation but not aneuploidy or ouabain-resistant mutations or sister chromatid exchange in cultured mammalian cells. It did not induce gene mutations in bacteria.

5.5 Evaluation

There is *inadequate evidence* in humans for the carcinogenicity of phenolphthalein. There is *sufficient evidence* in experimental animals for the carcinogenicity of phenolphthalein.

Overall evaluation

Phenolphthalein is *possibly carcinogenic to humans (Group 2B)*.

6. References

Al-Shammary, F., Mian, M.S. & Mian, N.A.A (1991) Phenolphthalein. In: Florey, K., ed., *Analytical Profiles of Drug Substances*, New York, Academic Press, Vol. 20, pp. 627–664

American Hospital Formulary Service (1995) *AHFS Drug Information® 95*, Bethesda, MD, American Society of Health-System Pharmacists, pp. 1986–1995

American Hospital Formulary Service (1997) *AHFS Drug Information® 97*, Bethesda, MD, American Society of Health-System Pharmacists, pp. 2241–2242

Ayass, M., Bussing, R. & Mehta, P. (1993) Munchausen syndrome presenting as hemophilia: A convenient and economical 'steal' of disease and treatment. *Pediatr. Hematol. Oncol.*, **10**, 241–244

Bergan, T., Fotland, M.H. & Sund, R.B. (1982) Interaction between diphenolic laxatives and intestinal bacteria in vitro. *Acta pharmacol. toxicol.*, **51**, 165–172

Bishop, M.E., Aidoo, A., Domon, O.E., Morris, S.M. & Casciano, D.A. (1998) Phenolphthalein induces micronuclei in transgenic human lymphoblastoid cells. *Environ. mol. Mutag.*, **32**, 286–288

Bonin, A.M., Farqhuarson, J.B. & Baker, R.S.U. (1981) Mutagenicity of arylmethane dyes in *Salmonella. Mutat. Res.*, **89**, 21–34

British Pharmacopoeial Commission (1993) *British Pharmacopoeia 1993*, London, Her Majesty's Stationery Office, Vol. I, pp. 502–503

Budavari, S., ed. (1996) *The Merck Index*, 12th Ed., Whitehouse Station, NJ, Merck & Co., pp. 1248, 1726–1727

Canadian Pharmaceutical Association (1997) *CPS Compendium of Pharmaceuticals and Specialties*, 32nd Ed., Ottawa, Ontario, pp. 40, 490, 564

Canadian Pharmacists Association (1999) *Drug Brief—Phenolphthalein* [http://www.cdnpharm.ca/drugbrf2.htm]

Chapin, R., Gulati, D., Mounce, R. & Russell, S. (1997a) Phenolphthalein. *Environ. Health Perspectives*, **105**, 335–336

Chapin, R.E., Sloane, R.A. & Hasemen, J.K. (1997b) The relationships among reproductive endpoints in Swiss mice, using the Reproductive Assessment by Continuous Breeding database. *Fundam. appl. Toxicol.*, **38**, 129–142

CIS Information Services (1998) *Worldwide Bulk Drug Users Directory 1997/98 Edition*, Dallas, TX [CD-ROM]

Cleves, M. (1932) Poisoning by Exlax tablets. *J. Am. med. Assoc.*, **99**, 654–655

Colburn, W.A., Hirom, P.C., Parker, R.J. & Milburn, P. (1979) A pharmacokinetic model for enterohepatic recirculation in the rat: Phenolphthalein, a model drug. *Drug Metab. Dispos.*, **7**, 100–102

Cooke, W.T. (1977) Laxative abuse. *Clin. Gastroenterol.*, **6**, 659–673

Copeland, P.M. (1994) Renal failure associated with laxative abuse. *Psychother. Psychosom.*, **62**, 200–202

Cummings, J.H. (1974) Laxative abuse. *Gut*, **15**, 758–766

Cummings, J.H., Sladen, G.E., James, O.F.W., Sarner, M. & Misiewicz, J.J. (1974) Laxative-induced diarrhoea: A continuing clinical problem. *Br. med. J.*, **i**, 537–541

Davies, D.M., ed. (1985) *Textbook of Adverse Drug Reactions*, 3rd Ed., New York, Oxford University Press, pp. 110, 121, 475–479

Dietz, D.D., Elwell, M.R., Chapin, R.E., Shelby, M.D., Thompson, M.B., Filler, R. & Stedham, M.A. (1992) Subchronic (13 week) toxicity studies of phenolphthalein in Fischer 344 rats and B6C3F1 mice. *Fundam. appl. Toxicol.*, **18**, 48–58

Dunnick, J.K. & Hailey, J.R. (1996) Phenolphthalein exposure causes multiple carcinogenic effects in experimental model systems. *Cancer Res.*, **56**, 4922–4926

Dunnick, J.K., Hardisty, J.F., Herbert, R.A., Seely, J.C., Furedi-Machacek, E.M., Foley, J.F., Lacks, G.D., Stasiewicz, S. & French, J.E. (1997) Phenolphthalein induces thymic lymphomas accompanied by loss of the p53 wild type allele in heterozygous p53-deficient (±) mice. *Toxicol. Pathol.*, **25**, 533–540

Everhart, J.E., Go, V.L.W., Johannes, R.S., Fitzsimmons, S.C., Roth, H.P. & White, L.R. (1989) A longitudinal survey of self-reported bowel habits in the United States. *Dig. Dis. Sci.*, **34**, 1153–1162

Food & Drug Administration (1999) Laxative drug products for over-the-counter human use. *Fed. Regist.*, **64**, 4535–4540

Francesco International (1998) *Major Rx-to-OTC Switched Products: The Important Switches of 1997 in Major Markets* [http://www.rxtootcswitch.com/data.htm]

Furst, S.M., Blanchard, K.T., Lilly, P.D., Holden, H.E., Stoltz, J.H., Barthel, C. & Stoll, R.E. (1999) Six month oral gavage and diet carcinogenicity study with phenolphthalein in the heterozygous p53 +/– mouse (Abstract No. 1202). *Toxicologist*, **48**

Gennaro, A.R. (1995) *Remington: The Science and Practice of Pharmacy*, 19th Ed., Easton, PA, Mack Publishing, Vol. II, p. 897

Gibson, D.P., Brauninger, R., Shaffi, H.S., Kerckaert, G.A., LeBoeuf, R.A., Isfort, R.J. & Aardema, M.J. (1997) Induction of micronuclei in Syrian hamster embryo cells: Comparison to results in the SHE cell transformation assay for National Toxicology Program test chemicals. *Mutat. Res.*, **392**, 61–90

Griffin, R.J., Godfrey, V.B. & Burka, L.T. (1998) Metabolism and disposition of phenolphthalein in male and female F344 rats and B6C3F1 mice. *Toxicol. Sci.*, **42**, 73–81

Harari, D., Gurwitz, J.H., Avorn, J., Bohn, R. & Minaker, K.L. (1989) Bowel habit in relation to age and gender. Findings from the National Health Interview Survey and clinical implications. *Arch. intern. Med.*, **156**, 315–320

Hardman, J.G., Limbird, L.E., Molinoff, P.B. & Ruddon, R.W., eds (1996) *Goodman and Gilman's The Pharmacological Basis of Therapeutics*, 9th Ed., New York, McGraw-Hill, pp. 921–925

Harvey, M., McArthur, M.J., Montgomery, C.A., Jr, Butel, J.S., Bradley, A. & Donehower, L.A. (1993) Spontaneous and carcinogen-induced tumorigenesis in p53-deficient mice. *Nature Genet.*, **5**, 225–229

Hegi, M.E., Söderkvist, P., Foley, J.F., Schoonhoven, R., Swenberg, J.A., Kari, F., Maronpot, R., Anderson, M.W. & Wiseman, R.W. (1993) Characterization of *p53* mutations in methylene chloride-induced lung tumors from B6C3F1 mice. *Carcinogenesis*, **14**, 803–810

Heizer, W.D., Warshaw, A.L., Waldmann, T.A. & Laster, L. (1968) Protein-losing gastroenteropathy and malabsorption associated with factitious diarrhea. *Ann. intern. Med.*, **68**, 839–852

Hoyer, P.B., Boese, B. & Sipes, I.G. (1997) The effect of phenolphthalein on B6C3F1 mouse ovaries (Abstract No. 1825). *Toxicologist*, **36**, 359

Jacobs, E.J. & White, E. (1998) Constipation, laxative use, and colon cancer among middle-aged adults. *Epidemiology*, **9**, 385–391

Kada, T., Tutikawa, K. & Sadaie, Y. (1972) In vitro and host-mediated 'rec-assay' procedures for screening chemical mutagens; and phloxine, a mutagenic red dye detected. *Mutat. Res.*, **16**, 165–174

Kar, P.K., Dutta, R.K. & Shah, B.H. (1986) Toxic epidermal necrolysis in a patient induced by phenolphthalein. *J. Indian med. Assoc.*, **84**, 189–190, 193

Kendall, A.C. (1954) Fatal case of encephalitis after phenolphthalein ingestion. *Br. med. J.*, **ii**, 1461–1462

Kerckaert, G.A., Brauninger, R., LeBoeuf, R.A. & Isfort, R.J. (1996) Use of the Syrian hamster embryo cell transformation assay for carcinogenicity prediction of chemicals currently being tested by the National Toxicology Program in rodent bioassays. *Environ. Health Perspectives*, **104**, 1075–1084

Kune, G.A. (1993) Laxative use not a risk for colorectal cancer: Data from the Melbourne Colorectal Cancer Study. *Z. Gastroenterol.*, **31**, 140–143

Lambrianides, A.L. & Rosin, R.D. (1984) Acute pancreatitis complicating excessive intake of phenolphthalein. *Postgrad. med. J.*, **60**, 491–492

LaRusso, N.F. & McGill, D.B. (1975) Surreptitious laxative ingestion. Delayed recognition of a serious condition: A case report. *Mayo Clin. Proc.*, **50**, 706–708

Longnecker, M.P., Sandler, D.P., Haile, R.W. & Sandler, R.S. (1997) Phenolphthalein-containing laxative use in relation to adenomatous colorectal polyps in three studies. *Environ. Health Perspectives*, **105**, 1210–1212

Medical Economics (1998) *PDR®: Physicians' Desk Reference*, 52nd Ed., Montvale, NJ, Medical Economics Data Production, pp. 2601–2602, 2979

Mehendale, H.M. (1990) Assessment of hepatobiliary function with phenolphthalein and phenolphthalein glucuronide. *Clin. Chem. Enzyme Commun.*, **2**, 195–204

Millburn, P., Smith, R.L. & Williams, R.T. (1967) Biliary excretion of foreign compounds. Biphenyl, stilboestrol and phenolphthalein in the rat: Molecular weight, polarity and metabolism as factors in biliary excretion. *Biochem. J.*, **105**, 1275–1281

Mortelmans, K., Haworth, S., Lawlor, T., Speck, W., Tainer, B. & Zeiger, E. (1986) *Salmonella* mutagenicity tests. II. Results from the testing of 270 chemicals. *Environ. Mutag.*, **8** (Suppl. 7), 1–119

Mrvos, R., Swanson-Biearman, B., Dean, B.S. & Krenzelok, E.P. (1991) Acute phenolphthalein ingestion in children. A retrospective review. *J. pediatr. Health Care*, **5**, 147–151

National Toxicology Program (1996) *Toxicology and Carcinogenesis Studies of Phenolphthalein (CAS No. 77-09-8) in F344/N Rats and B6C3F$_1$ Mice (Feed Studies)* (Technical Report Series No. 465; NIH Publ. No. 97-3390), Research Triangle Park, NC

National Toxicology Program (1999) *NTP Report on Carcinogens. Background Document for Phenolphthalein (Final, March 1999)*, Research Triangle Park, NC, NTP Board of Scientific Counselors

Nieto, A., Garciá, C. & López de Haro, S. (1990) In vivo estrogenic and antiestrogenic activity of phenolphthalein and derivative compounds. *Biochem. int.*, **2**, 305–311

Nishikawa, J. (1981) Effects of sodium picosulfate and other laxatives in cultured Chang cells. *Arzneimittelforschung*, **31**, 1872–1875

Parker, R.J., Hirom, P.C. & Millburn, P. (1980) Enterohepatic recycling of phenolphthalein, morphine, lysergic acid diethylamide (LSD) and diphenylacetic acid in the rat. Hydrolysis of glucuronic acid conjugates in the gut lumen. *Xenobiotica*, **10**, 689–703

Pietrusko, R.G. (1977) Use and abuse of laxatives. *Am. J. Hosp. Pharm.*, **34**, 291–300

Pohl, A. & Lowe, J.P. (1978) Phenolphthalein poisoning—four cases. *Proc. Mine med. Off. Assoc. S.A.*, **57**, 84–86

Pouchert, C.J. (1981) *The Aldrich Library of Infrared Spectra*, 3rd Ed., Milwaukee, WI, Aldrich Chemical Co., p. 1471

Pouchert, C.J. (1985) *The Aldrich Library of FT-IR Spectra*, Vol. 1-2-3, Milwaukee, WI, Aldrich Chemical Co., p. 1006

Ravdin, P.M., van Beurden, M. & Jordan, V.C. (1987) Estrogenic effects of phenolphthalein on human breast cancer cells *in vitro*. *Breast Cancer Res. Treat.*, **9**, 151–154

Rote Liste Sekretariat (1998) *Rote Liste 1998*, Frankfurt, Rote Liste Service GmbH, pp. 56–068

Royal Pharmaceutical Society of Great Britain (1999) *Martindale, The Extra Pharmacopoeia*, 13th Ed., London, The Pharmaceutical Press [MicroMedex Online: Health Care Series]

Sadtler Research Laboratories (1980) *Sadtler Standard Spectra, 1980 Cumulative Index*, Philadelphia, PA, p. 1048

Sarcinelli, L., Signore, L. & Malizia, E. (1970) Lethal phenolphthalein poisoning in a child. *Proc. Eur. Soc. Study Drug Toxicol.*, **50**, 261

Shelley, W.B., Schlappner, O.L.A. & Heiss, H.B. (1972) Demonstration of intercellular immunofluorescence and epidermal hysteresis in bullous fixed drug eruption due to phenolphthalein. *Br. J. Dermatol.*, **86**, 188–125

Sidhu, P.S., Wilkinson, M.L., Sladen, G.E., Filipe, M.I. & Toseland, P.A. (1989) Fatal phenolphthalein poisoning with fulminant hepatic failure and disseminated intravascular coagulation. *Hum. Toxicol.*, **8**, 381–384

Sipe, H.J., Jr, Corbett, J.T. & Mason, R.P. (1997) *In vitro* free radical metabolism of phenolphthalein by peroxidases. *Drug Metab. Dispos.*, **25**, 468–480

Steigmann, F., Barnard, R.D. & Dyniewicz, J.M. (1938) Phenolphthalein studies: Phenolphthalein in jaundice. *Am. J. med. Sci.*, **196**, 673–688

Stroud, M.B. & Rosio, T.J. (1987) A case of recurring painful red macules. *Arch. Dermatol.*, **123**, 1225–1230

Sugar, J.A., Belfer, M., Israel, E. & Herzog, D.B. (1991) A 3-year-old boy's chronic diarrhea and unexplained death. *J. Am. Acad. Child adolesc. Psychiatr.*, **30**, 1015–1021

Sund, R.B. & Hillestad, B. (1982) Uptake, conjugation and transport of laxative diphenols by everted sacs of the rat jejunum and stripped colon. *Acta pharmacol. toxicol.*, **51**, 377–387

Sund, R.B. & Lauterbach, F. (1986) Drug metabolism and metabolite transport in the small and large intestine: Experiments with 1-naphthol and phenolphthalein by luminal and contraluminal administration in the isolated guinea pig mucosa. *Acta pharmacol. toxicol.*, **58**, 74–83

Sund, R.B., Hetland, H.S. & Nafstad, I. (1986) Autoradiography in mice after intravenous and intragastric administration of phenolphthalein and desacetylated bisacodyl, two laxative diphenols of the diphenylmethane group. *Norw. pharm. Acta*, **48**, 57–73

Swiss Pharmaceutical Society, ed. (1999) *Index Nominum, International Drug Directory*, 16th Ed., Stuttgart, Medpharm Scientific Publishers [MicroMedex Online: Health Care Series]

Thomas, J., ed. (1998) *Australian Prescription Products Guide*, 27th Ed., Victoria, Australian Pharmaceutical Publishing, Vol. 1, pp. 286, 1190–1191, 1229, 1587, 1686

Tice, R.R., Furedi-Machacek, M., Satterfield, D., Udumudi, A., Vasquez, M. & Dunnick, J.K. (1998) Measurement of micronucleated erythrocytes and DNA damage during chronic ingestion of phenolphthalein in transgenic female mice heterozygous for the *p53* gene. *Environ. mol. Mutag.*, **31**, 113–124

Tsutsui, T., Tamura, Y., Yagi, E., Hasegawa, K., Tanaka, Y., Uehama, A., Someya, T., Hamaguchi, F., Yamamoto, H. & Barrett, J.C. (1997) Cell-transforming activity and genotoxicity of phenolphthalein in cultured Syrian hamster embryo cells. *Int. J. Cancer*, **73**, 697–701

Tyson, R.M., Shrader, E.A. & Perlman, H.H. (1937) Drugs transmitted through breast milk. Part I. Laxatives. *J. Pediatr.*, **11**, 824

US Pharmacopeial Convention (1994) *The 1995 US Pharmacopeia*, 23rd Rev./*The National Formulary*, 18th Rev., Rockville, MD, pp. 1205–1206

US Pharmacopeial Convention (1998) *USP Dispensing Information, Drug Information for the Health Care Professional*, 18th Ed., Rockville, MD, Vol. I, pp. 1798–1840

Velentzas, C.G. & Ikkos, D.G. (1971) Phenolphthalein as cause of factitious enteritis (Letter to the Editor). *J. Am. med. Assoc.*, **217**, 966

Visek, W.J., Liu, W.C. & Roth, L.J. (1956) Studies on the fate of carbon-14 labeled phenolphthalein. *J. Pharmacol. exp. Ther.*, **117**, 347–357

Weiss, B.D. & Wood, G.A. (1982) Laxative abuse causing gastrointestinal bleeding. *J. Fam. Pract.*, **15**, 177–181

WHO (1997) *Alert No. 65: Laxatives Containing Phenolphthalein—Proposed Ban on Sale of OTC Products: Risk of Carcinogenicity* [http://www.who.int/dmp/drugalert/alert65.htm]

WHO (1998) Regulatory matters: Phenolphthalein products withdrawn. *WHO Drug Inf.*, **12**, 13–14

Williams, R.T. (1959) *Detoxication Mechanisms. The Metabolism and Detoxication of Drugs, Toxic Substances and Other Organic Compounds*, 2nd Ed., New York, John Wiley & Sons, pp. 475–476

Witt, K.L., Gulati, D.K., Kaur, P. & Shelby, M.D. (1995) Phenolphthalein: Induction of micronucleated erythrocytes in mice. *Mutat. Res.*, **341**, 151–160

Wyatt, E., Greaves, M. & Søndergaard, J. (1972) Fixed drug eruption (phenolphthalein). Evidence for a blood-borne mediator. *Arch. Dermatol.*, **106**, 671–673

Zanolli, M.D., McAlvany, J. & Krowchuk, D.P. (1993) Phenolphthalein-induced fixed drug eruption: A cutaneous complication of laxative use in a child. *Pediatrics*, **91**, 1199–1201

VITAMIN K SUBSTANCES

Vitamin K comprises a group of substances, which are widespread in nature and are an essential co-factor in humans in the synthesis of several proteins that play a role in haemostasis and others that may be important in calcium homeostasis. The K vitamins all contain the 2-methyl-1,4-naphthoquinone (menadione) moiety, and the various naturally occurring forms differ in the alkyl substituent at the 3-position. Phylloquinone (vitamin K_1) is 2-methyl-3-phytyl-1,4-naphthoquinone and is widely found in higher plants, including green leafy vegetables, and in green and blue algae. The menaquinones (formerly vitamin K_2) have polyisoprenyl substituents at the 3-position and are produced by bacteria. The compound menadione (formerly vitamin K_3) lacks an alkyl group at the 3-position but can be alkylated *in vivo* in some species. Several synthetic water-soluble derivatives, such as the sodium diphosphate ester of menadiol and the addition product of menadione with sodium bisulfite, also have commercial applications (National Research Council, 1989; Gennaro, 1995; Weber & Rüttimann, 1996).

1. Exposure Data

1.1 Chemical and physical data

1.1.1 *Nomenclature, structural and molecular formulae and relative molecular masses*

Vitamin K (generic)

Chem. Abstr. Serv. Reg. No.: 12001-79-5
Chem. Abstr. Name: Vitamin K

Vitamin K_1 (generic)

Chem. Abstr. Serv. Reg. No.: 11104-38-4
Chem. Abstr. Name: Vitamin K_1

Phylloquinone

Chem. Abstr. Serv. Reg. No.: 84-80-0
Deleted CAS Reg. Nos.: 10485-69-5; 15973-57-6; 50926-17-5

Chem. Abstr. Name: 2-Methyl-3-[(2*E*,7*R*,11*R*)-3,7,11,15-tetramethyl-2-hexadecenyl]-1,4-naphthalenedione

IUPAC Systematic Name: [*R*-[*R**,*R**-(*E*)]]-2-Methyl-3-(3,7,11,15-tetramethyl-2-hexadecenyl)-1,4-naphthalenedione

Synonyms: Antihaemorrhagic vitamin; 2-methyl-3-phytyl-1,4-naphthoquinone; 2-methyl-3-(3,7,11,15-tetramethyl-2-hexadecenyl)-1,4-naphthalenedione; α-phylloquinone; *trans*-phylloquinone; phylloquinone K_1; phytomenadione; phytonadione; phytylmenadione; 3-phytylmenadione; phytylmenaquinone; vitamin K_1; vitamin $K_{1(20)}$; 2′,3′-*trans*-vitamin K_1 [Note: The IUPAC recommends use of the name 'phylloquinone' and the abbreviation 'K' (rather than 'K_1'). Both phylloquinone and vitamin K_1 are in common use. The *United States Pharmacopeia* uses the name 'phytonadione'; *The European Pharmacopoeia* uses the name 'phytomenadione', which is a synonym occasionally found in the pharmaceutical and pharmacological literature.]

$C_{31}H_{46}O_2$ Relative molecular mass: 450.71

Menaquinone-4

Chem. Abstr. Serv. Reg. No.: 863-61-6

Deleted CAS Reg. Nos.: 15261-37-7; 20977-31-5; 39776-41-5

Chem. Abstr. Name: 2-Methyl-3-[(2*E*,6*E*,10*E*)-3,7,11,15-tetramethyl-2,6,10,14-hexadecatetraenyl]-1,4-naphthalenedione

IUPAC Systematic Name: 2-Methyl-3-(3,7,11,15-tetramethyl-2,6,10,14-hexadecatetraenyl)-1,4-naphthoquinone

Synonyms: Menaquinone-K4; menatetrenone; (*E*,*E*,*E*)-2-methyl-3-(3,7,11,15-tetramethyl-2,6,10,14-hexadecatetraenyl]-1,4-naphthalenedione; MK4; vitamin $K_{2(20)}$; vitamin MK4

$C_{31}H_{40}O_2$ Relative molecular mass: 444.66

Vitamin K₂ (generic)

Chem. Abstr. Serv. Reg. No.: 11032-49-8
Chem. Abstr. Name: Vitamin K_2

Menadione

Chem. Abstr. Serv. Reg. No.: 58-27-5
Chem. Abstr. Name: 1,4-Naphthalenedione, 2-methyl-
IUPAC Systematic Name: 1,4-Naphthoquinone, 2-methyl-
Synonyms: 1,4-Dihydro-1,4-dioxo-2-methylnaphthalene; 2-methyl-1,4-naphthalenedione; 2-methylnaphthoquinone; β-methyl-1,4-naphthoquinone; 2-methyl-1,4-naphthoquinone; 3-methyl-1,4-naphthoquinone; MK-0; vitamin K_0; vitamin $K_{2(0)}$; vitamin K_3 [Note: 'Menadione' is the common name preferred by IUPAC for the chemical, previously called vitamin K_3]

$C_{11}H_8O_2$ Relative molecular mass: 172.18

Menadione sodium bisulfite

Chem. Abstr. Serv. Reg. No.: 130-37-0
Alternate CAS Reg. No.: 57414-02-5
Deleted CAS Reg. Nos.: 8012-53-1; 8017-97-8; 8028-24-8; 8053-08-5
Chem. Abstr. Name: 1,2,3,4-Tetrahydro-2-methyl-1,4-dioxo-2-naphthalenesulfonic acid, sodium salt
IUPAC Systematic Name: 1,2,3,4-Tetrahydro-2-methyl-1,4-dioxo-2-naphthalenesulfonic acid, sodium salt
Synonyms: 3,3-Dihydro-2-methyl-1,4-naphthoquinone-2-sulfonate sodium; menadione sodium hydrogen sulfite; menaphthone sodium bisulfite; menaphthone sodium bisulphite; 2-methyl-1,4-naphthalenedione, sodium bisulfite deriv.; 2-methyl-1,4-naphthoquinone sodium bisulfite; 2-methylnaphthoquinone sodium hydrogen sulfite; 2-methyl-1,4-naphthoquinone sodium hydrogen sulfite; MSBC; sodium menadione bisulfite; vitamin K injection; vitamin K_3 sodium bisulfite

$C_{11}H_9NaO_5S$ Relative molecular mass: 276.24

Menadione sodium bisulfite trihydrate

Chem. Abstr. Serv. Reg. No.: 6147-37-1
Chem. Abstr. Name: 1,2,3,4-Tetrahydro-2-methyl-1,4-dioxo-2-naphthalenesulfonic acid, sodium salt, trihydrate

$C_{11}H_9NaO_5S \cdot 3H_2O$ Relative molecular mass: 330.28

Menadiol

Chem. Abstr. Serv. Reg. No.: 481-85-6
Chem. Abstr. Name: 2-Methyl-1,4-naphthalenediol
IUPAC Systematic Name: 2-Methyl-1,4-naphthalenediol
Synonyms: Dihydrovitamin K_3; menaquinol; 2-methyl-1,4-dihydroxynaphthalene; 2-methylhydronaphthoquinone; 2-methylnaphthalene-1,4-diol; 2-methyl-1,4-naphthohydroquinone; 2-methyl-1,4-naphthoquinol; reduced menadione; reduced vitamin K_3; vitamin K_3H_2

$C_{11}H_{10}O_2$ Relative molecular mass: 174.19

Menadiol sodium phosphate

Chem. Abstr. Serv. Reg. No.: 131-13-5
Chem. Abstr. Name: 2-Methyl-1,4-naphthalenediol, bis(dihydrogen phosphate), tetrasodium salt

IUPAC Systematic Name: 2-Methyl-1,4-naphthalenediol, diphosphate, tetrasodium salt
Synonyms: Menadiol diphosphate tetrasodium salt; menadiol sodium diphosphate; menadiol tetrasodium diphosphate; menadione diphosphate tetrasodium salt; 2-methyl-1,4-naphthoquinol bis(disodium phosphate); tetrasodium 2-methyl-1,4-naphthalenediol bis(dihydrogen phosphate)

$C_{11}H_8Na_4O_8P_2$ Relative molecular mass: 422.09

Menadiol sodium phosphate hexahydrate

Chem. Abstr. Serv. Reg. No.: 6700-42-1
Chem. Abstr. Name: 2-Methyl-1,4-naphthalenediol, bis(dihydrogen phosphate), tetrasodium salt, hexahydrate
IUPAC Systematic Name: 2-Methyl-1,4-naphthalenediol, diphosphate, tetrasodium salt, hexahydrate
Synonyms: Menadiol sodium diphosphate hexahydrate

$C_{11}H_8Na_4O_8P_2 \cdot 6H_2O$ Relative molecular mass: 530.18

Acetomenaphthone

Chem. Abstr. Serv. Reg. No.: 573-20-6
Chem. Abstr. Name: 2-Methyl-1,4-naphthalenediol, diacetate
IUPAC Systematic Name: 2-Methyl-1,4-naphthalenediol, diacetate
Synonyms: 1,4-Diacetoxy-2-methylnaphthalene; menadiol diacetate; 2-methyl-1,4-naphthohydroquinone diacetate; 2-methyl-1,4-naphthoquinol diacetate; 2-methyl-1,4-naphthylene diacetate; vitamin K diacetate; vitamin K_4

$C_{15}H_{14}O_4$ Relative molecular mass: 258.27

IUPAC recommends that 2-methyl-3-polyprenyl-1,4-naphthoquinone be referred to as menaquinone-*n*, previously vitamin K_2, *n* being the number of prenyl residues. Vitamin $K_{2(20)}$ is so named because it contains 20 carbon atoms in the chain. In the biological literature, vitamin K_2 is frequently referred to as menaquinone and is further designated by the number of isoprene units in the side-chain. For example, vitamin $K_{2(20)}$ is also called menaquinone-4 for the four isoprene units in the side-chain. The compound originally isolated from rotting fish meal and named vitamin K_2 was later identified as menaquinone-7 (2-methyl-3-farnesylgeranyl-geranyl-1,4-naphthoquinone). In the older literature, the designation vitamin $K_{2(35)}$ is used for menaquinone-7, but this is no longer used. Menaquinones found in nature have side-chains of 4–13 isoprenoid residues and are usually in the all-*trans* configuration; however, menaquinones with the *cis* configuration and partially saturated side-chains also exist (Suttie, 1985, 1991; Weber & Rüttimann, 1996; Van Arnum, 1998).

1.1.2 *Chemical and physical properties of the pure substances*

Phylloquinone

(a) *Description*: Clear, yellow to amber, very viscous, odourless liquid (Gennaro, 1995; Budavari, 1996)
(b) *Spectroscopy data*: Ultraviolet, infrared, nuclear magnetic resonance (proton and ^{13}C) and mass spectral data have been reported (Hassan *et al.*, 1988).
(c) *Solubility*: Insoluble in water; sparingly soluble in methanol; soluble in acetone, benzene, chloroform, diethyl ether, dioxane, ethanol, hexane, petroleum ether and other fat solvents and vegetable oils (Budavari, 1996)
(d) *Stability*: Stable to air and moisture; decomposes in sunlight; unaffected by dilute acids; destroyed by solutions of alkali hydroxides and by reducing agents (Gennaro, 1995; Budavari, 1996)
(e) *Optical rotation*: $[\alpha]_D^{25}$, $-28°$ (Budavari, 1996)

Menaquinone-4

From Japan Medical Products Trade Association (1996)
(a) *Description*: Yellow crystals or an oily substance
(b) *Melting-point*: 34–38 °C
(c) *Solubility*: Practically insoluble in water; very soluble in diethyl ether, chloroform and hexane; freely soluble in isooctane; sparingly soluble in ethanol and isopropanol; slightly soluble in methanol
(d) *Stability*: Decomposed by light or alkalis

Menadione

(a) *Description*: Bright-yellow crystals with a very faint acrid odour (Budavari, 1996)
(b) *Melting-point*: 105–107 °C (Budavari, 1996)
(c) *Spectroscopy data*: Infrared (prism [8077]; grating [8522]), ultraviolet [2183] and nuclear magnetic resonance (proton [3217]; ^{13}C [6002]) spectral data have been reported (Sadtler Research Laboratories, 1980; British Pharmacopoeial Commission, 1993).
(d) *Solubility*: Insoluble in water; soluble in benzene (1 g/10 mL), ethanol (1 g/60 mL), and vegetable oils (1 g/50 mL); moderately soluble in carbon tetrachloride and chloroform (Budavari, 1996)
(e) *Stability*: Stable in air; decomposed by sunlight; destroyed by alkalis and reducing agents (Budavari, 1996)

Menadione sodium bisulfite (trihydrate)

(a) *Description*: White, crystalline, odourless, hygroscopic powder (Gennaro, 1985; Budavari, 1996)
(b) *Solubility*: Soluble in water (~0.5 g/mL); slightly soluble in chloroform and ethanol; practically insoluble in benzene and diethyl ether (Gennaro, 1985; Budavari, 1996)
(c) *Stability*: Discolours and may turn purple under light (Budavari, 1996)

Menadiol

(a) *Description*: White needles (Budavari, 1996)
(b) *Melting-point*: 168–170 °C (Budavari, 1996)
(c) *Solubility*: Very soluble in acetone and ethanol; slightly soluble in benzene and chloroform (Budavari, 1996)

Menadiol sodium phosphate (hexahydrate)

(a) *Description*: White to pinkish, hygroscopic powder with a salty taste (Gennaro, 1995; Budavari, 1996)

(b) *Spectroscopy data*: Infrared spectral data have been reported (British Pharmacopoeial Commission, 1993).

(c) *Solubility*: Very soluble in water; practically insoluble in acetone, diethyl ether, ethanol and methanol (Budavari, 1996)

Acetomenaphthone

(a) *Description*: Crystalline solid (Budavari, 1996)
(b) *Melting-point*: 112–114 °C (Budavari, 1996)
(c) *Solubility*: Practically insoluble in water; slightly soluble in ethanol; soluble in acetic acid (Budavari, 1996)
(d) *Spectroscopy data*: Infrared (prism [20206]; grating [32489]), ultraviolet [6761] and nuclear magnetic resonance (proton [2298]; ^{13}C [2451]) spectral data have been reported (Sadtler Research Laboratories, 1980).

1.1.3 *Technical products and impurities*

Commercially available phylloquinone is prepared synthetically and may contain not only 2′,3′-*trans*-phylloquinone (not less than 75%) but also 2′,3′-*cis*-phylloquinone and *trans*-epoxyphylloquinone (not more than 4.0%). Phylloquinone occurs in nature only as the 2′,3′-*trans*-phylloquinone stereoisomer (Weber & Rüttimann, 1996; American Hospital Formulary Service, 1997; Council of Europe, 1997).

Phylloquinone is available as a 5- and 10-mg tablet (chewable), a 2- and 10 mg/mL injection solution, a 10- and 20-mg/mL oral solution and a 20-mg/mL emulsion. The tablet may also contain carmellose, carob bean flour, carob gum, cocoa butter, cocoa powder, ethyl cellulose, ethyl vanillin, glucose, glycerol, gum arabic, hard and viscous paraffin, lactose, rice starch, sugar, silicic acid, silicon dioxide, skim-milk powder, sodium cyclamate, talc and titanium dioxide. The injection solution may also contain benzyl alcohol, dextrose, glacial acetic acid, glucose, glycocholic acid, hydrochloric acid, macrogol ricinoleate, phenol, phosphatidylcholine from soya beans, polyethoxylated fatty acid derivative (castor oil), polysorbate 80, propylene glycol, sodium acetate, sodium hydroxide and water. A widely used injectable formulation, Konakion®, formerly contained a polyethoxylated castor oil as an emulsifying agent, but has been reformulated as a mixed micellar preparation, Konakion MM®, containing glycocholic acid, lecithin and buffered to pH 6. The oral solution may also contain benzoic acid, glycocholic acid, hydrochloric acid, lecithin, macrogol ricinoleate, methyl 4-hydroxybenzoate, propyl 4-hydroxybenzoate, sodium hydroxide and water. The emulsion may also contain polysorbate 80, purified water and sorbic acid.

Phylloquinone is also available as a component (200 µg) of a multivitamin lyophilized, sterile powder intended for reconstitution and dilution in intravenous infusions, as a component (0.075 mg) of an effervescent multivitamin tablet, and as a component (5.5 µg) of a multivitamin infant formula (Gennaro, 1995; American Hospital Formulary Service, 1997; Canadian Pharmaceutical Association, 1997; British Medical Association/Royal Pharmaceutical Society of Great Britain, 1998; Editions du Vidal, 1998; LINFO Läkemedelsinformation AB, 1998; Rote Liste Sekretariat, 1998; Thomas, 1998; US Pharmacopeial Convention, 1998).

Trade names for phylloquinone include AquaMEPHYTON, AquaMephyton, AquaMephyton R, Combinal K_1, Hymeron, Kanakion, Kanavit, Kaywan, Kephton, Kinadion, K1 Delagrange, Konakion, Konakion MM, Menadion 'Dak', Mephyton, Monodion, Synthex P, Vitacon, Vita-K1, Vitamina K1 Biol, Vitamine K1 Roche and Vitamin K_1 (CIS Information Services, 1998; Royal Pharmaceutical Society of Great Britain, 1999; Swiss Pharmaceutical Society, 1999).

Menaquinone-4 is available in Japan as 5- and 15-mg capsules and as a 2-mg/mL syrup. The capsules may also contain ethyl parahydroxybenzoate, propyl paraoxyhydroxybenzoate, sodium lauryl sulfate and FD&C Yellow No. 6 (Sunset Yellow). The syrup may also contain polyoxyethylene hydrogenated castor oil 60, propylene glycol, ethyl parahydroxybenzoate, sodium benzoate and flavouring (Japan Medical Products Trade Association, 1996).

Trade names for menaquinone-4 include Glakay and Kaytwo (Japan Medical Products Trade Association, 1996).

Menadione is available as a 2-, 5- and 10-mg tablet and as a 2- and 10-mg/mL injection (in oil). Menadione sodium bisulfite is available as a 10-mg tablet and as a 5- and 10-mg/mL and 72-mg/10 mL injection (Gennaro, 1985).

Trade names for menadione include Aquakay, Aquinone, Austrovit-K Depot, Hemodal, K-Thrombyl, K-Vitan, Kaergona, Kanone, Kaom Belgarum, Kappaxan, Kappaxin, Karanum, Karcon, Kareon, Kativ-G, Kavitamin, Kayklot, Kaykot, Kayquinone, Kipca, Kipca-Oil Soluble, Klottone, Koaxin, Kolklot, Menadion, Menaphthon, Menaphthone, Menaquinone 0, Mitenon, Mitenone, MNQ, Neo-Zimema-K, Panosine, Prokayvit, Synkay, Thyloquinone, Vikaman, Vita-Noxi K and Vitavel-K (Swiss Pharmaceutical Society, 1999).

Trade names for menadione sodium bisulfite include Austrovit-K, Golagen K, Hemoklot, Hetrogen K, Hetrogen K Premix, Hykinone, Ido-K, K-Thrombin, K-Trombina, Kalzon, Kareon, Kavitamin, Kavitan, Kavitol, Kawitan, Klotogen, Libavit K, Nuvit K, Vikaman, Vikasol, Vitaminum K and Zimema K (Swiss Pharmaceutical Society, 1999).

Menadiol sodium phosphate (as the hexahydrate) is available as a 5-mg and 10 mg (equivalent of menadiol phosphate) tablet and as 5- and 10-mg/mL and 75-mg/2 mL injections (Gennaro, 1995; British Medical Association/Royal Pharmaceutical Society of Great Britain, 1998; US Pharmacopeial Convention, 1998).

Acetomenaphthone is available in a chilblain formula tablet containing 30 mg nicotinamide and 5 mg acetomenaphthone and as a component (10 mg) of a multivitamin injection solution, which may also contain butyl hydroxyanisole, butyl hydroxytoluene, peanut oil, medium-chain triglycerides and olive oil (Rote Liste Sekretariat, 1998; Thomas, 1998).

Trade names for menadiol sodium phosphate hexahydrate include Kappadione, Kativ (injection), Kipca water soluble, Naphthidone, Procoagulo, Synkavit, Synka-Vit, Synkavite, Synkayvite and Thylokay (Swiss Pharmaceutical Society, 1999).

Trade names for acetomenaphthone include Adaprin, Davitamon-K, Davitamon-K-oral, Kapathrom, Kapilin, Kapilon, Kappaxan, Kativ powder, Kayvite, Pafavit, Prokayvit Oral and Vitavel K.

1.1.4 Analysis

Several international pharmacopoeias specify infrared (IR) and ultraviolet (UV) absorption spectrophotometry with comparison to standards as the methods for identifying phylloquinone; UV absorption spectrophotometry and liquid chromatography are used to assay its purity. Phylloquinone is identified in pharmaceutical preparations by IR and UV absorption spectrophotometry and liquid chromatography; liquid chromatography is used to assay for its content (British Pharmacopoeial Commission, 1993; US Pharmacopeial Convention, 1994; Society of Japanese Pharmacopoeia, 1996; Council of Europe, 1997). AOAC International (1996) has developed a liquid chromatographic method with UV detection for the determination of phylloquinone in ready-to-feed milk-based infant formulae.

As a result of its high selectivity and sensitivity, high-performance liquid chromatography (HPLC) is the method of choice for the determination of phylloquinone and menaquinones in blood, tissues, milk and foods. Various procedures for extraction and preliminary purification, normal or reversed-phase HPLC and UV, electrochemical and fluorescence detection (both after electrochemical or chemical reduction and after photochemical decomposition) of the various vitamin K substances have been described. The limit of detection of phylloquinone is 25–500 pg, depending on the detection method used. Similar values, which vary according to the length of the side-chain, apply to the menaquinones. HPLC methods are also available for the determination of menadione and water-soluble derivatives in feedstuffs, premixes and vitamin concentrates (Weber & Rüttimann, 1996).

Alternative methods are thin-layer chromatography, high-performance thin-layer chromatography and gas chromatography. The spectrophotometric, fluorimetric and colorimetric methods previously used without chromatographic purification of the samples to be analysed are frequently less sensitive and less specific than HPLC, for instance allowing no distinction between phylloquinone and menaquinones (Weber & Rüttimann, 1996).

Several international pharmacopoeias specify IR absorption spectrophotometry with comparison to standards and colorimetry as the methods for identifying menadiol sodium phosphate hexahydrate; potentiometric titration with ceric sulfate is used to assay its purity. In pharmaceutical preparations, menadiol sodium phosphate is identified by IR absorption spectrophotometry and colorimetry; potentiometric titration with ceric sulfate and UV absorption spectrophotometry are used to assay for its content (British Pharmacopoeial Commission, 1993; US Pharmacopeial Convention, 1994; Council of Europe, 1997).

Several international pharmacopoeias specify IR and UV absorption spectrophotometry with comparison to standards as the methods for identifying menadione; titration with ammonium and cerium nitrate or ceric sulfate is used to assay its purity. Visible (635 nm) absorption spectrophotometry is used to assay for its content in pharmaceutical preparations (British Pharmacopoeial Commission, 1993; US Pharmacopeial Convention, 1994; Council of Europe, 1997).

1.2 Production

Although the predominant commercial form of phylloquinone is the synthetic racemate, natural phylloquinone is accessible either by extraction from a natural source or from condensation of menadione with natural phytol. The stability of phylloquinone to heat made possible the use of commercially dehydrated alfalfa meal, for example, as a natural source (Hassan et al., 1988). The synthesis and spectral properties of all four stereoisomers of (E)-phylloquinone have been described and their biological potencies determined. When natural phylloquinone was used as a standard in bioassays, it was concluded that all four stereoisomers have essentially identical activity (Van Arnum, 1998).

The first syntheses and structural elucidation of phylloquinone were published in 1939 almost simultaneously by four groups. The starting materials were menadione or menadiol as the aromatic component and natural phytol or one of its derivatives. A breakthrough in commercial synthesis was achieved in the 1950s, when it was found that monoacylated menadiols (e.g. the monoacetate or the monobenzoate) could be used advantageously in the alkylation step and that natural phytol could be replaced by isophytol, which is easy to synthesize (Weber & Rüttimann, 1996).

In the Isler-Lindlar method, excess menadiol monobenzoate is condensed with isophytol in the presence of boron trifluoride etherate as a catalyst. The alkylation product is obtained as a 70:30 *trans*/*cis* mixture. The *trans* form can be enriched by recrystallization. The *trans*-enriched alkylation product (*trans*:*cis* 9:1) is saponified with potassium hydroxide and oxidized to phylloquinone with oxygen (Weber & Rüttimann, 1996).

The industrial synthesis of menaquinones parallels that of phylloquinone and involves as a key step alkylation of monosubstituted menadione with an appropriate (all-*trans*) polyisoprenyl derivative. Considerably more work has been done on fermentative approaches to menaquinones than for phylloquinone. Menaquinones of varying chain lengths, from C_5 to C_{65}, have been produced and isolated from bacteria. Menaquinone-4 is produced and used extensively in Japan (Van Arnum, 1998).

Menadione can be prepared by oxidizing 2-methylnaphthalene with chromic acid or hydrogen peroxide (Weber & Rüttimann, 1996). A process based on biotechnological techniques has been reported in Japan (Van Arnum, 1998).

Menadione sodium bisulfite can be prepared by reacting menadione with sodium bisulfite. The reaction may be visualized as consisting of the typical addition of sodium bisulfite to a ketone, forming the $R(OH)(SO_3Na)$ compound, which then rearranges at the expense of one degree of unsaturation of the quinoid nucleus. The compound readily regenerates menadione on treatment with mild alkali and behaves as a typical ketone–sodium bisulfite addition compound (Gennaro, 1985; Van Arnum, 1998).

Menadiol sodium phosphate can be prepared by reducing menadione to the diol, followed by double esterification with hydriodic acid, metathesis of the resulting 1,4-diiodo compound with silver phosphate and neutralization of the bis(dihydrogen phosphate) ester with sodium hydroxide (Gennaro, 1995).

Information available in 1999 indicated that phylloquinone was manufactured and/or formulated in 41 countries, menadione in 26 countries, menadione sodium bisulfite in 21 countries, menadiol and menadiol sodium phosphate (as the hexahydrate) in two countries each and acetomenaphthone in seven countries (CIS Information Services, 1998; Royal Pharmaceutical Society of Great Britain; 1999; Swiss Pharmaceutical Society, 1999).

1.3 Use

1.3.1 *Physiological function*

The only established biochemical role for vitamin K is as a cofactor in a unique post-translational chemical modification in which selective glutamate (Glu) residues on certain specialized calcium-binding proteins are transformed to γ-carboxyglutamate (Gla) residues (Suttie, 1991; Shearer, 1997). The modification is catalysed by a microsomal enzyme called γ-glutamyl or vitamin K-dependent carboxylase, which is present in most tissues. The best-known vitamin K-dependent proteins are those synthesized in the liver, which play a role in the maintenance of normal haemostasis. They comprise four proteins (II, VII, IX and X) that promote coagulation and two proteins (C and S) that act in the regulatory feedback control of coagulation. Vitamin K-dependent proteins, of uncertain function, are also known to occur in a variety of other tissues such as bone, kidney, pancreas, placenta, spleen and lungs. They include the bone protein osteocalcin (also called bone Gla protein) and matrix Gla protein; there is growing evidence that these proteins may be important for bone health and other regulatory functions in calcium metabolism. In those proteins with well-established functions, such as coagulation proteins, the Gla groups are essential for the biological activity (Thijssen & Drittij-Reijnders, 1996; Shearer, 1997).

Naturally occurring phylloquinone and menaquinones all γ-carboxylate the vitamin K-dependent coagulation proteins. Synthetic forms of menadione (and related water-soluble salts) that lack a side-chain at the 3-position have biological activity *in vivo* only after side-chain alkylation, which results in the specific synthesis of menaquinone-4 (Suttie, 1991; see also section 4).

1.3.2 Supplementation and therapy

Vitamin K is given as a supplement to prevent or cure vitamin K deficiency when the endogenous vitamin K supply from the diet is likely to become or has proven to be insufficient. Neonates are born with very limited vitamin K stores, but most infants do not show relevant hypoprothrombinaemia at birth (von Kries *et al.*, 1987a, 1988; von Kries, 1991). Biochemical signs of vitamin K deficiency are common during the first week of life, however, unless sufficient amounts of vitamin K are ingested. The natural diet of newborns is human milk, which contains vitamin K at concentrations of 0.69–9.2 ng/mL (see Table 1). [The Working Group noted that some of the high values in the Table may reflect methodological problems with analysis and milk collection.] Bleeding, the classical clinical manifestation of vitamin K deficiency, is extremely rare on the first day of life, and the typical time of onset is during the first week, with bleeding from mucous membranes, the umbilicus, following circumcision, and rarely, into the central nervous system (von Kries *et al.*, 1988; von Kries, 1991). This condition was originally called 'classical haemorrhagic disease of the newborn'; the present nomenclature is 'classical vitamin K deficiency bleeding' (Sutor *et al.*, 1999).

During the first three months of life, exclusively breast-fed infants remain at risk for vitamin K deficiency bleeding. In many of these infants, the bleeding episode, which is often intracranial haemorrhage, is the first perceived symptom of an underlying cholestatic disease. In 10–30% of the cases, however, no underlying disease can be found (von Kries *et al.*, 1988).

After the first three months of life, vitamin K deficiency is almost completely confined to patients with cholestatic diseases (congenital or acquired obstruction of the bile duct), malabsorption syndromes or cystic fibrosis (Houwen *et al.*, 1987; van den Anker & Sinaasappel, 1993; O'Brien *et al.*, 1994; Kowdley *et al.*, 1997; Nowak *et al.*, 1997; see also section 1.3.4).

1.3.3 For prevention of vitamin K deficiency in newborns and early infancy

The use of vitamin K prophylaxis since the 1950s has varied widely over time, between countries and within countries between institutions. The predominant patterns were to give either selective intramuscular prophylaxis only to infants presumed to be at special risk for bleeding (mainly premature and low-birth-weight

Table 1. Concentrations of phylloquinone in human and cow's milk, infant formulae and various oils

Sample	Concentration of phylloquinone	Comments	Reference
Human milk	2.1 ng/mL (range, 1.1–6.5) 2.3 ng/mL (range, 0.7–4.2)	Mature milk Colostrum	Haroon et al. (1982)
Human milk	3.8 ng/mL (range, 1.1–8.3)	Mature milk	Motohara et al. (1984)
Human milk	1.2 ng/mL 1.8 ng/mL	Mature milk Colostrum	von Kries et al. (1987b)
Human milk	Median, 5.2 ng/mL (range, 3.1–11) Median, 8.9 ng/mL (range, 6.3–16) Median, 9.2 ng/mL (range, 4.8–13)	Day 3 of lactation (colostrum) Day 8 of lactation Day 10 of lactation (mature milk)	Fournier et al. (1987)
Human milk	1.6 ng/mL 0.9 ng/mL	Mature milk Colostrum	Canfield et al. (1988)
Human milk	Mean, 0.64 ng/mL Mean, 0.86 ng/mL Mean, 1.14 ng/mL Mean, 0.87 ng/mL	Week 1 of lactation (colostrum) Week 6 of lactation (mature milk) Week 12 of lactation Week 26 of lactation	Greer et al. (1991)
Human milk	0.69 ng/mL 76 ng/mL 75 ng/mL 82 ng/mL	Before supplements At 2 weeks with 5 mg/day supplement At 6 weeks with 5 mg/day supplement At 12 weeks with 5 mg/day supplement	Greer et al. (1997)
Human milk	0.11 μg/100 g milk		Indyk & Woollard (1997)
Cow's milk	Mean, 4.9 ng/mL (range, 3.6–8.9) Mean, 8.7 ng/mL (range, 3.8–18)	Holstein cows Jersey or Guernsey cows	Haroon et al. (1982)
Cow's milk	7.5 and 37 ng/mL	Measurements in January and July	Fournier et al. (1987)
Cow's milk	0.54 μg/100 g milk		Indyk & Woollard (1997)
Goat's milk	1.18 μg/100 g milk		Indyk & Woollard (1997)

Table 1 (contd)

Sample	Concentration of phylloquinone	Comments	Reference
Formula	79–118 ng/mL	Milk-substituted formulae with soya oil but without added vitamin K_1	Schneider et al. (1974)
	118–256 ng/mL	Milk-substituted formulae with various vegetable oils and with added vitamin K_1	
	19–69 ng/mL	Milk-based formulae with various vegetable oils but without added vitamin K_1	
Formula	Mean, 4.4 ng/mL	Unsupplemented infant formula containing only milkfat	Haroon et al. (1982)
	Mean, 11.5 ng/mL	Unsupplemented infant formula containing only vegetable oils	
Formula	~72–166 ng/mL	Ready-to-feed	Bueno & Villalobos (1983)
	~125–146 ng/mL	Concentrate	
	~129–175 ng/mL	Powder	
Formula	30–225 ng/mL (*trans* isomer); 2.8–25 ng/mL (*cis* isomer; 9.3–11% of total)	Ready-to-feed liquids	Hwang (1985)
	120–211 ng/mL (*trans* isomer); 7.2–31 ng/mL (*cis* isomer; 6.0–15% of total)	Concentrated liquids	
	90–195 ng/mL (*trans* isomer)	Powders	
Formula	0.87 µg/g	Powder (milk-based)	Schneiderman et al. (1988)
	0.95 µg/g	Powder (soya protein-based)	

Table 1 (contd)

Sample	Concentration of phylloquinone	Comments	Reference
Formula	37–130 µg/100 g	Powder (milk-based, predominantly milkfat containing < 5% corn oil)	Indyk & Woollard (1997)
	46–140 µg/100 g	Powder (milk-based, predominantly vegetable oil containing < 2% milkfat)	
	67–77 µg/100 g	Powder (goat milk-based, containing equivalent goat milkfat and vegetable oils)	
	72 µg/100 g	Powder (soya protein-based, containing exclusively vegetable oils)	
	110 µg/100 g	Powder (NIST SRM 1846 (standard reference milk))	
Soya bean oil	1.8 mg/kg (*trans* isomer)		Hwang (1985)
Corn oil	0.13 mg/kg (*trans* isomer)		
Coconut oil	< 0.06 mg/kg (*trans* isomer)		
Soya bean oil	1.9 µg/g		Haroon et al. (1982)
Palm oil	0.08 µg/g		
Oleo oil	0.06 µg/g		
Oleic oil	0.03 µg/g		
Corn oil	0.03 µg/g		
Coconut oil	< 0.01 µg/g		

Table 1 (contd)

Sample	Concentration of phylloquinone	Comments	Reference
Peanut oil	0.65 μg/100 g (range, 0.30–1.19)	Combined average	Ferland & Sadowski (1992)
Corn oil	2.91 μg/100 g (range, 1.63–4.18)	Combined average	
Almond oil	6.70 μg/100 g		
Sunflower oil	9.03 μg/100 g (range, 8.86–9.19)	Combined average	
Safflower oil	9.13 μg/100 g (range, 6.49–11.77)	Combined average	
Walnut oil	15.0 μg/100 g		
Sesame oil	15.5 μg/100 g (range, 12.1–18.7)	Combined average	
Olive oil	55.5 μg/100 g (range, 37.2–82.1)	Combined average	
Rapeseed oil	141 μg/100 g (range, 114–188)	Combined average	
Soya bean oil	193 μg/100 g (range, 139–290)	Combined average	

infants and those delivered surgically) or general prophylaxis for all infants. In the latter case, vitamin K was given either intramuscularly or orally.

Several preparations of fat-soluble vitamin K have been in use. In the early 1950s, water-soluble menadiol sodium phosphate was widely used, until haemolysis due to high doses of this preparation in neonates was identified (Meyer & Angus, 1956). In most countries, phylloquinone has been used since that time, although in some third-world countries water-soluble menadione sodium bisulfite still seems to be used (Sharma et al., 1995). Because it is technically difficult to dissolve phylloquinone, only a limited number of preparations became available. The Roche preparation (Konakion®) in which Cremophor (polyethoxylated castor oil) is used as an emulsifying vehicle has been widely available in Europe and North America. The manufacturer has recently replaced the Cremophor preparation by a new mixed micellar preparation Konakion–MM® (British Medical Association/Royal Pharmaceutical Society of Great Britain, 1998). In Japan, an oral preparation of menaquinone-4 is used instead of phylloquinone (Hanawa, 1992).

Almost all cases of vitamin K deficiency bleeding can be prevented by intramuscular administration of 1 mg of vitamin K at birth (von Kries & Hanawa, 1993). Clinical observations and laboratory investigations have also clearly shown that a single oral dose of vitamin K protects against classical vitamin K deficiency bleeding (Clark & James, 1995) but is less effective for prevention of this condition later in life (Tönz & Schubiger, 1988; Ekelund, 1991). Without vitamin K prophylaxis, the incidence of late vitamin K deficiency bleeding in Europe was estimated to be 40–100 per million livebirths, whereas in Asia the condition appears to be considerably more common (Hanawa, 1992; Choo et al., 1994).

Since intramuscular vitamin K prophylaxis has proven effective against late deficiency bleeding, 1 mg of vitamin K at birth was recommended in most western countries (von Kries, 1991). After reports of a potential association between vitamin K prophylaxis and the risk for childhood cancer (Golding et al., 1990, 1992), several countries switched to oral prophylaxis regimens with repeated doses of phylloquinone (Hill, 1994; Doran et al., 1995; Hansen & Ebbesen, 1996; Cornelissen et al., 1997). The optimal oral dose regimen remains to be established (von Kries, 1999).

1.3.4 Cholestatic and malabsorption syndromes

Vitamin K deficiency is observed in patients with cholestatic jaundice, cystic fibrosis, primary biliary cirrhosis and other diseases. In most cases, however, vitamin K deficiency is detectable only by measuring the plasma concentrations of vitamin K or with sensitive biochemical markers of vitamin K deficiency (Cornelissen et al., 1992; O'Brien et al., 1994; Kowdley et al., 1997). Bleeding is observed only rarely. Additional risk factors, such as therapy with antibiotics that interfere with vitamin K metabolism, may cause bleeding in patients with cystic fibrosis (Nowak et al., 1997). Some patients with this disease are given vitamin K supplements, although there are no uniform recommendations (Durie, 1994).

1.3.5 Vitamin supplementation to overcome side-effects of drugs that interfere with vitamin K metabolism

An important indication for vitamin K supplementation is the side-effects of drugs that interfere with its metabolism. Mothers on antiepileptic drugs, for example, are at high risk of delivering an infant with manifest vitamin K deficiency (Cornelissen et al., 1993a) and intracranial bleeding (Renzulli et al., 1998).

Hypoprothrombinaemia may be caused by some cephalosporins, especially those containing an N-methylthiotetrazole side-chain, and may require vitamin K supplementation (Breen & St Peter, 1997).

1.3.6 Vitamin K therapy

(a) Overdosage of vitamin K antagonists

The coumarin derivatives acenocoumarol, phenprocoumon and warfarin are among the most commonly used oral anticoagulants (Keller et al., 1999). The clinical symptom of overdosage of these drugs is bleeding. A tendency to bleed is also increased by individual susceptibility to one of these anticoagulants, interference with other drugs or poor dietary intake of vitamin K. The biochemical indicator for overdosage is an excessive prolongation of the prothrombin time. Minor bleeding is most commonly managed by temporarily discontinuing treatment and by giving vitamin K to counteract the effects of the coumarin derivative. In the case of major bleeding, especially intracranial haemorrhages, higher doses of vitamin K and use of prothrombin complex concentrates are recommended to induce immediate reversal of anticoagulation (Pindur et al., 1999). In the past, the oral or intravenous dose of phylloquinone used to counteract supratherapeutic anticoagulation was 10–50 mg (Fetrow et al., 1997). Much lower doses have been proposed recently. In asymptomatic patients, a 1-mg oral dose of vitamin K was shown to reduce the international normalized ratio effectively (Crowther et al., 1998). Low subcutaneous doses of phylloquinone are an effective alternative to intravenous administration of phylloquinone in the treatment of warfarin-induced hypoprothrombinaemia (Fetrow et al., 1997).

(b) Prevention of intracranial haemorrhage in very-low-birth-weight, premature infants

The effect of high doses of vitamin K given to women at imminent risk of early preterm parturition has been studied with the primary aim of preventing periventricular haemorrhage and the associated neurological injury in the infant. A first meta-analysis of the trials came to the conclusion, however, that it is ineffective (Thorp et al., 1995).

1.3.7 Other uses

Menadione is of industrial importance as an intermediate in the synthesis of phylloquinone, and salts of its bisulfite adduct are used as stabilized forms in the animal feed industry. Commercially significant forms are menadione sodium bisulfite and menadione dimethyl pyrimidinol (Van Arnum, 1998).

Menaquinone-4 has been used in Japan at high doses for the treatment of osteoporosis (Shearer, 1997).

1.4 Occurrence

Phylloquinone is widely distributed in higher plants and in some blue–green algae. It is present in many foods, especially leafy green vegetables and some vegetable oils. Table 2 shows the concentrations in some common foods (Booth *et al.*, 1995; Shearer *et al.*, 1996; Booth & Suttie, 1998).

The Total Diet Study of the US Food and Drug Administration is conducted periodically to monitor the safety and nutritional quality of the US food supply by assessing the levels of nutrients and contaminants in daily diets. It is based on the collection and analysis of 265 core foods. Intakes are estimated from the concentrations of individual nutrients and contaminants in the core foods and the mean consumption of the foods in each population group. The quantitative contributions of specific foods to the phylloquinone intake of the total population are presented in Table 3. Table 4 gives the estimated daily intake in 1990 for 14 categories of age and sex (Booth *et al.*, 1996).

Phylloquinone has been determined by several analytical methods in human milk, in cow's milk, in many brands of infant formula and in the oils that have been added to infant formulas for many years. Some of the concentrations found in each of these sources are presented in Table 1.

Menaquinones are synthesized by bacteria. They have a more restricted distribution in the diet than phylloquinone, and nutritionally significant amounts probably occur only in animal liver and some fermented foods, including cheese. Menaquinones are also synthesized by specific inhabitants of the human gut microflora. The major intestinal forms are MK-10 and MK-11 produced by *Bacteroides*, MK-8 by *Enterobacteria*, MK-7 by *Veillonella* genus and MK-6 by *Eubacterium lentum* (Shearer *et al.*, 1996). The total concentration of menaquinones in human distal colonic contents is about 20 µg/g dry weight, with MK-10 predominating (Conly & Stein, 1992; Shearer, 1995). It seems likely that menaquinones synthesized by the gut microflora make a significant contribution to human tissue stores and are used by the hepatic vitamin K-dependent carboxylase, but the extent of this contribution remains uncertain (Shearer, 1995; Suttie, 1995).

1.5 Regulations and guidelines

Phylloquinone is listed (as phytomenadione or phytonadione) in the British, Chinese, Czech Republic, European, French, German, International, Japanese, Swiss and US pharmacopoeias (Royal Pharmaceutical Society of Great Britain, 1999; Swiss Pharmaceutical Society, 1999).

Table 2. Phylloquinone content of common foods[a]

0.1–1.0 μg/100 g	1–10 μg/100 g	10–100 μg/100 g	100–1000 μg/100 g
Avocado [1]	Apple pie [11]	Asparagus [60]	Broccoli [179–180]
Banana [0.1]	Apples [6]	Beans, runner [26]	Brussels sprouts [147–177]
Beef, steak [0.8]	Aubergines [6]	Beans, French [39]	Cabbage [145–339]
Bread, white [0.4]	Baked beans [3]	Beans, broad [19]	Canola oil [127]
Chicken, thigh [0.1]	Barley [7]	Beef chow mein [31]	Collards [440]
Coconut oil [0.5]	Beef, corned [7]	Cabbage, red [19]	Kale [618]
Cod, fresh, fillet [< 0.1]	Beef, minced [2]	Cauliflower [20–31]	Lettuce [122–129]
Cornflakes [< 0.1]	Bilberries [4]	Chick peas [21]	Rapeseed oil [123]
Flour, white [0.8]	Bran, wheat [10]	Coleslaw [80]	Salad greens [315]
Grapefruit [< 0.1]	Bread [3]	Cottonseed oil [60]	Soya bean oil [173–193]
Ham, tinned [0.1]	Bread, wholemeal [2]	Cucumbers [20–21]	Spinach [380]
Maize [0.3]	Butter [7]	Dry lentils [22]	Watercress [315]
Mangoes [0.5]	Carrots [6–10]	Dry soya beans [47]	
Melon, yellow [0.1]	Cheeses, various [2–6]	Greengages [15]	
Melon, water [0.3]	Chocolate, plain [2]	Green beans [33]	
Milk, cows [0.6]	Corn oil [3]	Green peas [24]	
Mushrooms [0.3]	Courgettes [3]	Iceberg lettuce [35]	
Oranges [< 0.1]	Cranberries [2]	Margarine [42]	
Parsnips [< 0.1]	Cream, double [6]	Mayonnaise [41]	
Peanuts, roasted [0.4]	Dates, fresh [6]	Muffins [25]	
Pilchards, in brine [0.6]	Doughnuts [10]	Mustard greens, cress [88]	
Pineapple [0.2]	Egg yolk [2]	Okra [40]	
Pork, chop, lean [< 0.1]	Eggs [2]	Olive oil [55–80]	
Potatoes [0.9]	Figs, fresh [3]	Peas [34]	
Rice, white [0.1]	French fries [5]	Potato chips [15]	
Rice, brown [0.8]	Grapes, black [8]	Salad dressings [100]	
Salmon, tinned, in brine [0.1]	Grapes, green [9]	Tuna in oil [24]	
Sausage, pork or beef [0.2]	Hamburger and bun [4]		
Spaghetti [0.2]	Hot dog and bun [3]		
Tuna, tinned, in brine [0.3]	Lasagna [5]		
Turnips [0.2]	Leeks [10]		
Yoghurt [0.8]	Liver, lamb [7]		
	Liver, ox [4]		
	Macaroni with cheese [5]		
	Nectarines [3]		
	Oats [10]		
	Palm oil [8]		
	Peaches, fresh [4]		
	Pears [6]		
	Peppers, green [6]		
	Peppers, red [2]		
	Pizza [4]		
	Plums, red [8]		
	Potatoes [1]		
	Raisins [4]		
	Rhubarb [4]		
	Safflower oil [3]		
	Strawberries [3]		
	Sunflower oil [6]		
	Swedes [2]		
	Tomatoes [6]		
	Wheat [8]		

From Shearer et al. (1996); Booth & Suttie (1998)
[a] Numbers in brackets are actual levels measured. The phylloquinone content of oil-based preparations varies widely depending on the source of the oil used.

Table 3. Contribution of certain food groups to total adult intake (%) of phylloquinone in the USA, stratified by age and sex

Food group	Age group							
	25–30		40–45		60–65		≥ 70	
	Men	Women	Men	Women	Men	Women	Men	Women
Milk and cheese	1.7[a]	1.4	0.9	0.9	1.0	0.9	0.8	0.8
Eggs	3.6	2.5	2.1	1.7	2.4	1.3	1.7	1.4
Meat, poultry, fish	4.8	4.2	4.6	4.0	5.7	4.3	4.8	2.8
Legumes and nuts	1.3	0.5	0.5	0.6	0.7	0.4	0.7	0.6
Grain products	4.4	4.3	3.8	3.4	4.6	3.3	4.6	3.1
Fruits	1.3	1.4	1.4	1.6	1.7	2.0	2.5	2.2
Vegetables	51	56	60	61	59	67	63	73
Mixed dishes and meals	16	14	13	12	9.1	7.1	7.2	4.8
Desserts	4.9	4.2	4.3	3.8	4.6	5.1	5.2	3.9
Snacks	2.6	1.7	1.4	1.5	1.0	0.7	0.7	0.2
Condiments, sweeteners	1.3	1.0	0.6	1.0	1.0	1.0	1.2	0.9
Fats, dressings	6.8	8.7	7.7	8.1	9.1	6.3	7.3	5.1
Beverages	0.2	0.2	0.2	0.2	0.2	0.2	0.1	0.2

From Booth et al. (1996)
[a] Percentages in columns may not add up to 100% as values were rounded to the nearest 0.1.

The Food and Drug Administration (1999) requires that all infant formulae sold in the USA contain a minimum of 4 µg/100 kcal (0.2 mg/kg) vitamin K; and that any vitamin K added should be in the form of phylloquinone.

Menadione is listed in the Austrian, Belgian, British, Dutch, European, French, German, International, Italian, Portuguese, Swiss and US pharmacopoeias, and menadione sodium bisulfite is listed in the Belgian, International, Swiss and US pharmacopoeias (Royal Pharmaceutical Society of Great Britain, 1999; Swiss Pharmaceutical Society, 1999). Menadiol sodium phosphate is listed in the British, Czech Republic and US pharmacopoeias (Swiss Pharmaceutical Society, 1999).

2. Studies of Cancer in Humans

The association between childhood cancer and vitamin K administered during the perinatal period with a view to preventing haemorrhagic disease of the newborn has been investigated in a number of studies (summarized in Table 5). The prophylactic use of vitamin K in newborns has varied with time, geographical location and among hospitals within countries. Some hospitals during some periods have had a selective policy based on the indications low birth weight, prematurity and operative delivery.

Table 4. Estimated and recommended mean dietary intakes of phylloquinone in the USA, stratified by age and sex

Population group	Phylloquinone intake (μg/day)	
	Estimate[a]	Recommended
Infants		
6-month-old infants	77	10
Children		
2-year-old children	24	15
6-year-old children	46	20
10-year-old children	45	30
14–16-year-old girls	52	45–55
14–16-year-old boys	64	45–65
Younger adults		
25–30-year-old women	59	65
25–30-year-old men	66	80
40–45-year-old women	71	65
40–45-year-old men	86	80
Older adults		
60–65-year-old women	76	65
60–65-year-old men	80	80
> 70-year-old women	82	65
> 70-year-old men	80	80

From Booth et al. (1996)
[a] From Total Diet Study

The hypothesis that vitamin K might be a risk factor for childhood cancer was generated on the basis of the results of a cohort study of 16 193 infants delivered in Great Britain in one week of April 1970, who were followed up at ages five and 10. The 33 cases included in the study were in patients who had died from cancer or were identified through cancer registration as having a cancer diagnosed before the age of 10. An unexpected statistically significant association was found between childhood cancer and administration of any drug during the first week of life (Golding et al., 1990), and 16 of the 18 patients who had received drugs during the first week of life had received vitamin K. Within the cohort, a comparison was made between the 33 cases and 99 controls matched with the cases for the age of the mother at the time of the birth of the child, parity, social class, marital status at delivery and whether the birth was single or multiple. Statistically significant associations were identified not only with drug administration during the first week of life, but also with antenatal X-rays, antenatal smoking, non-term delivery and use of pethidine or pethilorfan (a pethidine-containing drug) during labour. Only two of the 33 cases had fewer than two of these risk factors, whereas

Table 5. Studies on childhood cancer and vitamin K administered during the perinatal period

Area and period of birth of children, period of diagnosis, reference	Age group	Type of preparation containing vitamin K	Method of determining route of administration	Route of administration	Prevalence of exposure to vitamin K in controls (%)	Group or subgroup	Total no. of cases	Total no. of controls	RR (95% CI)	Matching variables	Adjustment variables
Great Britain; birth, 1970; diagnosis, 1970–80 (Golding et al., 1990)	5 and 10 years	NR	NR	Oral, intravenous, intramuscular	31.2[a] (for drug to neonate) (28.1 for vitamin K to neonate)	All cancers	33	99 (96 with data on drug intake)	2.6 (1.3–5.2)[a] (drug to neonate)	Maternal age, parity, social class, marital status, multiplicity	Social class, smoking during pregnancy, X-ray in pregnancy, term delivery and pethidine in labour
Case–control studies											
United Kingdom, Bristol; birth, 1965–87; diagnosis, 1971–91 (Golding et al., 1992)	0–14 years[b]	Konakion[c]	Recorded in medical records or imputed on the basis of year of birth, type of delivery and whether or not infant admitted to special care	Intramuscular[d] Oral Intramuscular[d]	40.6[e] 35.1[e]	All cancers Leukaemia Cancers other than leukaemia	180 [g] [i]	544 544 544	2.2 (1.1–4.4)[f] 1.2 (0.5–2.7)[f] 2.7 (1.3–5.2)[h] 1.7 (1.0–2.8)[h]		Hospital and year of delivery
			Recorded in medical records	Intramuscular[j]	NR	All cancers	NR	NR	2.0 (1.2–3.3)[h] (route of administration clearly stated)		
USA, multicentre; birth, 1959–66; diagnosis, 1959–66 (Klebanoff et al., 1993)	1 day–8 years	Aquamephyton Konakion[k]	Review of records prospectively completed by labour and delivery room observers	Intramuscular[j]	71.2	All cancers Leukaemia Cancers other than leukaemia	44 15 29	226 NR NR	0.84 (0.41–1.7)[f] 0.47 (0.14–1.6)[f] 1.1 (0.45–2.6)[f]	Follow-up time	

Table 5 (contd)

Area and period of birth of children, period of diagnosis, reference	Age group	Type of preparation containing vitamin K	Method of determining route of administration	Route of administration	Prevalence of exposure to vitamin K in controls (%)	Group or subgroup	Total no. of cases	Total no. of controls	RR (95% CI)	Matching variables	Adjustment variables
Germany, Lower Saxony; birth, 1975–93; diagnosis, 1988–93 (von Kries et al., 1996)	30 days–15 years	Konakion[c]	Determined from medical records	Intramuscular or subcutaneous	61.4	Leukaemia, brain tumours, nephroblastoma, neuroblastoma and rhabdomyosarcoma	272	334	1.0 (0.74–1.5)[h]	Sex, date of birth, locality or state	Type of region (urban or rural), social class and prematurity
						Leukaemia	136	334	1.0 (0.64–1.5)[h]		
						Nephroblastoma, neuroblastoma, rhabdomyosarcoma, CNS tumours	136	334	1.2 (0.77–1.8)[h]		
Northern England; birth, 1960–91; diagnosis, 1968–92 (Parker et al., 1998)	3 months–14 years	Konakion[c]	Determined from medical records (obtained from case notes)	Intramuscular	NR	All cancers	438	NR	0.96 (0.67–1.4)		
						All cancers except ALL	306	NR	0.83 (0.54–1.3)		
						All ALL	132	NR	1.4 (0.71–1.7)		
						ALL diagnosed at 1–6 years	94	NR	2.3 (0.98–5.2)		
			Determined from medical records, route imputed from hospital records if not recorded	Intramuscular	NR	All cancers	664	3442	0.89 (0.69–1.15)		
						All cancers except ALL	457	NR	0.79 (0.59–1.1)		
						All ALL	207	NR	1.2 (0.75–1.9)		
						ALL diagnosed at 1–6 years	144	NR	1.8 (1.0–3.2)		

Table 5 (contd)

Area and period of birth of children, period of diagnosis, reference	Age group	Type of preparation containing vitamin K	Method of determining route of administration	Route of administration	Prevalence of exposure to vitamin K in controls (%)	Group or subgroup	Total no. of cases	Total no. of controls	RR (95% CI)	Matching variables	Adjustment variables
United Kingdom, Scotland; birth, 1976–94; diagnosis, 1991–94 (McKinney et al., 1998)	0–14 years	Konakion[c]	Determined from medical records, route imputed from hospital records if not recorded	Intramuscular (recorded)	48.9	Leukaemia	150	284	1.2 (0.77–2.0)	Sex, date of birth, health board of residence	Social class and type of delivery
					51.0	ALL	129	247	1.2 (0.70–2.0)		
					36.0	ALL diagnosed at 1–6 years	90	174	1.2 (0.62–2.2)		
					48.2	Lymphoma	46	86	1.7 (0.59–5.0)		
					51.5	CNS tumours	79	141	1.1 (0.55–2.1)		
					59.5	Other solid tumours	142	266	0.6 (0.36–1.0)		
				Intramuscular (imputed)	62.4	Leukaemia	150	284	1.3 (0.78–2.1)		
					50.0	ALL	129	247	1.1 (0.65–1.9)		
					59.6	ALL diagnosed at 1–6 years	NR	NR	1.3 (0.70–2.5)		
					59.4	Lymphoma	46	86	1.6 (0.49–4.9)		
						CNS tumours	79	141	1.0 (0.49–2.2)		
						Other solid tumours	142	266	1.0 (0.61–1.8)		
United Kingdom, 16 hospitals with large maternity units, 1969–86; born 1968 onwards; Cardiff births survey (3 more hospitals) (Passmore et al., 1998a)	1–14 years	Konakion[c]	Determined from medical records, route imputed from hospital records if not recorded	Intramuscular	NR	All cancers	597	NR	1.4 (1.0–2.1)	Sex, month of birth, hospital of birth	
						Leukaemia			1.5 (0.82–2.9)		
						All cancers except leukaemia			1.4 (0.88–2.2)		
						ALL			1.7 (0.89–3.3)		
						ALL diagnosed at 1–5 years			1.0 (0.48–2.2)		

Table 5 (contd)

RR, relative risk; CI, confidence interval; NR, not reported; ALL, acute lymphoblastic leukaemia; CNS, central nervous system
[a] Drug given to neonate; 16 of 18 case patients and 27 of 30 controls who received drugs were given vitamin K.
[b] Passmore et al. (1998a)
[c] Konakion contains phenol, Cremophor EL (polyoxyl 35 castor oil), propylene glycol and phytomenadione (vitamin K_1) (see Table 6).
[d] The authors reported a few instances of intravenous administration among those who received vitamin K intramuscularly.
[e] Calculated for 507 controls with information also on type of delivery and admission to special care. The frequency of intramuscularly administered vitamin K in one hospital was 59.4%, in the other 23.9%; that of oral administration was 13.8% and 54.1% respectively.
[f] Reference category is no vitamin K.
[g] 74 cases of leukaemia were ascertained; it is not stated how many were included in the analysis.
[h] Reference category is either no vitamin K or vitamin K administered only by the oral route.
[i] 143 cases of childhood cancer other than leukaemia were ascertained; it is not stated how many were included in the analysis.
[j] One child in the sample received vitamin K orally.
[k] When Konakion was used, the preparation contained polysorbate-80 as emulsifier (rather than Cremophor EL), phenol and propylene glycol and phytomenadione (Rennie & Kelsall, 1994) (see Table 6).

45/99 (47%) of the controls had either no or only one risk factor. All but four of the mothers of the 16 cases who had received vitamin K had received pethidine or pethilorfan during labour. In a logistic regression analysis carried out on the whole cohort, in which social class was included with the other variables already mentioned, the relative risk associated with drug administration during the first week of life was 2.6 (95% confidence interval [CI], 1.3–5.2). [The Working Group noted that Cremophor EL was the only emulsifier used in Great Britain for vitamin K injection at the time (Draper & Stiller, 1992; Rennie & Kelsall, 1994; see Table 6.]

Table 6. Brands of vitamin K and vehicle used in different countries

	Konakion[a]		Aquamephyton[a] (USA)
	Germany/United Kingdom/Sweden	USA	
Antimicrobial agent			
Phenol	+	+	
Emulsifier			
Cremophor EL	+		
Polysorbate-80		+	+
Propylene glycol	+	+	
Benzyl alcohol			+

From Rennie & Kelsall (1994)
[a] Trade name for phytomenadione

2.1 Case–control studies

In most of the case–control studies, the reference group comprised infants who had not received vitamin K and/or those who had received it orally. This combination is justified because the plasma concentrations after intramuscular administration are more than 10 times higher than those after oral administration (McNinch *et al.*, 1985).

In a second study (Golding *et al.*, 1992), 195 children with cancer diagnosed in the period 1971–91 who had been born at two major maternity hospitals in Bristol, England, in the period 1965–87 were compared with 558 controls identified from the delivery books of these hospitals. The cases were ascertained from the oncology register of the regional paediatric oncology unit and from the National Registry of Children's Tumours. The basic method of control selection was to select every 300th birth in each year in each hospital. In view of the observation that the immediate effects of identical oral and intramuscular doses of vitamin K are different, the investigators sought to distinguish the effects of administration by the two routes. When the route of vitamin K administration was not recorded in the neonatal notes, a route was imputed on the basis of year of birth, the type of delivery and whether or not the infant was admitted to special care; the imputed route was identified in the absence of knowledge of case or control status. On the basis of 180 cases (92% of those for which notes were available) and 544 controls (98% of those for which notes were available), the relative risk (adjusted for hospital and year of delivery) for childhood cancer associated with intramuscular vitamin K was 2.2 (95% CI, 1.1–4.4) when compared with no vitamin K and 1.2 (95% CI, 0.5–2.7) for oral vitamin K. In view of the absence of an association with oral vitamin K in these data, the authors conducted a subsequent analysis in which the reference group was defined to include infants who had not received vitamin K or who had received it orally. The relative risk for leukaemia associated with intramuscular vitamin K was 2.7 (95% CI, 1.3–5.2) and that for other types of childhood cancer was 1.7 (95% CI, 1.0–2.8). Thus, there was no clear difference in the association by type of childhood cancer. When the analysis was confined to records in which the route was clearly stated, the odds ratio for all childhood cancer was 2.0 (95% CI, 1.2–3.3). These results could not be accounted for by other factors associated with the administration of intramuscular vitamin K, such as type of delivery or admission to a special care unit. Data were collected on 319 variables for all controls and for 111 cases of cancer ascertained from the oncology register of the regional paediatric oncology unit; these data were not obtained for the remaining 84 cancer cases. Of these variables, the presence of rubella antibody, resuscitation by intermittent positive pressure and paediatric estimate of gestation were statistically significant at the 1% level, which is what would be expected by chance. Adjustment for these and other variables reported to be associated with childhood cancer or known to be indicators for administering intramuscular vitamin K had little effect on the odds ratio for childhood cancer associated with vitamin K. Nineteen of the cases were diagnosed in the first year of life, and the possibility was considered that these cancers might have been present before the child was born and could therefore not have been initiated by an injection of vitamin K; however, the association persisted after exclusion of these 19 cases from the analysis. When the analysis was restricted to subjects who would have been followed for at least 10 years, by considering only those born in the period 1971–80, the relative risk for all childhood cancer associated with intramuscular vitamin K was 1.9 (95% CI, 1.1–3.4), similar to that assessed for all subjects. [The Working Group noted, as acknowledged by the authors, a large number of instances in which the information on potentially confounding variables was not available, for example on smoking in pregnancy. Medical records are not necessarily reliable sources of information about pregnancy and childbirth (Hewson & Bennett, 1987; Oakley *et al.*, 1990), and this, together with the fact that potential confounding was assessed only for a subset of cases, constitutes a limitation of the study. The relationship between the type of delivery and intramuscular administration of vitamin K differed markedly between the two maternity hospitals in Bristol in which the case and control subjects in the study had been born (Carstensen, 1992; Draper & Stiller, 1992). The association with childhood cancer is largely accounted for by data from one of the hospitals in which virtually all of the control infants who received intramuscular vitamin K had been born by an assisted delivery. This raises the issue as to whether bias arose in control selection in that hospital.]

A study in the USA was reported by Klebanoff *et al.* (1993) which was based on follow-up to the age of seven or eight years of 54 795 liveborn children of women enrolled between 1959 and 1966 in 12 centres contributing to the National Collaborative Perinatal Project. Neonates whose cancer was diagnosed or strongly suspected during the first day of life were excluded because vitamin K could not have been a factor in those cases. Vitamin K was administered in the delivery room or the nursery, and information about the administration was recorded with other events during and after delivery by observers who were not involved in the clinical care of the mother or the infant. Cancer was diagnosed in 48 of 54 795 liveborn children after the first day of life. For each case, five controls were selected and matched with the index case on length of follow-up. In spite of the prospective recording by the observers, the data on vitamin K administration were not recorded unambiguously for 43 infants; a review of hospital records without knowledge of case or control status resulted in data for 25 (58%) of these. The exposure status was unknown for four case children. The relative risk for all childhood cancer associated with vitamin K was 0.84 (95% CI, 0.41–1.7), and that for leukaemia was 0.47 (95% CI, 0.14–1.6; based on 15 cases). In the USA, only two brands, Aquamephyton and Konakion, have been approved for use (see Table 6). Konakion in the USA contains polysorbate-80 rather than Cremophor EL as an emulsifier and phenol as an antrimicrobial agent. In the study of Klebanoff *et al.* (1993), the relative risk for total childhood cancer associated with the two brands together was 0.6, whereas that for children who had received the phenol-containing preparation alone was 0.7. In this study, only one child had received vitamin K orally.

von Kries *et al.* (1996) carried out a case–control study of children born in 162 obstetric hospitals in Lower Saxony (Germany) during the period 1975–93 when only one vitamin K preparation, Konakion, the same as that used in the United Kingdom, was licensed for neonatal vitamin K prophylaxis. Of a total of 218 children with leukaemia identified as eligible, information on vitamin K prophylaxis was obtained for 136 (62%). For each leukaemia case, one control was selected from the municipality where the patient lived at the time of diagnosis (local control), and a second one (state control) from a municipality selected at random in Lower Saxony by means of a population-weighted sampling scheme. These controls were matched with cases by sex and date of birth. Case and control families were contacted initially by being sent a questionnaire. If a control family refused to collaborate in the study or did not return the questionnaire within three months, another control family was invited; control families that returned the questionnaire after more than three months were also included. Thus, a total of 305 local and 308 state controls were invited to participate. Information on vitamin K prophylaxis was obtained for 174 (57%) of the local controls and 160 (52%) of the state controls. As the study was performed as part of a population-based case–control study to explore possible causes of childhood leukaemia in Lower

Saxony, a third control group for the leukaemia study was identified which comprised cases of brain tumours, nephroblastoma, neuroblastoma and rhabdomyosarcoma. No population-based controls were selected for these cases, but they were used as additional cases in the study of vitamin K. Of a total of 246 potentially eligible cases of this type, information on vitamin K prophylaxis was obtained for 136 (55%). Data on vitamin K prophylaxis were abstracted from the birth report with no knowledge of the case or control status of each child. Information on the dose and route of vitamin K prophylaxis was obtained from the birth record or in the delivery book for 72% of the 272 cases of leukaemia and other cancers and 64% of the 334 controls. When this information was not available, the index child was assumed to have had the same exposure to vitamin K as the child nearest to the index infant in the delivery book with the same route of delivery and same perinatal morbidity (nine cases and six controls). When this could not be established, staff who worked in the delivery unit at the time when the index child was born were asked what kind of vitamin K prophylaxis the index infant would have received, given the birth weight and route of delivery (63 cases and 109 controls). Finally, similar information was sought from medical staff who did not work in the delivery unit at the time the index child was born (four cases and four controls). In the comparison with local controls ($n = 107$), the risk for leukaemia ($n = 107$) associated with intramuscular or subcutaneous administration of vitamin K relative to that for oral or no vitamin K prophylaxis was 1.2 (95% CI, 0.68–2.25). In the comparison with state controls ($n = 160$; leukaemia cases = 136), the relative risk was 0.82 (95% CI, 0.50–1.4). When the control groups were pooled ($n = 334$), the relative risk was close to unity (136 leukaemia cases), and the relative risk for brain tumours, nephroblastoma, neuroblastoma and rhabdomyosarcoma combined ($n = 136$) associated with vitamin K prophylaxis was 1.2 (95% CI, 0.77–1.8). When the analyses were repeated for subjects for whom vitamin K prophylaxis had been documented in birth records or delivery books, the results were almost unchanged, except in the comparison of leukaemia cases with local controls, which gave a relative risk of 2.0 (95% CI, 0.69–6.0). When the analyses were repeated for parenteral prophylaxis versus no prophylaxis, most of the relative risks were slightly decreased. The risk of the subgroup of cases of leukaemia in children aged 1–6 years was analysed as this was considered to be a relatively homogeneous subgroup, most of the cases having common acute lymphoblastic leukaemia. [The Working Group noted that it is not clear whether the decision to make this subgroup analysis was specified in the original study protocol or was made *post hoc*.] The risk relative to both control groups combined was 1.2 (95% CI, 0.69–2.15), in the comparison with state controls it was 0.99 (95% CI, 0.52–1.9) and in the comparison with local controls it was 2.3 (95% CI, 0.94–5.5). There was no difference between cases and controls in the source of information on vitamin K prophylaxis. The increased relative risk in the comparison with local controls could not be explained by any of the potential confounders. It would be expected that the policy of administration of vitamin K would be more likely to be similar for cases and local controls than for cases and state controls. Therefore, the relative risk would be expected to be closer to unity in the comparison between cases and local controls than in the other comparison, whereas the opposite was observed. The non-significantly increased risk relative to local controls may be a chance result in subgroup analysis with multiple testing, as acknowledged by the authors.

In a case–control study of childhood leukaemia based on births in three hospitals in England (Cambridge, Oxford and Reading), no association with intramuscular vitamin K, either as determined from hospital records (91 cases, 171 controls) or as imputed from hospital policy (132 cases, 264 controls), was found. In addition, no association was found specifically for acute lymphoblastic leukaemia (Ansell et al. 1996). Subsequently, Roman et al. (1997) reported a more detailed analysis of data on leukaemia and non-Hodgkin lymphoma diagnosed before the age of 30 years in subjects whose obstetric records were stored in the same three hospitals. Ninety-two per cent (132/143) of the cases of leukaemia were diagnosed at age 14 or less; these cases and their controls were included in the report of Ansell et al. (1996). There was no association between leukaemia and intramuscular vitamin K administration either recorded in the notes (relative risk, 1.2; 95% CI, 0.7–2.1) or imputed from information about hospital policy (relative risk, 1.2; 95% CI, 0.5–2.4). In view of the finding of von Kries et al. (1996), acute lymphoblastic leukaemia diagnosed between the ages of 1–6 years was considered; the relative risk associated with recorded administration (based on hospital notes) was 0.6 (95% CI, 0.3–1.4), and that based on hospital policy was again 0.6 (95% CI, 0.2–1.7).

Parker et al. (1998) identified 1432 children born in northern England between 1960 and 1991 from the regional Children's Malignant Disease Registry, in whom cancer was diagnosed in 1968–92 when they were aged between three months and 14 years while still resident in the region. The birth records of 701 of these children could not be traced, usually because the maternity unit had retained only its most recent records or because the unit had closed and the records could not be located. Thirty children who had been given vitamin K orally at birth and 16 cases in multiple births were excluded. The controls were selected by taking the fourth, eighth and 12th birth before and after the index birth from birth or admission registers for the hospital of birth of the index child. Towards the end of the study, the number of controls per case was reduced from six to three because of time constraints. When the birth notes for control children could not be located, or when the child selected was found to be on the Malignant Disease Register, the next possible control was selected. The fact of intramuscular administration of vitamin K or non-administration of vitamin K was recorded in the maternity unit records for 438 of 685 cases (case notes). [The Working Group noted that the corresponding proportion for controls was not specified.] There was no association between intramuscular vitamin K administration and either all cancers or all cancers other than acute lymphoblastic leukaemia. The relative risk for acute lymphoblastic leukaemia associated with vitamin K administration based on case notes was 1.4 (95% CI, 0.71–1.7; 132 cases). Two secondary analyses were conducted to consider cases typical of the peak incidence of leukaemia in early childhood. When the 51 children in the case note analysis who had T-cell leukaemia or for whom subtype characterization was not available were excluded, the relative risk for the 81 cases of non-T-cell lymphoblastic leukaemia was 1.8 (95% CI, 0.82–3.9). In an analysis of 94 children aged 1–6 years at diagnosis, the relative risk was 2.3 (95% CI, 0.98–5.2). In all of these analyses, adjusted relative risks were calculated separately for the specified potential confounding factors—sex, gestation, birth weight, opiates during labour, assisted delivery, signs of asphyxia at birth, admission to special care or neonatal blood transfusions. Except for adjustment for assisted delivery, admission to special care or opiate exposure in labour, none of these changed any of the relative risks by more than 10%. Adjustment for assisted delivery or admission to special care caused a larger rise in the relative risk. The relative risk for acute lymphoblastic leukaemia diagnosed at ages 1–6 was 2.4 (95% CI, 1.0–5.7) after adjustment for exposure to opiates and 3.6 (95% CI, 1.3–9.7) after adjustment for assisted delivery based on case note analysis. As in many of the other studies, information on hospital policy was obtained in order to impute exposure when this was unclear from medical records. This information was obtained by a research midwife and neonatal staff in each unit in the region and by a paediatrician from current and recently retired medical staff, and this independently obtained information was then cross-validated. When inconsistencies were identified, the case notes were sampled to determine what policy had actually been followed. This enabled a further 226 cases to be included at the analysis; 21 cases were excluded because the policy of the local unit could not be ascertained. The relative risks were similar to but somewhat lower than those in the analysis based exclusively on subjects for whom data on vitamin K exposure was obtained only from medical records. [The Working Group noted that it was unclear which hypotheses about subgroups had been pre-specified. Bias may have arisen from the fact that while a large proportion of cases had to be excluded there was a mechanism for adding controls when a control record was unobtainable. Availability of records might have associations with both perinatal health problems and subsequent development of childhood cancer.]

McKinney *et al.* (1998) carried out a case–control study on childhood cancer in Scotland using data abstracted from 76 hospital records. A total of 500 cases of cancer diagnosed in children aged 0–14 years during the period 1991–94 while resident in Scotland were identified. Controls matched on age, sex and health board of residence were randomly selected from among all eligible children registered for primary care within each health board. A total of 1338 eligible controls was identified. A total of 460 mothers of cases (92%) and 861 mothers of controls (64%) were interviewed, and medical notes were abstracted for 440 cases and 802 controls. The data set for statistical analysis was restricted to matched sets, and information was lost for 23 cases without matched controls and 25 controls without a matched case. Therefore, 417 cases and 777 controls were included in the matched case–control analysis. Vitamin K was recorded as given or definitely not given only when this was mentioned in the notes. Similarly, the route of administration was classified as intramuscular, oral or not recorded. None of the relative risks reported for leukaemias, acute lymphoblastic leukaemia, lymphomas, central nervous system tumours or other solid tumours, either crude or adjusted for social class and type of delivery, was statistically significantly different from unity. The adjusted relative risk for leukaemia associated with vitamin K given intramuscularly (recorded) in the neonatal period was 1.2 (95% CI, 0.77–2.0) and that for acute lymphoblastic leukaemia was 1.2 (95% CI, 0.70–2.0). In view of the findings of Parker *et al.* (1998, see above), the subset of acute lymphoblastic leukaemia diagnosed in children aged 1–6 years (90 cases, 174 controls) was also analysed, and the adjusted relative risk was found to be 1.2 (95% CI, 0.62–2.2). As nothing about vitamin K had been written in the medical records for a substantial proportion of children (37% of cases and 35% of controls), the authors also sought to impute exposure on the basis of hospital policies. Information on the vitamin K policies of hospitals in which over 500 infants were delivered annually was validated by abstraction of a sample of medical records and through consultations with hospital pharmacies and senior labour room midwives. For 100 (24%) cases and 191 (25%) controls, no hospital policy was available for any imputation. The relative risks for the specific diagnostic categories associated with intramuscular vitamin K administration in the neonatal period either as recorded in medical records or imputed from hospital policy were very similar to those calculated for subjects for whom only data from medical records were included. The adjusted relative risk for leukaemia was 1.3 (95% CI, 0.78–2.1), that for acute lymphoblastic leukaemia was 1.1 (95% CI, 0.65–1.9) and that for acute lymphoblastic leukaemia in children aged 1–6 years was 1.3 (95% CI, 0.70–2.5). Very few subjects were recorded as having or imputed to have been given vitamin K orally in the neonatal period (12 cases, 2.9%; and 33 controls, 4.3%).

Passmore *et al.* (1998a) identified cases of childhood cancer diagnosed at ages up to 14 years in persons who were resident in Great Britain and had been born in 16 hospitals with large maternity units in 1968 or later and diagnosed by the end of 1986 from the National Registry of Childhood Tumours (excluding retinoblastoma, Down syndrome or neurofibromatosis). The 16 hospitals were selected on the basis of a survey which showed that they had a selective policy for the use of vitamin K prophylaxis. Of 1092 cases initially identified as born in these hospitals, 523 were born in the years for which a policy was known and for whom the medical records were found. Four controls matched on sex, month of birth and hospital of birth were selected randomly from these registers. Medical records departments were asked to locate the records for each case and for one control. Initially, two out of each of the four potentially eligible controls were selected randomly for location by the medical records department. If the records department was unable to locate the notes of either of these, details were supplied of the other two. Controls with illegible records, twins, stillbirths and neonatal deaths were excluded. In addition, infants with severe neural tube defects or a birth weight of less than 1000 g were excluded, as they were unlikely to have survived to the age at which the case patient developed cancer. For these, an alternative control was selected by using the next suitable birth in the hospital birth register. [The numbers of control replacements were not specified.] A second group of cases from the same period was chosen from records of the National Registry of Childhood Tumours in order to identify cases of cancer among children included in a survey of more than 100 000 births in South Glamorgan, Wales. For each case, two controls matched for sex, month of birth and hospital were selected, applying the same set of exclusions. Medical records were sought for all cases and controls, and information on vitamin K administration taken from these records was supplemented by data from the birth survey, which was available for most but not all of the period of study. This added three further hospitals to the study, all of which had selective policies of vitamin K administration, and 74 cases. In the combined data (16 maternity units in England and Wales and the three hospitals included in the survey in South Glamorgan), the relative risk for childhood cancer of all types associated with intramuscular vitamin K administration was 1.4 (95% CI, 1.0–2.1). In the data for the 16 maternity units in England and Wales, the relative risk was 1.2 (95% CI, 0.77–1.9), while in the data from South Glamorgan, the relative risk was 2.1 (95% CI, 1.1–4.1). For the combined data and for the data from South Glamorgan, mode of delivery (forceps, vacuum extraction, breech or caesarean) was a statistically significant confounding variable, and adjustment for this reduced the relative risks to 1.1 for the combined data and 1.3 for the South Glamorgan data. In the combined data, the relative risk for leukaemia was 1.5 (95% CI, 0.82–2.85), that for acute lymphoblastic leukaemia was 1.7 (95% CI, 0.89–3.3) and that for acute lymphoblastic leukaemia diagnosed at ages 1–5 years was 1.0 (95% CI, 0.48–2.2). Again, adjustment for mode of delivery reduced the relative risks. [The Working Group noted that the substantially lower relative risk for the 1–5 year-old group than for all ages combined implies that the effect for children of other ages is higher than that for this group, in contrast to the observations of von Kries *et al.* (1996) and Parker *et al.* (1998).] The relative risk for non-leukaemia cancers was 1.4 (95% CI, 0.88–2.2) in the combined data and 2.4 (95% CI, 1.1–5.4) in the data from South Glamorgan. In the South Glamorgan data, none of the potential confounders that were adjusted for reduced the magnitude of the relative risk. [The Working Group noted that in the absence of an effect in the data from the 16 maternity units in England and Wales, the South Glamorgan finding may reflect an unidentified bias or be a chance finding.]

[The Working Group noted that in the subgroup analyses of acute lymphoblastic leukaemia diagnosed at 1–6 years carried out by Parker *et al.* (1998) and 1–5 years by Passmore *et al.* (1998a), adjustment for mode of delivery had contrasting effects. In the study of Passmore *et al.* it attenuated the relative risk associated with vitamin K, while in the study of Parker *et al.* the relative risk was increased.]

2.2 Ecological studies

These studies are summarized in Table 7.

Ekelund *et al.* (1993) investigated the association between childhood cancer and intramuscular administration of vitamin K in a study in Sweden based on linkage of the medical birth registry to the national cancer registry. The study was restricted to full-

Table 7. Ecological studies on childhood cancer and vitamin K administered intramuscularly during the perinatal period as Konakian[a]

Area and period of birth of children, period of diagnosis, reference	Age group	Method of determining route of administration	Prevalence of exposure in all children (%)	Group or subgroup	Total no. of cases	No. of patients	RR (95% CI)	Reference category
Sweden; full-term non-instrumental deliveries; birth, 1973–89 (follow-up, 1992); birth, 1982–89 (Ekelund et al., 1993)	30 days–17 years 30 days–9 years	Imputed on the basis of hospital policy	78.4 66.2	All cancers Leukaemia All cancers Leukaemia	2287 708 722 250	Nos of patients given vitamin K intramuscularly and orally 1 357 734 1 357 734 655 454 655 454	1.0 (0.88–1.2)[b] 0.90 (0.70–1.2)[b] 1.1 (0.88–1.4) 1.2 (0.69–2.1)	Vitamin K orally
Denmark, 1945–54, 1975–84; (Olsen et al., 1994)	1–12 years	Imputed from recommended practice as: no vitamin K for births 1945–54; intramuscular administration for births 1975–84	NR	All cancers Leukaemia	NR	No. of patients given vitamin K intramuscularly and not given vitamin K 1 421 808 1 421 808	1.3 (1.2–1.4) 1.0 (0.9–1.1) at age 13	No vitamin K

RR, relative risk; CI, confidence interval; NR, not reported
[a] Konakion contains phenol, Cremophor EL (polyoxyl 35 castor oil), propylene glycol and phytomenadione (see Table 6).
[b] Adjusted for year of birth

term infants (gestation, 37–42 weeks) who had survived and who were born in 1973–89 after a delivery without use of forceps or vacuum extraction. The infants were followed up to 1 January 1992. Cancers diagnosed within 30 days of birth were regarded as congenital and were excluded from the analysis. Routines for administration of vitamin K were obtained from all 95 maternity hospitals and validated for a subset of 102 children with cancer and 100 control children randomly selected from among those who, according to the information on routine exposure, received intramuscular vitamin K, and 94 children with cancer and 100 control children from among those who should have received oral vitamin K. The doses of vitamin K given in Sweden were similar to those given in the United Kingdom, and the same preparation was used (phylloquinone, Konakion, see Table 6). When the method of administration of vitamin K was recorded, it agreed with the stated routine method of administration in 92% of the 235 cases for which individual information could be found. The relative risk for all childhood cancer associated with a hospital policy of intramuscular administration of vitamin K as compared with oral administration was 1.0 (95% CI, 0.88–1.2, after stratification for year of birth). The relative risk for leukaemia was 0.90 (95% CI, 0.70–1.2).

Olsen *et al.* (1994) compared the cumulative risk of childhood cancer among children aged 1–15 years who were born during the period 1945–54 ($n = 835\,430$), in which no vitamin K was administered, those aged 1–15 years born during the period 1960–69 ($n = 797\,472$), in which pregnant women received oral vitamin K, and those aged 1–13 years born during the period 1975–84 ($n = 586\,378$), in which virtually all newborns received vitamin K intramuscularly. There was a small increase in risk for all tumour types combined, due mainly to lymphoma in boys and neuroblastoma in boys and girls. There was no trend for childhood leukaemia. The preparation was the same as that used in the United Kingdom (Draper & McNinch, 1994).

In addition to the case–control study in northern England described above, Parker *et al.* (1998) compared the incidence of acute lymphoblastic leukaemia diagnosed in children aged up to 14 years who were born in hospital units in which all infants received vitamin K, with those born in units where less than a third received this prophylaxis. As described above, information on hospital policy was obtained separately and independently by two people and then cross-validated. In units with a policy of selective prophylaxis, less than 30% of infants received intramuscular vitamin K at birth, while in units offering universal prophylaxis, sampling of case notes showed that more than 95% of babies received vitamin K. The risk for acute lymphoblastic leukaemia in children born in hospitals with a policy of universal prophylaxis relative to those born in hospitals with a policy of selective prophylaxis was 0.95 (95% CI, 0.78–1.2). The relative risk of the subgroup diagnosed at 1–6 years was 1.05 (95% CI, 0.82–1.35). [The Working Group noted that the cases included in this analysis overlapped with those included in the case–control study, so that the results are not independent].

Passmore *et al.* (1998b) carried out a similar comparison of cancers of all types other than retinoblastoma or associated with Down syndrome or neurofibromatosis diagnosed in children aged 1–14 years who were born in 94 hospital units in Great

Britain. Information on hospital policy for neonatal vitamin K was obtained during the case–control studies of Passmore *et. al.* (1998a) and Ansell *et al.* (1996), described above, for 30 hospitals in Scotland from members of the Scottish Neonatal Network and from paediatricians for 41 of a further 80 hospitals in England and Wales in which more than 25 children who subsequently developed cancer had been born in the period 1968–85. The observed numbers of cases in hospitals with universal and selective policies were compared with the numbers expected on the basis of national rates. Separate analyses were carried out for births in hospitals that followed one policy throughout the period of study and births in hospitals in which the policy changed during the period of study. A large number of observed:expected ratios were calculated. The ratio for all cancers was 0.97, that for leukaemia at 1–14 years was 1.03, and that for acute lymphoblastic leukaemia at 1–5 years was 1.01 for hospitals with a consistent, non-selective policy. The ratio tended to be smaller in hospitals with a selective policy than in those offering universal prophylaxis. The only statistically significant ($p < 0.05$, two-tailed test) departure from unity indicated a lower risk for cancer other than leukaemia among children born in hospitals offering universal prophylaxis that those born in hospitals consistently offering selective prophylaxis in Scotland. [The Working Group noted that the cases included in this analysis overlapped with those in the case–control studies of Parker *et al.* (1998) and Ansell *et al.* (1996), so that the results are not independent.]

3. Studies of Cancer in Experimental Animals

No reports of studies specifically designed to investigate the carcinogenicity of vitamin K substances were available to the Working Group. One study on the initiating effects of menadione in an assay of liver foci in rats was available (Denda *et al.*, 1991) but could not be evaluated owing to methodological limitations.

4. Other Data Relevant to an Evaluation of Carcinogenicity and its Mechanisms

The studies summarized in this section should be considered in the light of the differences between naturally occurring forms of vitamin K that have a lipophilic side-chain at the 3-position of the 2-methyl-1,4-naphthoquinone (menadione) ring structure (phylloquinone and menaquinones) and the synthetic forms which lack this side-chain (menadione and its water-soluble derivatives). Lack of this side-chain results in profound differences in the absorption, tissue distribution and metabolism of natural K vitamins. Importantly, the lack of a lipophilic side-chain is the reason for the increased chemical reactivity and greater toxicity of menadione when compared with phylloquinone and menaquinones. In the strict sense, menadione is a provitamin K, because it is biologically active for the synthesis of vitamin K-dependent proteins only after conversion to the naturally occurring menaquinone-4 (four prenyl units) *in vivo*.

4.1 Absorption, distribution, metabolism and excretion

4.1.1 *Humans*

(*a*) *Intestinal absorption and plasma transport in adults*

The major dietary form of vitamin K is phylloquinone (Shearer *et al.*, 1996). It is absorbed chemically unchanged from the proximal intestine after solubilization into mixed micelles composed of bile salts and the products of pancreatic lipolysis. In healthy adults, the efficiency of absorption of phylloquinone in its free form is about 80% (Shearer *et al.*, 1974), but the efficiency of absorption from green leafy vegetables such as spinach is < 10% (Gijsbers *et al.*, 1996).

Within the intestinal mucosa, phylloquinone is incorporated into chylomicrons, is secreted into the lymph and enters the blood via the lacteals (Shearer *et al.*, 1970, 1974). After a phylloquinone-containing meal, the plasma concentration peaks between 3 and 6 h (Shearer *et al.*, 1970; Lamon-Fava *et al.*, 1998). Once in the circulation, phylloquinone is rapidly cleared at a rate consistent with its continuing association with chylomicrons and the chylomicron remnants that are produced by lipoprotein lipase hydrolysis at the surface of capillary endothelial cells. During the postprandial phase and after an overnight fast, more than half of the circulating phylloquinone is associated with triglyceride-rich lipoproteins, and the remainder is carried by low-density and high-density lipoproteins (Kohlmeier *et al.*, 1996; Lamon-Fava *et al.*, 1998). Although phylloquinone is the major circulating form of vitamin K, menaquinone-7 is present in plasma at lower concentrations and has a similar lipoprotein distribution to phylloquinone. While phylloquinone in blood is derived exclusively from the diet, it is not known what proportion of circulating menaquinones such as menaquinone-7 derives from the diet or the intestinal flora (Shearer *et al.*, 1996).

(*b*) *Plasma pharmacokinetics of phylloquinone in adults*

The plasma clearance of an intravenous dose of 1 mg [^{3}H]phylloquinone during the first 6 h resolved approximately into two exponential functions, the first with a half-time of 20–24 min and the second with a half-time of 121–150 min (Shearer *et al.*, 1972). The curves for clearance up to 12 h after an intravenous injection of a 10-mg dose of phylloquinone (Konakion MM) were similar to those after 1 mg and were consistent with a two-compartment (sometimes three-compartment) model in which the log-linear terminal phase over 3–12 h had a half-time of about 3 h (Soedirman *et al.*, 1996). A gradual slowing of the clearance rate was seen after the first 6 h (Shearer *et al.*, 1972, 1974), as was also found in a study of the clearance of pharmacological doses of 10–60 mg by Øie *et al.* (1988), who reported that the log-linear terminal elimination phase was not reached before 8–12 h and that the average half-time was 14 h (range, 8–22 h). This slowing of the clearance rate may be explained by the complexity of the plasma transport of phylloquinone, in which the proportion of phylloquinone associated with low-density and high-density lipoproteins increases progressively (Lamon-Fava *et al.*, 1998).

The plasma disposition of oral doses of 5–60 mg phylloquinone (Konakion or AquaMephyton) is similar to that found after a more physiological dose (≤ 1 mg), with peak plasma concentrations at 4–6 h followed by a rapid clearance phase (Shearer *et al.*, 1974; Park *et al.*, 1984; Øie *et al.*, 1988; Hagstrom *et al.*, 1995). After an oral dose of 10 or 50 mg Konakion, the plasma concentration declined from the peak absorptive level at a similar log-linear rate as that seen after intravenous administration, with a terminal half-time of about 2 h for measurements up to 9–12 h (Park *et al.*, 1984). The absorption of oral preparations of phylloquinone shows inter- and intra-individual variation and, for doses of Konakion ranging from 10 to 60 mg, the bioavailability was 10–63% (Park *et al.*, 1984) and 3.5–60% (Øie *et al.*, 1988).

The pharmacokinetics of phylloquinone after an intramuscular dose is completely different, showing sustained, slow release from the muscle site over many hours and marked inter-individual variation (Hagstrom *et al.*, 1995; Soedirman *et al.*, 1996). The pharmacokinetics may also be influenced by the solubilizing agent. The systemic availability of intramuscularly injected Konakion MM, which is a mixed-micellar solution of phylloquinone in natural solubilizers, the bile acid glycocholic acid and the phospholipid lecithin (Schubiger *et al.*, 1997; see Table 6), was irregular and < 65% in 20% of subjects (Soedirman *et al.*, 1996). After intramuscular injection of phylloquinone (AquaMephyton R), most of the substance was carried by low-density and high-density lipoproteins instead of by triglyceride-rich (very-low-density) lipoproteins as found after oral administration (Hagstrom *et al.*, 1995).

(c)   *Plasma pharmacokinetics of phylloquinone in neonates*

The pharmacokinetics of phylloquinone during the early clearance phase up to 6 h in neonates (of low birth weight) after intravenous injection was very similar to that of adults (Shearer *et al.*, 1972), declining bi-exponentially with median half-times of 23 and 109 min (Sann *et al.*, 1985).

An early study of the plasma disposition of 1 mg Konakion given orally or intramuscularly at birth showed wide inter-individual differences during the first 24 h, especially after oral administration (McNinch *et al.*, 1985). The peak plasma concentration after an oral dose occurred after 4 h; the median concentration was 73 ng/mL, which fell to 23 ng/mL after 24 h. The plasma concentration after administration of 1 mg of Konakion intramuscularly exceeded those after oral administration at all times, and after 24 h the median was 444 ng/mL. Physiologically, these concentrations compare with adult endogenous levels of about 0.5 ng/mL (Shearer, 1992).

In a comparison of the plasma concentrations of Konakion and Konakion MM in exclusively breast-fed infants at 24 h and 4 and 24 days after a single oral dose of 2 mg at birth (Schubiger et al., 1997), the mixed-micellar Konakion MM preparation resulted in higher median concentrations at all times, suggesting greater bioavailability. The largest difference was seen after four days, with median concentrations of 41 ng/mL Konakion MM and 12 ng/mL Konakion. By 24 days, the concentrations in both groups were mainly within the adult physiological range (0.3–0.4 ng/mL). An earlier study by the same group (Schubiger et al., 1993) had shown that a single oral dose of 3 mg Konakion MM resulted in higher plasma concentrations than a single dose of 1.5 mg of the same preparation given intramuscularly after four days. In this study, however, the plasma concentrations after 24 days were significantly higher after intramuscular injection, consistent with the hypothesis of the depot effect of intramuscular phylloquinone (Loughnan & McDougall, 1996; see also section 4.1.1(f)).

Stoeckel et al. (1996) pointed out that the terminal elimination plasma half-time of phylloquinone in neonates is probably longer than that in adults. They calculated from published studies that a realistic estimate of the terminal plasma half-time in neonates was 26–193 h (median, 76 h), as compared with 8–22 h (median, 14 h) in adults after intravenous administration (Øie et al., 1988). This longer terminal half-time may reflect the poorly developed organ systems of neonates and a reduced capacity to metabolize and excrete vitamin K (Stoeckel et al., 1996).

(d)   Plasma pharmacokinetics of menaquinone-4

Oral preparations of menaquinone-4 are used in Japan for the prophylaxis of vitamin K deficiency bleeding. The plasma profile of an oral dose of this preparation in five-day-old infants appeared to be similar to that of phylloquinone; after a 4-mg dose, a peak concentration of about 100 ng/mL was achieved after 3–4 h, before declining to about 30 ng/mL by 12 h (Shinzawa et al., 1989). The half-time of menaquinone-4 was not calculated.

(e)   Adult tissue reserves and distribution of vitamin K

Dietary vitamin K is delivered to the liver and possibly other tissues, including bone marrow, in the form of chylomicron remnants (Kohlmeier et al., 1996). The liver has often been assumed to be a major depot for vitamin K because it is the site of synthesis of the vitamin K-dependent coagulation proteins. Measurements of phylloquinone in livers obtained at autopsy from 32 adults in the United Kingdom revealed hepatic concentrations ranging from 1.1 to 21 ng/g wet tissue [2.4–47 pmol/g], with a median concentration of 5.5 ng/g [12 pmol/g]. The corresponding total liver stores of phylloquinone were 1.7–38 µg [3.8–85 pmol/g], with a median total store of 7.8 µg [17 pmol/g] (Shearer et al., 1988). Similar hepatic concentrations of phylloquinone were found in a smaller number of analyses of post-mortem samples from adults in Japan (10 ng/g) (Uchida & Komeno, 1988) and in The Netherlands (11 ng/g) (Thijssen & Drittij-Reijnders, 1996). The limited ability of the liver to store vitamin K is illustrated by the observation that the phylloquinone reserves are about 40 000-fold lower than those of vitamin A despite a daily dietary intake of vitamin K (~100 µg) which is only about 10-fold lower than that of vitamin A (~1000 µg). The distribution of the various forms of vitamin K in the liver is quite different from that in plasma in that the major transport form, phylloquinone, represents the minority of total hepatic stores (about 10%); the remainder comprises bacterial menaquinones, mainly menaquinones-6–13 (Shearer et al., 1988; Shearer, 1992; Shearer et al., 1996). The pattern of individual menaquinones in the liver varies considerably between individuals (Shearer et al., 1988; Uchida & Komeno, 1988; Thijssen & Drittij-Reijnders, 1996), perhaps reflecting their origin from the intestinal microflora (Shearer et al., 1996). This proposal is supported by the finding that two menaquinones, -10 and -11, which are major forms in most liver samples (Uchida & Komeno, 1988; Thijssen & Drittij-Reijnders, 1996), are known to be synthesized by *Bacteroides* species which are predominant members of the human intestinal flora (Conly & Stein, 1992); yet menaquinone-10 and menaquinone-11 do not make appreciable contributions to normal diets (Shearer et al., 1996).

Phylloquinone is also present in other human tissues. The concentration in the heart (~5 ng/g) [~10 pmol/g] is comparable to those in the liver, and even higher concentrations (~13 ng/g) [~25 pmol/g] are found in the pancreas, but lower concentrations (< 1 ng/g) [< 2 pmol/g] were detected in brain, kidney and lung. These tissues do not appear to contain appreciable concentrations of menaquinones except for the short-chain menaquinone-4. Particularly high concentrations of menaquinone-4 relative to phylloquinone are present in the kidney, brain and pancreas. Although these and other tissues contain the enzymes of the vitamin K epoxide cycle (see Figure 1) and carry out vitamin K-dependent carboxylation of protein precursors, this would not appear to account for the tissue-specific accumulation of menaquinone-4 and may suggest a hitherto unrecognized physiological role for menaquinone-4 in certain tissues (Shearer, 1992; Thijssen & Drittij-Reijnders, 1996). Indeed, menaquinone-4 may arise by tissue synthesis from phylloquinone itself (Davidson et al., 1998).

Osteocalcin is a major vitamin K-dependent bone protein synthesized by osteoblasts and therefore requires a source of vitamin K for γ-glutamyl carboxylation. Both trabecular and cortical bone contain ample reserves of vitamin K, with phylloquinone predominating and smaller amounts of shorter-chain menaquinones (Hodges et al., 1993; Shearer, 1997). With the absence of the typical hepatic forms menaquinones-10–13, the vitamin K content of bone resembles that of other extrahepatic tissues.

(f)   *Tissue stores and blood concentrations in neonates and infants*

Information on liver stores (the site of synthesis of vitamin K-dependent clotting proteins) in infants and their response to vitamin K prophylaxis is limited (Shearer et al., 1988; Guillaumont et al., 1993). The endogenous stores of vitamin K in the liver of the newborn differ both quantitatively and qualitatively from those of adults because the concentrations and total reserves of phylloquinone are lower than those of adults (Shearer et al., 1988) and because bacterial menaquinones are undetectable (Shearer et al., 1988; Guillaumont et al., 1993). The endogenous hepatic concentrations of

Figure 1. Cyclic metabolism of vitamin K for conversion of glutamate (Glu) residues to γ-carboxy glutamate (Gla) residues in vitamin K-dependent proteins

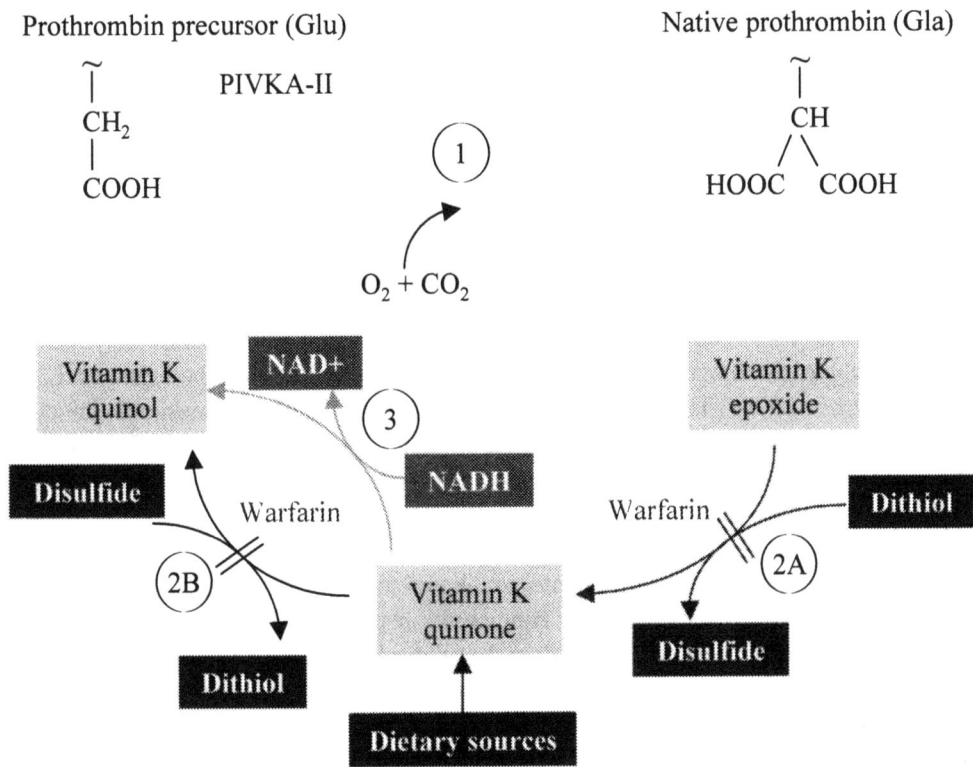

Adapted from Shearer (1992) and Suttie (1987)
PIVKA-II, protein induced by vitamin K absence factor II
The active form of vitamin K needed for carboxylation is the reduced form, vitamin K quinol. The carboxylation reaction is driven by a vitamin K-dependent carboxylase activity (1) coupled to vitamin K-epoxidase activity (1) which simultaneously converts vitamin K quinol to vitamin K 2,3-epoxide. Vitamin K 2,3-epoxide is reduced back to the quinone by vitamin K epoxide reductase (2A). The cycle is completed by the reduction of recycled vitamin K quinone by vitamin K reductase activity (2B). The activities of both vitamin K epoxide (2A) and vitamin K reductase (2B) are dithiol-dependent (dithiol and disulfide denote reduced and oxidized dithiols) and are inhibited by coumarin anticoagulants such as warfarin. Exogenous vitamin K may enter the cycle via an NAD(P)H-dependent vitamin K reductase activity (3) which is not inhibited by warfarin.

phylloquinone ranged from 0.3 to 6.0 ng/g (median, 1.4 ng/g) in preterm infants and from 0.1 to 8.8 ng/g (median, 1.0 ng/g) in term infants. The median hepatic concentration of 1 ng/g in term infants is equivalent to a total liver pool of about 0.1 µg phylloquinone, whereas the concentration is 5.5 ng/g and the pool 7.8 µg in adult liver. In infants who had received 0.5 or 1 mg phylloquinone at birth by intramuscular injection, these liver reserves were raised by some two to three orders of magnitude within 24 h. Hepatic phylloquinone concentrations may remain elevated for several weeks after injection: in two infants known to have received 1 mg phylloquinone by the intramuscular route and who survived 13 and 28 days, the total hepatic stores were 24 and 15 µg, respectively (Shearer *et al.*, 1988). Guillaumont *et al.* (1993) measured hepatic concentrations in post-mortem liver samples obtained within the first 48 h of death from infants who had received 2 mg phylloquinone intravenously or orally (in some cases combined with extra intravenous or oral doses of 1, 5 or 10 mg). In three newborns who survived < 24 h, the hepatic concentrations of phylloquinone ranged from 63 to 94 µg/g (total liver stores, 2800–7300 µg), which were four orders of magnitude higher than the endogenous concentrations of 0.002–0.008 µg/g (total liver stores, 0.1–0.9 µg). Between 24 and 48 h, the hepatic concentrations in 10 infants had fallen to a median of 8.4 µg/g (total liver stores, 550 µg), and in one infant who survived for five days it was 2.9 µg/g (110 µg). The quite rapid fall in hepatic stores presumably reflects the relatively rapid metabolism and excretion of vitamin K via the urine and bile (Shearer *et al.*, 1974). The lower hepatic concentration after intramuscular injection (Shearer *et al.*, 1988) compared with intravenous injection (Guillaumont *et al.*, 1993) is consistent with the idea that phylloquinone injected intramuscularly is released relatively slowly from the injection site (Loughnan & McDougall, 1996).

The reduced hepatic reserves of vitamin K in the human neonate are best explained by the existence of a barrier to placental uptake or transfer. This suggestion was originally made on the basis of the large concentration gradient of physiological concentrations of phylloquinone between maternal and cord blood plasma and the inefficient maternal–fetal transfer of pharmacological doses administered as an intravenous injection to the mother just before delivery (Shearer *et al.*, 1982). The poor placental transport of phylloquinone has been confirmed by others (Mandelbrot *et al.*, 1988; Yang *et al.*, 1989). There is now general agreement that the cord plasma concentration of phylloquinone is < 50 pg/mL [110 pmol/L] and that the average maternal–fetal concentration gradient is within the range 20:1 to 40:1 (Shearer, 1992).

Few longitudinal studies have been conducted of plasma concentrations in infants who were not given vitamin K prophylaxis. In one such study, cord plasma concentrations were compared for breast-fed and formula-fed infants and in blood on days 3, 7 and 28 after birth (Pietersma-de Bruyn *et al.*, 1990). In entirely breast-fed infants, the blood concentration rose from undetectable (< 20 pg/mL) at birth to mean values of 0.76, 0.49 and 0.49 ng/mL [1.7, 1.1 and 1.1 pmol/mL] on days 3, 7 and 28, respectively. In infants fed a milk formula containing 68 ng/mL phylloquinone, the plasma concentration rose steadily, with mean values of 1.4, 3.1 and 4.4 ng/mL [3.2, 6.8, and 9.9 pmol/mL] on days 3, 7 and 28, respectively. In another group of infants, Pietersma-de Bruyn *et al.* (1990) found that phylloquinone was undetectable in cord blood and in venous blood taken at 30 min but became measurable in venous blood after 12 h in 30% of infants (range, 0.04–0.40 ng/mL) and after 24 h in 60% of infants (range, 0.04–0.63 ng/mL).

A more detailed longitudinal comparison of plasma concentrations in breast-fed and formula-fed infants at 6, 12 and 26 weeks was made by Greer *et al.* (1991). This study is of special interest because the intakes of phylloquinone were also estimated at each time by measuring the vitamin K content of the milk and the volume of milk ingested (by weighing the infant). Such an assessment of the intake of phylloquinone depends on both the analytical accuracy of the measurements in breast milk and validation of the milk collection and sampling technique; both have proved problematical. The study of Greer *et al.* (1991) seems to have met the requisite criteria, and, although the concentrations were at the lower end of published values, they were in the same range as those in a carefully designed longitudinal study of the phylloquinone content of breast milk over the first five weeks of lactation (1–2 ng/mL) (von Kries *et al.*, 1987b). The results, summarized in Table 8, illustrate the extreme differences in intakes between breast-fed and formula-fed infants, which are also reflected in the plasma concentrations. The plasma concentrations in the formula-fed infants agree with those found by Pietersma-de Bruyn *et al.* (1990) after 28 days (4.5 ng/mL), and suggest that they plateau at around one month. The concentrations in entirely breast-fed infants aged one month and beyond tend, as in this study, to be at the lower end of the normal range in adults (~0.15–1.0 ng/mL; mean, ~0.5 ng/mL), even when the infants have received prophylaxis during the first week of life (Cornelissen *et al.*, 1992; Schubiger *et al.*, 1993, 1997). In contrast, the plasma concentrations in formula-fed infants are about 10-fold higher than the average values in adults (Pietersma-de Bruyn *et al.*, 1990; Greer *et al.*, 1991).

Table 8. Dietary intakes and plasma concentrations of phylloquinone in breast-fed and formula-fed infants aged 0–6 months in the USA

Age (weeks)	Phylloquine intake (µg/day)		Plasma phylloquinone (µg/L)	
	Breast-fed[a]	Formula-fed[b]	Breast-fed	Formula-fed
6	0.55	45	0.13	6.0
12	0.74	56	0.20	5.6
26	0.56	52	0.24	4.4

From Greer *et al.* (1991)
[a] The average breast-milk concentrations were 0.86, 1.1 and 0.87 µg/L (ng/mL) at 6, 12 and 26 weeks, respectively.
[b] All infants were fed a formula containing 55 µg/L (ng/mL) phylloquinone.

(g) *Hepatic catabolism*

The liver plays an exclusive role in the metabolic transformations leading to the elimination of vitamin K from the body. After intravenous doses of 45 µg to 1 mg [^{3}H]phylloquinone, about 20% of the radiolabel was excreted in the urine within three days, and 35–50% was excreted as metabolites in the faeces via the bile (Shearer *et al.*, 1974). Rapid depletion of hepatic reserves of phylloquinone was also seen in surgical patients placed on a low-phylloquinone diet (Usui *et al.*, 1990). These results suggest that the body stores of vitamin K are replenished constantly.

The route of hepatic catabolism leading to urinary excretion of vitamin K proceeds by oxidative degradation of the phytyl side-chain, probably involving the same enzymes used for ω-methyl and β-oxidation of fatty acids, steroids and prostaglandins. Two major metabolites or aglycones have been identified, which are carboxylic acids with five- and seven-carbon atom side-chains and are excreted in the urine as glucuronide conjugates (McBurney *et al.*, 1980). The biliary metabolites have not been clearly identified but are initially excreted as water-soluble conjugates and become lipid-soluble during their passage through the gut, probably through deconjugation by the gut flora. There is no evidence that the body stores of vitamin K are conserved by enterohepatic circulation. Vitamin K itself is too lipophilic to be excreted in the bile, and the side-chain-shortened carboxylic acid metabolites are not biologically active.

(*h*)   *Vitamin K-epoxide cycle*

In all tissues and cells found to carry out vitamin K-dependent carboxylation, the reaction has been shown to be intimately linked to a metabolic sequence known as the vitamin K-epoxide cycle. This cycle and the associated enzyme activities are shown in Figure 1. Its function seems to be to serve as a salvage pathway to conserve tissue reserves of vitamin K. In the course of γ-glutamyl carboxylation, vitamin K quinol is transformed into vitamin K epoxide, and the epoxide product is recycled in two steps; firstly by vitamin K epoxide reductase activity to produce vitamin K quinone and secondly by quinone reductase activity to produce the co-enzyme vitamin K quinol. Both these activities are thiol-dependent and are probably effected by the same enzyme (Suttie, 1987).

An important property of the dithiol-dependent epoxide and quinone reductase is their sensitivity to certain antagonists, especially those based on 4-hydroxycoumarin (e.g. warfarin) or indandione structures, which have long been used as oral anticoagulants. It is now clear that their anticoagulant action is based on their ability to inhibit epoxide reductase activity and block the recycling of the vitamin. The dithiol-dependent quinone reductase is also sensitive to warfarin, but the activity of a second quinone reductase catalysed by an NAD(P)H-dependent enzyme is less sensitive to warfarin inhibition and provides an alternative pathway for the reduction of vitamin K quinone to quinol in the presence of warfarin and other oral anticoagulant drugs (Shearer, 1992).

(i)   *Menadione and related water-soluble derivatives*

No studies appear to have been conducted on the absorption, distribution, metabolism or excretion of menadione and related compounds in humans. Water-soluble salts of menadione (vitamin K_3) were introduced for vitamin K prophylaxis in newborns in the early 1940s and, until their use was almost entirely superseded by phylloquinone in the early 1960s, there were no suitable techniques for measuring menadione, its salts or their metabolites other than by radioisotopic techniques.

4.1.2 Experimental systems

(a) Absorption

The route and mechanism of absorption of menadione is different from that of natural K vitamins such as phylloquinone. Jaques *et al.* (1954) fed [^{14}C]menadione to rats and measured the radiolabel in faeces, bile, lymph and urine. They deduced that all the absorbed menadione was transported exclusively via the portal vein to the liver, unlike phylloquinone which is transported by the lymphatic pathway. Also unlike phylloquinone, menadione participated in rapid entero-hepatic circulation after excretion in the bile. Mezick *et al.* (1968) suggested that, while the portal route is important in rats, menadione could also be transported via the lymphatic system. Direct evidence for some lymphatic transport was found by experiments in dogs, showing that about 10% of the absorbed menadione was recovered in thoracic duct lymph. In studies with bile exclusion, the absorption of menadione in rats was found not to be dependent on bile, as would be expected if menadione is absorbed predominantly via the portal vein.

(b) Tissue distribution, metabolism and excretion

Early experiments with [^{14}C]menadione in mice showed rapid clearance from the intramuscular injection site of doses of 0.1 and 1.0 mg (about 4–40 mg/kg bw) within the first hour and excretion in the urine. Radiolabel was initially detectable in blood, but the concentrations later declined. No significant accumulation was seen in tissues. Small amounts of activity were sometimes detected in liver, lung and kidney, but no significant amounts were found in skin, bone or muscle (Solvonuk *et al.*, 1952). A comparison of the tissue distribution of [^{14}C]menadione and [^{14}C]phylloquinone in rats after intravenous administration of a pharmacological dose (5 mg/kg bw) showed a much higher (24-fold) concentration of radiolabel in the livers of animals given phylloquinone than in those given menadione, and a fivefold greater accumulation of phylloquinone was found in the spleen. As in the studies of Solvonuk *et al.* (1952), no organ-specific accumulation of radiolabel was found in rats given labelled menadione, the highest proportions of radioactivity being found in urine and faeces (Taylor *et al.*, 1957). The rapid, extensive excretion of [^{14}C]menadione in the urine was confirmed by Losito *et al.* (1968) who found that rats excreted about 70% of an intravenous dose in the urine within 24 h compared with only about 10% of a dose of phylloquinone. They also showed that the urinary excretion of menadione (again unlike phylloquinone) was not dependent on an intact liver, as hepatectomized rats excreted the same amount of the dose (70%) as normal rats.

Rats given intracardial injections of a more physiological total dose (10 µg [30 µg/kg bw]) of high-activity 6,7-[^{3}H]menadione showed a pattern of excretion and tissue distribution similar to that of pharmacological doses, with recovery of 78–83% of the label in the urine after 18 h (Taggart & Matschiner, 1969). A similar pattern was seen in rats given an intraperitoneal injection of about 2 µg of the water-soluble salt menadiol diphosphate; 17 h later, some 43% of the radiolabel had been excreted in urine and about 4% in faeces. The compound was not concentrated in any tissue but was distributed throughout all body organs, and the distribution was the same in vitamin K-replete and -deficient animals. This water-soluble compound underwent rapid conversion to lipid-soluble forms, and the compound and its metabolites were found generally to be associated with the membranous fractions of cells (Thierry & Suttie, 1969).

Three major metabolites of menadione have been isolated from urine. After oral administration of menadione to rabbits, Richert (1951) isolated the sulfated compound 2-methyl-4-hydroxy-1-naphthyl sulfate and noted increased excretion of glucuronic acid. Hoskin et al. (1954) resolved three metabolites from rat urine, of which the major product was tentatively identified as 2-methyl-1,4-dihydroxynaphthalene-1,4-diglucuronide and another as the monosulfate conjugate found by Richert (1951). A third, minor metabolite appears to be a phosphate conjugate (Hart, 1958).

Losito et al. (1967) showed in an isolated perfused rat liver system that menadione glucuronide or sulfate conjugates are excreted but that the glucuronide is confined to bile and the sulfate to the perfusing blood. In rats in vivo, Losito et al. (1968) separated three major urinary metabolites, two of which were identified as the same glucuronide and sulfate conjugates as those found in their liver perfusion system (Losito et al. 1967). The chromatographic pattern in hepatectomized rats was different, but the major peak was shown to be a glucuronide conjugate, showing that animals have the capacity for extrahepatic conjugation of menadione with glucuronic acid (Losito et al., 1968).

(c)   Conversion of menadione to menaquinone-4

The vitamin K activity of menadione and its water-soluble salts depends on its specific metabolic conversion to menaquinone-4 (Suttie, 1985, 1991). The early evidence that both menadione and phylloquinone could be converted in birds and rats has been reviewed (Martius, 1967). The enzymic alkylation of menadione to menaquinone-4 was subsequently confirmed by more sophisticated techniques both in vivo in rats (Taggart & Matschiner, 1969) and in vitro in chick liver homogenates (Dialameh et al., 1970). The greatest alkylating activity was found in the microsomal fraction and was six to seven times higher in chick liver microsomes than in rat liver microsomes (Dialameh et al., 1970).

4.2 Toxic effects

4.2.1 *Humans*

(a) *Phylloquinone*

Reports of acute toxicity associated with pharmaceutical preparations of vitamin K as phylloquinone are rare and are often attributed to the vehicle of solubilization or other component of the preparation rather than to vitamin K itself. Adverse events associated with two products (Konakion and Konakion MM, currently representing about 50% of the market share worldwide) were monitored in a post-marketing surveillance programme, and the results were analysed and reviewed by Pereira and Williams (1998). During the period 1974 to July 1995, an estimated 635 million adults and 728 million children were prescribed Konakion or Konakion MM, and only 404 adverse events in 286 subjects were reported. Of these, the majority (96%) were associated with the older, Cremophor EL-based Konakion, which accounted for 95% of sales during this period. 'Skin, hair and nail disorders' were the most common adverse effects, accounting for about 25% of those reported. Rare cutaneous reactions to another vitamin K preparation, AquaMephyton, have been reported and are suspected to be immunologically mediated (Sanders & Winkelmann, 1988). This preparation contains a polyoxyethylated fatty acid derivative as the emulsifying agent (Rich & Drage, 1982).

The most serious reaction to vitamin K is anaphylactoid reactions after parenteral administration, but evidence that this effect is due to the polyethoxylated castor oil emulsifier (non-ionic detergent) Cremophor EL (polyethyleneglycolglycerol riconoleate) rather than vitamin K is twofold. Firstly, during the last 12 months of post-marketing surveillance (1994–95), 14 serious adverse events were reported from an estimated 21 million individuals receiving the Cremophor EL-based Konakion but none from the 13 million who received Konakion MM (Pereira & Williams, 1998). Secondly, anaphylactoid reactions in humans have been reported with other drugs solubilized with Cremophor EL, and there is experimental evidence in dogs that Cremophor EL and its components cause histamine release and hypotensive reactions (Lorenz *et al.*, 1982). The mixed-micellar Konakion MM preparation in which the vitamin K is solubilized by the naturally occurring components glycocholic acid and phosphatidylcholine appears to have far fewer anaphylactoid properties, only one probable anaphylactoid reaction having been reported in an estimated 66 million adults and 1–2 million infants and children who received this preparation (Pereira & Williams, 1998). Severe complications resulting in cardiopulmonary arrest were reported after intravenous injection of AquaMephyton (Rich & Drage, 1982).

(b) *Menadione*

The potential toxicity of preparations of menadione and its water-soluble derivatives to newborn infants is well established and has been reviewed (Vest, 1966).

The toxic reactions commonly include haemolytic symptoms evidenced by increased reticulocyte counts and Heinz body formation. In severe cases, overt haemolytic anaemia with haemoglobinuria may occur. The increased erythrocyte breakdown may lead to hyperbilirubinaemia and kernicterus. These effects are clearly dose-dependent, as premature infants given 30 mg of menadiol sodium phosphate had higher serum bilirubin concentrations, more Heinz bodies, lower haemoglobin concentrations and lower erythrocyte counts than those given 1 mg. The toxic reactions are more pronounced and may lead to severe haemolysis in premature infants and in infants with a congenital defect of glucose 6-phosphate dehydrogenase.

An explanation for the haemolytic toxicity of menadione is provided by studies showing the high reactivity of the 3-position of menadione with sulfhydryl compounds. Canady and Roe (1956) showed that when menadione is added to blood, it combines directly with blood proteins, probably by forming a thio ether at the 3-position. A later study showed that menadione reacts with both the haem groups and the β-93 thiol groups of haemoglobin and that it oxidizes the haem groups of oxyhaemoglobin, resulting in the formation of methaemoglobin (Winterbourn et al., 1979).

With elucidation of the toxic properties of menadione in newborn infants and, in the 1960s, the industrial synthesis of natural K vitamins, use of menadione for vitamin K prophylaxis in the newborn was discontinued in most countries (Vest, 1966).

4.2.2 Experimental systems

(a) Phylloquinone

Israels et al. (1983) suggested that vitamin K compounds may have a regulatory function in the metabolism of benzo[a]pyrene and possibly other compounds that are metabolized through the mixed-function oxidase system. This suggestion stemmed from their studies with menadione, which was shown to inhibit the conversion of benzo[a]pyrene to its more polar metabolites in rat liver microsomes in vitro. The inhibition showed a plateau (25% of control) at a concentration of 100 μmol/L [17 μg/mL]. With phylloquinone, no inhibition to polar metabolites was evident at concentrations up to 50 μmol/L [8.6 μg/mL], but at concentrations of 50–200 μmol/L [34 μg/mL] the inhibition increased rapidly, and at 500 μmol/L [86 μg/mL] the degree of inhibition was similar to that produced by menadione. The authors concluded that menadione acted as an electron acceptor. The weaker effect of phylloquinone at lower concentrations is perhaps due to its much greater lipophilicity and reduced penetration and solubility in microsomal membranes as compared with menadione; this explanation would also be consistent with the absence of a difference in solubility at higher concentrations of phylloquinone. In a later paper, Israels et al. (1985) found that microsomal metabolism of benzo[a]pyrene to polar metabolites in vitro was actually increased when the concentration of phylloquinone was reduced to 25 μmol/L [11.3 μg/mL] but, as in their earlier paper, was decreased at a concentration of 200 μmol/L [90 μg/mL].

In studies of the effects of menadione and phylloquinone on tumorigenesis in mice *in vivo*, the rate of tumour appearance and the death rate of mice given an intraperitoneal injection of benzo[*a*]pyrene were slowed by menadione but increased by phylloquinone. In parallel studies, tumorigenesis was inhibited in mice treated with the vitamin K antagonist warfarin and in mice made vitamin K-deficient by dietary deprivation. In these experiments, the compounds were given either before or both before and after benzo[*a*]pyrene (Israels *et al.*, 1983).

(*b*)   *Menadione*

Menadione also causes haemolytic anaemia in animals. The results of studies conducted in the 1940s were confirmed by Munday *et al.* (1991), who gave menadione (in 2% Tween 80) to Sprague-Dawley rats at a single dose of 750 μmol/kg bw per day [equivalent to about 100 mg/kg bw per day] for six consecutive days. This dose resulted in significant increases in splenic weight and decreased blood packed cell volume and haemoglobin concentration. Heinz bodies were observed in stained erythrocytes. There was no evidence that menadione caused haemaglobinaemia, suggesting that the haemolysis is not intravascular but is due to the destruction of damaged erythrocytes by cells of the reticuloendothelial system. Haemolysis was the only toxic change identified in rats dosed with menadione.

Melgar *et al.* (1991) examined the toxicity of menadione by giving Sprague-Dawley rats gradually increasing oral doses of menadione for six weeks, starting at 5 mg/kg bw per day and increasing to 20 mg/kg bw per day in the third week and 40 mg/kg bw per day in the fifth week of treatment. This dose regime was generally well tolerated with no relevant haematological changes, although there was a significant increase in spleen weight.

Many studies have been reported of the cytotoxicity of menadione in isolated and cultured cells of several types, including isolated rat hepatocytes (Mirabelli *et al.*, 1988; Shertzer *et al.*, 1992; Toxopeus *et al.*, 1993), rat renal epithelial cells (Brown *et al.*, 1991), bovine heart microvascular endothelial cells (Kossenjans *et al.*, 1996), Chinese hamster V79 cells (Ochi, 1996) and human hepatoma and leukaemia cell lines (Chiou *et al.*, 1998). The cytotoxicity of menadione has also been studied in isolated rat platelets (Chung *et al.*, 1997).

A characteristic finding in isolated rat hepatocytes treated with menadione is the appearance of numerous protrusions in the plasma membrane, known as blebs. Menadione produced a dose- and time-dependent increase in the frequency of cytoskeletal abnormalities; protein thiol oxidation seems to be intimately related to the appearance of surface blebs (Mirabelli *et al.*, 1988).

4.3 Reproductive and prenatal effects

4.3.1 *Humans*

No formal investigations of the safety of vitamin K in pregnancy have been found, although it has been proposed that vitamin K deficiency causes congenital malformations (Menger *et al.*, 1997). In a study of the efficacy of vitamin K for the prevention of the vitamin K deficiency induced by antiepileptic drugs, 16 women receiving antiepileptic drugs known to induce hepatic microsomal enzymes were treated orally with phylloquinone (Konakion) at 10 mg/day from the 36th week of pregnancy until delivery (mean, 29 days; range, 10–46). A control group of 20 epileptic women on similar antiepileptic drugs did not receive supplemental vitamin K. No adverse effects were observed in the infants of women given vitamin K supplementation. The median maternal plasma concentration of phylloquinone was raised 60-fold and the cord blood concentration was raised 15-fold, for a median maternal:cord blood ratio of 44 (Cornelissen *et al.*, 1993b).

4.3.2 *Experimental systems*

The offspring of mice treated with phylloquinone by injection had cleft lip and exencephaly (Schardein, 1993). Six pregnant Sprague-Dawley rats were dosed with 10 mg/kg bw phylloquinone (Konakion) daily on days 9–20 of gestation, and the fetuses were delivered on day 21 and examined for external malformations and the presence of haemorrhages only. No adverse effects were noted when compared with a group of five untreated controls (Howe & Webster, 1990). [The Working Group noted the small numbers of animals and the restricted fetal examination.]

Oral administration of menadione to groups of 10 pregnant Wistar rats throughout gestation at a dose of 0.15, 15 or 150 mg/day [approximately 0.6, 60 or 600 mg/kg bw per day] had no adverse effect on maternal body-weight gain, pregnancy rate or litter size, but the fetuses showed slightly retarded growth and delayed ossification at the high dose. No abnormalities were observed (Kosuge, 1973).

4.4 Genetic and related effects

4.4.1 *Humans*

Cornelissen *et al.* (1991) observed no difference in sister chromatid exchange or chromosomal aberration frequency in peripheral blood lymphocytes from six neonates given intramuscular phylloquinone prophylaxis and in those from six control neonates. The blood was taken 24 h after an intramuscular dose of 1 mg, at which time the plasma concentrations of phylloquinone ranged from 115 to 1150 ng/mL (mean, 536 ng/mL), compared with about 0.15 ng/mL in the control neonates.

Pizer et al. (1995) used the glycophorin A mutation assay to assess the risk for somatic mutations of NO and NN variant red cells of 64 infants aged 10 days to six months heterozygous for the MN blood group, who had received either oral, intramuscular or intravenous phylloquinone prophylaxis at birth. All three groups showed a lower variant frequency than a reference group of children aged 1–15 years. For ethical reasons, there was no control group of infants who had not received vitamin K prophylaxis, and the conclusion was therefore limited to a lack of association between the route of vitamin K administration and somatic mutation.

4.4.2 Experimental systems

Limited data are available on the genetic and related effects of phylloquinone and menaquinones (Table 9). Phylloquinone did not induce mutation in *Salmonella typhimurium*. It enhanced the frequency of sister chromatid exchange in cultured human maternal lymphocytes at concentrations that are relevant *in vivo*, and a similar increase in sister chromatid exchange frequency was observed in cultured lymphocytes from human placental blood. In fetal sheep that received a catheter in the femoral vein 10–15 days before term, phylloquinone significantly increased the frequency of sister chromatid exchange in peripheral blood lymphocytes sampled 24 h later.

Menaquinone-4 but not phylloquinone inhibited osteoclastic bone resorption by inducing osteoclast apoptosis (Kameda *et al.*, 1996). Menaquinone-4 and its derivatives also induced apoptosis in various human leukaemic cell lines (Yaguchi *et al.*, 1997).

In preincubation protocols with Ames *Salmonella* tester strains, menadione did not induce reverse mutation in strains TA100, TA102, TA1535, TA1537, TA1538 or TA2638 in the presence or absence of an exogenous metabolic activation system. It was mutagenic in TA98 with metabolic activation and in TA2637 with or without activation. Menadione also induced mutation in strain TA104, but only with metabolic activation by purified NADPH–cytochrome P450 reductase; in another study it was mutagenic in this strain without activation. Menadione did not induce reverse mutation in *Escherichia coli* WP2/pKM101 or WP2*uvr*A/pkM101 in the absence of metabolic activation.

In tests with derivatives of *E. coli* WP2s (*uvr*A *trp*E) that are defective in 7,8-dihydro-8-oxoguanine DNA glycosylase activity (*mut*M) or MutY glycosylase activity on an A:7,8-dihydro-8-oxoguanine mispair (*mut*Y) or give an adaptive response to oxidative stress by superoxide (*sox*RS), to compare the mutability of various reactive oxygen-generating compounds, menadione was not mutagenic; however, it was mutagenic in two strains of *E. coli* WP2 that contain deficiencies in the oxyR function. Menadione induced forward mutation to L-arabinose resistance (Ara^R) in *E. coli* K-12 strains with diminished concentrations of superoxide dismutase and induced a SOS response in PQ37.

This agent induced concentration-dependent single-strand and double-strand DNA breaks in a human breast cancer MCF-7 cell line, in cultured rat hepatocytes, in

Table 9. Genetic and related effects of phylloquinone and menadione

Test system	Result[a] Without exogenous metabolic system	Result[a] With exogenous metabolic system	Dose[b] (LED or HID)	Reference
Phylloquinone				
Salmonella typhimurium TA98, TA100, TA2637, reverse mutation	–	–	100 µg/plate	Tikkanen et al. (1983)
Sister chromatid exchange, human peripheral blood lymphocytes *in vitro*	+	NT	0.45	Israels et al. (1987)
Sister chromatid exchange, fetal sheep peripheral blood lymphocytes *in vivo*	+		1 mg/animal	Israels et al. (1987)
Menadione				
Escherichia coli K12, forward mutation, arabinose resistance	(+)[c]	NT	43 µg/plate	Prieto-Alamo et al. (1993)
Escherichia coli WP2s (ZA570, ZA580, ZA590, ZA700, ZA770, ZA780), reverse mutation	–	–	300 µg/plate	Kato et al. (1994)
Escherichia coli WP2/pKM101, WPS*avrA*/pkM101, reverse mutation	–[d]	NT	30 µg/plate	Blanco et al. (1998)
Escherichia coli WP2/pKM101, WP2*uvrA*/pkM101, reverse mutation	–	NT	300 µg/plate	Watanabe et al. (1998)
Salmonella typhimurium TA102, TA2638, reverse mutation	–	NT	300 µg/plate	Watanabe et al. (1998)
Salmonella typhimurium TA102, TA1535, TA1537, TA1538, reverse mutation	–	–	NR	Hakura et al. (1994)
Salmonella typhimurium TA2637, reverse mutation	+	+	NR	Hakura et al. (1994)
Salmonella typhimurium TA98, reverse mutation	–	–	NR	Hakura et al. (1994)
Salmonella typhimurium TA97, TA100, TA104, reverse mutation	+	+	NR	Hakura et al. (1994)
Salmonella typhimurium TA104, reverse mutation	NT	+	0.17	Chesis et al. (1984)
Salmonella typhimurium TA100, reverse mutation	–	–	140 µg/plate	Tikkanen et al. (1983)
Salmonella typhimurium TA98, reverse mutation	–	(+)	140 µg/plate	Tikkanen et al. (1983)
Salmonella typhimurium TA2637, reverse mutation	–	+	80	Tikkanen et al. (1983)
Drosophila melanogaster, genetic crossing-over or recombination (*white–ivory* assay)	–		10 mmol/L in feed	Ferreiro et al. (1997)
lacI Mutation, rat embryonic fibroblasts (λ*lacI*-transfected)	+	NT	0.85	Andrew et al. (1999)
DNA single-strand breaks, rat primary hepatocytes *in vitro*	+	NT	4.3	Morrison et al. (1984)

Table 9 (contd)

Test system	Result[a] Without exogenous metabolic system	Result[a] With exogenous metabolic system	Dose[b] (LED or HID)	Reference
Menadione (contd)				
DNA single-strand breaks, rat primary hepatocytes *in vitro*	+	NT	1.7	Morrison et al. (1985)
DNA single-strand breaks, rat primary hepatocytes *in vitro*	+	NT	8.5	Morgan et al. (1992)
DNA fragmentation, rat hepatocytes *in vitro*	+	NT	4.3	Fischer-Nielsen et al. (1995)
Cell transformation, BALB/c 3T3 cells (followed by TPA treatment)	+[e]	NT	0.5	Sakai et al. (1995)
DNA single-strand breaks, human breast cancer MCF-7 cells *in vitro*	+[f]	NT	0.85	Ngo et al. (1991)
DNA single-strand breaks, human primary fibroblasts *in vitro*	+	NT	3.4	Morrison et al. (1985)
DNA strand breaks (alkaline single-cell gel electrophoresis assay, comet), human lymphocytes *in vitro*	+	NT	0.17	Woods et al. (1997)
DNA single-strand breaks, human chronic myeloid leukaemic K562 cells *in vitro*	+	NT	2.6	Morgan et al. (1992); Morgan (1995)
Menaquinone				
Escherichia coli PQ37, SOS response	+	NT	50 µg/plate	Cook et al. (1991)

TPA, 12-*O*-tetradecanoylphorbol 13-acetate

[a] +, positive; (+), weak positive; –, negative; NT, not tested
[b] LED, lowest effective dose; HID, highest ineffective dose; in-vitro tests, µg/mL; NR, not reported
[c] LEDs in *E. coli* K12 lacking superoxide dismutase or catalase were ~25 and ~5 times lower, respectively.
[d] Response in cells deficient in OxyR function (WP2 oxyR/pKM101 and WP2*uvrA* oxyR/pKM101) was positive at 10 µg/plate.
[e] Menadione acted as an initiator.
[f] DNA double-strand breaks were induced at 4.3 µg/mL.

human fibroblasts, in human chronic myeloid leukaemic K562 cells and in a single-cell gel electrophoresis assay to measure DNA strand breaks in human lymphocytes at doses as low as 1 μmol/L. At concentrations of 15–100 μmol/L, menadione induced extensive DNA fragmentation in human chronic myeloid leukaemic K562 cells which could be measured in alkaline elution assays. At these doses, no oxidative stress appeared to occur in these cells.

Cantoni *et al.* (1991) reported that hydrogen peroxide produced during the metabolism of menadione does not contribute to the cytotoxic action of the quinone. In isolated rat hepatocytes, menadione induced DNA fragmentation consistent with apoptosis. These effects occurred in the absence of 8-oxo-2′-deoxyguanosine production, and the authors concluded that oxidative modification of DNA bases was unlikely to be involved (Fischer-Nielsen *et al.*, 1995). Menadione induced protein-linked DNA breaks in the presence of purified human DNA topoisomerase II but not DNA topoisomerase I (Frydman *et al.*, 1997), and it seems likely that DNA topoisomerase II poisoning is involved in DNA breakage by menadione at the lower concentrations, at which oxygen stress does not occur.

Menadione induced morphological transformation of BALB/c 3T3 cells, but only when tested in the presence of the tumour promotor 12-*O*-tetradecanoylphorbol 13-acetate.

Andrew *et al.* (1999) found that menadione enhanced the spontaneous mutation frequency and induced a novel mutation spectrum of *lac*I genes recovered from a rat embryonic fibroblast line transfected with a λ-phage shuttle vector, in both the traditional plaque assay and a positive selection assay.

4.5 Mechanistic considerations

(a) *Phylloquinone*

On the basis of studies of microsomal metabolism *in vitro* and studies in rats and mice *in vivo*, Israels *et al.* (1983, 1985) suggested that vitamin K may be mutagenic by affecting the mixed-function oxidase system which metabolizes benzo[*a*]pyrene. Phylloquinone at a high concentration (200 μmol/L) inhibited the conversion of benzo-[*a*]pyrene to its more polar metabolites, a property it shares with menadione. Paradoxically, at a lower concentration of phylloquinone (25 μmol/L), but not with menadione, the metabolism of benzo[*a*]pyrene was increased. In this system, therefore, whereas menadione consistently acts as a potential inhibitor of carcinogenesis, phylloquinone could either potentiate or inhibit it, depending on the concentration. The overall weaker inhibitory effect of phylloquinone could be due to the low solubility of this lipophilic compound, but it is difficult to explain the mechanism of the enhanced metabolism of benzo[*a*]pyrene at lower concentrations of phylloquinone.

In studies *in vivo*, Israels and co-workers found that menadione and vitamin K deficiency (nutritional or induced by the vitamin K antagonist, warfarin) both inhibited the rates of benzo[*a*]pyrene-induced tumour appearance and death, whereas phylloquinone increased the rate of carcinogenesis. They concluded that vitamin K deficiency confers a protective effect against benzo[*a*]pyrene-induced tumour formation. They subsequently tendered the hypothesis that the low vitamin K status of normal newborns confers a biological advantage by reducing the risk of mutagenic events during a period of rapid cell proliferation (Israels *et al.*, 1987; Saxena *et al.*, 1997).

Vervoort *et al.* (1997) reported that metabolic cycling of vitamin K compounds via the vitamin K cycle (Figure 1) confers potent antioxidant activity against lipid peroxidation. They concluded that the antioxidant effect is probably due to radical chain-breaking by vitamin K quinol and that dietary intake of vitamin K may strengthen cellular defences against oxidative stress.

(*b*) Menadione

In many of the studies of the cytotoxicity of menadione in cultured cells and blood platelets, menadione was used as a model compound for induction of cellular damage either by arylating protein-bound and soluble thiols or by inducing oxidative stress. The relative importance of these two mechanisms is difficult to determine. The toxicity may result directly from binding of menadione to a critical protein thiol (such as a membrane cation transporter) or indirectly from binding to and decreasing concentrations of reduced glutathione, thereby predisposing the cell to oxidative stress. An alternative mechanism whereby menadione may produce oxidative stress is by redox cycling, which ultimately results in the production of reactive oxygen species. Oxidative stress results when the production of reactive oxygen species exceeds the antioxidant defence mechanisms, which in turn may result in cellular injury and death through a variety of mechanisms. In human cancer cells, menadione-induced cell degeneration was considered to result mainly from lipid peroxidative damage rather than from other mechanisms such as a depleted glutathione content (Chiou *et al.*, 1998).

It has been proposed that menadione causes mutations by generating active oxygen species from semiquinone radicals (e.g. Chesis *et al.*, 1984; Smith *et al.*, 1987; Hakura *et al.*, 1994; Morgan *et al.*, 1998). Semiquinones can generate superoxide anion, which itself produces other active species, such as hydrogen peroxide and hydroxyl radical, through enzyme- and metal-catalysed reactions (Chesis *et al.*, 1984).

It now seems likely that menadione has an additional mode of action as a mutagen, by acting as a poison of DNA topoisomerase II enzymes. This could well be responsible for the DNA breakage, chromosomal aberrations and apoptosis observed in mammalian cells under conditions that did not lead to oxidative stress (e.g. Sawada *et al.*, 1987; Fischer-Nielsen *et al.*, 1995; Morgan, 1995). Cells in culture can, however, convert menadione to menaquinone-4, and there is already evidence that this plays a role in apoptosis.

5. Summary of Data Reported and Evaluation

5.1 Exposure data

The term 'vitamin K' refers to a group of 2-methyl-1,4-naphthoquinone derivatives which can fulfil an essential co-factor function in humans in the biosynthesis of a number of calcium-binding proteins, some of which are essential for haemostasis. In nature, vitamin K occurs as phylloquinone in plants and as menaquinones produced by bacteria. The major dietary sources of vitamin K are green leafy vegetables and certain vegetable oils. Clinically, vitamin K is used primarily to prevent or cure deficiency-related bleeding in newborns and patients with malabsorption syndromes and to reverse the anticoagulative effects of vitamin K antagonists.

5.2 Human carcinogenicity data

An association between childhood leukaemia and vitamin K prophylaxis given by the intramuscular route was found in two reports but was not confirmed in a number of studies in various countries. A major limitation of most of the studies is that the fact of intramuscular administration of vitamin K was difficult to establish retrospectively for a substantial proportion of subjects, although the results of the analyses based on individual records and on imputed hospital policies for vitamin K administration are similar. In the studies in which a suggestion of an association was observed, selection bias may have accounted for the result. The possibility cannot be entirely excluded of a small increase in the risk for acute lymphoblastic leukaemia occurring at ages around those of the peak incidence in childhood in children given intramuscular administration of vitamin K.

The few studies that investigated oral administration of vitamin K found no increase in the relative risk for leukaemia.

5.3 Animal carcinogenicity data

No adequate study on the carcinogenicity of vitamin K substances was available to the Working Group.

5.4 Other relevant data

Phylloquinone and menaquinones are absorbed from food into the lymphatic system and carried by triglyceride-rich lipoproteins in the blood. Menaquinones synthesized by the gut microflora may also be absorbed. Phylloquinone is rapidly cleared from the circulation by the liver, metabolized to metabolites with shortened side-chains and excreted in the bile and urine. In animals, menadione is absorbed predominantly by the portal route, does not accumulate in specific organs and is extensively excreted unchanged in the urine. A fraction of menadione is converted in tissues to menaquinone-4.

Phylloquinone rarely has toxic effects, and the few serious immunological complications observed have been attributed to the vehicle of solubilization. Menadione may cause haemolytic anaemia and induce cellular damage by arylating protein-bound and soluble thiols or by inducing oxidative stress.

No adverse effects have been reported in mothers or infants after administration of vitamin K during pregnancy, whereas vitamin K deficiency is teratogenic. The safety of vitamin K in pregnancy has not been adequately studied experimentally.

Neither phylloquinone nor menaquinones have been adequately studied for mutagenicity. Menadione acts as a bacterial mutagen in several specific strains of *Salmonella typhimurium* and *Escherichia coli*. In mammalian cells, menadione leads to DNA breakage, and there are isolated reports of chromosomal aberrations and sister chromatid exchange.

5.5 Evaluation

There is *inadequate evidence* in humans for the carcinogenicity of vitamin K substances.

There is *inadequate evidence* in experimental animals for the carcinogenicity of vitamin K substances.

Overall evaluation

Vitamin K substances are *not classifiable as to their carcinogenicity to humans (Group 3)*.

6. References

American Hospital Formulary Service (1997) *AHFS Drug Information® 97*, Bethesda, MD, American Society of Health-System Pharmacists, pp. 2834–2836

Andrew, S.E., Hsiao, L., Milhausen, K. & Jirik, F.R. (1999) Comparison of selectable and plaque assay systems to detect menadione- and UV-induced *lacI* mutations in mammalian cells. *Mutat. Res.*, **427**, 89–97

van den Anker, J.N. & Sinaasappel, M. (1993) Bleeding as presenting symptom of cholestasis. *J. Pernatol.*, **13**, 322–324

Ansell, P., Bull, D. & Roman, E. (1996) Childhood leukaemia and intramuscular vitamin K: Findings from a case–control study. *Br. med. J.*, **313**, 204–205

AOAC International (1996) AOAC Official Method 992.27. *trans*-Vitamin K_1 (phylloquinone) in ready-to-feed milk-based infant formula. In: *Official Methods of Analysis of AOAC International*, 16th Ed., 4th rev., Gaithersburg, MD [CD-ROM edition]

Blanco, M., Urios, A. & Martínez, A. (1998) New *Escherichia coli* WP2 tester strains highly sensitive to reversion by oxidative mutagens. *Mutat. Res.*, **413**, 95–101

Booth, S.L & Suttie, J.W. (1998) Dietary intake and adequacy of vitamin K_1. *J. Nutr.*, **128**, 785–788

Booth, S.L., Sadowski, J.A. & Pennington, J.A.T. (1995) Phylloquinone (vitamin K_1) content in the US Food and Drug Administration's Total Diet Study. *J. agric. Food Chem.*, **43**, 1574–1579

Booth, S.L., Pennington, J.A.T. & Sadowski, J.A. (1996) Food sources and dietary intakes of vitamin K-1 (phylloquinone) in the American diet: Data from the FDA Total Diet Study. *J. Am. diet. Assoc.*, **96**, 149–154

Breen, G.A. & St Peter, W.L. (1997) Hypoprothombinemia associated with cefmetazole. *Ann. Pharmacother.*, **31**, 180–184

British Medical Association/Royal Pharmaceutical Society of Great Britain (1998) *British National Formulary*, No. 36, London, pp. 422–423

British Pharmacopoeial Commission (1993) *British Pharmacopoeia 1993*, London, Her Majesty's Stationery Office, Vols I & II, pp. 409–411, 516–517, 999–1000, 1059–1060, S79–S80

Brown, P.C., Dulik, D.M. & Jones, T.W. (1991) The toxicity of menadione (2-methyl-1,4-naphthoquinone) and two thioether conjugates studied with isolated renal epithelial cells. *Arch. Biochem. Biophys.*, **285**, 187–196

Budavari, S., ed. (1996) *The Merck Index*, 12th Ed., Whitehouse Station, NJ, Merck & Co., pp. 994, 1269–1270

Bueno, M.P. & Villalobos, M.C. (1983) Reverse phase high pressure liquid chromatographic determination of vitamin K_1 in infant formulas. *J. Assoc. off. anal. Chem.*, **66**, 1063–1066

Canadian Pharmaceutical Association (1997) *CPS Compendium of Pharmaceuticals and Specialties*, 32nd Ed., Ottawa, Ontario, p. 1730

Canady, W.J. & Roe, J.H. (1956) Studies on the reaction of menadione with blood and denatured proteins. *J. biol. Chem.*, **220**, 571–582

Canfield, L.M., Martin, G.S. & Sugimoto, K. (1988) Vitamin K in human milk. In: Suttie, J.W., ed., *Current Advances in Vitamin K Research*, New York, Elsevier, pp. 499–504

Cantoni, O., Fiorani, M., Cattabeni, F. & Bellomo, G. (1991) DNA breakage caused by hydrogen peroxide produced during the metabolism of 2-methyl-1,4-naphthoquinone (menadione) does not contribute to the cytotoxic action of the quinone. *Biochem. Pharmacol.*, **42**, S220–S222

Carstensen, J. (1992) Intramuscular vitamin K and childhood cancer (Letter to the Editor). *Br. med. J.*, **305**, 709–710

Chesis, P.L., Levin, D.E., Smith, M.T., Ernster, L. & Ames, B.N. (1984) Mutagenicity of quinones: Pathways of metabolic activation and detoxification. *Proc. natl Acad. Sci. USA*, **81**, 1696–1700

Chiou, T.-J., Chou, Y.-T. & Tzeng, W.-F. (1998) Menadione-induced cell degeneration is related to lipid peroxidation in human cancer cells. *Proc. natl Sci. Counc., ROC, Part B: Life Sci.*, **22**, 13–21

Choo, K.E., Tan, K.K., Chuah, S.P., Ariffin, W.A. & Gururaj, A. (1994) Haemorrhagic disease in newborn and older infants: A study in hospitalized children in Kelantan, Malaysia. *Ann. trop. Paediatr.*, **14**, 231–237

Chung, J.-H., Seo, D.-C., Chung, S.-H., Lee, J.-Y. & Seung, S.-A. (1997) Metabolism and cytotoxicity of menadione and its metabolite in rat platelets. *Toxicol. appl. Pharmacol.*, **142**, 378–385

CIS Information Services (1998) *Worldwide Bulk Drug Users Directory 1997/98 Edition*, Dallas, TX [CD-ROM]

Clark, F.I. & James, E.J. (1995) Twenty-seven years of experience with oral vitamin K_1 therapy in neonates. *J. Pediatr.*, **127**, 301–304

Conly, J.M. & Stein, K. (1992) Quantitative and qualitative measurements of K vitamins in human intestinal contents. *Am. J. Gastroenterol.*, **87**, 311–316

Cook, A., Stovicek, R., D'Odorico, A., Tkac, A. & Bilton, R.F. (1991) Menaquinone mediated free radical generation: A possible mutagenic mechanism. *Biochem. Soc. Trans.*, **19**, 426S

Cornelissen, M., Smeets, D., Merkx, G., De Abreu, R., Kollée, L. & Monnens, L. (1991) Analysis of chromosome aberrations and sister chromatid exchanges in peripheral blood lymphocytes of newborns after vitamin K prophylaxis at birth. *Pediatr. Res.*, **30**, 550–553

Cornelissen, E.A.M., Kollée, L.A.A., De Abreu, R.A., van Baal, J.M., Motohara, K., Verbruggen, B. & Monnens, L.A.H. (1992) Effects of oral and intramuscular vitamin K prophylaxis on vitamin K_1, PIVKA-II, and clotting factors in breast fed infants. *Arch. Dis. Child.*, **67**, 1250–1254

Cornelissen, E.A.M., van Lieburg, A.F., Motohara, K. & van Oostrom, C.G. (1992) Vitamin K status in cystic fibrosis. *Acta paediatr.*, **81**, 658–661

Cornelissen, M., Steegers-Theunissen, R., Kollée, L., Eskes, T., Vogels-Mentink, G., Motohara, K., De Abreu, R. & Monnens, L. (1993a) Increased incidence of neonatal vitamin K deficience resulting from maternal anticonvulsant therapy. *Am. J. Obstet. Gynecol.*, **168**, 923–928

Cornelissen, M., Steegers-Theunissen, R., Kollée, L., Eskes, T., Motohara, K. & Monnens, L. (1993b) Supplementation of vitamin K in pregnant women receiving anticonvulsant therapy prevents neonatal vitamin K deficiency. *Am. J. Obstet. Gynecol.*, **168**, 884–888

Cornelissen, M., von Kries, R., Loughnan, P. & Schubiger, G. (1997) Prevention of vitamin K deficiency bleeding: Efficacy of different multiple oral dose schedules of vitamin K. *Eur. J. Pediatr.*, **156**, 126–130

Council of Europe (1997) *European Pharmacopoeia*, 3rd Ed., Strasbourg, pp. 1154–1155, 1332–1333

Crowther, M.A., Donovan, D., Harrison, L., McGinnis, J. & Ginsberg, J. (1998) Low-dose oral vitamin K reliably reverses over-anticoagulation due to warfarin. *Thromb. Haemostasis*, **79**, 1116–1118

Davidson, R.T., Foley, A.L., Engelke, J.A. & Suttie, J.W. (1998) Conversion of dietary phylloquinone to tissue menaquinone-4 in rats is not dependent on gut bacteria. *J. Nutr.*, **128**, 220–223

Denda, A., Sai, K.M., Tang, Q., Tsujiuchi, T., Tsutsumi, M., Amanuma, T., Murata, Y., Nakae, D., Maruyama, H., Kurokawa, Y. & Konishi, Y. (1991) Induction of 8-hydroxydeoxyguanosine but not initiation of carcinogenesis by redox enzyme modulations with or without menadione in rat liver. *Carcinogenesis*, **12**, 719–726

Dialameh, G.H., Yekundi, K.G. & Olson, R.E. (1970) Enzymatic alkylation of menaquinone-0 to menaquinones by microsomes from chick liver. *Biochim. biophys. Acta*, **223**, 332–338

Doran, O., Austic, N.C. & Taylor, B.J. (1995) Vitamin K administration in neonates: Survey of compliance with recommended practices in the Dunedin area. *N.Z. J. Med.*, **108**, 337–339

Draper, G. & McNinch, A. (1994) Vitamin K for neonates: The controversy. *Br. med. J.*, **308**, 867–868

Draper, G.J. & Stiller, C.A. (1992) Intramuscular vitamin K and childhood cancer (Letter to the Editor). *Br. med. J.*, **305**, 709

Durie, P.R. (1994) Vitamin K and the management of patients with cystic fibrosis. *Can. med. Assoc. J.*, **151**, 933–936

Editions du Vidal (1998) *Dictionnaire Vidal 1998*, 74th Ed., Paris, OVP, pp. 1989–1990

Ekelund, H. (1991) Late haemorrhagic disease in Sweden 1987–89. *Acta paediatr. scand.*, **80**, 966–968

Ekelund, H., Finnström, O., Gunnarskog, J., Källén, B. & Larsson, Y. (1993) Administration of vitamin K to newborn infants and childhood cancer. *Br. med. J.*, **307**, 89–91

Ferland, G. & Sadowski, J.A. (1992) Vitamin K_1 (phylloquinone) content of edible oils: Effects of heating and light exposure. *J. agric. Food Chem.*, **40**, 1869–1873

Fetrow, C.W., Overlock, T. & Leff, L. (1997) Antagonism of warfarin-induced hypoprothrombinemia with use of low-dose subcutaneous vitamin K1. *J. clin. Pharmacol.*, **37**, 751–757

Fischer-Nielsen, A., Corcoran, G.B., Poulsen, H.E., Kamendulis, L.M. & Loft, S. (1995) Menadione-induced DNA fragmentation without 8-oxo-2′-deoxyguanosine formation in isolated rat hepatocytes. *Biochem. Pharmacol.*, **49**, 1469–1474

Food & Drug Administration (1999) Food and drugs. *US Code Fed. Regul.*, **Title 21**, Part 107.100, Subpart D, pp. 186–187

Fournier, B., Sann, L., Guillaumont, M. & Leclercq, M. (1987) Variations of phylloquinone concentration in human milk at various stages of lactation and in cow's milk at various seasons. *Am. J. clin. Nutr.*, **45**, 551–558

Frydman, B., Marton, L.J., Sun, J.S., Neder, K., Witiak, D.T., Liu, A.A., Wang, H.-M., Mao, Y., Wu, H.-Y., Sanders, M.M. & Liu, L.F. (1997) Induction of DNA topoisomerase II-mediated DNA cleavage by beta-lapachone and related naphthoquinones. *Cancer Res.*, **57**, 620–627

Gennaro, A.R. (1985) *Remington's Pharmaceutical Sciences*, 17th Ed., Easton, PA, Mack Publishing Co., pp. 1010–1011

Gennaro, A.R. (1995) *Remington: The Science and Practice of Pharmacy*, 19th Ed., Easton, PA, Mack Publishing Co., Vol. II, pp. 1114–1115

Gijsbers, B.L.M.G., Jie, K.-S.G. & Vermeer, C. (1996) Effect of food composition on vitamin K absorption in human volunteers. *Br. J. Nutr.*, **76**, 223–229

Golding, J., Paterson, M. & Kinlen, L.J. (1990) Factors associated with childhood cancer in a national cohort study. *Br. J. Cancer*, **62**, 304–308

Golding, J., Greenwood, R., Birmingham, K. & Mott, M. (1992) Childhood cancer, intramuscular vitamin K, and pethidine given during labour. *Br. med. J.*, **305**, 341–346

Greer, F.R., Marshall, S., Cherry, J. & Suttie, J.W. (1991) Vitamin K status of lactating mothers, human milk, and breast-feeding infants. *Pediatrics*, **88**, 751–756

Greer, F.R., Marshall, S.P., Foley, A.L. & Suttie, J.W. (1997) Improving the vitamin K status of breastfeeding infants with maternal vitamin K supplements. *Pediatrics*, **99**, 88–92

Guillaumont, M., Sann, L., Leclercq, M., Dostalova, L., Vignal, B. & Frederich, A. (1993) Changes in hepatic vitamin K1 levels after prophylactic administration to the newborn. *J. pediatr. Gastroenterol. Nutr.*, **16**, 10–14

Hagstrom, J.N., Bovill, E.G., Soll, R.F., Davidson, K.W. & Sadowski, J.A. (1995) The pharmacokinetics and lipoprotein fraction distribution of intramuscular vs. oral vitamin K_1 supplementation in women of childbearing age: Effects on hemostasis. *Thromb. Haemostasis*, **74**, 1486–1490

Hakura, A., Mochida, H., Tsutsui, Y. & Yamatsu, K. (1994) Mutagenicity and cytotoxicity of naphthoquinones for Ames *Salmonella* tester strains. *Chem. Res. Toxicol.*, **7**, 559–567

Hanawa, Y. (1992) Vitamin K deficiency in infancy: The Japanese experience. *Acta paediatr. jpn.*, **34**, 107–116

Hansen, K.B. & Ebbesen, F. (1996) Neonatal vitamin K prophylaxis in Denmark: Three years' experience with oral administration during the first three months of life compared with one oral administration at birth. *Acta pediatr.*, **85**, 1137–1139

Haroon, Y., Shearer, M.J., Rahin, S., Gunn, W.G., McEnery, G. & Barkhan, P. (1982) The content of phylloquinone (vitamin K_1) in human milk, cows' milk and infant formula foods determined by high-performance liquid chromatography. *J. Nutr.*, **112**, 1105–1117

Hart, K.T. (1958) Study of hydrolysis of urinary metabolites of 2-methyl-1,4-naphthoquinone. *Proc. Soc. exp. Biol. Med.*, **97**, 848–851

Hassan, M.M.A., Mossa, J.S. & Taragan, A.H.U.K. (1988) Analytical profile of phytonadione. In: Florey, K., ed., *Analytical Profiles of Drug Substances*, New York, Academic Press, Vol. 17, pp. 449–531

Hewson, D. & Bennett, A. (1987) Childbirth research data: Medical records or women's reports? *Am. J. Epidemiol.*, **125**, 484–491

Hill, R.J. (1994) The uptake of the third oral vitamin K dose in general practice. *N.Z. Med. J.*, **107**, 177–178

Hodges, S.J., Bejui, J., Leclercq, M. & Delmas, P.D. (1993) Detection and measurement of vitamins K_1 and K_2 in human cortical and trabecular bone. *J. Bone Min. Res.*, **8**, 1005–1008

Hoskin, F.C.G., Spinks, J.W.T. & Jaques, L.B. (1954) Urinary excretion products of menadione (vitamin K_3). *Can. J. Biochem. Physiol.*, **32**, 240–250

Houwen, R.H.J., Bouquet, J. & Bijleveld, C.M.A. (1987) Bleeding as the first symptom of extra-hepatic biliary atresia. *Eur. J. Pediatr.*, **146**, 425–426

Howe, A.M. & Webster, W.S. (1990) Exposure of the pregnant rat to warfarin and vitamin K1: An animal model of intraventricular hemorrhage in the fetus. *Teratology*, **42**, 413–420

Hwang, S.-M. (1985) Liquid chromatographic determination of vitamin K_1 *trans-* and *cis-*isomers in infant formula. *J. Assoc. off. anal. Chem.*, **68**, 684–689

Indyk, H.E. & Woollard, D.C. (1997) Vitamin K in milk and infant formulas: Determination and distribution of phylloquinone and menaquinone-4. *Analyst*, **122**, 465–469

Israels, L.G., Walls, G.A., Ollmann, D.J., Friesen, E. & Israels, E.D. (1983) Vitamin K as a regulator of benzo(a)pyrene metabolism, mutagenesis, and carcinogenesis. Studies with rat microsomes and tumorigenesis in mice. *J. clin. Invest.*, **71**, 1130–1140

Israels, L.G., Ollmann, D.J. & Israels, E.D. (1985) Vitamin K_1 as a modulator of benzo(a)-pyrene metabolism as measured by *in vitro* metabolite formation and *in vivo* DNA-adduct formation. *Int. J. Biochem.*, **17**, 1263–1266

Israels, L.G., Friesen, E., Jansen, A.H. & Israels, E.D. (1987) Vitamin K1 increases sister chromatid exchange *in vitro* in human leukocytes and *in vivo* in fetal sheep cells: A possible role for 'vitamin K deficiency' in the fetus. *Pediatr. Res.*, **22**, 405–408

Japan Medical Products Trade Association (1996) *Japan Pharmaceutical Reference (JPR). Products and Administration in Japan*, 4th Ed., Tokyo, pp. 161–164, 181–186

Jaques, L.B., Millar, G.J. & Spinks, J.W.T. (1954) The metabolism of the K vitamins. *Schweiz. med. Wochenschr.*, **84**, 792–796

Kameda, T., Miyazawa, K., Mori, Y., Yuasa, T., Shiokawa, M., Nakamaru, Y., Mano, H., Hakeda, Y., Kameda, A. & Kumegawa, M. (1996) Vitamin K2 inhibits osteoclastic bone resorption by inducing osteoclast apoptosis. *Biochem. biophys. Res. Commun.*, **220**, 515–519

Kato, T., Watanabe, M. & Ohta, T. (1994) Induction of the SOS response and mutations by reactive oxygen-generating compounds in various *Escherichia coli* mutants defective in the *mutM, mutY* or *soxRS* loci. *Mutagenesis*, **9**, 245–251

Keller, C., Matzdorff, C. & Kemkes-Matthes, B. (1999) Pharmacology of warfarin and clinical implication. *Semin. Thromb. Hemostasis*, **25**, 13–16

Klebanoff, M.A., Read, J.S., Mills, J.L. & Shiono, P.H. (1993) The risk of childhood cancer after neonatal exposure to vitamin K. *New Engl. J. Med.*, **329**, 905–908

Kohlmeier, M., Salomon, A., Saupe, J. & Shearer, M.J. (1996) Transport of vitamin K to bone in humans. *J. Nutr.*, **126**, 1192S–1196S

Kossenjans, W., Rymaszewski, Z., Barankiewicz, J., Bobst, A. & Ashraf, M. (1996) Menadione-induced oxidative stress in bovine heart microvascular endothelial cells. *Microcirculation*, **3**, 39–47

Kosuge, Y. (1973) [Study of developmental pharmacology on vitamin K3. Part 1. Effect of vitamin K3 on the rat fetus.] *Folia pharmacol. jpn.*, **69**, 285–291 (in Japanese)

Kowdley, K.V., Emond, M.J., Sadowski, J.A. & Kaplan, M.M. (1997) Plasma vitamin K_1 level is decreased in primary biliary cirrhosis. *Am. J. Gastroenterol.*, **92**, 2059–2061

von Kries, R. (1991) Neonatal vitamin K—Prophylaxis for all. *Br. med. J.*, **303**, 1083–1084

von Kries, R. (1999) Oral versus intramuscular phytomenadione: Safety and efficacy compared. *Drug Saf.*, **21**, 1–6

von Kries, R. & Hanawa, Y. (1993) Neonatal vitamin K prophylaxis. Report of Scientific and Standardization Subcommittee on Perinatal Haemostasis. *Thromb. Haemostasis*, **69**, 293–295

von Kries, R., Becker, A. & Göbel, U. (1987a) Vitamin K in the newborn: Influence of nutritional factors on acarboxy-prothrombin detectability and factor II and VII clotting activity. *Eur. J. Pediatr.*, **146**, 123–127

von Kries, R., Shearer, M., McCarthy, P.T., Haug, M., Harzer, G. & Göbel, U. (1987b) Vitamin K_1 content of maternal milk: Influence of the stage of lactation, lipid composition, and vitamin K_1 supplements given to the mother. *Pediatr. Res.*, **22**, 513–517

von Kries, R., Shearer, M.J. & Gobel, U. (1988) Vitamin K in infancy. *Eur. J. Pediatr.*, **147**, 106–112

von Kries, R., Göbel, U., Hachmeister, A., Kaletsch, U. & Michaelis, J. (1996) Vitamin K and childhood cancer: A population based case–control study in Lower Saxony, Germany. *Br. med. J.*, **313**, 199–203

Lamon-Fava, S., Sadowski, J.A., Davidson, K.W., O'Brien, M.E., McNamara, J.R. & Schaefer, E.J. (1998) Plasma lipoproteins as carriers of phylloquinone (vitamin K_1) in humans. *Am. J. clin. Nutr.*, **67**, 1226–1231

LINFO Läkemedelsinformation AB (1998) *FASS 1998 Läkemedel i Sverige*, Stockholm, pp. 694–695

Lorenz, W., Schmal, A., Schult, H., Lang, S. Ohmann, C., Weber, D., Kapp, B., Lüben, L. & Doenicke, A. (1982) Histamine release and hypotensive reactions in dogs by solubilizing agents and fatty acids: Analysis of various components in Cremophor EL and development of a compound with reduced toxicity. *Agents Actions*, **12**, 64–80

Losito, R., Owen, C.A., Jr & Flock, E.V. (1967) Metabolism of [^{14}C]menadione. *Biochemistry*, **6**, 62–68

Losito, R., Owen, C.A., Jr & Flock, E.V. (1968) Metabolic studies of vitamin K_1-^{14}C and menadione-^{14}C in the normal and hepatectomized rats. *Thromb. Diath. Haemorrh.*, **19**, 383–388

Loughnan, P.M. & McDougall, P.N. (1996) Does intramuscular vitamin K_1 act as an unintended depot preparation? *J. paediatr. Child Health*, **32**, 251–254

Mandelbrot, L., Guillaumont, M., Leclercq, M., Lefrère, J.J., Gozin, D., Daffos, F. & Forestier, F. (1988) Placental transfer of vitamin K_1 and its implications in fetal hemostasis. *Thromb. Haemostasis*, **60**, 39–43

Martius, C. (1967) Chemistry and function of vitamin K. In: Seegers W.H., ed., *Blood Clotting Enzymology*, New York, Academic Press, pp. 551–575

McBurney, A., Shearer, M.J. & Barkhan, P. (1980) Preparative isolation and characterization of the urinary aglycones of vitamin K_1 (phylloquinone) in man. *Biochem. Med.*, **24**, 250–267

McKinney, P.A., Juszczak, E., Findlay, E. & Smith, K. (1998) Case–control study of childhood leukaemia and cancer in Scotland: Findings for neonatal intramuscular vitamin K. *Br. med. J.*, **316**, 173–177

McNinch, A.W., Upton, C., Samuels, M., Shearer, M.J., McCarthy, P., Tripp, J.H. & Orme, R.L.'E. (1985) Plasma concentrations after oral or intramuscular vitamin K_1 in neonates. *Arch. Dis. Child.*, **60**, 814–818

Melgar, M.J., Anadon, A. & Bello, J. (1991) Effects of menadione on the cardiovascular system. *Vet. hum. Toxicol.*, **33**, 110–114

Menger, H., Lin, A.E., Toriello, H.V., Bernert, G. & Spranger, J.W. (1997) Vitamin K deficiency embryopathy: A phenocopy of the warfarin embryopathy due to a disorder of embryonic vitamin K metabolism. *Am. J. med. Genet.*, **72**, 129–134

Meyer, T.C. & Angus, J. (1956) The effect of large doses of 'Synkavit' in the newborn. *Arch. Dis. Child.*, **31**, 212–215

Mezick, J.A., Tomkins, R.K. & Cornwell, D.G. (1968) Absorption and intestinal lymphatic transport of ^{14}C-menadione. *Life Sci.*, **7**, 153–158

Mirabelli, F., Salis, A., Marinoni, V., Finardi, G., Bellomo, G., Thor, H. & Orrenius, S. (1988) Menadione-induced bleb formation in hepatocytes is associated with the oxidation of thiol groups in actin. *Arch. Biochem. Biophys.*, **264**, 261–269

Morgan, W.A. (1995) DNA single-strand breakage in mammalian cells induced by redox cycling quinones in the absence of oxidative stress. *J. biochem. Toxicol.*, **10**, 227–232

Morgan, W.A., Hartley, J.A. & Cohen, G.M. (1992) Quinone-induced DNA single strand breaks in rat hepatocytes and human chronic myelogenous leukaemic K562 cells. *Biochem. Pharmacol.*, **44**, 215–221

Morgan, W.A., Kaler, B. & Bach, P.H. (1998) The role of reactive oxygen species in adriamycin and menadione-induced glomerular toxicity. *Toxicol. Lett.*, **94**, 209–215

Morrison, H., Jernström, B., Nordenskjöld, M., Thor, H. & Orrenius, S. (1984) Induction of DNA damage by menadione (2-methyl-1,4-naphthoquinone) in primary cultures of rat hepatocytes. *Biochem. Pharmacol.*, **33**, 1763–1769

Morrison, H., Di Monte, D., Nordenskjöld, M. & Jernström, B. (1985) Induction of cell damage by menadione and benzo(a)pyrene-3,6-quinone in cultures of adult rat hepatocytes and human fibroblasts. *Toxicol. Lett.*, **28**, 37–47

Motohara, K., Matsukura, M., Matsuda, I., Iribe, K., Ikeda, T., Kondo, Y., Yonekubo, A., Yamamoto, Y. & Tsuchiya, F. (1984) Severe vitamin K deficiency in breast-fed infants. *J. Pediatr.*, **105**, 943–945

Munday, R., Smith, B.L. & Fowke, E.A. (1991) Haemolytic activity and nephrotoxicity of 2-hydroxy-1,4-naphthoquinone in rats. *J. appl. Toxicol.*, **11**, 85–90

National Research Council (1989) *Recommended Dietary Allowances*, 10th Ed., Washington DC, National Academy Press, pp. 107–114

Ngo, E.O., Sun, T.-P., Chang, J.-Y., Wang, C.-C., Chi, K.-H., Cheng, A.-L. & Nutter, L.M. (1991) Menadione-induced DNA damage in a human tumor cell line. *Biochem. Pharmacol.*, **42**, 1961–1968

Nowak, D., Chudzik, J., Pietras, T. & Bialasiewicz, P. (1997) Severe haemorrhagic diathesis in an adult patient with cystic fibrosis after long-term antibiotic treatment of pulmonary infection. *Monaldi Arch. Chest Dis.*, **52**, 343–345

Oakley, A., Rajan, L. & Robertson, P. (1990) A comparison of different sources of information about pregnancy and childbirth. *J. biosoc. Sci.*, **22**, 477–487

O'Brien, D.P., Shearer, M.J., Waldron, R.P., Horgan, P.G. & Given, H.F. (1994) The extent of vitamin K deficiency in patients with cholestatic jaundice: A preliminary communication. *J. R. Soc. Med.*, **87**, 320–322

Ochi, T. (1996) Menadione causes increases in the level of glutathione and in the activity of γ-glutamylcysteine synthetase in cultured Chinese hamster V79 cells. *Toxicology*, **112**, 45–55

Øie, S., Trenk, D., Guentert, T.W., Mosberg, H. & Jähnchen, E. (1988) Disposition of vitamin K_1 after intravenous and oral administration to subjects on phenprocoumon therapy. *Int. J. Pharm.*, **48**, 223–230

Olsen, J.H., Hertz, H., Blinkenberg, K. & Verder, H. (1994) Vitamin K regimens and incidence of childhood cancer in Denmark. *Br. med. J.*, **308**, 895–896

Park, B.K., Scott, A.K., Wilson, A.C., Haynes, B.P. & Breckenridge, A.M. (1984) Plasma disposition of vitamin K_1 in relation to anticoagulant poisoning. *Br. J. clin. Pharmacol.*, **18**, 655–662

Parker, L., Cole, M., Craft, A.W. & Hey, E.N. (1998) Neonatal vitamin K administration and childhood cancer in the north of England: Retrospective case–control study. *Br. med. J.*, **316**, 189–193

Passmore, S.J., Draper, G., Brownbill, P. & Kroll, M. (1998a) Case–control studies of relation between childhood cancer and neonatal vitamin K administration. *Br. med. J.*, **316**, 178–184

Passmore, S.J., Draper, G., Brownbill, P. & Kroll, M. (1998b) Ecological studies of relation between hospital policies on neonatal vitamin K administration and subsequent occurrence of childhood cancer. *Br. med. J.*, **316**, 184–189

Pereira, S.P. & Williams, R. (1998) Adverse events associated with vitamin K_1: Results of a worldwide postmarketing surveillance programme. *Pharmacoepidemiol. Drug Saf.*, **7**, 173–182

Pietersma-de Bruyn, A.L.J.M., van Haard, P.M.M., Beunis, M.H., Hamulyák, K. & Kuijpers, J.C. (1990) Vitamin K_1 levels and coagulation factors in healthy newborns till 4 weeks after birth. *Haemostasis*, **20**, 8–14

Pindur, G., Mörsdorf, S., Schenk, J.F., Krischek, B., Heinrich, W. & Wenzel, E. (1999) The overdosed patient and bleeding with oral anticoagulation. *Semin. Thromb. Hemostasis*, **25**, 85–88

Pizer, B., Boyse, J., Hunt, L. & Mott, M. (1995) Neonatal vitamin K administration and in vivo somatic mutation. *Mutat. Res.*, **347**, 135–139

Prieto-Alamo, M.J., Abril, N. & Pueyo, C. (1993) Mutagenesis in *Escherichia coli* K-12 mutants defective in superoxide dismutase or catalase. *Carcinogenesis*, **14**, 237–244

Rennie, J.M. & Kelsall, A.W.R. (1994) Vitamin K prophylaxis in the newborn—again. *Arch. Dis. Child.*, **70**, 248–251

Renzulli, P., Tuchschmid, P., Eich, G., Fanconi, S. & Schwobel, M.G. (1998) Early vitamin K deficiency bleeding after maternal phenobarbital intake: Management of massive intracranial haemorrhage by minimal surgical intervention. *Eur. J. Pediatr.*, **157**, 663–665

Rich, E.C. & Drage, C.W. (1982) Severe complications of intravenous phytonadione therapy. *Postgrad. Med.*, **72**, 303–306

Richert, D.A. (1951) Studies on the detoxification of 2-methyl-1,4-naphthoquinone in rabbits. *J. biol. Chem.*, **189**, 763–768

Roman, E., Ansell, P. & Bull, D. (1997) Leukaemia and non-Hodgkin's lymphoma in children and young adults: Are prenatal and neonatal factors important determinants of disease? *Br. J. Cancer*, **76**, 406–415

Rote Liste Sekretariat (1998) *Rote Liste 1998*, Frankfurt, Rote Liste Service GmbH, pp. 84-171, 84-177, 84-180

Royal Pharmaceutical Society of Great Britain (1999) *Martindale, The Extra Pharmacopoeia*, 13th Ed., London, The Pharmaceutical Press [MicroMedex Online: Health Care Series]

Sadtler Research Laboratories (1980) *Sadtler Standard Spectra, 1980 Cumulative Index*, Philadelphia, PA, p. 881

Sakai, A., Miyata, N. & Takahashi, A. (1995) Initiating activity of quinones in the two-stage transformation of BALB/3T3 cells. *Carcinogenesis*, **16**, 477–481

Sanders, M.N. & Winkelmann, R.K. (1988) Cutaneous reactions to vitamin K. *J. Am. Acad. Dermatol.*, **19**, 699–704

Sann, L., Leclercq, M., Frederich, A., Bourgeois, J., Bethenod, M. & Bourgeay-Causse, M. (1985) Pharmacokinetics of vitamin K_1 in low-birth-weight neonates. *Dev. Pharmacol. Ther.*, **8**, 269–279

Sawada, M., Sofuni, T., Hatanaka, M. & Ishidate, M., Jr (1987) Induction of chromosome aberrations in active oxygen-generating systems. 4. Studies with hydrogen peroxide-resistant cells in culture (Abstract No. 52). *Mutat. Res.*, **182**, 376

Saxena, S.P., Fan, T., Li, M., Israels, E.D. & Israels, L.G. (1997) A novel role for vitamin K_1 in a tyrosine phosphorylation cascade during chick embryogenesis. *J. clin. Invest.*, **99**, 602–607

Schardein, J.L. (1993) *Chemically Induced Birth Defects*, 2nd Ed., New York, Marcel Dekker, p. 552

Schneider, D.L., Fluckiger, H.B. & Manes, J.D. (1974) Vitamin K_1 content of infant formula products. *Pediatrics*, **53**, 273–275

Schneiderman, M.A., Sharma, A.K., Mahanama, K.R.R. & Locke, D.C. (1988) Determination of vitamin K1 in powdered infant formulas, using supercritical fluid extraction and liquid chromatography with electrochemical detection. *J. Assoc. off. anal. Chem.*, **71**, 815–817

Schubiger, G., Tönz, O., Grüter, J. & Shearer, M.J. (1993) Vitamin K_1 concentration in breast-fed neonates after oral or intramuscular administration of a single dose of a new mixed-micellar preparation of phylloquinone. *J. pediatr. Gastroenterol. Nutr.*, **16**, 435–439

Schubiger, G., Grüter, J. & Shearer, M.J. (1997) Plasma vitamin K_1 and PIVKA-II after oral administration of mixed-micellar or Cremophor EL-solubilized preparations of vitamin K_1 to normal breast-fed newborns. *J. pediatr. Gastroenterol. Nutr.*, **24**, 280–284

Sharma, R.K., Marwaha, N., Kumar, P. & Narang, A. (1995) Effect of oral water soluble vitamin K on PIVKA-II levels in newborns. *Indian Pediatr.*, **32**, 863–867

Shearer, M.J. (1992) Vitamin K metabolism and nutriture. *Blood Rev.*, **6**, 92–104

Shearer, M.J. (1995) Fat-soluble vitamins. Vitamin K. *Lancet*, **345**, 229–234

Shearer, M.J. (1997) The roles of vitamins D and K in bone health and osteoporosis prevention. *Proc. Nutr. Soc.*, **56**, 915–937

Shearer, M.J., Barkhan, P. & Webster, G.R. (1970) Absorption and excretion of an oral dose of tritiated vitamin K_1 in man. *Br. J. Haematol.*, **18**, 297–308

Shearer, M.J., Mallinson, C.N., Webster, G.R. & Barkhan, P. (1972) Clearance from plasma and excretion in urine, faeces and bile of an intravenous dose of tritiated vitamin K_1 in man. *Br. J. Haematol.*, **22**, 579–588

Shearer, M.J., McBurney, A. & Barkhan, P. (1974) Studies on the absorption and metabolism of phylloquinone (vitamin K_1) in man. In: Harris, R.S., Munson, P.L., Diczfalusy, E. & Glover, J., *Vitamins and Hormones, Advances in Research and Applications*, New York, Academic Press, Vol. 32, pp. 513–542

Shearer, M.J., Rahm, S., Barkhan, P. & Stimmler, L. (1982) Plasma vitamin K_1 in mothers and their newborn babies. *Lancet*, **ii**, 460–463

Shearer, M.J., McCarthy, P.T., Crampton, O.E. & Mattock, M.B. (1988) The assessment of human vitamin K status from tissue measurements. In: Suttie J.W., ed., *Current Advances in Vitamin K Research*, New York, Elsevier, pp. 437–452

Shearer, M.J., Bach, A. & Kohlmeier, M. (1996) Chemistry, nutritional sources, tissue distribution and metabolism of vitamin K with special reference to bone health. *J. Nutr.*, **126** (Suppl. 4), 1181S–1186S

Shertzer, H.G., Låstbom, L., Sainsbury, M. & Moldéus, P. (1992) Menadione-mediated membrane fluidity alterations and oxidative damage in rat hepatocytes. *Biochem. Pharmacol.*, **43**, 2135–2142

Shinzawa, T., Mura, T., Tsunei, M. & Shiraki, K. (1989) Vitamin K absorption capacity and its association with vitamin K deficiency. *Am. J. Dis. Child.*, **143**, 686–689

Smith, P.F., Alberts, D.W. & Rush, G.F. (1987) Menadione-induced oxidative stress in hepatocytes isolated from fed and fasted rats: The role of NADPH-regenerating pathways. *Toxicol. appl. Pharmacol.*, **89**, 190–201

Society of Japanese Pharmacopoeia (1996) *The Japanese Pharmacopoeia JP XIII*, 13th Ed., Tokyo, p. 569

Soedirman, J.R., De Bruijn, E.A., Maes, R.A.A., Hanck, A. & Grüter, J. (1996) Pharmacokinetics and tolerance of intravenous and intramuscular phylloquinone (vitamin K_1) mixed micelles formulation. *Br. J. clin. Pharmacol.*, **41**, 517–523

Solvonuk, P.F., Jaques, L.B., Leddy, J.E., Trevoy, L.W. & Spinks, J.W.T. (1952) Experiments with C^{14}-menadione (vitamin K_3). *Proc. Soc. exp. Biol. Med.*, **79**, 597–604

Stoeckel, K., Joubert, P.H. & Grüter, J. (1996) Elimination half-life of vitamin K_1 in neonates is longer than is generally assumed: Implications for the prophylaxis of haemorrhagic disease of the newborn. *Eur. J. clin. Pharmacol.*, **49**, 421–423

Sutor, A.H., von Kries, R., Cornelissen, M., McNinch, A.W. & Andrew, M. (1999) Vitamin K deficiency bleeding (VKDB) in infancy. *Thromb. Haemostasis*, **81**, 456–461

Suttie, J.W. (1985) Vitamin K. In: Diplock, A.T., ed., *Fat-soluble Vitamins. Their Biochemistry and Applications*, Lancaster, PA, Technomic Publishing Co., pp. 225–233, 295–311

Suttie, J.W. (1987) Recent advances in hepatic vitamin K metabolism and function. *Hepatology*, **7**, 367–376

Suttie, J.W. (1991) Vitamin K. In: Machlin, L.J., ed., *Handbook of Vitamins*, 2nd Ed., New York, Marcel Dekker, pp. 145–194

Suttie, J.W. (1995) The importance of menaquinones in human nutrition. *Ann. Rev. Nutr.*, **15**, 399–417

Swiss Pharmaceutical Society, ed. (1999) *Index Nominum, International Drug Directory*, 16th Ed., Stuttgart, Medpharm Scientific Publishers [MicroMedex Online: Health Care Series]

Taggart, W.V. & Matschiner, J.T. (1969) Metabolism of menadione-6,7-^{3}H in the rat. *Biochemistry*, **8**, 1141–1146

Taylor, J.D., Millar, G.J. & Wood, R.J. (1957) A comparison of the concentration of C^{14} in the tissues of pregnant and nonpregnant female rats following the intravenous administration of vitamin K_1-C^{14} and vitamin K_3-C^{14}. *Can. J. Biochem. Physiol.*, **35**, 691–697

Thierry, M.J. & Suttie, J.W. (1969) Distribution and metabolism of menadiol diphosphate in the rat. *J. Nutr.*, **97**, 512–516

Thijssen, H.H.W. & Drittij-Reijnders, M.J. (1996) Vitamin K status in human tissues: Tissue-specific accumulation of phylloquinone and menaquinone-4. *Br. J. Nutr.*, **75**, 121–127

Thomas, J., ed. (1998) *Australian Prescription Products Guide*, 27th Ed., Victoria, Australian Pharmaceutical Publishing Co., Vol. 1, pp. 687, 1562–1563, 1566, 1570, 1908–1909

Thorp, J.A., Gaston, L., Caspers, D.R. & Pal, M.L. (1995) Current concepts and controversies in the use of vitamin K. *Drugs*, **49**, 376–387

Tikkanen, L., Matsushima, T., Natori, S. & Yoshihira, K. (1983) Mutagenicity of natural naphthoquinones and benzoquinones in the *Salmonella*/microsome test. *Mutat. Res.*, **124**, 25–34

Tönz, O. & Schubiger, G. (1988) [Neonatal vitamin K prophylaxis and vitamin K deficiency hemorrhage in Switzerland 1986–1988.] *Schweiz. med. Wochenschr.*, **118**, 1747–1752 (in German)

Toxopeus, C., van Holsteijn, I., Thuring, J.W.F., Blaauboer, B.J. & Noordhoek, J. (1993) Cytotoxicity of menadione and related quinones in freshly isolated rat hepatocytes: Effects on thiol homeostasis and energy charge. *Arch. Toxicol.*, **67**, 674–679

Uchida, K. & Komeno, T. (1988) Relationships between dietary and intestinal vitamin K, clotting factor levels, plasma vitamin K, and urinary Gla. In: Suttie J.W., ed., *Current Advances in Vitamin K Research*, New York, Elsevier, pp. 477–492

US Pharmacopeial Convention (1994) *The 1995 US Pharmacopeia*, 23rd Rev./*The National Formulary*, 18th Rev., Rockville, MD, pp. 946–948, 1224–1226

US Pharmacopeial Convention (1998) *USP Dispensing Information*, Vol. I, *Drug Information for the Health Care Professional*, 18th Ed., Rockville, MD, pp. 2984–2986

Usui, Y., Tanimura, H., Nishimura, N., Kobayashi, N., Okanoue, T. & Ozawa, K. (1990) Vitamin K concentrations in the plasma and liver of surgical patients. *Am. J. clin. Nutr.*, **51**, 846–852

Van Arnum, S.D. (1998) Vitamin K. In: Kroschwitz, J.I. & Howe-Grant, M., eds, *Kirk-Othmer Encyclopedia of Chemical Technology*, 4th Ed., New York, John Wiley & Sons, Vol. 25, pp. 269–283

Vervoort, L.M.T., Ronden, J.E. & Thijssen, H.H.W. (1997) The potent antioxidant activity of the vitamin K cycle in microsomal lipid peroxidation. *Biochem. Pharmacol.*, **54**, 871–876

Vest, M. (1966) Vitamin K in medical practice: Pediatrics. *Vitam. Horm.*, **24**, 644–663

Watanabe, K., Sakamoto, K. & Sasaki, T. (1998) Comparisons on chemically-induced mutation among four bacterial strains, *Salmonella typhimurium* TA102 and TA2638, and *Escherichia coli* WP2/pKM101 and WP2 *uvrA*/pKM101: Collaborative study II. *Mutat. Res.*, **412**, 17–31

Weber, F. & Rüttimann, A. (1996) Vitamins. 5. Vitamin K. In: Elvers, B. & Hawkins, S., eds, *Ullmann's Encyclopedia of Chemical Technology*, 5th Ed., Weinheim, VCH Verlagsgesellschaft, Vol. A27, pp. 488–506

Winterbourn, C.C., French, J.K. & Claridge, R.F.C. (1979) The reaction of menadione with haemoglobin. Mechanism and effect of superoxide dismutase. *Biochem. J.*, **179**, 665–673

Woods, J.A., Young, A.J., Gilmore, I.T., Morris, A. & Bilton, R.F. (1997) Measurement of menadione-mediated DNA damage in human lymphocytes using the comet assay. *Free Radic. Res.*, **26**, 113–124

Yaguchi, M., Miyazawa, K., Katagiri, T., Nishimaki, J., Kizaki, M., Tohyama, K. & Toyama, K. (1997) Vitamin K2 and its derivatives induce apoptosis in leukemia cells and enhance the effect of all-*trans* retinoic acid. *Leukemia*, **11**, 779–787

Yang, Y.-M., Simon, N., Maertens, P., Brigham, S. & Liu, P. (1989) Maternal–fetal transport of vitamin K_1 and its effect on coagulation in premature infants. *J. Pediatr.*, **115**, 1009–1013

SUMMARY OF FINAL EVALUATIONS

Agent	Degree of evidence of carcinogenicity		Overall evaluation of carcinogenicity to humans
	Human	Animal	
Aciclovir	I	I	3
Amsacrine	I (ND)	S	2B
Didanosine	I	I (ND)	3
Etoposide	L	I	2A*
Etoposide in combination with cisplatin and bleomycin	S	I (ND)	1
Hydroxyurea	I	I	3
Mitoxantrone	L	I (ND)	2B
Phenolphthalein	I	S	2B
Teniposide	L	I (ND)	2A*
Vitamin K substances	I	I	3
Zalcitabine	I	S	2B
Zidovudine (AZT)	I	S	2B

I, inadequate evidence; L, limited evidence; S, sufficient evidence; ND, no data; group 1, carcinogenic to humans; group 2A, probably carcinogenic to humans; group 2B, possibly carcinogenic to humans; group 3, not classifiable as to its carcinogenicity to humans; for definitions of criteria for degrees of evidence and groups, see preamble, pp. 23–27.
*Other relevant data taken into consideration in making the overall evaluation.

CUMULATIVE CROSS INDEX TO *IARC MONOGRAPHS ON THE EVALUATION OF CARCINOGENIC RISKS TO HUMANS*

The volume, page and year of publication are given. References to corrigenda are given in parentheses.

A

A-α-C	40, 245 (1986); *Suppl.* 7, 56 (1987)
Acetaldehyde	36, 101 (1985) (*corr.* 42, 263); *Suppl.* 7, 77 (1987); 71, 319 (1999)
Acetaldehyde formylmethylhydrazone (*see* Gyromitrin)	
Acetamide	7, 197 (1974); *Suppl.* 7, 389 (1987); 71, 1211 (1999)
Acetaminophen (*see* Paracetamol)	
Aciclovir	76, 47 (2000)
Acridine orange	16, 145 (1978); *Suppl.* 7, 56 (1987)
Acriflavinium chloride	13, 31 (1977); *Suppl.* 7, 56 (1987)
Acrolein	19, 479 (1979); 36, 133 (1985); *Suppl.* 7, 78 (1987); 63, 337 (1995) (*corr.* 65, 549)
Acrylamide	39, 41 (1986); *Suppl.* 7, 56 (1987); 60, 389 (1994)
Acrylic acid	19, 47 (1979); *Suppl.* 7, 56 (1987); 71, 1223 (1999)
Acrylic fibres	19, 86 (1979); *Suppl.* 7, 56 (1987)
Acrylonitrile	19, 73 (1979); *Suppl.* 7, 79 (1987); 71, 43 (1999)
Acrylonitrile-butadiene-styrene copolymers	19, 91 (1979); *Suppl.* 7, 56 (1987)
Actinolite (*see* Asbestos)	
Actinomycin D (*see also* Actinomycins)	*Suppl.* 7, 80 (1987)
Actinomycins	10, 29 (1976) (*corr.* 42, 255)
Adriamycin	10, 43 (1976); *Suppl.* 7, 82 (1987)
AF-2	31, 47 (1983); *Suppl.* 7, 56 (1987)
Aflatoxins	1, 145 (1972) (*corr.* 42, 251); 10, 51 (1976); *Suppl.* 7, 83 (1987); 56, 245 (1993)
Aflatoxin B_1 (*see* Aflatoxins)	
Aflatoxin B_2 (*see* Aflatoxins)	
Aflatoxin G_1 (*see* Aflatoxins)	
Aflatoxin G_2 (*see* Aflatoxins)	
Aflatoxin M_1 (*see* Aflatoxins)	
Agaritine	31, 63 (1983); *Suppl.* 7, 56 (1987)
Alcohol drinking	44 (1988)
Aldicarb	53, 93 (1991)
Aldrin	5, 25 (1974); *Suppl.* 7, 88 (1987)

Allyl chloride	36, 39 (1985); *Suppl. 7*, 56 (1987); 71, 1231 (1999)
Allyl isothiocyanate	36, 55 (1985); *Suppl. 7*, 56 (1987); 73, 37 (1999)
Allyl isovalerate	36, 69 (1985); *Suppl. 7*, 56 (1987); 71, 1241 (1999)
Aluminium production	34, 37 (1984); *Suppl. 7*, 89 (1987)
Amaranth	8, 41 (1975); *Suppl. 7*, 56 (1987)
5-Aminoacenaphthene	16, 243 (1978); *Suppl. 7*, 56 (1987)
2-Aminoanthraquinone	27, 191 (1982); *Suppl. 7*, 56 (1987)
para-Aminoazobenzene	8, 53 (1975); *Suppl. 7*, 390 (1987)
ortho-Aminoazotoluene	8, 61 (1975) (*corr.* 42, 254); *Suppl. 7*, 56 (1987)
para-Aminobenzoic acid	16, 249 (1978); *Suppl. 7*, 56 (1987)
4-Aminobiphenyl	*1*, 74 (1972) (*corr.* 42, 251); *Suppl. 7*, 91 (1987)
2-Amino-3,4-dimethylimidazo[4,5-*f*]quinoline (*see* MeIQ)	
2-Amino-3,8-dimethylimidazo[4,5-*f*]quinoxaline (*see* MeIQx)	
3-Amino-1,4-dimethyl-5*H*-pyrido[4,3-*b*]indole (*see* Trp-P-1)	
2-Aminodipyrido[1,2-*a*:3′,2′-*d*]imidazole (*see* Glu-P-2)	
1-Amino-2-methylanthraquinone	27, 199 (1982); *Suppl. 7*, 57 (1987)
2-Amino-3-methylimidazo[4,5-*f*]quinoline (*see* IQ)	
2-Amino-6-methyldipyrido[1,2-*a*:3′,2′-*d*]imidazole (*see* Glu-P-1)	
2-Amino-1-methyl-6-phenylimidazo[4,5-*b*]pyridine (*see* PhIP)	
2-Amino-3-methyl-9*H*-pyrido[2,3-*b*]indole (*see* MeA-α-C)	
3-Amino-1-methyl-5*H*-pyrido[4,3-*b*]indole (*see* Trp-P-2)	
2-Amino-5-(5-nitro-2-furyl)-1,3,4-thiadiazole	7, 143 (1974); *Suppl. 7*, 57 (1987)
2-Amino-4-nitrophenol	57, 167 (1993)
2-Amino-5-nitrophenol	57, 177 (1993)
4-Amino-2-nitrophenol	16, 43 (1978); *Suppl. 7*, 57 (1987)
2-Amino-5-nitrothiazole	31, 71 (1983); *Suppl. 7*, 57 (1987)
2-Amino-9*H*-pyrido[2,3-*b*]indole (*see* A-α-C)	
11-Aminoundecanoic acid	39, 239 (1986); *Suppl. 7*, 57 (1987)
Amitrole	7, 31 (1974); *41*, 293 (1986) (*corr.* 52, 513; *Suppl. 7*, 92 (1987)
Ammonium potassium selenide (*see* Selenium and selenium compounds)	
Amorphous silica (*see also* Silica)	42, 39 (1987); *Suppl. 7*, 341 (1987); 68, 41 (1997)
Amosite (*see* Asbestos)	
Ampicillin	50, 153 (1990)
Amsacrine	76, 317 (2000)
Anabolic steroids (*see* Androgenic (anabolic) steroids)	
Anaesthetics, volatile	*11*, 285 (1976); *Suppl. 7*, 93 (1987)
Analgesic mixtures containing phenacetin (*see also* Phenacetin)	*Suppl. 7*, 310 (1987)
Androgenic (anabolic) steroids	*Suppl. 7*, 96 (1987)
Angelicin and some synthetic derivatives (*see also* Angelicins)	40, 291 (1986)
Angelicin plus ultraviolet radiation (*see also* Angelicin and some synthetic derivatives)	*Suppl. 7*, 57 (1987)
Angelicins	*Suppl. 7*, 57 (1987)
Aniline	4, 27 (1974) (*corr.* 42, 252); 27, 39 (1982); *Suppl. 7*, 99 (1987)
ortho-Anisidine	27, 63 (1982); *Suppl. 7*, 57 (1987); 73, 49 (1999)
para-Anisidine	27, 65 (1982); *Suppl. 7*, 57 (1987)

Anthanthrene	32, 95 (1983); *Suppl. 7*, 57 (1987)
Anthophyllite (*see* Asbestos)	
Anthracene	32, 105 (1983); *Suppl. 7*, 57 (1987)
Anthranilic acid	16, 265 (1978); *Suppl. 7*, 57 (1987)
Antimony trioxide	47, 291 (1989)
Antimony trisulfide	47, 291 (1989)
ANTU (*see* 1-Naphthylthiourea)	
Apholate	9, 31 (1975); *Suppl. 7*, 57 (1987)
para-Aramid fibrils	68, 409 (1997)
Aramite®	5, 39 (1974); *Suppl. 7*, 57 (1987)
Areca nut (*see* Betel quid)	
Arsanilic acid (*see* Arsenic and arsenic compounds)	
Arsenic and arsenic compounds	1, 41 (1972); 2, 48 (1973); 23, 39 (1980); *Suppl. 7*, 100 (1987)
Arsenic pentoxide (*see* Arsenic and arsenic compounds)	
Arsenic sulfide (*see* Arsenic and arsenic compounds)	
Arsenic trioxide (*see* Arsenic and arsenic compounds)	
Arsine (*see* Arsenic and arsenic compounds)	
Asbestos	2, 17 (1973) (*corr.* 42, 252); 14 (1977) (*corr.* 42, 256); *Suppl. 7*, 106 (1987) (*corr.* 45, 283)
Atrazine	53, 441 (1991); 73, 59 (1999)
Attapulgite (*see* Palygorskite)	
Auramine (technical-grade)	1, 69 (1972) (*corr.* 42, 251); *Suppl. 7*, 118 (1987)
Auramine, manufacture of (*see also* Auramine, technical-grade)	*Suppl. 7*, 118 (1987)
Aurothioglucose	13, 39 (1977); *Suppl. 7*, 57 (1987)
Azacitidine	26, 37 (1981); *Suppl. 7*, 57 (1987); 50, 47 (1990)
5-Azacytidine (*see* Azacitidine)	
Azaserine	10, 73 (1976) (*corr.* 42, 255); *Suppl. 7*, 57 (1987)
Azathioprine	26, 47 (1981); *Suppl. 7*, 119 (1987)
Aziridine	9, 37 (1975); *Suppl. 7*, 58 (1987); 71, 337 (1999)
2-(1-Aziridinyl)ethanol	9, 47 (1975); *Suppl. 7*, 58 (1987)
Aziridyl benzoquinone	9, 51 (1975); *Suppl. 7*, 58 (1987)
Azobenzene	8, 75 (1975); *Suppl. 7*, 58 (1987)
AZT (*see* Zidovudine)	

B

Barium chromate (*see* Chromium and chromium compounds)	
Basic chromic sulfate (*see* Chromium and chromium compounds)	
BCNU (*see* Bischloroethyl nitrosourea)	
Benz[*a*]acridine	32, 123 (1983); *Suppl. 7*, 58 (1987)
Benz[*c*]acridine	3, 241 (1973); 32, 129 (1983); *Suppl. 7*, 58 (1987)
Benzal chloride (*see also* α-Chlorinated toluenes and benzoyl chloride)	29, 65 (1982); *Suppl. 7*, 148 (1987); 71, 453 (1999)
Benz[*a*]anthracene	3, 45 (1973); 32, 135 (1983); *Suppl. 7*, 58 (1987)

Benzene	7, 203 (1974) (*corr. 42*, 254); *29*, 93, 391 (1982); *Suppl. 7*, 120 (1987)
Benzidine	*1*, 80 (1972); *29*, 149, 391 (1982); *Suppl. 7*, 123 (1987)
Benzidine-based dyes	*Suppl. 7*, 125 (1987)
Benzo[*b*]fluoranthene	*3*, 69 (1973); *32*, 147 (1983); *Suppl. 7*, 58 (1987)
Benzo[*j*]fluoranthene	*3*, 82 (1973); *32*, 155 (1983); *Suppl. 7*, 58 (1987)
Benzo[*k*]fluoranthene	*32*, 163 (1983); *Suppl. 7*, 58 (1987)
Benzo[*ghi*]fluoranthene	*32*, 171 (1983); *Suppl. 7*, 58 (1987)
Benzo[*a*]fluorene	*32*, 177 (1983); *Suppl. 7*, 58 (1987)
Benzo[*b*]fluorene	*32*, 183 (1983); *Suppl. 7*, 58 (1987)
Benzo[*c*]fluorene	*32*, 189 (1983); *Suppl. 7*, 58 (1987)
Benzofuran	*63*, 431 (1995)
Benzo[*ghi*]perylene	*32*, 195 (1983); *Suppl. 7*, 58 (1987)
Benzo[*c*]phenanthrene	*32*, 205 (1983); *Suppl. 7*, 58 (1987)
Benzo[*a*]pyrene	*3*, 91 (1973); *32*, 211 (1983) (*corr. 68*, 477); *Suppl. 7*, 58 (1987)
Benzo[*e*]pyrene	*3*, 137 (1973); *32*, 225 (1983); *Suppl. 7*, 58 (1987)
1,4-Benzoquinone (see *para*-Quinone)	
1,4-Benzoquinone dioxime	*29*, 185 (1982); *Suppl. 7*, 58 (1987); *71*, 1251 (1999)
Benzotrichloride (*see also* α-Chlorinated toluenes and benzoyl chloride)	*29*, 73 (1982); *Suppl. 7*, 148 (1987); *71*, 453 (1999)
Benzoyl chloride (*see also* α-Chlorinated toluenes and benzoyl chloride)	*29*, 83 (1982) (*corr. 42*, 261); *Suppl. 7*, 126 (1987); *71*, 453 (1999)
Benzoyl peroxide	*36*, 267 (1985); *Suppl. 7*, 58 (1987); *71*, 345 (1999)
Benzyl acetate	*40*, 109 (1986); *Suppl. 7*, 58 (1987); *71*, 1255 (1999)
Benzyl chloride (*see also* α-Chlorinated toluenes and benzoyl chloride)	*11*, 217 (1976) (*corr. 42*, 256); *29*, 49 (1982); *Suppl. 7*, 148 (1987); *71*, 453 (1999)
Benzyl violet 4B	*16*, 153 (1978); *Suppl. 7*, 58 (1987)
Bertrandite (*see* Beryllium and beryllium compounds)	
Beryllium and beryllium compounds	*1*, 17 (1972); *23*, 143 (1980) (*corr. 42*, 260); *Suppl. 7*, 127 (1987); *58*, 41 (1993)
Beryllium acetate (*see* Beryllium and beryllium compounds)	
Beryllium acetate, basic (*see* Beryllium and beryllium compounds)	
Beryllium-aluminium alloy (*see* Beryllium and beryllium compounds)	
Beryllium carbonate (*see* Beryllium and beryllium compounds)	
Beryllium chloride (*see* Beryllium and beryllium compounds)	
Beryllium-copper alloy (*see* Beryllium and beryllium compounds)	
Beryllium-copper-cobalt alloy (*see* Beryllium and beryllium compounds)	
Beryllium fluoride (*see* Beryllium and beryllium compounds)	
Beryllium hydroxide (*see* Beryllium and beryllium compounds)	
Beryllium-nickel alloy (*see* Beryllium and beryllium compounds)	
Beryllium oxide (*see* Beryllium and beryllium compounds)	
Beryllium phosphate (*see* Beryllium and beryllium compounds)	
Beryllium silicate (*see* Beryllium and beryllium compounds)	

Beryllium sulfate (see Beryllium and beryllium compounds)
Beryl ore (see Beryllium and beryllium compounds)
Betel quid 37, 141 (1985); Suppl. 7, 128
(1987)
Betel-quid chewing (see Betel quid)
BHA (see Butylated hydroxyanisole)
BHT (see Butylated hydroxytoluene)
Bis(1-aziridinyl)morpholinophosphine sulfide 9, 55 (1975); Suppl. 7, 58 (1987)
Bis(2-chloroethyl)ether 9, 117 (1975); Suppl. 7, 58 (1987); 71, 1265 (1999)
N,N-Bis(2-chloroethyl)-2-naphthylamine 4, 119 (1974) (corr. 42, 253); Suppl. 7, 130 (1987)
Bischloroethyl nitrosourea (see also Chloroethyl nitrosoureas) 26, 79 (1981); Suppl. 7, 150 (1987)
1,2-Bis(chloromethoxy)ethane 15, 31 (1977); Suppl. 7, 58 (1987); 71, 1271 (1999)
1,4-Bis(chloromethoxymethyl)benzene 15, 37 (1977); Suppl. 7, 58 (1987); 71, 1273 (1999)
Bis(chloromethyl)ether 4, 231 (1974) (corr. 42, 253); Suppl. 7, 131 (1987)
Bis(2-chloro-1-methylethyl)ether 41, 149 (1986); Suppl. 7, 59 (1987); 71, 1275 (1999)
Bis(2,3-epoxycyclopentyl)ether 47, 231 (1989); 71, 1281 (1999)
Bisphenol A diglycidyl ether (see also Glycidyl ethers) 71, 1285 (1999)
Bisulfites (see Sulfur dioxide and some sulfites, bisulfites and metabisulfites)
Bitumens 35, 39 (1985); Suppl. 7, 133 (1987)
Bleomycins (see also Etoposide) 26, 97 (1981); Suppl. 7, 134 (1987)
Blue VRS 16, 163 (1978); Suppl. 7, 59 (1987)
Boot and shoe manufacture and repair 25, 249 (1981); Suppl. 7, 232 (1987)
Bracken fern 40, 47 (1986); Suppl. 7, 135 (1987)
Brilliant Blue FCF, disodium salt 16, 171 (1978) (corr. 42, 257); Suppl. 7, 59 (1987)
Bromochloroacetonitrile (see also Halogenated acetonitriles) 71, 1291 (1999)
Bromodichloromethane 52, 179 (1991); 71, 1295 (1999)
Bromoethane 52, 299 (1991); 71, 1305 (1999)
Bromoform 52, 213 (1991); 71, 1309 (1999)
1,3-Butadiene 39, 155 (1986) (corr. 42, 264 Suppl. 7, 136 (1987); 54, 237 (1992); 71, 109 (1999)
1,4-Butanediol dimethanesulfonate 4, 247 (1974); Suppl. 7, 137 (1987)
n-Butyl acrylate 39, 67 (1986); Suppl. 7, 59 (1987); 71, 359 (1999)
Butylated hydroxyanisole 40, 123 (1986); Suppl. 7, 59 (1987)
Butylated hydroxytoluene 40, 161 (1986); Suppl. 7, 59 (1987)
Butyl benzyl phthalate 29, 193 (1982) (corr. 42, 261); Suppl. 7, 59 (1987); 73, 115 (1999)
β-Butyrolactone 11, 225 (1976); Suppl. 7, 59 (1987); 71, 1317 (1999)
γ-Butyrolactone 11, 231 (1976); Suppl. 7, 59 (1987); 71, 367 (1999)

C

Cabinet-making (*see* Furniture and cabinet-making)
Cadmium acetate (*see* Cadmium and cadmium compounds)
Cadmium and cadmium compounds   2, 74 (1973); *11*, 39 (1976) (*corr.* 42, 255); *Suppl. 7*, 139 (1987); *58*, 119 (1993)

Cadmium chloride (*see* Cadmium and cadmium compounds)
Cadmium oxide (*see* Cadmium and cadmium compounds)
Cadmium sulfate (*see* Cadmium and cadmium compounds)
Cadmium sulfide (*see* Cadmium and cadmium compounds)
Caffeic acid   *56*, 115 (1993)
Caffeine   *51*, 291 (1991)
Calcium arsenate (*see* Arsenic and arsenic compounds)
Calcium chromate (see Chromium and chromium compounds)
Calcium cyclamate (*see* Cyclamates)
Calcium saccharin (*see* Saccharin)
Cantharidin   *10*, 79 (1976); *Suppl. 7*, 59 (1987)
Caprolactam   *19*, 115 (1979) (*corr.* 42, 258); *39*, 247 (1986) (*corr.* 42, 264); *Suppl. 7*, 390 (1987); *71*, 383 (1999)
Captafol   *53*, 353 (1991)
Captan   *30*, 295 (1983); *Suppl. 7*, 59 (1987)
Carbaryl   *12*, 37 (1976); *Suppl. 7*, 59 (1987)
Carbazole   *32*, 239 (1983); *Suppl. 7*, 59 (1987); *71*, 1319 (1999)
3-Carbethoxypsoralen   *40*, 317 (1986); *Suppl. 7*, 59 (1987)
Carbon black   *3*, 22 (1973); *33*, 35 (1984); *Suppl. 7*, 142 (1987); *65*, 149 (1996)
Carbon tetrachloride   *1*, 53 (1972); *20*, 371 (1979); *Suppl. 7*, 143 (1987); *71*, 401 (1999)
Carmoisine   *8*, 83 (1975); *Suppl. 7*, 59 (1987)
Carpentry and joinery   *25*, 139 (1981); *Suppl. 7*, 378 (1987)
Carrageenan   *10*, 181 (1976) (*corr.* 42, 255); *31*, 79 (1983); *Suppl. 7*, 59 (1987)
Catechol   *15*, 155 (1977); *Suppl. 7*, 59 (1987); *71*, 433 (1999)
CCNU (*see* 1-(2-Chloroethyl)-3-cyclohexyl-1-nitrosourea)
Ceramic fibres (see Man-made mineral fibres)
Chemotherapy, combined, including alkylating agents (*see* MOPP and other combined chemotherapy including alkylating agents)
Chloral   *63*, 245 (1995)
Chloral hydrate   *63*, 245 (1995)
Chlorambucil   *9*, 125 (1975); *26*, 115 (1981); *Suppl. 7*, 144 (1987)
Chloramphenicol   *10*, 85 (1976); *Suppl. 7*, 145 (1987); *50*, 169 (1990)
Chlordane (*see also* Chlordane/Heptachlor)   *20*, 45 (1979) (*corr.* 42, 258)
Chlordane/Heptachlor   *Suppl. 7*, 146 (1987); *53*, 115 (1991)

Chlordecone	20, 67 (1979); Suppl. 7, 59 (1987)
Chlordimeform	30, 61 (1983); Suppl. 7, 59 (1987)
Chlorendic acid	48, 45 (1990)
Chlorinated dibenzodioxins (other than TCDD) (see also Polychlorinated dibenzo-*para*-dioxins)	15, 41 (1977); Suppl. 7, 59 (1987)
Chlorinated drinking-water	52, 45 (1991)
Chlorinated paraffins	48, 55 (1990)
α-Chlorinated toluenes and benzoyl chloride	Suppl. 7, 148 (1987); 71, 453 (1999)
Chlormadinone acetate	6, 149 (1974); 21, 365 (1979); Suppl. 7, 291, 301 (1987); 72, 49 (1999)
Chlornaphazine (see *N,N*-Bis(2-chloroethyl)-2-naphthylamine)	
Chloroacetonitrile (see also Halogenated acetonitriles)	71, 1325 (1999)
para-Chloroaniline	57, 305 (1993)
Chlorobenzilate	5, 75 (1974); 30, 73 (1983); Suppl. 7, 60 (1987)
Chlorodibromomethane	52, 243 (1991); 71, 1331 (1999)
Chlorodifluoromethane	41, 237 (1986) (corr. 51, 483); Suppl. 7, 149 (1987); 71, 1339 (1999)
Chloroethane	52, 315 (1991); 71, 1345 (1999)
1-(2-Chloroethyl)-3-cyclohexyl-1-nitrosourea (see also Chloroethyl nitrosoureas)	26, 137 (1981) (corr. 42, 260); Suppl. 7, 150 (1987)
1-(2-Chloroethyl)-3-(4-methylcyclohexyl)-1-nitrosourea (see also Chloroethyl nitrosoureas)	Suppl. 7, 150 (1987)
Chloroethyl nitrosoureas	Suppl. 7, 150 (1987)
Chlorofluoromethane	41, 229 (1986); Suppl. 7, 60 (1987); 71, 1351 (1999)
Chloroform	1, 61 (1972); 20, 401 (1979); Suppl. 7, 152 (1987); 73, 131 (1999)
Chloromethyl methyl ether (technical-grade) (see also Bis(chloromethyl)ether)	4, 239 (1974); Suppl. 7, 131 (1987)
(4-Chloro-2-methylphenoxy)acetic acid (see MCPA)	
1-Chloro-2-methylpropene	63, 315 (1995)
3-Chloro-2-methylpropene	63, 325 (1995)
2-Chloronitrobenzene	65, 263 (1996)
3-Chloronitrobenzene	65, 263 (1996)
4-Chloronitrobenzene	65, 263 (1996)
Chlorophenols (see also Polychlorophenols and their sodium salts)	Suppl. 7, 154 (1987)
Chlorophenols (occupational exposures to)	41, 319 (1986)
Chlorophenoxy herbicides	Suppl. 7, 156 (1987)
Chlorophenoxy herbicides (occupational exposures to)	41, 357 (1986)
4-Chloro-*ortho*-phenylenediamine	27, 81 (1982); Suppl. 7, 60 (1987)
4-Chloro-*meta*-phenylenediamine	27, 82 (1982); Suppl. 7, 60 (1987)
Chloroprene	19, 131 (1979); Suppl. 7, 160 (1987); 71, 227 (1999)
Chloropropham	12, 55 (1976); Suppl. 7, 60 (1987)
Chloroquine	13, 47 (1977); Suppl. 7, 60 (1987)
Chlorothalonil	30, 319 (1983); Suppl. 7, 60 (1987); 73, 183 (1999)
para-Chloro-*ortho*-toluidine and its strong acid salts (see also Chlordimeform)	16, 277 (1978); 30, 65 (1983); Suppl. 7, 60 (1987); 48, 123 (1990)

Chlorotrianisene (*see also* Nonsteroidal oestrogens)	*21*, 139 (1979); *Suppl. 7*, 280 (1987)
2-Chloro-1,1,1-trifluoroethane	*41*, 253 (1986); *Suppl. 7*, 60 (1987); *71*, 1355 (1999)
Chlorozotocin	*50*, 65 (1990)
Cholesterol	*10*, 99 (1976); *31*, 95 (1983); *Suppl. 7*, 161 (1987)
Chromic acetate (*see* Chromium and chromium compounds)	
Chromic chloride (*see* Chromium and chromium compounds)	
Chromic oxide (*see* Chromium and chromium compounds)	
Chromic phosphate (*see* Chromium and chromium compounds)	
Chromite ore (*see* Chromium and chromium compounds)	
Chromium and chromium compounds (*see also* Implants, surgical)	*2*, 100 (1973); *23*, 205 (1980); *Suppl. 7*, 165 (1987); *49*, 49 (1990) (*corr. 51*, 483)
Chromium carbonyl (*see* Chromium and chromium compounds)	
Chromium potassium sulfate (*see* Chromium and chromium compounds)	
Chromium sulfate (*see* Chromium and chromium compounds)	
Chromium trioxide (*see* Chromium and chromium compounds)	
Chrysazin (*see* Dantron)	
Chrysene	*3*, 159 (1973); *32*, 247 (1983); *Suppl. 7*, 60 (1987)
Chrysoidine	*8*, 91 (1975); *Suppl. 7*, 169 (1987)
Chrysotile (*see* Asbestos)	
CI Acid Orange 3	*57*, 121 (1993)
CI Acid Red 114	*57*, 247 (1993)
CI Basic Red 9 (*see also* Magenta)	*57*, 215 (1993)
Ciclosporin	*50*, 77 (1990)
CI Direct Blue 15	*57*, 235 (1993)
CI Disperse Yellow 3 (see Disperse Yellow 3)	
Cimetidine	*50*, 235 (1990)
Cinnamyl anthranilate	*16*, 287 (1978); *31*, 133 (1983); *Suppl. 7*, 60 (1987)
CI Pigment Red 3	*57*, 259 (1993)
CI Pigment Red 53:1 (*see* D&C Red No. 9)	
Cisplatin (*see also* Etoposide)	*26*, 151 (1981); *Suppl. 7*, 170 (1987)
Citrinin	*40*, 67 (1986); *Suppl. 7*, 60 (1987)
Citrus Red No. 2	*8*, 101 (1975) (*corr. 42*, 254); *Suppl. 7*, 60 (1987)
Clinoptilolite (*see* Zeolites)	
Clofibrate	*24*, 39 (1980); *Suppl. 7*, 171 (1987); *66*, 391 (1996)
Clomiphene citrate	*21*, 551 (1979); *Suppl. 7*, 172 (1987)
Clonorchis sinensis (infection with)	*61*, 121 (1994)
Coal dust	*68*, 337 (1997)
Coal gasification	*34*, 65 (1984); *Suppl. 7*, 173 (1987)
Coal-tar pitches (*see also* Coal-tars)	*35*, 83 (1985); *Suppl. 7*, 174 (1987)
Coal-tars	*35*, 83 (1985); *Suppl. 7*, 175 (1987)
Cobalt[III] acetate (*see* Cobalt and cobalt compounds)	
Cobalt-aluminium-chromium spinel (*see* Cobalt and cobalt compounds)	
Cobalt and cobalt compounds (*see also* Implants, surgical)	*52*, 363 (1991)
Cobalt[II] chloride (*see* Cobalt and cobalt compounds)	

Cobalt-chromium alloy (see Chromium and chromium compounds)
Cobalt-chromium-molybdenum alloys (see Cobalt and cobalt compounds)
Cobalt metal powder (see Cobalt and cobalt compounds)
Cobalt naphthenate (see Cobalt and cobalt compounds)
Cobalt[II] oxide (see Cobalt and cobalt compounds)
Cobalt[II,III] oxide (see Cobalt and cobalt compounds)
Cobalt[II] sulfide (see Cobalt and cobalt compounds)

Coffee	*51*, 41 (1991) (*corr. 52*, 513)
Coke production	*34*, 101 (1984); *Suppl. 7*, 176 (1987)

Combined oral contraceptives (see Oral contraceptives, combined)

Conjugated equine oestrogens	*72*, 399 (1999)
Conjugated oestrogens (see also Steroidal oestrogens)	*21*, 147 (1979); *Suppl. 7*, 283 (1987)

Contraceptives, oral (see Oral contraceptives, combined; Sequential oral contraceptives)

Copper 8-hydroxyquinoline	*15*, 103 (1977); *Suppl. 7*, 61 (1987)
Coronene	*32*, 263 (1983); *Suppl. 7*, 61 (1987)
Coumarin	*10*, 113 (1976); *Suppl. 7*, 61 (1987)
Creosotes (see also Coal-tars)	*35*, 83 (1985); *Suppl. 7*, 177 (1987)
meta-Cresidine	*27*, 91 (1982); *Suppl. 7*, 61 (1987)
para-Cresidine	*27*, 92 (1982); *Suppl. 7*, 61 (1987)

Cristobalite (see Crystalline silica)
Crocidolite (see Asbestos)

Crotonaldehyde	*63*, 373 (1995) (*corr. 65*, 549)
Crude oil	*45*, 119 (1989)
Crystalline silica (see also Silica)	*42*, 39 (1987); *Suppl. 7*, 341 (1987); *68*, 41 (1997)
Cycasin (see also Methylazoxymethanol)	*1*, 157 (1972) (*corr. 42*, 251); *10*, 121 (1976); *Suppl. 7*, 61 (1987)
Cyclamates	*22*, 55 (1980); *Suppl. 7*, 178 (1987); *73*, 195 (1999)

Cyclamic acid (see Cyclamates)

Cyclochlorotine	*10*, 139 (1976); *Suppl. 7*, 61 (1987)
Cyclohexanone	*47*, 157 (1989); *71*, 1359 (1999)

Cyclohexylamine (see Cyclamates)

Cyclopenta[*cd*]pyrene	*32*, 269 (1983); *Suppl. 7*, 61 (1987)

Cyclopropane (see Anaesthetics, volatile)

Cyclophosphamide	*9*, 135 (1975); *26*, 165 (1981); *Suppl. 7*, 182 (1987)
Cyproterone acetate	*72*, 49 (1999)

D

2,4-D (see also Chlorophenoxy herbicides; Chlorophenoxy herbicides, occupational exposures to)	*15*, 111 (1977)
Dacarbazine	*26*, 203 (1981); *Suppl. 7*, 184 (1987)
Dantron	*50*, 265 (1990) (*corr. 59*, 257)
D&C Red No. 9	*8*, 107 (1975); *Suppl. 7*, 61 (1987); *57*, 203 (1993)
Dapsone	*24*, 59 (1980); *Suppl. 7*, 185 (1987)
Daunomycin	*10*, 145 (1976); *Suppl. 7*, 61 (1987)

DDD (see DDT)	
DDE (see DDT)	
DDT	5, 83 (1974) (corr. 42, 253); Suppl. 7, 186 (1987); 53, 179 (1991)
Decabromodiphenyl oxide	48, 73 (1990); 71, 1365 (1999)
Deltamethrin	53, 251 (1991)
Deoxynivalenol (see Toxins derived from *Fusarium graminearum*, *F. culmorum* and *F. crookwellense*)	
Diacetylaminoazotoluene	8, 113 (1975); Suppl. 7, 61 (1987)
N,N'-Diacetylbenzidine	16, 293 (1978); Suppl. 7, 61 (1987)
Diallate	12, 69 (1976); 30, 235 (1983); Suppl. 7, 61 (1987)
2,4-Diaminoanisole	16, 51 (1978); 27, 103 (1982); Suppl. 7, 61 (1987)
4,4'-Diaminodiphenyl ether	16, 301 (1978); 29, 203 (1982); Suppl. 7, 61 (1987)
1,2-Diamino-4-nitrobenzene	16, 63 (1978); Suppl. 7, 61 (1987)
1,4-Diamino-2-nitrobenzene	16, 73 (1978); Suppl. 7, 61 (1987); 57, 185 (1993)
2,6-Diamino-3-(phenylazo)pyridine (see Phenazopyridine hydrochloride)	
2,4-Diaminotoluene (see also Toluene diisocyanates)	16, 83 (1978); Suppl. 7, 61 (1987)
2,5-Diaminotoluene (see also Toluene diisocyanates)	16, 97 (1978); Suppl. 7, 61 (1987)
ortho-Dianisidine (see 3,3'-Dimethoxybenzidine)	
Diatomaceous earth, uncalcined (see Amorphous silica)	
Diazepam	13, 57 (1977); Suppl. 7, 189 (1987); 66, 37 (1996)
Diazomethane	7, 223 (1974); Suppl. 7, 61 (1987)
Dibenz[a,h]acridine	3, 247 (1973); 32, 277 (1983); Suppl. 7, 61 (1987)
Dibenz[a,j]acridine	3, 254 (1973); 32, 283 (1983); Suppl. 7, 61 (1987)
Dibenz[a,c]anthracene	32, 289 (1983) (corr. 42, 262); Suppl. 7, 61 (1987)
Dibenz[a,h]anthracene	3, 178 (1973) (corr. 43, 261); 32, 299 (1983); Suppl. 7, 61 (1987)
Dibenz[a,j]anthracene	32, 309 (1983); Suppl. 7, 61 (1987)
7H-Dibenzo[c,g]carbazole	3, 260 (1973); 32, 315 (1983); Suppl. 7, 61 (1987)
Dibenzodioxins, chlorinated (other than TCDD) (see Chlorinated dibenzodioxins (other than TCDD))	
Dibenzo[a,e]fluoranthene	32, 321 (1983); Suppl. 7, 61 (1987)
Dibenzo[h,rst]pentaphene	3, 197 (1973); Suppl. 7, 62 (1987)
Dibenzo[a,e]pyrene	3, 201 (1973); 32, 327 (1983); Suppl. 7, 62 (1987)
Dibenzo[a,h]pyrene	3, 207 (1973); 32, 331 (1983); Suppl. 7, 62 (1987)
Dibenzo[a,i]pyrene	3, 215 (1973); 32, 337 (1983); Suppl. 7, 62 (1987)
Dibenzo[a,l]pyrene	3, 224 (1973); 32, 343 (1983); Suppl. 7, 62 (1987)
Dibenzo-*para*-dioxin	69, 33 (1997)
Dibromoacetonitrile (see also Halogenated acetonitriles)	71, 1369 (1999)

1,2-Dibromo-3-chloropropane	*15*, 139 (1977); *20*, 83 (1979); Suppl. 7, 191 (1987); *71*, 479 (1999)
1,2-Dibromoethane (*see* Ethylene dibromide)	
Dichloroacetic acid	*63*, 271 (1995)
Dichloroacetonitrile (*see also* Halogenated acetonitriles)	*71*, 1375 (1999)
Dichloroacetylene	*39*, 369 (1986); Suppl. 7, 62 (1987); *71*, 1381 (1999)
ortho-Dichlorobenzene	*7*, 231 (1974); *29*, 213 (1982); Suppl. 7, 192 (1987); *73*, 223 (1999)
meta-Dichlorobenzene	*73*, 223 (1999)
para-Dichlorobenzene	*7*, 231 (1974); *29*, 215 (1982); Suppl. 7, 192 (1987); *73*, 223 (1999)
3,3'-Dichlorobenzidine	*4*, 49 (1974); *29*, 239 (1982); Suppl. 7, 193 (1987)
trans-1,4-Dichlorobutene	*15*, 149 (1977); Suppl. 7, 62 (1987); *71*, 1389 (1999)
3,3'-Dichloro-4,4'-diaminodiphenyl ether	*16*, 309 (1978); Suppl. 7, 62 (1987)
1,2-Dichloroethane	*20*, 429 (1979); Suppl. 7, 62 (1987); *71*, 501 (1999)
Dichloromethane	*20*, 449 (1979); *41*, 43 (1986); Suppl. 7, 194 (1987); *71*, 251 (1999)
2,4-Dichlorophenol (*see* Chlorophenols; Chlorophenols, occupational exposures to; Polychlorophenols and their sodium salts)	
(2,4-Dichlorophenoxy)acetic acid (*see* 2,4-D)	
2,6-Dichloro-*para*-phenylenediamine	*39*, 325 (1986); Suppl. 7, 62 (1987)
1,2-Dichloropropane	*41*, 131 (1986); Suppl. 7, 62 (1987); *71*, 1393 (1999)
1,3-Dichloropropene (technical-grade)	*41*, 113 (1986); Suppl. 7, 195 (1987); *71*, 933 (1999)
Dichlorvos	*20*, 97 (1979); Suppl. 7, 62 (1987); *53*, 267 (1991)
Dicofol	*30*, 87 (1983); Suppl. 7, 62 (1987)
Dicyclohexylamine (*see* Cyclamates)	
Didanosine	*76*, 153 (2000)
Dieldrin	*5*, 125 (1974); Suppl. 7, 196 (1987)
Dienoestrol (*see also* Nonsteroidal oestrogens)	*21*, 161 (1979); Suppl. 7, 278 (1987)
Diepoxybutane (*see also* 1,3-Butadiene)	*11*, 115 (1976) (*corr. 42*, 255); Suppl. 7, 62 (1987); *71*, 109 (1999)
Diesel and gasoline engine exhausts	*46*, 41 (1989)
Diesel fuels	*45*, 219 (1989) (*corr. 47*, 505)
Diethyl ether (*see* Anaesthetics, volatile)	
Di(2-ethylhexyl)adipate	*29*, 257 (1982); Suppl. 7, 62 (1987)
Di(2-ethylhexyl)phthalate	*29*, 269 (1982) (*corr. 42*, 261); Suppl. 7, 62 (1987)
1,2-Diethylhydrazine	*4*, 153 (1974); Suppl. 7, 62 (1987); *71*, 1401 (1999)
Diethylstilboestrol	*6*, 55 (1974); *21*, 173 (1979) (*corr. 42*, 259); Suppl. 7, 273 (1987)
Diethylstilboestrol dipropionate (*see* Diethylstilboestrol)	

Diethyl sulfate	4, 277 (1974); *Suppl. 7*, 198 (1987); *54*, 213 (1992); *71*, 1405 (1999)
Diglycidyl resorcinol ether	*11*, 125 (1976); *36*, 181 (1985); *Suppl. 7*, 62 (1987); *71*, 1417 (1999)
Dihydrosafrole	*1*, 170 (1972); *10*, 233 (1976) *Suppl. 7*, 62 (1987)
1,8-Dihydroxyanthraquinone (*see* Dantron)	
Dihydroxybenzenes (*see* Catechol; Hydroquinone; Resorcinol)	
Dihydroxymethylfuratrizine	*24*, 77 (1980); *Suppl. 7*, 62 (1987)
Diisopropyl sulfate	*54*, 229 (1992); *71*, 1421 (1999)
Dimethisterone (*see also* Progestins; Sequential oral contraceptives)	*6*, 167 (1974); *21*, 377 (1979))
Dimethoxane	*15*, 177 (1977); *Suppl. 7*, 62 (1987)
3,3'-Dimethoxybenzidine	*4*, 41 (1974); *Suppl. 7*, 198 (1987)
3,3'-Dimethoxybenzidine-4,4'-diisocyanate	*39*, 279 (1986); *Suppl. 7*, 62 (1987)
para-Dimethylaminoazobenzene	*8*, 125 (1975); *Suppl. 7*, 62 (1987)
para-Dimethylaminoazobenzenediazo sodium sulfonate	*8*, 147 (1975); *Suppl. 7*, 62 (1987)
trans-2-[(Dimethylamino)methylimino]-5-[2-(5-nitro-2-furyl)-vinyl]-1,3,4-oxadiazole	*7*, 147 (1974) (*corr. 42*, 253); *Suppl. 7*, 62 (1987)
4,4'-Dimethylangelicin plus ultraviolet radiation (*see also* Angelicin and some synthetic derivatives)	*Suppl. 7*, 57 (1987)
4,5'-Dimethylangelicin plus ultraviolet radiation (*see also* Angelicin and some synthetic derivatives)	*Suppl. 7*, 57 (1987)
2,6-Dimethylaniline	*57*, 323 (1993)
N,N-Dimethylaniline	*57*, 337 (1993)
Dimethylarsinic acid (*see* Arsenic and arsenic compounds)	
3,3'-Dimethylbenzidine	*1*, 87 (1972); *Suppl. 7*, 62 (1987)
Dimethylcarbamoyl chloride	*12*, 77 (1976); *Suppl. 7*, 199 (1987); *71*, 531 (1999)
Dimethylformamide	*47*, 171 (1989); *71*, 545 (1999)
1,1-Dimethylhydrazine	*4*, 137 (1974); *Suppl. 7*, 62 (1987); *71*, 1425 (1999)
1,2-Dimethylhydrazine	*4*, 145 (1974) (*corr. 42*, 253); *Suppl. 7*, 62 (1987); *71*, 947 (1999)
Dimethyl hydrogen phosphite	*48*, 85 (1990); *71*, 1437 (1999)
1,4-Dimethylphenanthrene	*32*, 349 (1983); *Suppl. 7*, 62 (1987)
Dimethyl sulfate	*4*, 271 (1974); *Suppl. 7*, 200 (1987); *71*, 575 (1999)
3,7-Dinitrofluoranthene	*46*, 189 (1989); *65*, 297 (1996)
3,9-Dinitrofluoranthene	*46*, 195 (1989); *65*, 297 (1996)
1,3-Dinitropyrene	*46*, 201 (1989)
1,6-Dinitropyrene	*46*, 215 (1989)
1,8-Dinitropyrene	*33*, 171 (1984); *Suppl. 7*, 63 (1987); *46*, 231 (1989)
Dinitrosopentamethylenetetramine	*11*, 241 (1976); *Suppl. 7*, 63 (1987)
2,4-Dinitrotoluene	*65*, 309 (1996) (*corr. 66*, 485)
2,6-Dinitrotoluene	*65*, 309 (1996) (*corr. 66*, 485)
3,5-Dinitrotoluene	*65*, 309 (1996)
1,4-Dioxane	*11*, 247 (1976); *Suppl. 7*, 201 (1987); *71*, 589 (1999)
2,4'-Diphenyldiamine	*16*, 313 (1978); *Suppl. 7*, 63 (1987)
Direct Black 38 (*see also* Benzidine-based dyes)	*29*, 295 (1982) (*corr. 42*, 261)
Direct Blue 6 (*see also* Benzidine-based dyes)	*29*, 311 (1982)

Direct Brown 95 (*see also* Benzidine-based dyes)	*29*, 321 (1982)
Disperse Blue 1	*48*, 139 (1990)
Disperse Yellow 3	*8*, 97 (1975); *Suppl. 7*, 60 (1987); *48*, 149 (1990)
Disulfiram	*12*, 85 (1976); *Suppl. 7*, 63 (1987)
Dithranol	*13*, 75 (1977); *Suppl. 7*, 63 (1987)
Divinyl ether (*see* Anaesthetics, volatile)	
Doxefazepam	*66*, 97 (1996)
Droloxifene	*66*, 241 (1996)
Dry cleaning	*63*, 33 (1995)
Dulcin	*12*, 97 (1976); *Suppl. 7*, 63 (1987)

E

Endrin	*5*, 157 (1974); *Suppl. 7*, 63 (1987)
Enflurane (*see* Anaesthetics, volatile)	
Eosin	*15*, 183 (1977); *Suppl. 7*, 63 (1987)
Epichlorohydrin	*11*, 131 (1976) (*corr. 42*, 256); *Suppl. 7*, 202 (1987); *71*, 603 (1999)
1,2-Epoxybutane	*47*, 217 (1989); *71*, 629 (1999)
1-Epoxyethyl-3,4-epoxycyclohexane (*see* 4-Vinylcyclohexene diepoxide)	
3,4-Epoxy-6-methylcyclohexylmethyl 3,4-epoxy-6-methyl-cyclohexane carboxylate	*11*, 147 (1976); *Suppl. 7*, 63 (1987); *71*, 1441 (1999)
cis-9,10-Epoxystearic acid	*11*, 153 (1976); *Suppl. 7*, 63 (1987); *71*, 1443 (1999)
Epstein-Barr virus	*70*, 47 (1997)
d-Equilenin	*72*, 399 (1999)
Equilin	*72*, 399 (1999)
Erionite	*42*, 225 (1987); *Suppl. 7*, 203 (1987)
Estazolam	*66*, 105 (1996)
Ethinyloestradiol	*6*, 77 (1974); *21*, 233 (1979); *Suppl. 7*, 286 (1987); *72*, 49 (1999)
Ethionamide	*13*, 83 (1977); *Suppl. 7*, 63 (1987)
Ethyl acrylate	*19*, 57 (1979); *39*, 81 (1986); *Suppl. 7*, 63 (1987); *71*, 1447 (1999)
Ethylene	*19*, 157 (1979); *Suppl. 7*, 63 (1987); *60*, 45 (1994); *71*, 1447 (1999)
Ethylene dibromide	*15*, 195 (1977); *Suppl. 7*, 204 (1987); *71*, 641 (1999)
Ethylene oxide	*11*, 157 (1976); *36*, 189 (1985) (*corr. 42*, 263); *Suppl. 7*, 205 (1987); *60*, 73 (1994)
Ethylene sulfide	*11*, 257 (1976); *Suppl. 7*, 63 (1987)
Ethylene thiourea	*7*, 45 (1974); *Suppl. 7*, 207 (1987)
2-Ethylhexyl acrylate	*60*, 475 (1994)
Ethyl methanesulfonate	*7*, 245 (1974); *Suppl. 7*, 63 (1987)
N-Ethyl-*N*-nitrosourea	*1*, 135 (1972); *17*, 191 (1978); *Suppl. 7*, 63 (1987)
Ethyl selenac (*see also* Selenium and selenium compounds)	*12*, 107 (1976); *Suppl. 7*, 63 (1987)

Ethyl tellurac	12, 115 (1976); Suppl. 7, 63 (1987)
Ethynodiol diacetate	6, 173 (1974); 21, 387 (1979); Suppl. 7, 292 (1987); 72, 49 (1999)
Etoposide	76, 177 (2000)
Eugenol	36, 75 (1985); Suppl. 7, 63 (1987)
Evans blue	8, 151 (1975); Suppl. 7, 63 (1987)

F

Fast Green FCF	16, 187 (1978); Suppl. 7, 63 (1987)
Fenvalerate	53, 309 (1991)
Ferbam	12, 121 (1976) (corr. 42, 256); Suppl. 7, 63 (1987)
Ferric oxide	1, 29 (1972); Suppl. 7, 216 (1987)
Ferrochromium (see Chromium and chromium compounds)	
Fluometuron	30, 245 (1983); Suppl. 7, 63 (1987)
Fluoranthene	32, 355 (1983); Suppl. 7, 63 (1987)
Fluorene	32, 365 (1983); Suppl. 7, 63 (1987)
Fluorescent lighting (exposure to) (see Ultraviolet radiation)	
Fluorides (inorganic, used in drinking-water)	27, 237 (1982); Suppl. 7, 208 (1987)
5-Fluorouracil	26, 217 (1981); Suppl. 7, 210 (1987)
Fluorspar (see Fluorides)	
Fluosilicic acid (see Fluorides)	
Fluroxene (see Anaesthetics, volatile)	
Foreign bodies	74 (1999)
Formaldehyde	29, 345 (1982); Suppl. 7, 211 (1987); 62, 217 (1995) (corr. 65, 549; corr. 66, 485)
2-(2-Formylhydrazino)-4-(5-nitro-2-furyl)thiazole	7, 151 (1974) (corr. 42, 253); Suppl. 7, 63 (1987)
Frusemide (see Furosemide)	
Fuel oils (heating oils)	45, 239 (1989) (corr. 47, 505)
Fumonisin B_1 (see Toxins derived from Fusarium moniliforme)	
Fumonisin B_2 (see Toxins derived from Fusarium moniliforme)	
Furan	63, 393 (1995)
Furazolidone	31, 141 (1983); Suppl. 7, 63 (1987)
Furfural	63, 409 (1995)
Furniture and cabinet-making	25, 99 (1981); Suppl. 7, 380 (1987)
Furosemide	50, 277 (1990)
2-(2-Furyl)-3-(5-nitro-2-furyl)acrylamide (see AF-2)	
Fusarenon-X (see Toxins derived from Fusarium graminearum, F. culmorum and F. crookwellense)	
Fusarenone-X (see Toxins derived from Fusarium graminearum, F. culmorum and F. crookwellense)	
Fusarin C (see Toxins derived from Fusarium moniliforme)	

G

γ-radiation	75, 121 (2000)

Gasoline	45, 159 (1989) (corr. 47, 505)
Gasoline engine exhaust (see Diesel and gasoline engine exhausts)	
Gemfibrozil	66, 427 (1996)
Glass fibres (see Man-made mineral fibres)	
Glass manufacturing industry, occupational exposures in	58, 347 (1993)
Glasswool (see Man-made mineral fibres)	
Glass filaments (see Man-made mineral fibres)	
Glu-P-1	40, 223 (1986); Suppl. 7, 64 (1987)
Glu-P-2	40, 235 (1986); Suppl. 7, 64 (1987)
L-Glutamic acid, 5-[2-(4-hydroxymethyl)phenylhydrazide] (see Agaritine)	
Glycidaldehyde	11, 175 (1976); Suppl. 7, 64 (1987); 71, 1459 (1999)
Glycidyl ethers	47, 237 (1989); 71, 1285, 1417, 1525, 1539 (1999)
Glycidyl oleate	11, 183 (1976); Suppl. 7, 64 (1987)
Glycidyl stearate	11, 187 (1976); Suppl. 7, 64 (1987)
Griseofulvin	10, 153 (1976); Suppl. 7, 391 (1987)
Guinea Green B	16, 199 (1978); Suppl. 7, 64 (1987)
Gyromitrin	31, 163 (1983); Suppl. 7, 391 (1987)

H

Haematite	1, 29 (1972); Suppl. 7, 216 (1987)
Haematite and ferric oxide	Suppl. 7, 216 (1987)
Haematite mining, underground, with exposure to radon	1, 29 (1972); Suppl. 7, 216 (1987)
Hairdressers and barbers (occupational exposure as)	57, 43 (1993)
Hair dyes, epidemiology of	16, 29 (1978); 27, 307 (1982);
Halogenated acetonitriles	52, 269 (1991); 71, 1325, 1369, 1375, 1533 (1999)
Halothane (see Anaesthetics, volatile)	
HC Blue No. 1	57, 129 (1993)
HC Blue No. 2	57, 143 (1993)
α-HCH (see Hexachlorocyclohexanes)	
β-HCH (see Hexachlorocyclohexanes)	
γ-HCH (see Hexachlorocyclohexanes)	
HC Red No. 3	57, 153 (1993)
HC Yellow No. 4	57, 159 (1993)
Heating oils (see Fuel oils)	
Helicobacter pylori (infection with)	61, 177 (1994)
Hepatitis B virus	59, 45 (1994)
Hepatitis C virus	59, 165 (1994)
Hepatitis D virus	59, 223 (1994)
Heptachlor (see also Chlordane/Heptachlor)	5, 173 (1974); 20, 129 (1979)
Hexachlorobenzene	20, 155 (1979); Suppl. 7, 219 (1987)
Hexachlorobutadiene	20, 179 (1979); Suppl. 7, 64 (1987); 73, 277 (1999)
Hexachlorocyclohexanes	5, 47 (1974); 20, 195 (1979) (corr. 42, 258); Suppl. 7, 220 (1987)

Hexachlorocyclohexane, technical-grade (see Hexachlorocyclohexanes)
Hexachloroethane   20, 467 (1979); Suppl. 7, 64 (1987);
                                                                  73, 295 (1999)
Hexachlorophene   20, 241 (1979); Suppl. 7, 64 (1987)
Hexamethylphosphoramide   15, 211 (1977); Suppl. 7, 64
                                                                  (1987); 71, 1465 (1999)
Hexoestrol (see also Nonsteroidal oestrogens)   Suppl. 7, 279 (1987)
Hormonal contraceptives, progestogens only   72, 339 (1999)
Human herpesvirus 8   70, 375 (1997)
Human immunodeficiency viruses   67, 31 (1996)
Human papillomaviruses   64 (1995) (corr. 66, 485)
Human T-cell lymphotropic viruses   67, 261 (1996)
Hycanthone mesylate   13, 91 (1977); Suppl. 7, 64 (1987)
Hydralazine   24, 85 (1980); Suppl. 7, 222 (1987)
Hydrazine   4, 127 (1974); Suppl. 7, 223
                                                                  (1987); 71, 991 (1999)
Hydrochloric acid   54, 189 (1992)
Hydrochlorothiazide   50, 293 (1990)
Hydrogen peroxide   36, 285 (1985); Suppl. 7, 64
                                                                  (1987); 71, 671 (1999)
Hydroquinone   15, 155 (1977); Suppl. 7, 64
                                                                  (1987); 71, 691 (1999)
4-Hydroxyazobenzene   8, 157 (1975); Suppl. 7, 64 (1987)
17α-Hydroxyprogesterone caproate (see also Progestins)   21, 399 (1979) (corr. 42, 259)
8-Hydroxyquinoline   13, 101 (1977); Suppl. 7, 64 (1987)
8-Hydroxysenkirkine   10, 265 (1976); Suppl. 7, 64 (1987)
Hydroxyurea   76, 347 (2000)
Hypochlorite salts   52, 159 (1991)

I

Implants, surgical   74, 1999
Indeno[1,2,3-cd]pyrene   3, 229 (1973); 32, 373 (1983);
                                                                  Suppl. 7, 64 (1987)
Inorganic acids (see Sulfuric acid and other strong inorganic acids,
    occupational exposures to mists and vapours from)
Insecticides, occupational exposures in spraying and application of   53, 45 (1991)
Ionizing radiation (see Neutrons, γ- and X-radiation)
IQ   40, 261 (1986); Suppl. 7, 64
                                                                  (1987); 56, 165 (1993)
Iron and steel founding   34, 133 (1984); Suppl. 7, 224
                                                                  (1987)
Iron-dextran complex   2, 161 (1973); Suppl. 7, 226 (1987)
Iron-dextrin complex   2, 161 (1973) (corr. 42, 252);
                                                                  Suppl. 7, 64 (1987)
Iron oxide (see Ferric oxide)
Iron oxide, saccharated (see Saccharated iron oxide)
Iron sorbitol-citric acid complex   2, 161 (1973); Suppl. 7, 64 (1987)
Isatidine   10, 269 (1976); Suppl. 7, 65 (1987)
Isoflurane (see Anaesthetics, volatile)
Isoniazid (see Isonicotinic acid hydrazide)
Isonicotinic acid hydrazide   4, 159 (1974); Suppl. 7, 227 (1987)
Isophosphamide   26, 237 (1981); Suppl. 7, 65 (1987)

Isoprene	*60*, 215 (1994); *71*, 1015 (1999)
Isopropanol	*15*, 223 (1977); *Suppl. 7*, 229 (1987); *71*, 1027 (1999)
Isopropanol manufacture (strong-acid process) *(see also* Isopropanol; Sulfuric acid and other strong inorganic acids, occupational exposures to mists and vapours from)	*Suppl. 7*, 229 (1987)
Isopropyl oils	*15*, 223 (1977); *Suppl. 7*, 229 (1987); *71*, 1483 (1999)
Isosafrole	*1*, 169 (1972); *10*, 232 (1976); *Suppl. 7*, 65 (1987)

J

Jacobine	*10*, 275 (1976); *Suppl. 7*, 65 (1987)
Jet fuel	*45*, 203 (1989)
Joinery *(see* Carpentry and joinery)	

K

Kaempferol	*31*, 171 (1983); *Suppl. 7*, 65 (1987)
Kaposi's sarcoma herpesvirus	*70*, 375 (1997)
Kepone *(see* Chlordecone)	

L

Lasiocarpine	*10*, 281 (1976); *Suppl. 7*, 65 (1987)
Lauroyl peroxide	*36*, 315 (1985); *Suppl. 7*, 65 (1987); *71*, 1485 (1999)
Lead acetate *(see* Lead and lead compounds)	
Lead and lead compounds *(see also* Foreign bodies)	*1*, 40 (1972) *(corr. 42*, 251); *2*, 52, 150 (1973); *12*, 131 (1976); *23*, 40, 208, 209, 325 (1980); *Suppl. 7*, 230 (1987)
Lead arsenate *(see* Arsenic and arsenic compounds)	
Lead carbonate *(see* Lead and lead compounds)	
Lead chloride *(see* Lead and lead compounds)	
Lead chromate *(see* Chromium and chromium compounds)	
Lead chromate oxide *(see* Chromium and chromium compounds)	
Lead naphthenate *(see* Lead and lead compounds)	
Lead nitrate *(see* Lead and lead compounds)	
Lead oxide *(see* Lead and lead compounds)	
Lead phosphate *(see* Lead and lead compounds)	
Lead subacetate *(see* Lead and lead compounds)	
Lead tetroxide *(see* Lead and lead compounds)	
Leather goods manufacture	*25*, 279 (1981); *Suppl. 7*, 235 (1987)
Leather industries	*25*, 199 (1981); *Suppl. 7*, 232 (1987)
Leather tanning and processing	*25*, 201 (1981); *Suppl. 7*, 236 (1987)
Ledate *(see also* Lead and lead compounds)	*12*, 131 (1976)

Levonorgestrel	72, 49 (1999)
Light Green SF	16, 209 (1978); Suppl. 7, 65 (1987)
d-Limonene	56, 135 (1993); 73, 307 (1999)
Lindane (see Hexachlorocyclohexanes)	
Liver flukes (see Clonorchis sinensis, Opisthorchis felineus and Opisthorchis viverrini)	
Lumber and sawmill industries (including logging)	25, 49 (1981); Suppl. 7, 383 (1987)
Luteoskyrin	10, 163 (1976); Suppl. 7, 65 (1987)
Lynoestrenol	21, 407 (1979); Suppl. 7, 293 (1987); 72, 49 (1999)

M

Magenta	4, 57 (1974) (corr. 42, 252); Suppl. 7, 238 (1987); 57, 215 (1993)
Magenta, manufacture of (see also Magenta)	Suppl. 7, 238 (1987); 57, 215 (1993)
Malathion	30, 103 (1983); Suppl. 7, 65 (1987)
Maleic hydrazide	4, 173 (1974) (corr. 42, 253); Suppl. 7, 65 (1987)
Malonaldehyde	36, 163 (1985); Suppl. 7, 65 (1987); 71, 1037 (1999)
Malondialdehyde (see Malonaldehyde)	
Maneb	12, 137 (1976); Suppl. 7, 65 (1987)
Man-made mineral fibres	43, 39 (1988)
Mannomustine	9, 157 (1975); Suppl. 7, 65 (1987)
Mate	51, 273 (1991)
MCPA (see also Chlorophenoxy herbicides; Chlorophenoxy herbicides, occupational exposures to)	30, 255 (1983)
MeA-α-C	40, 253 (1986); Suppl. 7, 65 (1987)
Medphalan	9, 168 (1975); Suppl. 7, 65 (1987)
Medroxyprogesterone acetate	6, 157 (1974); 21, 417 (1979) (corr. 42, 259); Suppl. 7, 289 (1987); 72, 339 (1999)
Megestrol acetate	Suppl. 7, 293 (1987); 72, 49 (1999)
MeIQ	40, 275 (1986); Suppl. 7, 65 (1987); 56, 197 (1993)
MeIQx	40, 283 (1986); Suppl. 7, 65 (1987); 56, 211 (1993)
Melamine	39, 333 (1986); Suppl. 7, 65 (1987); 73, 329 (1999)
Melphalan	9, 167 (1975); Suppl. 7, 239 (1987)
6-Mercaptopurine	26, 249 (1981); Suppl. 7, 240 (1987)
Mercuric chloride (see Mercury and mercury compounds)	
Mercury and mercury compounds	58, 239 (1993)
Merphalan	9, 169 (1975); Suppl. 7, 65 (1987)
Mestranol	6, 87 (1974); 21, 257 (1979) (corr. 42, 259); Suppl. 7, 288 (1987); 72, 49 (1999)
Metabisulfites (see Sulfur dioxide and some sulfites, bisulfites and metabisulfites)	

Metallic mercury (*see* Mercury and mercury compounds)	
Methanearsonic acid, disodium salt (*see* Arsenic and arsenic compounds)	
Methanearsonic acid, monosodium salt (*see* Arsenic and arsenic compounds	
Methotrexate	26, 267 (1981); *Suppl. 7*, 241 (1987)
Methoxsalen (*see* 8-Methoxypsoralen)	
Methoxychlor	5, 193 (1974); 20, 259 (1979); *Suppl. 7*, 66 (1987)
Methoxyflurane (*see* Anaesthetics, volatile)	
5-Methoxypsoralen	40, 327 (1986); *Suppl. 7*, 242 (1987)
8-Methoxypsoralen (*see also* 8-Methoxypsoralen plus ultraviolet radiation)	24, 101 (1980)
8-Methoxypsoralen plus ultraviolet radiation	*Suppl. 7*, 243 (1987)
Methyl acrylate	19, 52 (1979); 39, 99 (1986); *Suppl. 7*, 66 (1987); 71, 1489 (1999)
5-Methylangelicin plus ultraviolet radiation (*see also* Angelicin and some synthetic derivatives)	*Suppl. 7*, 57 (1987)
2-Methylaziridine	9, 61 (1975); *Suppl. 7*, 66 (1987); 71, 1497 (1999)
Methylazoxymethanol acetate (*see also* Cycasin)	1, 164 (1972); 10, 131 (1976); *Suppl. 7*, 66 (1987)
Methyl bromide	41, 187 (1986) (*corr.* 45, 283); *Suppl. 7*, 245 (1987); 71, 721 (1999)
Methyl *tert*-butyl ether	73, 339 (1999)
Methyl carbamate	12, 151 (1976); *Suppl. 7*, 66 (1987)
Methyl-CCNU (*see* 1-(2-Chloroethyl)-3-(4-methylcyclohexyl)-1-nitrosourea)	
Methyl chloride	41, 161 (1986); *Suppl. 7*, 246 (1987); 71, 737 (1999)
1-, 2-, 3-, 4-, 5- and 6-Methylchrysenes	32, 379 (1983); *Suppl. 7*, 66 (1987)
N-Methyl-N,4-dinitrosoaniline	1, 141 (1972); *Suppl. 7*, 66 (1987)
4,4'-Methylene bis(2-chloroaniline)	4, 65 (1974) (*corr.* 42, 252); *Suppl. 7*, 246 (1987); 57, 271 (1993)
4,4'-Methylene bis(N,N-dimethyl)benzenamine	27, 119 (1982); *Suppl. 7*, 66 (1987)
4,4'-Methylene bis(2-methylaniline)	4, 73 (1974); *Suppl. 7*, 248 (1987)
4,4'-Methylenedianiline	4, 79 (1974) (*corr.* 42, 252); 39, 347 (1986); *Suppl. 7*, 66 (1987)
4,4'-Methylenediphenyl diisocyanate	19, 314 (1979); *Suppl. 7*, 66 (1987); 71, 1049 (1999)
2-Methylfluoranthene	32, 399 (1983); *Suppl. 7*, 66 (1987)
3-Methylfluoranthene	32, 399 (1983); *Suppl. 7*, 66 (1987)
Methylglyoxal	51, 443 (1991)
Methyl iodide	15, 245 (1977); 41, 213 (1986); *Suppl. 7*, 66 (1987); 71, 1503 (1999)
Methylmercury chloride (*see* Mercury and mercury compounds)	
Methylmercury compounds (*see* Mercury and mercury compounds)	
Methyl methacrylate	19, 187 (1979); *Suppl. 7*, 66 (1987); 60, 445 (1994)

Methyl methanesulfonate	7, 253 (1974); *Suppl. 7*, 66 (1987); 71, 1059 (1999)
2-Methyl-1-nitroanthraquinone	27, 205 (1982); *Suppl. 7*, 66 (1987)
N-Methyl-N'-nitro-N-nitrosoguanidine	4, 183 (1974); *Suppl. 7*, 248 (1987)
3-Methylnitrosaminopropionaldehyde [*see* 3-(N-Nitrosomethylamino)-propionaldehyde]	
3-Methylnitrosaminopropionitrile [*see* 3-(N-Nitrosomethylamino)-propionitrile]	
4-(Methylnitrosamino)-4-(3-pyridyl)-1-butanal [*see* 4-(N-Nitrosomethyl-amino)-4-(3-pyridyl)-1-butanal]	
4-(Methylnitrosamino)-1-(3-pyridyl)-1-butanone [*see* 4-(-Nitrosomethyl-amino)-1-(3-pyridyl)-1-butanone]	
N-Methyl-N-nitrosourea	1, 125 (1972); 17, 227 (1978); *Suppl. 7*, 66 (1987)
N-Methyl-N-nitrosourethane	4, 211 (1974); *Suppl. 7*, 66 (1987)
N-Methylolacrylamide	60, 435 (1994)
Methyl parathion	30, 131 (1983); *Suppl. 7*, 392 (1987)
1-Methylphenanthrene	32, 405 (1983); *Suppl. 7*, 66 (1987)
7-Methylpyrido[3,4-c]psoralen	40, 349 (1986); *Suppl. 7*, 71 (1987)
Methyl red	8, 161 (1975); *Suppl. 7*, 66 (1987)
Methyl selenac (*see also* Selenium and selenium compounds)	12, 161 (1976); *Suppl. 7*, 66 (1987)
Methylthiouracil	7, 53 (1974); *Suppl. 7*, 66 (1987)
Metronidazole	13, 113 (1977); *Suppl. 7*, 250 (1987)
Mineral oils	3, 30 (1973); 33, 87 (1984) (*corr.* 42, 262); *Suppl. 7*, 252 (1987)
Mirex	5, 203 (1974); 20, 283 (1979) (*corr.* 42, 258); *Suppl. 7*, 66 (1987)
Mists and vapours from sulfuric acid and other strong inorganic acids	54, 41 (1992)
Mitomycin C	10, 171 (1976); *Suppl. 7*, 67 (1987)
Mitoxantrone	76, 289 (2000)
MNNG (*see* N-Methyl-N'-nitro-N-nitrosoguanidine)	
MOCA (*see* 4,4'-Methylene bis(2-chloroaniline))	
Modacrylic fibres	19, 86 (1979); *Suppl. 7*, 67 (1987)
Monocrotaline	10, 291 (1976); *Suppl. 7*, 67 (1987)
Monuron	12, 167 (1976); *Suppl. 7*, 67 (1987); 53, 467 (1991)
MOPP and other combined chemotherapy including alkylating agents	*Suppl. 7*, 254 (1987)
Mordanite (*see* Zeolites)	
Morpholine	47, 199 (1989); 71, 1511 (1999)
5-(Morpholinomethyl)-3-[(5-nitrofurfurylidene)amino]-2-oxazolidinone	7, 161 (1974); *Suppl. 7*, 67 (1987)
Musk ambrette	65, 477 (1996)
Musk xylene	65, 477 (1996)
Mustard gas	9, 181 (1975) (*corr.* 42, 254); *Suppl. 7*, 259 (1987)
Myleran (*see* 1,4-Butanediol dimethanesulfonate)	

N

Nafenopin	*24*, 125 (1980); *Suppl. 7*, 67 (1987)
1,5-Naphthalenediamine	*27*, 127 (1982); *Suppl. 7*, 67 (1987)
1,5-Naphthalene diisocyanate	*19*, 311 (1979); *Suppl. 7*, 67 (1987); *71*, 1515 (1999)
1-Naphthylamine	*4*, 87 (1974) (*corr. 42*, 253); *Suppl. 7*, 260 (1987)
2-Naphthylamine	*4*, 97 (1974); *Suppl. 7*, 261 (1987)
1-Naphthylthiourea	*30*, 347 (1983); *Suppl. 7*, 263 (1987)
Neutrons	*75*, 361 (2000)
Nickel acetate (*see* Nickel and nickel compounds)	
Nickel ammonium sulfate (*see* Nickel and nickel compounds)	
Nickel and nickel compounds (*see also* Implants, surgical)	*2*, 126 (1973) (*corr. 42*, 252); *11*, 75 (1976); *Suppl. 7*, 264 (1987) (*corr. 45*, 283); *49*, 257 (1990) (*corr. 67*, 395)
Nickel carbonate (*see* Nickel and nickel compounds)	
Nickel carbonyl (*see* Nickel and nickel compounds)	
Nickel chloride (*see* Nickel and nickel compounds)	
Nickel-gallium alloy (*see* Nickel and nickel compounds)	
Nickel hydroxide (*see* Nickel and nickel compounds)	
Nickelocene (*see* Nickel and nickel compounds)	
Nickel oxide (*see* Nickel and nickel compounds)	
Nickel subsulfide (*see* Nickel and nickel compounds)	
Nickel sulfate (*see* Nickel and nickel compounds)	
Niridazole	*13*, 123 (1977); *Suppl. 7*, 67 (1987)
Nithiazide	*31*, 179 (1983); *Suppl. 7*, 67 (1987)
Nitrilotriacetic acid and its salts	*48*, 181 (1990); *73*, 385 (1999)
5-Nitroacenaphthene	*16*, 319 (1978); *Suppl. 7*, 67 (1987)
5-Nitro-*ortho*-anisidine	*27*, 133 (1982); *Suppl. 7*, 67 (1987)
2-Nitroanisole	*65*, 369 (1996)
9-Nitroanthracene	*33*, 179 (1984); *Suppl. 7*, 67 (1987)
7-Nitrobenz[*a*]anthracene	*46*, 247 (1989)
Nitrobenzene	*65*, 381 (1996)
6-Nitrobenzo[*a*]pyrene	*33*, 187 (1984); *Suppl. 7*, 67 (1987); *46*, 255 (1989)
4-Nitrobiphenyl	*4*, 113 (1974); *Suppl. 7*, 67 (1987)
6-Nitrochrysene	*33*, 195 (1984); *Suppl. 7*, 67 (1987); *46*, 267 (1989)
Nitrofen (technical-grade)	*30*, 271 (1983); *Suppl. 7*, 67 (1987)
3-Nitrofluoranthene	*33*, 201 (1984); *Suppl. 7*, 67 (1987)
2-Nitrofluorene	*46*, 277 (1989)
Nitrofural	*7*, 171 (1974); *Suppl. 7*, 67 (1987); *50*, 195 (1990)
5-Nitro-2-furaldehyde semicarbazone (*see* Nitrofural)	
Nitrofurantoin	*50*, 211 (1990)
Nitrofurazone (*see* Nitrofural)	
1-[(5-Nitrofurfurylidene)amino]-2-imidazolidinone	*7*, 181 (1974); *Suppl. 7*, 67 (1987)
N-[4-(5-Nitro-2-furyl)-2-thiazolyl]acetamide	*1*, 181 (1972); *7*, 185 (1974); *Suppl. 7*, 67 (1987)
Nitrogen mustard	*9*, 193 (1975); *Suppl. 7*, 269 (1987)
Nitrogen mustard *N*-oxide	*9*, 209 (1975); *Suppl. 7*, 67 (1987)

1-Nitronaphthalene	*46*, 291 (1989)
2-Nitronaphthalene	*46*, 303 (1989)
3-Nitroperylene	*46*, 313 (1989)
2-Nitro-*para*-phenylenediamine (*see* 1,4-Diamino-2-nitrobenzene)	
2-Nitropropane	*29*, 331 (1982); *Suppl. 7*, 67 (1987); *71*, 1079 (1999)
1-Nitropyrene	*33*, 209 (1984); *Suppl. 7*, 67 (1987); *46*, 321 (1989)
2-Nitropyrene	*46*, 359 (1989)
4-Nitropyrene	*46*, 367 (1989)
N-Nitrosatable drugs	*24*, 297 (1980) (*corr. 42*, 260)
N-Nitrosatable pesticides	*30*, 359 (1983)
N'-Nitrosoanabasine	*37*, 225 (1985); *Suppl. 7*, 67 (1987)
N'-Nitrosoanatabine	*37*, 233 (1985); *Suppl. 7*, 67 (1987)
N-Nitrosodi-*n*-butylamine	*4*, 197 (1974); *17*, 51 (1978); *Suppl. 7*, 67 (1987)
N-Nitrosodiethanolamine	*17*, 77 (1978); *Suppl. 7*, 67 (1987)
N-Nitrosodiethylamine	*1*, 107 (1972) (*corr. 42*, 251); *17*, 83 (1978) (*corr. 42*, 257); *Suppl. 7*, 67 (1987)
N-Nitrosodimethylamine	*1*, 95 (1972); *17*, 125 (1978) (*corr. 42*, 257); *Suppl. 7*, 67 (1987)
N-Nitrosodiphenylamine	*27*, 213 (1982); *Suppl. 7*, 67 (1987)
para-Nitrosodiphenylamine	*27*, 227 (1982) (*corr. 42*, 261); *Suppl. 7*, 68 (1987)
N-Nitrosodi-*n*-propylamine	*17*, 177 (1978); *Suppl. 7*, 68 (1987)
N-Nitroso-*N*-ethylurea (*see* *N*-Ethyl-*N*-nitrosourea)	
N-Nitrosofolic acid	*17*, 217 (1978); *Suppl. 7*, 68 (1987)
N-Nitrosoguvacine	*37*, 263 (1985); *Suppl. 7*, 68 (1987)
N-Nitrosoguvacoline	*37*, 263 (1985); *Suppl. 7*, 68 (1987)
N-Nitrosohydroxyproline	*17*, 304 (1978); *Suppl. 7*, 68 (1987)
3-(*N*-Nitrosomethylamino)propionaldehyde	*37*, 263 (1985); *Suppl. 7*, 68 (1987)
3-(*N*-Nitrosomethylamino)propionitrile	*37*, 263 (1985); *Suppl. 7*, 68 (1987)
4-(*N*-Nitrosomethylamino)-4-(3-pyridyl)-1-butanal	*37*, 205 (1985); *Suppl. 7*, 68 (1987)
4-(*N*-Nitrosomethylamino)-1-(3-pyridyl)-1-butanone	*37*, 209 (1985); *Suppl. 7*, 68 (1987)
N-Nitrosomethylethylamine	*17*, 221 (1978); *Suppl. 7*, 68 (1987)
N-Nitroso-*N*-methylurea (*see* *N*-Methyl-*N*-nitrosourea)	
N-Nitroso-*N*-methylurethane (*see* *N*-Methyl-*N*-nitrosourethane)	
N-Nitrosomethylvinylamine	*17*, 257 (1978); *Suppl. 7*, 68 (1987)
N-Nitrosomorpholine	*17*, 263 (1978); *Suppl. 7*, 68 (1987)
N'-Nitrosonornicotine	*17*, 281 (1978); *37*, 241 (1985); *Suppl. 7*, 68 (1987)
N-Nitrosopiperidine	*17*, 287 (1978); *Suppl. 7*, 68 (1987)
N-Nitrosoproline	*17*, 303 (1978); *Suppl. 7*, 68 (1987)
N-Nitrosopyrrolidine	*17*, 313 (1978); *Suppl. 7*, 68 (1987)
N-Nitrososarcosine	*17*, 327 (1978); *Suppl. 7*, 68 (1987)
Nitrosoureas, chloroethyl (*see* Chloroethyl nitrosoureas)	
5-Nitro-*ortho*-toluidine	*48*, 169 (1990)
2-Nitrotoluene	*65*, 409 (1996)
3-Nitrotoluene	*65*, 409 (1996)
4-Nitrotoluene	*65*, 409 (1996)
Nitrous oxide (*see* Anaesthetics, volatile)	
Nitrovin	*31*, 185 (1983); *Suppl. 7*, 68 (1987)

Nivalenol (see Toxins derived from *Fusarium graminearum*,
   F. culmorum and *F. crookwellense*)
NNA (see 4-(*N*-Nitrosomethylamino)-4-(3-pyridyl)-1-butanal)
NNK (see 4-(*N*-Nitrosomethylamino)-1-(3-pyridyl)-1-butanone)

Nonsteroidal oestrogens	*Suppl. 7*, 273 (1987)
Norethisterone	*6*, 179 (1974); *21*, 461 (1979); *Suppl. 7*, 294 (1987); *72*, 49 (1999)
Norethisterone acetate	*72*, 49 (1999)
Norethynodrel	*6*, 191 (1974); *21*, 461 (1979) (*corr. 42*, 259); *Suppl. 7*, 295 (1987); *72*, 49 (1999)
Norgestrel	*6*, 201 (1974); *21*, 479 (1979); *Suppl. 7*, 295 (1987); *72*, 49 (1999)
Nylon 6	*19*, 120 (1979); *Suppl. 7*, 68 (1987)

O

Ochratoxin A	*10*, 191 (1976); *31*, 191 (1983) (*corr. 42*, 262); *Suppl. 7*, 271 (1987); *56*, 489 (1993)
Oestradiol	*6*, 99 (1974); *21*, 279 (1979); *Suppl. 7*, 284 (1987); *72*, 399 (1999)

Oestradiol-17β (see Oestradiol)
Oestradiol 3-benzoate (see Oestradiol)
Oestradiol dipropionate (see Oestradiol)

Oestradiol mustard	*9*, 217 (1975); *Suppl. 7*, 68 (1987)

Oestradiol valerate (see Oestradiol)

Oestriol	*6*, 117 (1974); *21*, 327 (1979); *Suppl. 7*, 285 (1987); *72*, 399 (1999)

Oestrogen-progestin combinations (see Oestrogens,
   progestins (progestogens) and combinations)
Oestrogen-progestin replacement therapy (see Post-menopausal
   oestrogen-progestogen therapy)
Oestrogen replacement therapy (see Post-menopausal oestrogen
   therapy)
Oestrogens (see Oestrogens, progestins and combinations)
Oestrogens, conjugated (see Conjugated oestrogens)
Oestrogens, nonsteroidal (see Nonsteroidal oestrogens)

Oestrogens, progestins (progestogens) and combinations	*6* (1974); *21* (1979); *Suppl. 7*, 272 (1987); *72*, 49, 339, 399, 531 (1999)

Oestrogens, steroidal (see Steroidal oestrogens)

Oestrone	*6*, 123 (1974); *21*, 343 (1979) (*corr. 42*, 259); *Suppl. 7*, 286 (1987); *72*, 399 (1999)

Oestrone benzoate (see Oestrone)

Oil Orange SS	*8*, 165 (1975); *Suppl. 7*, 69 (1987)
Opisthorchis felineus (infection with)	*61*, 121 (1994)
Opisthorchis viverrini (infection with)	*61*, 121 (1994)
Oral contraceptives, combined	*Suppl. 7*, 297 (1987); *72*, 49 (1999)

Oral contraceptives, sequential (*see* Sequential oral contraceptives)
Orange I   *8*, 173 (1975); *Suppl. 7*, 69 (1987)
Orange G   *8*, 181 (1975); *Suppl. 7*, 69 (1987)
Organolead compounds (*see also* Lead and lead compounds) *Suppl. 7*, 230 (1987)
Oxazepam   *13*, 58 (1977); *Suppl. 7*, 69 (1987); *66*, 115 (1996)
Oxymetholone (*see also* Androgenic (anabolic) steroids)   *13*, 131 (1977)
Oxyphenbutazone   *13*, 185 (1977); *Suppl. 7*, 69 (1987)

P

Paint manufacture and painting (occupational exposures in)   *47*, 329 (1989)
Palygorskite   *42*, 159 (1987); *Suppl. 7*, 117 (1987); *68*, 245 (1997)
Panfuran S (*see also* Dihydroxymethylfuratrizine) *24*, 77 (1980); *Suppl. 7*, 69 (1987)
Paper manufacture (*see* Pulp and paper manufacture)
Paracetamol   *50*, 307 (1990); *73*, 401 (1999)
Parasorbic acid   *10*, 199 (1976) (*corr. 42*, 255); *Suppl. 7*, 69 (1987)
Parathion   *30*, 153 (1983); *Suppl. 7*, 69 (1987)
Patulin   *10*, 205 (1976); *40*, 83 (1986); *Suppl. 7*, 69 (1987)
Penicillic acid   *10*, 211 (1976); *Suppl. 7*, 69 (1987)
Pentachloroethane   *41*, 99 (1986); *Suppl. 7*, 69 (1987); *71*, 1519 (1999)
Pentachloronitrobenzene (see Quintozene)
Pentachlorophenol (*see also* Chlorophenols; Chlorophenols,   *20*, 303 (1979); *53*, 371 (1991)
    occupational exposures to; Polychlorophenols and their sodium salts)
Permethrin   *53*, 329 (1991)
Perylene   *32*, 411 (1983); *Suppl. 7*, 69 (1987)
Petasitenine   *31*, 207 (1983); *Suppl. 7*, 69 (1987)
Petasites japonicus (*see also* Pyrrolizidine alkaloids) *10*, 333 (1976)
Petroleum refining (occupational exposures in)   *45*, 39 (1989)
Petroleum solvents   *47*, 43 (1989)
Phenacetin   *13*, 141 (1977); *24*, 135 (1980); *Suppl. 7*, 310 (1987)
Phenanthrene   *32*, 419 (1983); *Suppl. 7*, 69 (1987)
Phenazopyridine hydrochloride   *8*, 117 (1975); *24*, 163 (1980) (*corr. 42*, 260); *Suppl. 7*, 312 (1987)
Phenelzine sulfate   *24*, 175 (1980); *Suppl. 7*, 312 (1987)
Phenicarbazide   *12*, 177 (1976); *Suppl. 7*, 70 (1987)
Phenobarbital   *13*, 157 (1977); *Suppl. 7*, 313 (1987)
Phenol   *47*, 263 (1989) (*corr. 50*, 385); *71*, 749 (1999)
Phenolphthalein   *76*, 387 (2000)
Phenoxyacetic acid herbicides (*see* Chlorophenoxy herbicides)
Phenoxybenzamine hydrochloride   *9*, 223 (1975); *24*, 185 (1980); *Suppl. 7*, 70 (1987)
Phenylbutazone   *13*, 183 (1977); *Suppl. 7*, 316 (1987)

meta-Phenylenediamine	*16*, 111 (1978); *Suppl. 7*, 70 (1987)
para-Phenylenediamine	*16*, 125 (1978); *Suppl. 7*, 70 (1987)
Phenyl glycidyl ether (*see also* Glycidyl ethers)	*71*, 1525 (1999)
N-Phenyl-2-naphthylamine	*16*, 325 (1978) (*corr. 42*, 257); *Suppl. 7*, 318 (1987)
ortho-Phenylphenol	*30*, 329 (1983); *Suppl. 7*, 70 (1987); *73*, 451 (1999)
Phenytoin	*13*, 201 (1977); *Suppl. 7*, 319 (1987); *66*, 175 (1996)
Phillipsite (*see* Zeolites)	
PhIP	*56*, 229 (1993)
Pickled vegetables	*56*, 83 (1993)
Picloram	*53*, 481 (1991)
Piperazine oestrone sulfate (*see* Conjugated oestrogens)	
Piperonyl butoxide	*30*, 183 (1983); *Suppl. 7*, 70 (1987)
Pitches, coal-tar (*see* Coal-tar pitches)	
Polyacrylic acid	*19*, 62 (1979); *Suppl. 7*, 70 (1987)
Polybrominated biphenyls	*18*, 107 (1978); *41*, 261 (1986); *Suppl. 7*, 321 (1987)
Polychlorinated biphenyls	*7*, 261 (1974); *18*, 43 (1978) (*corr. 42*, 258); *Suppl. 7*, 322 (1987)
Polychlorinated camphenes (*see* Toxaphene)	
Polychlorinated dibenzo-*para*-dioxins (other than 2,3,7,8-tetrachlorodibenzodioxin)	*69*, 33 (1997)
Polychlorinated dibenzofurans	*69*, 345 (1997)
Polychlorophenols and their sodium salts	*71*, 769 (1999)
Polychloroprene	*19*, 141 (1979); *Suppl. 7*, 70 (1987)
Polyethylene (*see also* Implants, surgical)	*19*, 164 (1979); *Suppl. 7*, 70 (1987)
Poly(glycolic acid) (*see* Implants, surgical)	
Polymethylene polyphenyl isocyanate (*see also* 4,4'-Methylenediphenyl diisocyanate)	*19*, 314 (1979); *Suppl. 7*, 70 (1987)
Polymethyl methacrylate (*see also* Implants, surgical)	*19*, 195 (1979); *Suppl. 7*, 70 (1987)
Polyoestradiol phosphate (*see* Oestradiol-17β)	
Polypropylene (*see also* Implants, surgical)	*19*, 218 (1979); *Suppl. 7*, 70 (1987)
Polystyrene (*see also* Implants, surgical)	*19*, 245 (1979); *Suppl. 7*, 70 (1987)
Polytetrafluoroethylene (*see also* Implants, surgical)	*19*, 288 (1979); *Suppl. 7*, 70 (1987)
Polyurethane foams (*see also* Implants, surgical)	*19*, 320 (1979); *Suppl. 7*, 70 (1987)
Polyvinyl acetate (*see also* Implants, surgical)	*19*, 346 (1979); *Suppl. 7*, 70 (1987)
Polyvinyl alcohol (*see also* Implants, surgical)	*19*, 351 (1979); *Suppl. 7*, 70 (1987)
Polyvinyl chloride (*see also* Implants, surgical)	*7*, 306 (1974); *19*, 402 (1979); *Suppl. 7*, 70 (1987)
Polyvinyl pyrrolidone	*19*, 463 (1979); *Suppl. 7*, 70 (1987); *71*, 1181 (1999)
Ponceau MX	*8*, 189 (1975); *Suppl. 7*, 70 (1987)
Ponceau 3R	*8*, 199 (1975); *Suppl. 7*, 70 (1987)
Ponceau SX	*8*, 207 (1975); *Suppl. 7*, 70 (1987)
Post-menopausal oestrogen therapy	*Suppl. 7*, 280 (1987); *72*, 399 (1999)
Post-menopausal oestrogen-progestogen therapy	*Suppl. 7*, 308 (1987); *72*, 531 (1999)
Potassium arsenate (*see* Arsenic and arsenic compounds)	
Potassium arsenite (*see* Arsenic and arsenic compounds)	
Potassium bis(2-hydroxyethyl)dithiocarbamate	*12*, 183 (1976); *Suppl. 7*, 70 (1987)

Potassium bromate	40, 207 (1986); *Suppl. 7*, 70 (1987); 73, 481 (1999)
Potassium chromate (*see* Chromium and chromium compounds)	
Potassium dichromate (*see* Chromium and chromium compounds)	
Prazepam	66, 143 (1996)
Prednimustine	50, 115 (1990)
Prednisone	26, 293 (1981); *Suppl. 7*, 326 (1987)
Printing processes and printing inks	65, 33 (1996)
Procarbazine hydrochloride	26, 311 (1981); *Suppl. 7*, 327 (1987)
Proflavine salts	24, 195 (1980); *Suppl. 7*, 70 (1987)
Progesterone (*see also* Progestins; Combined oral contraceptives)	6, 135 (1974); 21, 491 (1979) (*corr.* 42, 259)
Progestins (*see* Progestogens)	
Progestogens	*Suppl. 7*, 289 (1987); 72, 49, 339, 531 (1999)
Pronetalol hydrochloride	13, 227 (1977) (*corr.* 42, 256); *Suppl. 7*, 70 (1987)
1,3-Propane sultone	4, 253 (1974) (*corr.* 42, 253); *Suppl. 7*, 70 (1987); 71, 1095 (1999)
Propham	12, 189 (1976); *Suppl. 7*, 70 (1987)
β-Propiolactone	4, 259 (1974) (*corr.* 42, 253); *Suppl. 7*, 70 (1987); 71, 1103 (1999)
n-Propyl carbamate	12, 201 (1976); *Suppl. 7*, 70 (1987)
Propylene	19, 213 (1979); *Suppl. 7*, 71 (1987); 60, 161 (1994)
Propyleneimine (*see* 2-Methylaziridine)	
Propylene oxide	11, 191 (1976); 36, 227 (1985) (*corr.* 42, 263); *Suppl. 7*, 328 (1987); 60, 181 (1994)
Propylthiouracil	7, 67 (1974); *Suppl. 7*, 329 (1987)
Ptaquiloside (*see also* Bracken fern)	40, 55 (1986); *Suppl. 7*, 71 (1987)
Pulp and paper manufacture	25, 157 (1981); *Suppl. 7*, 385 (1987)
Pyrene	32, 431 (1983); *Suppl. 7*, 71 (1987)
Pyrido[3,4-*c*]psoralen	40, 349 (1986); *Suppl. 7*, 71 (1987)
Pyrimethamine	13, 233 (1977); *Suppl. 7*, 71 (1987)
Pyrrolizidine alkaloids (*see* Hydroxysenkirkine; Isatidine; Jacobine; Lasiocarpine; Monocrotaline; Retrorsine; Riddelliine; Seneciphylline; Senkirkine)	

Q

Quartz (*see* Crystalline silica)	
Quercetin (*see also* Bracken fern)	31, 213 (1983); *Suppl. 7*, 71 (1987); 73, 497 (1999)
para-Quinone	15, 255 (1977); *Suppl. 7*, 71 (1987); 71, 1245 (1999)
Quintozene	5, 211 (1974); *Suppl. 7*, 71 (1987)

R

Radon	43, 173 (1988) (corr. 45, 283)
Reserpine	10, 217 (1976); 24, 211 (1980) (corr. 42, 260); Suppl. 7, 330 (1987)
Resorcinol	15, 155 (1977); Suppl. 7, 71 (1987); 71, 1119 (1990)
Retrorsine	10, 303 (1976); Suppl. 7, 71 (1987)
Rhodamine B	16, 221 (1978); Suppl. 7, 71 (1987)
Rhodamine 6G	16, 233 (1978); Suppl. 7, 71 (1987)
Riddelliine	10, 313 (1976); Suppl. 7, 71 (1987)
Rifampicin	24, 243 (1980); Suppl. 7, 71 (1987)
Ripazepam	66, 157 (1996)
Rockwool (see Man-made mineral fibres)	
Rubber industry	28 (1982) (corr. 42, 261); Suppl. 7, 332 (1987)
Rugulosin	40, 99 (1986); Suppl. 7, 71 (1987)

S

Saccharated iron oxide	2, 161 (1973); Suppl. 7, 71 (1987)
Saccharin and its salts	22, 111 (1980) (corr. 42, 259); Suppl. 7, 334 (1987); 73, 517 (1999)
Safrole	1, 169 (1972); 10, 231 (1976); Suppl. 7, 71 (1987)
Salted fish	56, 41 (1993)
Sawmill industry (including logging) (see Lumber and sawmill industry (including logging))	
Scarlet Red	8, 217 (1975); Suppl. 7, 71 (1987)
Schistosoma haematobium (infection with)	61, 45 (1994)
Schistosoma japonicum (infection with)	61, 45 (1994)
Schistosoma mansoni (infection with)	61, 45 (1994)
Selenium and selenium compounds	9, 245 (1975) (corr. 42, 255); Suppl. 7, 71 (1987)
Selenium dioxide (see Selenium and selenium compounds)	
Selenium oxide (see Selenium and selenium compounds)	
Semicarbazide hydrochloride	12, 209 (1976) (corr. 42, 256); Suppl. 7, 71 (1987)
Senecio jacobaea L. (see also Pyrrolizidine alkaloids)	10, 333 (1976)
Senecio longilobus (see also Pyrrolizidine alkaloids)	10, 334 (1976)
Seneciphylline	10, 319, 335 (1976); Suppl. 7, 71 (1987)
Senkirkine	10, 327 (1976); 31, 231 (1983); Suppl. 7, 71 (1987)
Sepiolite	42, 175 (1987); Suppl. 7, 71 (1987); 68, 267 (1997)
Sequential oral contraceptives (see also Oestrogens, progestins and combinations)	Suppl. 7, 296 (1987)
Shale-oils	35, 161 (1985); Suppl. 7, 339 (1987)
Shikimic acid (see also Bracken fern)	40, 55 (1986); Suppl. 7, 71 (1987)

Shoe manufacture and repair (*see* Boot and shoe manufacture and repair)
Silica (*see also* Amorphous silica; Crystalline silica)   42, 39 (1987)
Silicone (*see* Implants, surgical)
Simazine   53, 495 (1991); 73, 625 (1999)
Slagwool (*see* Man-made mineral fibres)
Sodium arsenate (*see* Arsenic and arsenic compounds)
Sodium arsenite (*see* Arsenic and arsenic compounds)
Sodium cacodylate (*see* Arsenic and arsenic compounds)
Sodium chlorite   52, 145 (1991)
Sodium chromate (*see* Chromium and chromium compounds)
Sodium cyclamate (*see* Cyclamates)
Sodium dichromate (*see* Chromium and chromium compounds)
Sodium diethyldithiocarbamate   12, 217 (1976); *Suppl. 7*, 71 (1987)
Sodium equilin sulfate (*see* Conjugated oestrogens)
Sodium fluoride (*see* Fluorides)
Sodium monofluorophosphate (*see* Fluorides)
Sodium oestrone sulfate (*see* Conjugated oestrogens)
Sodium *ortho*-phenylphenate (*see also ortho*-Phenylphenol)   30, 329 (1983); *Suppl. 7*, 392 (1987); 73, 451 (1999)
Sodium saccharin (*see* Saccharin)
Sodium selenate (*see* Selenium and selenium compounds)
Sodium selenite (*see* Selenium and selenium compounds)
Sodium silicofluoride (*see* Fluorides)
Solar radiation   55 (1992)
Soots   3, 22 (1973); 35, 219 (1985); *Suppl. 7*, 343 (1987)
Spironolactone   24, 259 (1980); *Suppl. 7*, 344 (1987)
Stannous fluoride (*see* Fluorides)
Steel founding (*see* Iron and steel founding)
Steel, stainless (*see* Implants, surgical)
Sterigmatocystin   1, 175 (1972); 10, 245 (1976); *Suppl. 7*, 72 (1987)
Steroidal oestrogens   *Suppl. 7*, 280 (1987)
Streptozotocin   4, 221 (1974); 17, 337 (1978); *Suppl. 7*, 72 (1987)
Strobane® (*see* Terpene polychlorinates)
Strong-inorganic-acid mists containing sulfuric acid (*see* Mists and vapours from sulfuric acid and other strong inorganic acids)
Strontium chromate (*see* Chromium and chromium compounds)
Styrene   19, 231 (1979) (*corr.* 42, 258); *Suppl. 7*, 345 (1987); 60, 233 (1994) (*corr.* 65, 549)
Styrene-acrylonitrile-copolymers   19, 97 (1979); *Suppl. 7*, 72 (1987)
Styrene-butadiene copolymers   19, 252 (1979); *Suppl. 7*, 72 (1987)
Styrene-7,8-oxide   11, 201 (1976); 19, 275 (1979); 36, 245 (1985); *Suppl. 7*, 72 (1987); 60, 321 (1994)
Succinic anhydride   15, 265 (1977); *Suppl. 7*, 72 (1987)
Sudan I   8, 225 (1975); *Suppl. 7*, 72 (1987)
Sudan II   8, 233 (1975); *Suppl. 7*, 72 (1987)
Sudan III   8, 241 (1975); *Suppl. 7*, 72 (1987)
Sudan Brown RR   8, 249 (1975); *Suppl. 7*, 72 (1987)

Sudan Red 7B	8, 253 (1975); Suppl. 7, 72 (1987)
Sulfafurazole	24, 275 (1980); Suppl. 7, 347 (1987)
Sulfallate	30, 283 (1983); Suppl. 7, 72 (1987)
Sulfamethoxazole	24, 285 (1980); Suppl. 7, 348 (1987)
Sulfites (see Sulfur dioxide and some sulfites, bisulfites and metabisulfites)	
Sulfur dioxide and some sulfites, bisulfites and metabisulfites	54, 131 (1992)
Sulfur mustard (see Mustard gas)	
Sulfuric acid and other strong inorganic acids, occupational exposures to mists and vapours from	54, 41 (1992)
Sulfur trioxide	54, 121 (1992)
Sulphisoxazole (see Sulfafurazole)	
Sunset Yellow FCF	8, 257 (1975); Suppl. 7, 72 (1987)
Symphytine	31, 239 (1983); Suppl. 7, 72 (1987)

T

2,4,5-T (see also Chlorophenoxy herbicides; Chlorophenoxy herbicides, occupational exposures to)	15, 273 (1977)
Talc	42, 185 (1987); Suppl. 7, 349 (1987)
Tamoxifen	66, 253 (1996)
Tannic acid	10, 253 (1976) (corr. 42, 255); Suppl. 7, 72 (1987)
Tannins (see also Tannic acid)	10, 254 (1976); Suppl. 7, 72 (1987)
TCDD (see 2,3,7,8-Tetrachlorodibenzo-para-dioxin)	
TDE (see DDT)	
Tea	51, 207 (1991)
Temazepam	66, 161 (1996)
Teniposide	76, 259 (2000)
Terpene polychlorinates	5, 219 (1974); Suppl. 7, 72 (1987)
Testosterone (see also Androgenic (anabolic) steroids)	6, 209 (1974); 21, 519 (1979)
Testosterone oenanthate (see Testosterone)	
Testosterone propionate (see Testosterone)	
2,2',5,5'-Tetrachlorobenzidine	27, 141 (1982); Suppl. 7, 72 (1987)
2,3,7,8-Tetrachlorodibenzo-para-dioxin	15, 41 (1977); Suppl. 7, 350 (1987); 69, 33 (1997)
1,1,1,2-Tetrachloroethane	41, 87 (1986); Suppl. 7, 72 (1987); 71, 1133 (1999)
1,1,2,2-Tetrachloroethane	20, 477 (1979); Suppl. 7, 354 (1987); 71, 817 (1999)
Tetrachloroethylene	20, 491 (1979); Suppl. 7, 355 (1987); 63, 159 (1995) (corr. 65, 549)
2,3,4,6-Tetrachlorophenol (see Chlorophenols; Chlorophenols, occupational exposures to; Polychlorophenols and their sodium salts)	
Tetrachlorvinphos	30, 197 (1983); Suppl. 7, 72 (1987)
Tetraethyllead (see Lead and lead compounds)	
Tetrafluoroethylene	19, 285 (1979); Suppl. 7, 72 (1987); 71, 1143 (1999)
Tetrakis(hydroxymethyl)phosphonium salts	48, 95 (1990); 71, 1529 (1999)
Tetramethyllead (see Lead and lead compounds)	

Tetranitromethane	65, 437 (1996)
Textile manufacturing industry, exposures in	48, 215 (1990) (corr. 51, 483)
Theobromine	51, 421 (1991)
Theophylline	51, 391 (1991)
Thioacetamide	7, 77 (1974); Suppl. 7, 72 (1987)
4,4'-Thiodianiline	16, 343 (1978); 27, 147 (1982); Suppl. 7, 72 (1987)
Thiotepa	9, 85 (1975); Suppl. 7, 368 (1987); 50, 123 (1990)
Thiouracil	7, 85 (1974); Suppl. 7, 72 (1987)
Thiourea	7, 95 (1974); Suppl. 7, 72 (1987)
Thiram	12, 225 (1976); Suppl. 7, 72 (1987); 53, 403 (1991)
Titanium (see Implants, surgical)	
Titanium dioxide	47, 307 (1989)
Tobacco habits other than smoking (see Tobacco products, smokeless)	
Tobacco products, smokeless	37 (1985) (corr. 42, 263; 52, 513); Suppl. 7, 357 (1987)
Tobacco smoke	38 (1986) (corr. 42, 263); Suppl. 7, 359 (1987)
Tobacco smoking (see Tobacco smoke)	
ortho-Tolidine (see 3,3'-Dimethylbenzidine)	
2,4-Toluene diisocyanate (see also Toluene diisocyanates)	19, 303 (1979); 39, 287 (1986)
2,6-Toluene diisocyanate (see also Toluene diisocyanates)	19, 303 (1979); 39, 289 (1986)
Toluene	47, 79 (1989); 71, 829 (1999)
Toluene diisocyanates	39, 287 (1986) (corr. 42, 264); Suppl. 7, 72 (1987); 71, 865 (1999)
Toluenes, α-chlorinated (see α-Chlorinated toluenes and benzoyl chloride)	
ortho-Toluenesulfonamide (see Saccharin)	
ortho-Toluidine	16, 349 (1978); 27, 155 (1982) (corr. 68, 477); Suppl. 7, 362 (1987)
Toremifene	66, 367 (1996)
Toxaphene	20, 327 (1979); Suppl. 7, 72 (1987)
T-2 Toxin (see Toxins derived from Fusarium sporotrichioides)	
Toxins derived from Fusarium graminearum, F. culmorum and F. crookwellense	11, 169 (1976); 31, 153, 279 (1983); Suppl. 7, 64, 74 (1987); 56, 397 (1993)
Toxins derived from Fusarium moniliforme	56, 445 (1993)
Toxins derived from Fusarium sporotrichioides	31, 265 (1983); Suppl. 7, 73 (1987); 56, 467 (1993)
Tremolite (see Asbestos)	
Treosulfan	26, 341 (1981); Suppl. 7, 363 (1987)
Triaziquone (see Tris(aziridinyl)-para-benzoquinone)	
Trichlorfon	30, 207 (1983); Suppl. 7, 73 (1987)
Trichlormethine	9, 229 (1975); Suppl. 7, 73 (1987); 50, 143 (1990)
Trichloroacetic acid	63, 291 (1995) (corr. 65, 549)
Trichloroacetonitrile (see also Halogenated acetonitriles)	71, 1533 (1999)
1,1,1-Trichloroethane	20, 515 (1979); Suppl. 7, 73 (1987); 71, 881 (1999)

1,1,2-Trichloroethane	20, 533 (1979); *Suppl. 7*, 73 (1987); *52*, 337 (1991); *71*, 1153 (1999)
Trichloroethylene	*11*, 263 (1976); *20*, 545 (1979); *Suppl. 7*, 364 (1987); *63*, 75 (1995) (*corr. 65*, 549)
2,4,5-Trichlorophenol (*see also* Chlorophenols; Chlorophenols occupational exposures to; Polychlorophenols and their sodium salts)	20, 349 (1979)
2,4,6-Trichlorophenol (*see also* Chlorophenols; Chlorophenols, occupational exposures to; Polychlorophenols and their sodium salts)	20, 349 (1979)
(2,4,5-Trichlorophenoxy)acetic acid (*see* 2,4,5-T)	
1,2,3-Trichloropropane	63, 223 (1995)
Trichlorotriethylamine-hydrochloride (*see* Trichlormethine)	
T_2-Trichothecene (*see* Toxins derived from *Fusarium sporotrichioides*)	
Tridymite (*see* Crystalline silica)	
Triethylene glycol diglycidyl ether	*11*, 209 (1976); *Suppl. 7*, 73 (1987); *71*, 1539 (1999)
Trifluralin	53, 515 (1991)
4,4',6-Trimethylangelicin plus ultraviolet radiation (*see also* Angelicin and some synthetic derivatives)	*Suppl. 7*, 57 (1987)
2,4,5-Trimethylaniline	*27*, 177 (1982); *Suppl. 7*, 73 (1987)
2,4,6-Trimethylaniline	*27*, 178 (1982); *Suppl. 7*, 73 (1987)
4,5',8-Trimethylpsoralen	*40*, 357 (1986); *Suppl. 7*, 366 (1987)
Trimustine hydrochloride (*see* Trichlormethine)	
2,4,6-Trinitrotoluene	65, 449 (1996)
Triphenylene	*32*, 447 (1983); *Suppl. 7*, 73 (1987)
Tris(aziridinyl)-*para*-benzoquinone	*9*, 67 (1975); *Suppl. 7*, 367 (1987)
Tris(1-aziridinyl)phosphine-oxide	*9*, 75 (1975); *Suppl. 7*, 73 (1987)
Tris(1-aziridinyl)phosphine-sulphide (*see* Thiotepa)	
2,4,6-Tris(1-aziridinyl)-*s*-triazine	*9*, 95 (1975); *Suppl. 7*, 73 (1987)
Tris(2-chloroethyl) phosphate	*48*, 109 (1990); *71*, 1543 (1999)
1,2,3-Tris(chloromethoxy)propane	*15*, 301 (1977); *Suppl. 7*, 73 (1987); *71*, 1549 (1999)
Tris(2,3-dibromopropyl) phosphate	*20*, 575 (1979); *Suppl. 7*, 369 (1987); *71*, 905 (1999)
Tris(2-methyl-1-aziridinyl)phosphine-oxide	*9*, 107 (1975); *Suppl. 7*, 73 (1987)
Trp-P-1	*31*, 247 (1983); *Suppl. 7*, 73 (1987)
Trp-P-2	*31*, 255 (1983); *Suppl. 7*, 73 (1987)
Trypan blue	*8*, 267 (1975); *Suppl. 7*, 73 (1987)
Tussilago farfara L. (*see also* Pyrrolizidine alkaloids)	10, 334 (1976)

U

Ultraviolet radiation	*40*, 379 (1986); *55* (1992)
Underground haematite mining with exposure to radon	*1*, 29 (1972); *Suppl. 7*, 216 (1987)
Uracil mustard	*9*, 235 (1975); *Suppl. 7*, 370 (1987)
Uranium, depleted (*see* Implants, surgical)	
Urethane	*7*, 111 (1974); *Suppl. 7*, 73 (1987)

V

Vat Yellow 4	*48*, 161 (1990)
Vinblastine sulfate	*26*, 349 (1981) (*corr. 42*, 261); *Suppl. 7*, 371 (1987)
Vincristine sulfate	*26*, 365 (1981); *Suppl. 7*, 372 (1987)
Vinyl acetate	*19*, 341 (1979); *39*, 113 (1986); *Suppl. 7*, 73 (1987); *63*, 443 (1995)
Vinyl bromide	*19*, 367 (1979); *39*, 133 (1986); *Suppl. 7*, 73 (1987); *71*, 923 (1999)
Vinyl chloride	*7*, 291 (1974); *19*, 377 (1979) (*corr. 42*, 258); *Suppl. 7*, 373 (1987)
Vinyl chloride-vinyl acetate copolymers	*7*, 311 (1976); *19*, 412 (1979) (*corr. 42*, 258); *Suppl. 7*, 73 (1987)
4-Vinylcyclohexene	*11*, 277 (1976); *39*, 181 (1986) *Suppl. 7*, 73 (1987); *60*, 347 (1994)
4-Vinylcyclohexene diepoxide	*11*, 141 (1976); *Suppl. 7*, 63 (1987); *60*, 361 (1994)
Vinyl fluoride	*39*, 147 (1986); *Suppl. 7*, 73 (1987); *63*, 467 (1995)
Vinylidene chloride	*19*, 439 (1979); *39*, 195 (1986); *Suppl. 7*, 376 (1987); *71*, 1163 (1999)
Vinylidene chloride-vinyl chloride copolymers	*19*, 448 (1979) (*corr. 42*, 258); *Suppl. 7*, 73 (1987)
Vinylidene fluoride	*39*, 227 (1986); *Suppl. 7*, 73 (1987); *71*, 1551 (1999)
N-Vinyl-2-pyrrolidone	*19*, 461 (1979); *Suppl. 7*, 73 (1987); *71*, 1181 (1999)
Vinyl toluene	*60*, 373 (1994)
Vitamin K substances	*76*, 417 (2000)

W

Welding	*49*, 447 (1990) (*corr. 52*, 513)
Wollastonite	*42*, 145 (1987); *Suppl. 7*, 377 (1987); *68*, 283 (1997)
Wood dust	*62*, 35 (1995)
Wood industries	*25* (1981); *Suppl. 7*, 378 (1987)

X

X-radiation	*75*, 121 (2000)
Xylenes	*47*, 125 (1989); *71*, 1189 (1999)
2,4-Xylidine	*16*, 367 (1978); *Suppl. 7*, 74 (1987)
2,5-Xylidine	*16*, 377 (1978); *Suppl. 7*, 74 (1987)
2,6-Xylidine (*see* 2,6-Dimethylaniline)	

Y

Yellow AB	8, 279 (1975); *Suppl. 7*, 74 (1987)
Yellow OB	8, 287 (1975); *Suppl. 7*, 74 (1987)

Z

Zalcitabine	76, 129 (2000)
Zearalenone (*see* Toxins derived from *Fusarium graminearum*, *F. culmorum* and *F. crookwellense*)	
Zectran	12, 237 (1976); *Suppl. 7*, 74 (1987)
Zeolites other than erionite	68, 307 (1997)
Zidovudine	76, 73 (2000)
Zinc beryllium silicate (*see* Beryllium and beryllium compounds)	
Zinc chromate (*see* Chromium and chromium compounds)	
Zinc chromate hydroxide (*see* Chromium and chromium compounds)	
Zinc potassium chromate (*see* Chromium and chromium compounds)	
Zinc yellow (*see* Chromium and chromium compounds)	
Zineb	12, 245 (1976); *Suppl. 7*, 74 (1987)
Ziram	12, 259 (1976); *Suppl. 7*, 74 (1987); *53, 423* (1991)

List of IARC Monographs on the Evaluation of Carcinogenic Risks to Humans*

Volume 1
Some Inorganic Substances, Chlorinated Hydrocarbons, Aromatic Amines, N-Nitroso Compounds, and Natural Products
1972; 184 pages (out-of-print)

Volume 2
Some Inorganic and Organometallic Compounds
1973; 181 pages (out-of-print)

Volume 3
Certain Polycyclic Aromatic Hydrocarbons and Heterocyclic Compounds
1973; 271 pages (out-of-print)

Volume 4
Some Aromatic Amines, Hydrazine and Related Substances, N-Nitroso Compounds and Miscellaneous Alkylating Agents
1974; 286 pages (out-of-print)

Volume 5
Some Organochlorine Pesticides
1974; 241 pages (out-of-print)

Volume 6
Sex Hormones
1974; 243 pages (out-of-print)

Volume 7
Some Anti-Thyroid and Related Substances, Nitrofurans and Industrial Chemicals
1974; 326 pages (out-of-print)

Volume 8
Some Aromatic Azo Compounds
1975; 357 pages

Volume 9
Some Aziridines, N-, S- and O-Mustards and Selenium
1975; 268 pages

Volume 10
Some Naturally Occurring Substances
1976; 353 pages (out-of-print)

Volume 11
Cadmium, Nickel, Some Epoxides, Miscellaneous Industrial Chemicals and General Considerations on Volatile Anaesthetics
1976; 306 pages (out-of-print)

Volume 12
Some Carbamates, Thiocarbamates and Carbazides
1976; 282 pages (out-of-print)

Volume 13
Some Miscellaneous Pharmaceutical Substances
1977; 255 pages

Volume 14
Asbestos
1977; 106 pages (out-of-print)

Volume 15
Some Fumigants, the Herbicides 2,4-D and 2,4,5-T, Chlorinated Dibenzodioxins and Miscellaneous Industrial Chemicals
1977; 354 pages (out-of-print)

Volume 16
Some Aromatic Amines and Related Nitro Compounds—Hair Dyes, Colouring Agents and Miscellaneous Industrial Chemicals
1978; 400 pages

Volume 17
Some N-Nitroso Compounds
1978; 365 pages

Volume 18
Polychlorinated Biphenyls and Polybrominated Biphenyls
1978; 140 pages (out-of-print)

Volume 19
Some Monomers, Plastics and Synthetic Elastomers, and Acrolein
1979; 513 pages (out-of-print)

Volume 20
Some Halogenated Hydrocarbons
1979; 609 pages (out-of-print)

Volume 21
Sex Hormones (II)
1979; 583 pages

Volume 22
Some Non-Nutritive Sweetening Agents
1980; 208 pages

Volume 23
Some Metals and Metallic Compounds
1980; 438 pages (out-of-print)

Volume 24
Some Pharmaceutical Drugs
1980; 337 pages

Volume 25
Wood, Leather and Some Associated Industries
1981; 412 pages

Volume 26
Some Antineoplastic and Immunosuppressive Agents
1981; 411 pages

Volume 27
Some Aromatic Amines, Anthraquinones and Nitroso Compounds, and Inorganic Fluorides Used in Drinking-water and Dental Preparations
1982; 341 pages

Volume 28
The Rubber Industry
1982; 486 pages

Volume 29
Some Industrial Chemicals and Dyestuffs
1982; 416 pages

Volume 30
Miscellaneous Pesticides
1983; 424 pages

---

*Certain older volumes, marked out-of-print, are still available directly from IARCPress. Further, high-quality photocopies of all out-of-print volumes may be purchased from University Microfilms International, 300 North Zeeb Road, Ann Arbor, MI 48106-1346, USA (Tel.: 313-761-4700, 800-521-0600).

Volume 31
Some Food Additives, Feed Additives and Naturally Occurring Substances
1983; 314 pages (out-of-print)

Volume 32
Polynuclear Aromatic Compounds, Part 1: Chemical, Environmental and Experimental Data
1983; 477 pages (out-of-print)

Volume 33
Polynuclear Aromatic Compounds, Part 2: Carbon Blacks, Mineral Oils and Some Nitroarenes
1984; 245 pages (out-of-print)

Volume 34
Polynuclear Aromatic Compounds, Part 3: Industrial Exposures in Aluminium Production, Coal Gasification, Coke Production, and Iron and Steel Founding
1984; 219 pages

Volume 35
Polynuclear Aromatic Compounds, Part 4: Bitumens, Coal-tars and Derived Products, Shale-oils and Soots
1985; 271 pages

Volume 36
Allyl Compounds, Aldehydes, Epoxides and Peroxides
1985; 369 pages

Volume 37
Tobacco Habits Other than Smoking; Betel-Quid and Areca-Nut Chewing; and Some Related Nitrosamines
1985; 291 pages

Volume 38
Tobacco Smoking
1986; 421 pages

Volume 39
Some Chemicals Used in Plastics and Elastomers
1986; 403 pages

Volume 40
Some Naturally Occurring and Synthetic Food Components, Furocoumarins and Ultraviolet Radiation
1986; 444 pages

Volume 41
Some Halogenated Hydrocarbons and Pesticide Exposures
1986; 434 pages

Volume 42
Silica and Some Silicates
1987; 289 pages

Volume 43
Man-Made Mineral Fibres and Radon
1988; 300 pages

Volume 44
Alcohol Drinking
1988; 416 pages

Volume 45
Occupational Exposures in Petroleum Refining; Crude Oil and Major Petroleum Fuels
1989; 322 pages

Volume 46
Diesel and Gasoline Engine Exhausts and Some Nitroarenes
1989; 458 pages

Volume 47
Some Organic Solvents, Resin Monomers and Related Compounds, Pigments and Occupational Exposures in Paint Manufacture and Painting
1989; 535 pages

Volume 48
Some Flame Retardants and Textile Chemicals, and Exposures in the Textile Manufacturing Industry
1990; 345 pages

Volume 49
Chromium, Nickel and Welding
1990; 677 pages

Volume 50
Pharmaceutical Drugs
1990; 415 pages

Volume 51
Coffee, Tea, Mate, Methyl-xanthines and Methylglyoxal
1991; 513 pages

Volume 52
Chlorinated Drinking-water; Chlorination By-products; Some Other Halogenated Compounds; Cobalt and Cobalt Compounds
1991; 544 pages

Volume 53
Occupational Exposures in Insecticide Application, and Some Pesticides
1991; 612 pages

Volume 54
Occupational Exposures to Mists and Vapours from Strong Inorganic Acids; and Other Industrial Chemicals
1992; 336 pages

Volume 55
Solar and Ultraviolet Radiation
1992; 316 pages

Volume 56
Some Naturally Occurring Substances: Food Items and Constituents, Heterocyclic Aromatic Amines and Mycotoxins
1993; 599 pages

Volume 57
Occupational Exposures of Hairdressers and Barbers and Personal Use of Hair Colourants; Some Hair Dyes, Cosmetic Colourants, Industrial Dyestuffs and Aromatic Amines
1993; 428 pages

Volume 58
Beryllium, Cadmium, Mercury, and Exposures in the Glass Manufacturing Industry
1993; 444 pages

Volume 59
Hepatitis Viruses
1994; 286 pages

Volume 60
Some Industrial Chemicals
1994; 560 pages

Volume 61
Schistosomes, Liver Flukes and *Helicobacter pylori*
1994; 270 pages

Volume 62
Wood Dust and Formaldehyde
1995; 405 pages

Volume 63
Dry Cleaning, Some Chlorinated Solvents and Other Industrial Chemicals
1995; 551 pages

Volume 64
Human Papillomaviruses
1995; 409 pages

Volume 65
Printing Processes and Printing Inks, Carbon Black and Some Nitro Compounds
1996; 578 pages

Volume 66
Some Pharmaceutical Drugs
1996; 514 pages

Volume 67
Human Immunodeficiency Viruses and Human T-Cell Lymphotropic Viruses
1996; 424 pages

Volume 68
Silica, Some Silicates, Coal Dust and *para*-Aramid Fibrils
1997; 506 pages

Volume 69
Polychlorinated Dibenzo-*para*-Dioxins and Polychlorinated Dibenzofurans
1997; 666 pages

Volume 70
Epstein-Barr Virus and Kaposi's Sarcoma Herpesvirus/Human Herpesvirus 8
1997; 524 pages

Volume 71
Re-evaluation of Some Organic Chemicals, Hydrazine and Hydrogen Peroxide
1999; 1586 pages

Volume 72
Hormonal Contraception and Post-menopausal Hormonal Therapy
1999; 660 pages

Volume 73
Some Chemicals that Cause Tumours of the Kidney or Urinary Bladder in Rodents and Some Other Substances
1999; 674 pages

Volume 74
Surgical Implants and Other Foreign Bodies
1999; 409 pages

Volume 75
Ionizing Radiation, Part 1, X-Radiation and γ-Radiation, and Neutrons
2000; 492 pages

Volume 76
Some Antiviral and Antineoplastic Drugs, and Other Pharmaceutical Agents
2000; 522 pages

Supplement No. 1
Chemicals and Industrial Processes Associated with Cancer in Humans (*IARC Monographs*, Volumes 1 to 20)
1979; 71 pages (out-of-print)

Supplement No. 2
Long-term and Short-term Screening Assays for Carcinogens: A Critical Appraisal
1980; 426 pages (out-of-print)

Supplement No. 3
Cross Index of Synonyms and Trade Names in Volumes 1 to 26 of the *IARC Monographs*
1982; 199 pages (out-of-print)

Supplement No. 4
Chemicals, Industrial Processes and Industries Associated with Cancer in Humans (*IARC Monographs*, Volumes 1 to 29)
1982; 292 pages (out-of-print)

Supplement No. 5
Cross Index of Synonyms and Trade Names in Volumes 1 to 36 of the *IARC Monographs*
1985; 259 pages (out-of-print)

Supplement No. 6
Genetic and Related Effects: An Updating of Selected *IARC Monographs* from Volumes 1 to 42
1987; 729 pages

Supplement No. 7
Overall Evaluations of Carcinogenicity: An Updating of *IARC Monographs* Volumes 1–42
1987; 440 pages

Supplement No. 8
Cross Index of Synonyms and Trade Names in Volumes 1 to 46 of the *IARC Monographs*
1990; 346 pages (out-of-print)

All IARC publications are available directly from
IARCPress, 150 Cours Albert Thomas, F-69372 Lyon cedex 08, France
(Fax: +33 4 72 73 83 02; E-mail: press@iarc.fr).

IARC Monographs and Technical Reports are also available from the
World Health Organization Distribution and Sales, CH-1211 Geneva 27
(Fax: +41 22 791 4857; E-mail: publications@who.int)
and from WHO Sales Agents worldwide.

IARC Scientific Publications, IARC Handbooks and IARC CancerBases are also available from
Oxford University Press, Walton Street, Oxford, UK OX2 6DP (Fax: +44 1865 267782).

www.ingramcontent.com/pod-product-compliance
Ingram Content Group UK Ltd.
Pitfield, Milton Keynes, MK11 3LW, UK
UKHW051117200426
11947UKWH00038B/1769